PSYCHOLOGICAL THEORIES
OF DRINKING AND ALCOHOLISM

THE GUILFORD SUBSTANCE ABUSE SERIES

Howard T. Blane and Thomas R. Kosten, Editors

Forthcoming Volume

Introduction to Addictive Behaviors, Second Edition
DENNIS L. THOMBS

Recent Volumes

Psychological Theories of Drinking and Alcoholism, Second Edition
KENNETH E. LEONARD and HOWARD T. BLANE, EDITORS

New Treatments for Opiate Dependence
THOMAS R. KOSTEN and SUSAN M. STINE, EDITORS

Couple Therapy for Alcoholism:
A Cognitive-Behavioral Treatment Manual
PHYLIS J. WAKEFIELD, REBECCA E. WILLIAMS,
ELIZABETH B. YOST, and KATHLEEN M. PATTERSON

Treating Substance Abuse: Theory and Technique
FREDERICK ROTGERS, DANIEL S. KELLER,
and JON MORGENSTERN, EDITORS

Clinical Guide to Alcohol Treatment:
The Community Reinforcement Approach
ROBERT K. MEYERS and JANE ELLEN SMITH

Psychotherapy and Substance Abuse:
A Practitioner's Handbook
ARNOLD M. WASHTON, EDITOR

Psychological Theories of Drinking and Alcoholism

Second Edition

Edited by

KENNETH E. LEONARD
HOWARD T. BLANE

THE GUILFORD PRESS
New York   London

© 1999 The Guilford Press
A Division of Guilford Publications, Inc.
72 Spring Street, New York, NY 10012
http://www.guilford.com

Printed in the United States of America

This book is printed on acid-free paper.

Last digit is print number: 9 8 7 6 5 4 3 2 1

Library of Congress Cataloging-in-Publication Data
available from the Publisher

ISBN 1-57230-410-3

About the Editors

Kenneth E. Leonard, PhD, is a Senior Research Scientist at the Research Institute on Addictions, the Director of the Division of Psychology in Psychiatry at the State University of New York at Buffalo Medical School, and a Fellow in the Division of Addictions (Division 50) of the American Psychological Association. He is co-editor (with R. Lorraine Collins and John S. Searles) of *Alcohol and the Family: Research and Clinical Perspectives* and has published extensively in the area of drinking and marital/family processes.

Howard T. Blane, PhD, is the former Director of the Research Institute on Addictions, a Research Professor Emeritus of Psychology, Psychiatry, and Social and Preventive Medicine at the State University of New York at Buffalo Medical School, and a Fellow in the Division of Clinical Psychology (Division 12) and in the Division of Addictions (Division 50) of the American Psychological Association. He is the author of *The Personality of the Alcoholic*, co-author (with M. E. Chafetz and M. J. Hill) of *Frontiers of Alcoholism*, and co-editor (with M. E. Chafetz) of *Youth, Alcohol, and Social Policy*.

Contributors

Bruce D. Bartholow, MS, Department of Psychology, University of Missouri, Columbia, Missouri

Howard T. Blane, PhD, Research Institute on Addictions, Buffalo, New York; Department of Psychology in Psychiatry, State University of New York at Buffalo Medical School, Buffalo, New York

Clara M. Bradizza, PhD, Research Institute on Addictions, Buffalo, New York

Kate B. Carey, PhD, Syracuse University, Syracuse, New York

Elizabeth J. D'Amico, PhD, Department of Psychology, University of California at San Diego, San Diego, California

Jack Darkes, PhD, Department of Psychology, University of South Florida, Tampa, Florida

Patrick T. Davies, PhD, Department of Clinical and Social Sciences in Psychology, University of Rochester, Rochester, New York

Frances K. Del Boca, PhD, Department of Psychology, University of South Florida, Tampa, Florida

Mark T. Fillmore, PhD, Department of Psychology, University of Waterloo, Waterloo, Ontario, Canada

Kim Fromme, PhD, Department of Psychology, The University of Texas at Austin, Austin, Texas

Mark S. Goldman, PhD, Department of Psychology, University of South Florida, Tampa, Florida

Janet Greeley, PhD, Faculty of Social Sciences, James Cook University of North Queensland, Townsville, Queensland, Australia

Alan R. Lang, PhD, Department of Psychology, Florida State University, Tallahassee, Florida

Kenneth E. Leonard, PhD, Research Institute on Addictions, Buffalo, New York; Division of Psychology in Psychiatry, State University of New York at Buffalo Medical School, Buffalo, New York

Stephen A. Maisto, PhD, Department of Psychology, Syracuse University, Syracuse, New York

Matt McGue, PhD, Department of Psychology, University of Minnesota, Minneapolis, Minnesota

Tian Oei, PhD, Department of Psychology, University of Queensland, Brisbane, Queensland, Australia

Christopher J. Patrick, PhD, Department of Psychology, University of Minnesota, Minneapolis, Minnesota

Michael A. Sayette, PhD, Department of Psychology, University of Pittsburgh, Pittsburgh, Pennsylvania

Werner G. K. Stritzke, PhD, University of Western Australia, Department of Psychology, Nedlands, Perth, Western Australia, Australia

Kenneth J. Sher, PhD, Department of Psychology, University of Missouri, Columbia, Missouri

Timothy J. Trull, PhD, Department of Psychology, University of Missouri, Columbia, Missouri

Angela Vieth, MA, Department of Psychology, University of Missouri, Columbia, Missouri

Muriel Vogel-Sprott, PhD, Department of Psychology, University of Waterloo, Waterloo, Ontario, Canada

Michael Windle, PhD, Department of Psychology, University of Alabama at Birmingham, Birmingham, Alabama

Contents

1

Introduction

KENNETH E. LEONARD
HOWARD T. BLANE

It is theory that decides what can be observed.
—ALBERT EINSTEIN

The value of theory to the understanding of a phenomenon, whether that phenomenon be alcoholism or some other psychological, sociological, or biological construct, is sometimes unappreciated. Theory represents our attempt to organize previous empirical observations into a series of logical rules that represent our hypotheses about the causal influences on the phenomenon of interest. Because those previous empirical observations were also collected in response to a previous set of logical rules, theory provides a historical record of the progress in understanding a phenomenon. In the best of circumstances, the current set of rules provides a new, more detailed and more sophisticated set of questions that can be addressed by further empirical observation. Consequently, theory represents the organizational structure of science.

Although the basis for scientific progress is often viewed as the ability to disconfirm a theory, it is, in fact, rarely the case that a formal psychological theory is discarded because its major hypotheses have been disproved. Because most new theories pick up where old theories left off and base the theory in the experience of empirical research, few theories entirely disappear because they are utterly incorrect. Instead, the theoretical landscape changes depending upon the pressures of accumulated data,

1

much the way the physical landscape is modified in response to various environmental pressures. Under the pressures of accumulating disconfirming data, some theories are gradually worn down and engender little interest because of their limited generalizability and utility. Sometimes the countervailing pressures of supportive and disconfirming data lead to further specification and qualification of a theory in a manner that enhances the value of the theory. Under still other pressures, a carefully qualified hypothesis may flourish and expand, and be adopted as an explanation for a phenomenon beyond that for which it was originally intended. This theoretical maturation is a gradual process driven by the slow accumulation of empirical observations.

In this context of gradual theoretical change fueled by the continued pressure of theoretically relevant research, we had long resisted the impulse to issue a second edition of *Psychological Theories of Drinking and Alcoholism*. Much of the first edition was devoted to detailing the historical development of psychological approaches to drinking and alcoholism, an aspect that we believed to be critical to further progress in the field. This material really did not require updating. Nor did the issuance of a second edition at this time come about because of the appearance or disappearance of any prominent feature of the landscape. Our motivation instead arose from an awareness that the accumulated pressures of theoretically driven research had exerted a noticeable difference: some theories had changed, still others expanded, and others disappeared. This awareness was driven home on numerous occasions by colleagues who, despite continued use of the first edition, indicated the need to supplement the book with other, more recent research. This edition represents our attempt to portray the current theoretical landscape and the empirical findings responsible for the changing landscape.

In the more than 10 years since the first edition of *Psychological Theories of Drinking and Alcoholism* appeared, the influence of psychology on the study of alcohol abuse and alcoholism has continued to expand. In 1986, we had noted the growth of an "invisible college" of psychologists interested in the area of substance abuse. This "invisible college" had been formalized as the Society of Psychologists in Substance Abuse in 1975. This name was subsequently changed to the Society of Psychologists in Addictive Behaviors (SPAB) to signify the broader interest of psychologists in this area. By 1986, there were over 500 members in SPAB, and a task force had been created to press for the creation of a division within the American Psychological Association (APA) devoted to addictive behaviors. By 1993, Division 50 had become a candidate division of APA with its own divisional journal, *Psychology of Addictive Behaviors,* and approximately 700 members. Full divisional status arrived a year later, and at present, there are over 1,000 members of Division 50. Although the interests of these professionals include substance abuse and other behavioral addictions, an interest in alcohol and alcoholism is shared by a large number of these researchers and practitioners. The "invisible college" has become visible in a major way.

In 1986, we also observed that the growth of research driving psychological formulations of drinking and alcoholism was directly related to the establishment of the National Institute on Alcohol Abuse and Alcoholism (NIAAA) in 1970, and the availability of federal funds for research accompanying that event. This impact became all the more evident in the past decade. Between 1986 and 1995, the federal dollars devoted to research grants at NIAAA grew from $43.6 million to $143.6 million. The National Institute on Drug Abuse, the other branch of the National Institutes of Health (NIH) providing major support to psychologists interested in substance abuse, increased from $57.9 million to $327.1 million. These increases of 329% and 565%, respectively, compare with a rough doubling of the research budget of NIH throughout this time. This reflects an increasing awareness of the overall impact that alcohol and drug abuse exert on the public health of the nation. Of course, these funds support a range of research activities, including research of a more biological and sociological nature, not simply those relating to psychology or to psychological theory. However, many of the research activities are devoted to psychological issues, and many of those not directly addressing psychological issues are nonetheless relevant to psychological theory.

With the continued expansion of research support and professional recognition of psychological approaches to drinking, alcoholism, and substance abuse, the ties between mainstream psychology and psychologists interested in addictive behaviors have changed. In the earliest days of psychological approaches to drinking and alcoholism, psychologists with mainstream interests would sometimes apply their expertise to alcoholism. This often took the form of assessing alcoholics with respect to some personality, social, or cognitive test, but the primary interest lay with that test or construct, not with furthering the understanding of alcoholism. Such endeavors tended to be atheoretical, and, with the many similar biomedical studies, paved the way for the formulation of Keller's Law—"The investigation of any trait in alcoholics will show that they have either more of it or less of it"—and the more pithy version—"Alcoholics are different in so many ways that it makes no difference" (Keller, 1972). The decades of the 1970s and 1980s saw a tightening connection between psychological approaches to behaviors in general and psychological approaches to alcoholism. This trend remains apparent to this day. For example, the psychological approaches that emphasize cognition have been greatly influenced by substantive and methodological advances in more basic cognitive research, adding the unique twist necessary to address the impact of a substance that can alter those basic processes.

It is particularly noteworthy that theoretical contributions originating among psychologists interested in alcoholism have been adopted more broadly by psychologists interested in other forms of psychopathology.

This is most apparent for the constructs of relapse prevention and the abstinence violation effect. Although originally developed in the context of alcoholism, these constructs were quickly applied to understanding other forms of substance abuse, such as cocaine dependence (McKay et al., 1997), smoking (Curry, Marlatt, & Gordon, 1987; Shiffman et al., 1997) and marijuana use (Stephens, Roffman, & Simpson, 1994). Given the nature of these constructs, they were soon applied to a variety of other behaviors involving impulse control, such as gambling (Sylvain, Ladouceur, & Boisvert, 1997), weight loss and eating disorders (Head & Brookhart, 1997; Ward, Hudson, & Bulik, 1993), sexual offenses (Ward, Hudson, & Marshall, 1994), and risky sexual behavior (Roffman et al., 1998).

Each of these trends, the development of a visible network of psychologists interested in drinking and alcoholism, the increased availability of federal funds for behavioral research in alcoholism, and the closer alignment and mutual influence between psychological approaches to alcoholism and psychological approaches to other behavioral phenomena, reflect the maturity of this area of inquiry. Alcoholism and drug abuse, long "stepchildren" of psychology, have been formally "adopted" by psychology. The process, occurring over approximately 50 years, culminated in the Policy Statement on Alcohol and Other Drug Abuse that was adopted by the APA Council of Representatives on February, 29, 1992. This document affirms the integration of the psychology of alcoholism and addictions into psychology, and affirms APA's commitment to the prevention, treatment, and research of alcohol and other drug abuse, and to the education of psychologists at the predoctoral, postdoctoral, and professional levels in these areas.

THE ORGANIZATION OF THIS VOLUME

In developing this edition, we were strongly influenced by the organizational approach that we had taken in the first edition. The first edition was organized around four "traditional" theoretical approaches and five "recent" theoretical approaches. The traditional theoretical approaches represented broad perspectives that served to organize the sometimes quite heterogeneous empirical data. It was our view that, particularly in view of many minitheories that focused on a single psychological construct and motivated a handful of empirical studies, that this broad perspective would best facilitate an understanding of the field as a whole. The topics that we chose were tension-reduction theory, social learning theory, personality theory, and interactional theory. We have maintained these four basic chapters, though interactional theory has been renamed developmental approaches (for reasons that will be explained). Rather than referring to these approaches as "traditional," more than 10 years of hindsight lead us to refer to these as "broad psychological perspectives."

TENSION-REDUCTION THEORY

One of the common criteria of a useful theory is the extent of research that the theory engenders. In this sense, tension-reduction theory (TRT) has clearly been the most successful of the psychological theories of alcoholism. Not only has TRT been successful in the amount and range of research that it has engendered, but also it is clearly the theoretical progenitor of many of the theories that have developed over the past 50 years. The progress and extensions of TRT encompass most of the psychological approaches to alcohol. As a field, we seem to have accepted the notion that alcohol is reinforcing because it reduces tension, and we have been undaunted in our pursuit of evidence of this basic precept, even in the face of a body of literature that is, at best, equivocal. In Chapter 2, Janet Greeley and Tian Oei describe the origins and early development of TRT, and recapitulate the findings of two earlier reviews (Cappell & Greeley, 1987; Cappell & Herman, 1972) that provided incisive appraisals of the theory, its generalizability, and its limitations. These authors document the continuing exploration of the TRT over the past decade and describe the progression of TRT from a broad, all-encompassing theory to a "minitheory" focusing on drinking as one of several alternatives for coping with stress, and tension reduction as one of several reinforcers for alcohol consumption.

PERSONALITY THEORY

Personality approaches to alcoholism represented a dominant theme in psychological research in the 1950s and 1960s. This research did not reflect a systematic theoretical approach to personality and alcoholism, but instead reflected an underlying assumption arising from psychoanalytic theory that certain personality types were prone to addiction. This notion of the addictive personality fueled the perspective that personality factors would prove critical to the development of alcoholism. As a consequence, alcoholics and nonalcoholics were examined with respect to nearly every personality assessment that had ever been devised. The observation that alcoholics and nonalcoholics differed on nearly every conceivable dimension and the recognition of the considerable heterogeneity within the alcoholic population led to the rejection of the concept of the "addictive personality." With the evolving prominence of behavioral approaches, the utility of the broad field of personality was questioned, and personality research in alcoholism declined. In Chapter 3, Kenneth J. Sher, Timothy J. Trull, Bruce D. Bartholow, and Angela Vieth describe the resurgence of interest in the broad field of personality and the current state of thinking with respect to overall models of personality. They argue that the etiological model that personality has a causal influence on the development of alcoholism is only one of a number of potential models, including spurious and consequential models, as well as models of mediation and moderation. One of the unique strengths of their contribution is the description of methodological concerns in the study of alcoholism and personality. With three broad models of how personality might influence the etiology of alcoholism as a framework, they review recent research and argue that personality processes must be integrated within broader, interdisciplinary investigations to forward our understanding of alcoholism.

SOCIAL LEARNING THEORY

Like TRT, social learning theory (SLT) has been enormously influential and has generated a tremendous amount of research activity. Some of this research reflects a broader philosophical agreement with the general tenets of SLT rather than any specific test of an SLT model of alcohol use or alcoholism. Arising from a SLT of general behavior and a rejection of the strict behaviorist approach, the SLT of alcohol use emphasized the role of the vicarious learning and social environment in the development of alcohol use and alcohol problems. Stephen A. Maisto, Kate B. Carey, and Clara M. Bradizza (Chapter 4) present a synopsis of Bandura's theoretical development of SLT and his initial hypotheses regarding an SLT approach to alcohol use and alcoholism. As shown by these authors, the later expositions of SLT by Bandura clearly emphasize the importance of the social environment (setting) and cognitive processes (person) as jointly influencing and being influenced by behavior. Given the broad and extensive literature arising from this perspective (some of which is reviewed in other chapters), this chapter focuses on three basic constructs that are critical to the SLT of alcohol use and alcoholism: the influence of the social environment; coping skills and cognitive variables, including self-efficacy; and outcome expectancies. The authors describe the rich, integrative nature of SLT and note that empirical attempts to address multiple SLT constructs in the context of reciprocal determinism have been sparse. The authors provide a thorough review of the few studies that have attempted to examine a broader SLT model and make a persuasive case for the emerging importance of integrative studies of SLT. Finally, these authors turn to the issue of relapse, arguably the most successful application of SLT. The SLT model described by Marlatt and Gordon (1985) and in this chapter represents the most sophisticated approach to relapse and one of the major achievements of SLT to date.

DEVELOPMENTAL THEORY

In the first edition of this book, Sadava (1987) described interactional approaches to drinking and alcoholism. These models viewed drinking as arising from the joint influence of person factors and the social environment. These models differed from SLT primarily in their emphasis on the person, and differed from the personality approaches in their focus on the interaction of person and environmental factors. More critically, these models often incorporated developmental constructs and longitudinal methodologies. Over the past decade, the developmental theme in these models has increased to such a degree that we believe these models should be viewed as developmental theories, or as the developmental psychopathology approach to alcoholism. Michael Windle and Patrick T. Davies (Chapter 5) describe the core elements of a lifespan developmental psychopathology approach and argue that these concepts are of critical importance in the study of drinking and alcoholism. Although there has been little research spanning developmental epochs, they describe the interplay of diathesis and stress, and its relevance to the development of alcoholism within infancy, childhood, adolescence, young adulthood, and middle and late adulthood. They explore the crucial methodological advances that have propelled this approach to prominence and point to critical empirical gaps in our understanding of drinking and alcoholism over the lifespan.

With regard to the "recent" theoretical approaches, the present volume includes several theoretical approaches that were in their formative periods in 1987 and have matured and expanded since that time: expectancy theory, cognitive theory, and learning theory. In addition, three areas of burgeoning interest to psychologists have gained attention as contributing to our understanding of drinking and alcoholism: the influence of alcohol on emotional processes, genetic influences on drinking and alcoholism, and neurobiological bases of the effects of alcohol.

EXPECTANCY THEORY

The construct of expectancies has played a critical role in psychological approaches to social behavior. In its initial application to alcohol research, alcohol expectancies were described more in terms of attitudes and beliefs, an approach that relied on the simple surface content of cognitions. Even within this early view, the power of alcohol expectancies to predict drinking patterns and alcohol-related behavior was impressive. As described by Mark S. Goldman, Frances K. Del Boca, and Jack Darkes (Chapter 6), this construct reflects the representation in memory of an individual's acquired information regarding the consequences of certain behaviors within general and specific contexts. These expectations may be acquired without direct experiences of those consequences either through observation or through any number of ways that humans acquire knowledge. They may also acquire these expectations on the basis of their own direct experience. These memories, in turn, structure the perception and interpretation of the environment, thereby directing behavior. With respect to drinking and alcoholism, expectancies about the positive and negative outcomes of drinking are viewed as one of the major proximal determinants of drinking behavior and as a mediator of many of the other psychological and pharmacological influences. In summary, these authors describe the substantial advances in alcohol expectancy theory, documenting its transition to a sophisticated cognitive model incorporating content, structure, and process to understand drinking and alcoholism.

COGNITIVE THEORIES

In the first edition, the self-awareness model of alcohol consumption reflected the field's initial foray into an approach explicitly focused on cognitive processes. Although the SLT model and the early alcohol expectancy approaches emphasized the content of cognition, the self-awareness model emphasized the psychopharmacological impact of alcohol on cognitive processes. In Chapter 7 of this volume, Michael A. Sayette describes the status of the self-awareness model and the development of alternative approaches to alcohol and cognitive processes, with particular emphasis on the alcohol myopia theory and the appraisal-disruption model. These theories not only provide an explanation of the variable effects of intoxication on social behavior, but also provide a compelling hypothesis regarding the reinforcing aspects of alcohol use: The disruption of cognitive processes in the presence of different social environments may be one source of a stress reduction due to alcohol.

Although much of the earlier cognitive research focused on the acute effect of alcohol on cognitive functioning, a second major thrust of this approach has been directed at the constructs of urges and craving. These constructs had been traditionally viewed as simply resulting from the absence of ethanol in a neurological system that had grown accustomed to its presence. Furthermore, craving was viewed as an important feature underlying the inability to abstain from drinking, and relapse after alcohol treatment. However, the empirical literature suggests that craving is not simply the psychological representation of physical withdrawal, nor is it the predominant trigger for alcohol relapses. Sayette presents a clear exposition of current views of craving that involves the interplay of motivation, and automatic and nonautomatic cognitive processing. Although this research is more advanced with respect to nicotine dependence and drug abuse, the application of these ideas to alcoholism is a promising avenue for future research.

LEARNING THEORY

Given the pivotal role of learning theory and its extensive applications in psychology, it is somewhat unusual that this should be referred to as a recent theoretical approach. Historically, learning theory played a more critical role in attempts to ameliorate alcohol problems (e.g., aversive conditioning, blood-alcohol-level discrimination) than in attempts to understand basic processes in the development of alcoholism. However, the work of Solomon and Corbit (1974) and Siegel (1983) suggested that critical aspects of drug dependence, specifically, tolerance and withdrawal, could be explained through classical conditioning models. The implication of these findings was that dependence was not solely a physiological adaptation to the continued presence of a drug, but rather, it was a learned response, the acquisition of a link between an environment stimulus and the pharmacological reaction to the drug.

In Chapter 8, Muriel Vogel-Sprott and Mark T. Fillmore elaborate on the earlier associative learning models of alcohol and substance use. They argue that three basic associations are acquired in the context of any drug use situation: the link between environmental cues of drug administration and the actual drug administration, the link between the drug administration and the pharmacological effect of the drug, and the link between the pharmacological effects and the external consequences. Within this associative expectancy framework, they review evidence that these links explain a variety of drug use effects that had previously been viewed in strict physiological terms, specifically, tolerance, withdrawal, and behavioral impairment. The chapter demonstrates convincingly that the physiological impacts of alcohol and drugs are modifiable, and that the traditional markers of dependency are, like all behaviors, modifiable by experience.

ALCOHOL AND EMOTIONAL RESPONSE

At the center of many theories of drinking and alcoholism is an explicit presumption that alcohol has an impact on mood. The central tenets of the TRT model, though not originally conceived of in terms of mood, have come to focus on the apparent anxiolytic effects of alcohol. Alcohol expectancy theory has been concerned with beliefs about the impact of alcohol, and the theme underlying many of those beliefs has been that alcohol influences affect in a largely positive fashion. In Chapter 9, Alan R. Lang, Christopher J. Patrick, and Werner G. K. Stritzke assert that much of the previous research addressing the alcohol–emotions link has been narrowly focused on the amelioration of negative affect. Moreover, this previous research was largely out of touch with the advances in contemporary theories of emotion that link emotions to neurological, motivational, and cognitive processes. After reviewing the progression of theory with respect to emotions and the methodological issues involved in its measurement, the authors briefly consider recent cognitive approaches that speak to the issue of alcohol and emotional responses. While these are viewed as important steps to a fuller understanding of alcohol and emotion, they present a sophisticated multidimensional and multilevel model of emotion that suggests that emotions are "action dispositions" that vary along dimensions of arousal and valence, and that these emotions influence and are influenced by higher cognitive processes. In contrast to the view that alcohol simply modifies a given emotion by its action on a specific brain system, this approach argues that the impact of alcohol on emotion is much more complicated. Lang, Patrick, and Stritzke make a strong case that this approach holds great promise for integrating the existing literature and will be of value in advancing our understanding of the role of affect and cognitions in the development of drinking and alcoholism.

GENETIC INFLUENCES ON DRINKING AND ALCOHOLISM

Although there was evidence in 1987 that alcoholism was heritable, the existing literature was marked by a variety of limitations and equivocal findings. Moreover, there were relatively few studies that had addressed the issue. At the present time, however, the evidence for a genetic component is very strong and persuasive. Matt McGue (Chapter 10) provides a thorough overview of behavioral genetic research addressing drinking behavior and alcoholism, and a review of the state of knowledge regarding different heritability between men and women, between more and less severe alcoholics, and between alcohol and other substance abuse. The behavioral genetic literature has been concerned not only with the heritability of alcoholism but also the heritability of other drinking behaviors, such as abstinence, frequency of drinking, and usual quantity of consumption. In addition, this literature has begun to address the extent of genetic influence at different developmental periods. McGue describes the research concerning possible location of genes contributing to alcoholism and concludes that there is considerable promise in these methods despite relatively slow progress to date. Of most importance to psychology, McGue argues that advances in genetics research will enable a more precise examination of the nature of mediating psychological and moderating environmental factors.

NEUROBIOLOGICAL BASES OF THE PSYCHOLOGICAL EFFECTS OF ALCOHOL

Similar to the chapter on genetics, this is not a topic that is traditionally within the purview of a psychological approach to alcoholism. However, recent research has begun to focus on the neurobiological substrates of different aspects of substance dependence and psychological disorders more generally. Although much of this research has traditionally been conducted by neurologists, psychologists interested in addictive behavior have become increasingly interested and involved in this endeavor. Consequently, it will become more and more important for psychologists to understand the neural substrates underlying alcohol effects.

The contribution by Kim Fromme and Elizabeth D'Amico (Chapter 11) provides a basic primer in neurotransmitter functions and processes, and in neurobiological methods. The authors also provide a thorough and accessible review of the effect of alcohol on neurotransmitters. Fromme and D'Amico cover both the acute and the chronic effects of alcohol on the key neurotransmitters. They emphasize two aspects of drinking—the reinforcing effects of alcohol and the impact of alcohol on cognitive processes and associative learning—and suggest that these effects may be mediated by two relatively distinct neuroanatomical and neurochemical response systems. The prospect of identifying neurological substrates underlying the reinforcement value of alcohol opens up numerous possibilities for further research directed at understanding the interface between psychosocial and biological influences on alcoholism, as well as for revealing potentially important insights with respect to psychosocial and psychopharmacological treatments of alcoholism.

As with the original *Psychological Theories of Drinking and Alcoholism,* we have designed the second edition to meet the needs of several diverse audiences. As the recognition of the magnitude of alcohol problems and of the co-occurrence of alcohol problems with other psychopathologies have increased, the importance of advanced training in alcoholism and addictive behaviors has become evident to many psychology departments. The first edition fostered and advanced the integration of addictive studies into the psychological curriculum. The second edition of this volume continues to fill a gap in instruction for advanced undergraduate and graduate studies in psychology. This volume consists of theoretical overviews, empirical observations, and methodological advances and limitations provided by recognized scholars in the area. These contemporary viewpoints are set within a historical framework that allows the student to see the continuity and significant advances of the field and the links to the broader field of psychological thought. While the most frequent use of the volume has been as a graduate psychology text, we hope that the expanded scope of the volume will make it appealing to both researchers and clinicians in fields such as psychiatry, sociology, and social work.

A second major niche that this book fills is the need for a comprehensive view of the current state of theory and research for behavioral scientists and practitioners. Over the past decade, we have heard from many such scientists, who indicated that the original volume was a vital day-to-day reference for their ongoing research activities. In a single volume, they were able to access clear and comprehensive analyses of the current research knowledge. Many of the chapters provide clear statements of the gaps in existent literature and opportunities for future research. These have proved invaluable. We have also heard from clinicians who valued the in-depth survey of the current advances in psychological approaches to alcoholism. This volume will help these readers to stay abreast of new knowledge and its potential implications for future treatment and prevention advances. Furthermore, the psychological approaches to drinking and alcoholism will prove informative to the broader audience of additions specialists, both researchers and clinicians. As we noted in our earlier discussion, many of the psychological principals that were developed with respect to alcoholism have been enthusiastically adopted by specialists addressing drug abuse, eating disorders, sexual addictions, and compulsive gambling. We believe that this volume will be a source for many of the future research and clinical developments in the area of addictive behaviors.

REFERENCES

Cappell, H., & Greeley, J. (1987). Alcohol and tension reduction: An update on research and theory. In H. T. Blane & K. E. Leonard (Eds.), *Psychological theories of drinking and alcoholism* (pp. 15–54). New York: Guilford Press.

Cappell, H., & Herman, C. P. (1972). Alcohol and tension reduction: A review. *Journal of Studies on Alcohol, 33*, 33–64.

Curry, S., Marlatt, G. A., & Gordon, J. R. (1987). Abstinence violation effect: Validation of an attributional construct with smoking cessation. *Journal of Consulting and Clinical Psychology, 55*(2), 145–149.

Head, S., & Brookhart, A. (1997). Lifestyle modification and relapse-prevention training during treatment for weight loss. *Behavior Therapy, 28*, 307–321.

Keller, M. (1972). Oddities of alcoholics. *Quarterly Journal of Studies on Alcohol, 33*(4), 1147–1148.

Marlatt, G. A., & Gordon, J. R. (Eds.). (1985). *Relapse prevention: Maintenance strategies in the treatment of addictive behaviors.* New York: Guilford Press.

McKay, J. R., Alterman, A. I., Cacciola, J. S., Rutherford, M. J., O'Brien, C. P., & Koppenhaver, J. (1997). Group counseling versus individualized relapse prevention aftercare following intensive outpatient treatment for cocaine dependence: Initial results. *Journal of Consulting and Clinical Psychology, 54*, 778–788.

Roffman, R. A., Stephens, R. S., Curtin, L., Gordon, J. R., Craver, J. N., Stern, M., Beadnell, B., & Downey, L. (1998). Relapse prevention as an interventive model for HIV risk reduction in gay and bisexual men. *AIDs Education and Prevention, 10*, 1–18.

Sadava, S. W. (1987). Interactional theory. In H. T. Blane & K. E. Leonard (Eds.), *Psychological theories of drinking and alcoholism* (pp. 90–130). New York: Guilford Press.

Shiffman, S., Hickcox, M., Paty, J. A., Gnys, M., Kassel, J. D., & Richards, T. J. (1997). The abstinence violation effect following smoking lapses and temptations. *Cognitive Therapy and Research, 21*, 497–523.

Siegel, S. (1983). Classical conditioning, drug tolerance and drug dependence. In Y. Israel, B. F. Glaser, H. Kalant, R. E. Popham, W. Schmidt, & R. G. Smart (Eds.), *Research advances in alcohol and drug problems* (Vol. 7, pp. 207–246). New York: Plenum.

Solomon, R. L., & Corbit, J. D. (1974). An opponent–process theory of motivation. *Psychological Review, 81,* 119–145.

Stephens, R. S., Roffman, R. A., & Simpson, E. E. (1994). Treating adult marijuana dependence: A test of the relapse prevention model. *Journal of Consulting and Clinical Psychology, 62,* 92–99.

Sylvain, C., Ladouceur, R., & Boisvert, J. M. (1997). Cognitive and behavioral treatment of pathological gambling: A controlled study. *Journal of Consulting and Clinical Psychology, 65,* 727–732.

Ward, T., Hudson, S. M., & Bulik, C. M. (1993). The abstinence violation effect in bulimia nervosa. *Addictive Behaviors, 18,* 671–680.

Ward, T., Hudson, S. M., & Marshall, W. L. (1994). The abstinence violation effect in child molesters. *Behaviour Research and Therapy, 32,* 431–437.

2

Alcohol and Tension Reduction

JANET GREELEY
TIAN OEI

INTRODUCTION

Historical Overview of the Tension-Reduction Concept

The tension-reduction theory of drinking and alcoholism asserts that people drink alcohol because it reduces tension. In its earliest conception, tension-reduction theory (TRT) exemplified the *Zeitgeist* of 1940s American psychology. Drive theory provided the dominant model of motivation and learning, and behaviorism was in its ascendance. Hull's (1943) drive reduction theory of learning was perhaps the most carefully formulated and well documented of the grand theories of the time. Drive reduction provided the impetus for behavior and was seen as the mechanism underlying reinforcement. For example, food deprivation increased the hunger drive, creating a buildup of tension within the organism that requires relief. Any behavior that led to the acquisition of food would reduce drive (tension) and thereby be reinforced.

Not surprisingly, researchers at the time began searching for the motives underlying the reinforcement of other behaviors. This was an important period in the development of addiction studies. Rather than conceive of alcoholism and other addictions as being mediated purely through a disease process or inherited physiological aberration, researchers began to consider how these self-destructive behaviors might be learned through experience. In the search for an explanation of why individuals would continue to engage in a behavior that could ultimately lead to their demise, focus was placed on trying to understand the immediate rewards gained from the behavior.

If an underlying hunger drive motivated eating, what engendered the drive that motivated alcohol consumption? Unlike food and water, alcohol is not essential to survival. Yet according to the theorizing of the time, alcohol must satisfy some internal drive state in order to be reinforcing. According to Kimble (1961), "An aversive state such as anxiety is conceived of as a drive, with anxiety reduction playing the role of reinforcer" (p. 447). The view that alcohol reduced tension was widely accepted by the research community. E. M. Jellinek (1945) went so far as to assert that this tension was generated by the increasing complexities of society, which served to subordinate the individual. If some other means of eliminating the cause of this tension were not available, then relief from tension would be sought. Alcohol was known to be one source of relief from tension. Jellinek did not presume that all drinking behavior was motivated by the need for tension reduction, but he did assume a widespread knowledge of this property of alcohol. Jellinek stated, "The emphasis on relief from tension is only to show the particular action of alcohol, through which it attained such social value as is attributed to it" (pp. 19–20). This statement could well be taken as a precursor to later cognitive accounts of learning and motivation.

Coincident with the development of drive theory, the experimental analysis of behavior by the use of animal models of human psychopathology was beginning to take its place in the annals of psychological research. Animal models of human psychopathology such as anxiety (Brady, 1956) and depression (Seligman, 1968) have been very useful in the development of behavioral and pharmaceutical therapies for these disorders. Masserman, Jacques, and Nicholson's (1945) studies of "experimental neurosis" and its relief by alcohol were a key development in the empirical analysis of the tension-reduction hypothesis that alcohol reduces tension. A number of studies proceeded in this vein, but it was not until 1956 that Conger drew together these and other data in his formulation of the tension-reduction theory of alcohol consumption. He wrote,

> From observation, we know that many people who have once made the response of drinking alcohol continue to do so, and that some of them do to excess. Through experience, the drinking response becomes learned. While this point seems clear, it is by no means as readily apparent that the drinking response is learned because it leads to a reduction in drive. But if we are to be consistent in applying a drive-reduction hypothesis, we must maintain that in those cases where the drinking response is learned, it is learned because it is rewarding. (p. 296)

Highlights from Earlier Reviews of the Literature

Cappell and Herman (1972)

In 1972, Cappell and Herman prepared a comprehensive and critical review of the experimental research that had been carried out since the

1940s, focusing on the question posed by the tension-reduction hypothesis (TRH)—does alcohol reduce tension? Logically, tension reduction cannot be the motive for alcohol consumption if it does not.

Until the 1970s, the majority of the experimental research on the TRH was carried out on laboratory animals (Cappell & Herman, 1972). The three main experimental procedures used to investigate alcohol's effects on what was termed "emotional behavior" were (1) escape–avoidance, (2) conflict and experimental neurosis, and (3) conditioned suppression. The fundamental rationale underpinning these procedures was similar: An aversive motivational state such as fear, anxiety, or frustration was deemed to have been produced by the introduction of aversive stimuli, the removal of appetitive stimuli, or a combination of both. For example, in a typical avoidance learning procedure, animals were trained to vacate an area or perform some behavior such as a bar press to avoid exposure to an aversive stimulus such as electric shock. In the tension-reduction hypothesis, it was predicted that alcohol would disrupt performance of avoidance and escape responding by reducing fear or anxiety produced by the anticipation of the aversive event (e.g., shock). Cappell and Herman concluded that research on the TRH using this procedure was equivocal. There were as many findings rejecting the hypothesis as supporting it.

In many experiments, there were difficulties ruling out other effects of alcohol as the underlying cause of behavior change when the doses required to affect avoidance behavior were high enough to produce sensory and motor impairment (e.g., Wallgren & Savolainen, 1962). Interpretation of research findings was made more difficult by the complexity of the relationship between fear and avoidance, which was described as nonmonotonic (Adamson & Black, 1959). It was also observed in some studies that alcohol actually facilitated avoidance responding (e.g., Reynolds & van Sommers, 1960). This, coupled with the fact that most experiments employed only one level of fear stimulus and one dose of alcohol, meant that negative results could indicate that either the TRH was not supported or that the experimenter had not used the appropriate test conditions. The observation of interactions between alcohol dose and avoidance response not only complicated the interpretation of experimental findings but also limited the generalizability of the TRH. These difficulties in interpretation were compounded by poor understanding of the underlying psychological processes that were being manipulated.

Failure to utilize balanced designs also compromised the interpretation of experimental tests of the TRH. For example, in many studies, subjects were given avoidance training in a nondrugged state, with the experimental group tested under the influence of alcohol and the control group given placebo. The test conditions more closely resembled the training conditions for the control subjects than for the experimental group. The internal conditions produced by alcohol may have served to produce a generalization decrement between training and test conditions that interfered with performance. If so, then there was no need to imply that there had been a change in motivation or fear levels produced by alcohol.

Experiments involving the production of conflict and "experimental neurosis" tended to generate results that were generally supportive of the TRH. These were exemplified by the studies of Masserman and colleagues, in which cats were trained to perform a complex response to obtain food. In the second phase of training, cats were given an airblast in the face when they contacted food. In response to the airblast, the cats inhibited feeding and developed what Masserman described as "neurotic behaviors" (e.g., cats avoided food, showed fear of the signal for food availability, and attempted to resist placement in the training apparatus) (Masserman, Jacques, & Nicholson, 1945; Masserman & Yum, 1946). When alcohol was administered prior to the second phase of training (when the airblast was introduced), the occurrence of neurotic behaviors was attenuated and the inhibition of feeding was blocked. When the same cats were retested without alcohol, they inhibited eating and developed neurotic behavior. It was assumed that conflict developed between two competing motives—the desire to eat and the fear of eating. In the TRH, alcohol is assumed to alleviate the tension or anxiety produced by this conflict, thereby preventing the development of neurotic behaviors. Early concerns that the introduction of alcohol in phase 2 of the conflict procedure may have merely interfered with the more recent learning experience (i.e., avoidance of the airblast) rather than the more well-established behavior were dispelled when a new procedure was introduced: By classically conditioning the fear response to a stimulus (i.e., a tone) before instrumental training to obtain food, the fear response was no longer the more recently learned event. The results from the revised method continued to support the TRH (Miller, 1961).

Conger's (1951) own work employed a similar type of approach–avoidance conflict procedure in which rats were trained to run to the end of an alley to obtain food as a reinforcer. There they also received electric shock as punishment. Conflict developed between the tendency to approach food and the tendency to avoid shock. The result was a reduction in running speed in the alley. Conger found that an intraperitoneal injection of a moderate dose of alcohol resulted in faster approach times. According to Conger, alcohol reduced the avoidance response by ameliorating fear motivation.

Tests of the TRH that employed the conditioned suppression procedure developed by Estes and Skinner (1941) did not support the hypothesis. Yet it was presumed aversive motivational/emotional states were elicited in this procedure, similar to those thought to underlie the conflict experiments. In this procedure, rats are trained to press a bar for food. They then receive classical conditioning of a conditioned stimulus (CS) with shock. The CS is then introduced when the rat is bar pressing for food, resulting in a suppression of bar pressing. The dependent measure is reflected as a ratio

$a/(a + b)$, where a is the number of bar presses in the presence of the CS for shock and b is the number of bar presses during a similar period in the absence of shock. Cappell and Herman (1972) found that criticisms that the procedure was flawed were not tenable, because inhibition of response suppression had been successfully produced using other drugs that were also effective in the conflict procedure. In a study in which alcohol did inhibit suppression, it was also observed to increase responding in the absence of the CS for shock (Goldman & Doctor, 1966). Thus, alcohol's effect was generally to increase responding for food irrespective of the prevailing motivational conditions. Ensuring that the effect of alcohol is specific to aversively motivated situations is another control condition that should be considered in investigations of the TRH.

According to Cappell and Herman's (1972) review, studies of the TRH involving humans were few, and these were not generally supportive of the hypothesis. They were often difficult to interpret because the measures of tension were unreliable (e.g., self-report), and the processes underlying the test procedures were not well understood. For example, human studies of the TRH measured psychophysiological indices of tension, such as the galvanic skin response (Lienert & Traxel, 1959), noradrenaline levels (Goddard, 1958), and self-reported anxiety (Williams, 1966). The relationships between these measures and tension are complex even without the addition of alcohol as a factor.

The general conclusion reached by Cappell and Herman (1972) regarding the status of the TRH in 1972 was "that while the TRH may be quite plausible intuitively, it has not been convincingly supported empirically" (p. 59). It was their view that even if the experimental results had been more positive, it would have been difficult to attribute the cause to a tension-reducing effect of alcohol. At best, tension reduction could be considered one of several plausible interpretations of many of the experimental findings. They expressed the view that although the tension reduction concept had been a useful stimulus for research, continued focus on it might be inhibiting research into more productive alternative areas.

Cappell and Greeley (1987)

Cappell and Herman (1972) had concluded that empirical support for the TRH was limited and most convincing in the approach–avoidance conflict procedure. Hodgson, Stockwell, and Rankin (1979) revisited this earlier review, providing a more positive appraisal of the data. They argued that Cappell and Herman had considered too broad a data base making the claim that tests using the passive–avoidance procedure were "the best test of the TRH because they represent the purest example of a behavior truly motivated by fear" (Cappell & Greeley, 1987, p. 20). Cappell and Greeley concluded that if Hodgson et al. were correct, then this interpretation might explain some of the contradictory findings reported in the literature.

However, by taking such a narrow view, they also constrained the generalizability of the theory and ignored a large body of contradictory data that other researchers considered germane. Studies of the TRH using conflict in animals have continued to support the TRH.

By the time of the later review by Cappell and Greeley (1987), more sophisticated experimental designs and measurement procedures had been developed, and many more studies had been carried out with human subjects. The strong behaviorist influences of the 1950s and 1960s had been supplanted by cognitive theories of behavior. The conditioned suppression procedure (described earlier) had become a standard for testing drugs for their anxiolytic properties. It was used in species as varied as mice, rats (Vogel et al., 1980), squirrel monkeys (Glowa & Barrett, 1976) and fish (Geller, Croy, & Ryback, 1974). Administration of alcohol increased responding that had been suppressed by the introduction of an aversive stimulus. Although results from these experiments generally supported the TRH, behavioral pharmacologists tended to interpret the results from a nonmotivational perspective, describing the increase in response rate under alcohol as an example of rate dependency (i.e., alcohol increased low rates of responding irrespective of how they were engendered). Some researchers did find that alcohol increased response rates in the nonpunished as well as the punished component of the procedure (Glowa & Barrett, 1976).

After 1976, more research with humans on the TRH began to appear. Some ingenious methodologies were devised. Lindman (1980) measured what he described as "behavioral fear" by having subjects traverse a floor to remove a ball from a jar containing electrolyte solution. When subjects placed their hand in the jar they received an unpleasant electric shock, and approach time was found to increase with increased probability of shock. When alcohol was administered at a dose of 0.9 g/kg, approach time was reduced. Two other studies were conducted in which handling of animals was used as the fear stimulus; for example, women were asked to transfer a mouse from one jar to another (Lindman, 1980) or subjects were asked to handle a 4-foot boa constrictor (Rimm, Briddell, Zimmerman, & Caddy, 1981). Response time for transferring the mouse was reduced by a 0.9 g/kg dose of alcohol but autonomic arousal, as measured by electrodermal activity, was not dampened. A lower dose of 0.5 g/kg had no effect on time taken approaching and handling the snake, but subjects did report feeling less fearful after drinking. These findings are difficult to interpret, as there was no attempt to compare the degree of fear engendered by these animal stimuli and the doses of alcohol used were markedly different. It is also possible that the reduction of self-reported fear in the study involving the snake may have been due to subjects' expectations of alcohol's effect rather than an actual pharmacologically induced change in perceived fear.

Steele, Southwick, and Critchlow (1981) employed a cognitive dissonance procedure in which students were asked to write an essay agreeing with an increase in tuition fees (a position that they did not endorse). Those who drank even small amounts of alcohol prior to the measurement of attitude change showed less change in their views. It was assumed that alcohol had alleviated the cognitive tension induced by writing an essay that expressed an opinion contrary to their beliefs. Subjects in the control group showed an increase in agreement with the tuition increase, as predicted by dissonance theory. It was questionable whether the effect observed in the alcohol group could be attributed to the pharmacological effects of alcohol given that it occurred at a dose as low as 0.3 g/kg. Subjects' expectations of alcohol's effects may have played a more important role in mediating this outcome.

Cappell and Greeley (1987) considered separately studies of responsiveness to "physically" noxious stimuli, such as electric shock, and social stressors, such as having subjects give a self-disclosing speech while being videotaped. The work of Sher, Levenson and colleagues on what they referred to as the stress-response dampening (SRD) effects of alcohol was instructive here. Levenson, Sher, Grossman, Newman, and Newlin (1980) measured psychophysiological and self-report indices of stress repeatedly during a baseline period, before the stressor was introduced, during a period while subjects anticipated delivery of the stressor, and immediately after its onset. Subjects were compared after consuming 1.0 g/kg of alcohol or a placebo. During the baseline period, alcohol produced both "stimulant" and "relaxant" effects on the physiological measures and reduced self-reported anxiety. During anticipation of the stressor and after its onset, physiological and self-report measures were dampened by the consumption of alcohol. These researchers identified several important principles to take into consideration when evaluating research on the TRH:

1. Stress-response dampening or tension reduction can only be tested if a validated stressor is used.
2. The effectiveness of alcohol as a stress-response dampening agent should be most pronounced during anticipation of and immediately after the onset of the stressor.
3. Stress-response dampening should be most evident at high doses of alcohol.

Some researchers suggested that the SRD effect of alcohol could be due to an analgesic effect that reduced the stressfulness of the stimulus (e.g., Brown & Cutter, 1977; Cutter, Maloof, Kurtz, & Jones, 1976). Investigations of the analgesic properties of alcohol indicated that there were individual differences in subjects' susceptibility to this effect, with "problem" drinkers showing greater analgesia after a high dose of alcohol (0.63 g/kg) than "moderate" drinkers. Moderate drinkers showed reduced pain at the lower dose (0.32 g/kg) and increased sensitivity to pain at the high dose (Brown & Cutter, 1977). Whether this different effect was a response acquired after years of drinking or due to some innate sensitivity to the analgesic properties of alcohol could not be determined from this study. Later studies began to investigate the basis for these individual differences.

Sher and Levenson (1982) reexamined their earlier study dividing subjects into high and low risk for alcoholism on the basis of results from preexisting personality inventories and not on current drinking behavior. Individuals with an alcoholic parent were excluded, and no differences were observed between risk groups on quantity and frequency of alcohol consumption. The SRD effects of alcohol were observed only in the high-risk group.

Another study by Dengerink and Fagan (1978) found that alcohol increased physiological and self-report measures of anxiety in college students who were exposed to an electric shock stressor. There was no information regarding the risk for alcoholism among this group. Why an increase in the stress response was observed in this study, even though the dose was similar to that used by Levenson and Sher (0.9 g/kg vs. 1.0 g/kg), has not been explained. If these subjects were at low risk for alcoholism, then an SRD effect may not have been expected.

Animal studies using physical stressors such as foot or tail shock, or immobilization provided some interesting findings using physiological and biochemical indicators of stress. Although some studies found alcohol to be a stressor (Ellis, 1966; Van Thiel, 1983), this was mainly when administered to animals who were in a nonstressed state (Cappell & Greeley, 1987). It also appeared that in a number of animal models of stress, alcohol was more effective in dampening the biochemical reactions to stress in lower rather than higher doses (Vogel & DeTurck, 1983 vs. Vogel et al., 1980). A dissociation was also observed between the behavioral and biochemical responses to stress. At higher doses (1.5 g/kg), alcohol produced a clear anticonflict effect on behavior but did not alter corticosterone levels in blood (Vogel et al., 1980). Yet in a later study, Vogel and DeTurck (1983) found that a dose of 0.5 g/kg of alcohol attenuated biochemical responses to stress caused by immobilization in rats bred for high sensitivity to this stressor. The same dose was without effect in rats low in sensitivity to the stressor. Cappell and Greeley (1987) noted that, like the studies with human subjects, data from research with other animals indicated that individual differences such as sensitivity to stress and the state of the organism at the time of alcohol administration can influence the outcome of investigations into the tension-reducing or stress-response dampening effects of alcohol.

Cappell and Greeley (1987) acknowledged that their separation of studies of the TRH using physically noxious stimuli from those using social stressors was arbitrary. Higgins and Marlatt (1975) suggested that these two types of stressor were psychically distinct: Social stressors would be more meaningful to the average drinker as a source of stress that could be alleviated by alcohol. Fear of electric shock, however, was something rarely experienced in everyday life and less likely to be associated with relief from alcohol consumption. Social stressors typically involve having subjects interact with, and attempt to make a favorable impression on, a member of the opposite sex (e.g., Wilson & Abrams, 1977), or having subjects videotaped while making a self-disclosing speech (e.g., Levenson et al., 1980). Cappell and Greeley found that reaching a consensus regarding the interpretation of findings from these studies was virtually impossible. This was due largely to the complexity of the procedures and experimental designs, and the number of variables manipulated (e.g., gender, expectancies, dose of alcohol). These were further complicated by dissociations in findings from different measures of stress (e.g., psychophysiological, self-report, and observer ratings). As indicated in the previous studies reviewed, individual differences emerged as particularly relevant factors in the interpretation of these results. Several studies suggested gender differences in the response to alcohol while under stress. Women tended to show increased rather than decreased stress after alcohol (Polivy, Scheuneman, & Carlson, 1976). Also, when subjects were tested on performance skills such as driving, alcohol tended to increase anxiety (Logue, Gentry, Linnoila, & Erwin, 1978) and impair performance. It was suggested that the anticipated and actual impairment of performance by alcohol might account for the increase in anxiety in these situations where people want to perform well but know they are disadvantaged.

Tension and Alcohol Self-Administration. Cappell and Greeley (1987) did not review the correlational research that examines the relationship between self-reports of drinking and measures of tension level. They reviewed only the previous 10 years of experimental reports in which tension was manipulated as the independent variable and alcohol consumption was measured as the dependent variable. They looked mainly at research with humans, as few investigations with other animals had been carried out during that period.

The classic study in the area was one by Higgins and Marlatt (1973). Subjects were exposed to what was described as low- and high-threat conditions (i.e., they were told they would receive either a weak or a strong shock). They were told that the purpose of the study was to assess the effect of a touch stimulus on the taste of alcohol. The amount of alcohol they consumed in this sham "taste test" was the dependent measure. There was no effect of the threat manipulation on alcohol consumption in either of two populations of drinkers—alcoholics and social drinkers. Subsequent studies employed a similar approach in that some form of taste test was introduced as a ruse to allow alcohol consumption. The types of stressors included social stressors, such as taking part in an evaluative personal interaction with a member of the opposite sex (Higgins & Marlatt, 1975), a 15-minute harassment over one's shortcomings (Miller, Hersen, Eisler, & Hilsman, 1974), slides of mutilation scenes (Gabel, Noel, Keane, & Lisman, 1980), and being told one performed poorly on a test of intelligence (Holroyd, 1978). Some studies attempted to compare alcohol consumption after exposure to positive and negative events (Pihl & Yankofsky, 1979) or to compare different populations of drinkers (Higgins & Marlatt, 1973). These studies revealed no strong trend in the data and were often subject to alternative explanations to the TRT.

From this historical account, we can see that the concept of tension reduction has its roots in motivation in drive-reduction theory. Although some writers have described tension-reduction as a basic need, two-factor avoidance learning provided the mechanism by which tension could become an "acquired need" or drive specific to alcohol (i.e., alcohol reduces tension). In other words, a state of tension provides the motive for action. Negative reinforcement based on the notion of drive reduction provides the mechanism for translating the drive state into action (i.e., people drink to reduce tension).

A number of major reviews of the literature have found that compelling evidence is lacking for either of the key tenets of TRT (Cappell, 1975; Cappell & Greeley, 1987; Cappell & Herman, 1972; Young, Oei, & Knight, 1990). The general consensus has been that alcohol, at certain dosages, is capable of reducing some signs of tension in some humans (and other animals) under certain contextual conditions. At the conclusion of their 1987 review, Cappell and Greeley advised that if tension-reduction theory were to be salvaged, future research would need to focus on delineating the conditions under which alcohol's tension-reducing effects were relatively strong and uncontaminated. They recommended a promising approach emerging at that time through the elegant work of Sher, Levenson, and colleagues on the stress-response dampening (SRD) effects of alcohol. Research since 1987 has followed this trend, and it is the past 10-year period in the history of TRT research on which this review focuses.

The Stress-Response Dampening Model

It was recognized in the 1970s that the concepts of tension and tension reduction proved too broad to be of much use in explaining how alcohol produces its effects (e.g., Cappell, 1975; Cappell & Herman, 1972). It was not until the 1980s that a formal alternative account was proposed by way of the stress-response dampening (SRD) model. The SRD model of alcohol's effects was more an offshoot of TRT than an alternative explanation. Its major advantages were its increased specificity in describing stress responses and its focus on individual differences in responsiveness to alcohol's stress-response dampening effects (Sher & Levenson, 1982). The TRT applied as a single-factor account of alcohol consumption would never receive unequivocal support. However, with the qualification that individual differences exist in responsiveness to stressors and to alcohol's SRD effects, the TRT might live again as part of a more constrained and testable theory.

Although the SRD model was a fertile ground for research in the early to mid-1980s, it has been largely subsumed under its predecessor, the TRT, in more recent times. The two accounts are used interchangeably by researchers to explain similar phenomena.

Although the SRD model seemed to hold promise, subsequent research findings on alcohol's SRD effects were as diverse and confusing as those surrounding the older TRT (Sayette, 1993a). So many different variables can influence whether an SRD effect will be observed that predicting when and under what conditions to expect one becomes very difficult. The power of a model rests in its utility as a predictor. The SRD model, in its basic form, has not proven particularly useful in this respect. Elaboration on precisely how alcohol's SRD effects are brought about, when they do occur, offers some hope of rescue for the model.

Paradoxical Effects of Alcohol as a Stressful Stimulus

Alcohol has been found to increase as well as decrease responses to stress. The SRD effects of alcohol tend to occur within moderate dosage levels (0.75–1.3 g/kg), while at lower doses, alcohol produces a sense of excitation and exhilaration (Mello, 1968) and at higher doses, increased anxiety and aggressiveness have been observed (Tamerin & Mendelson, 1969). At higher doses, alcohol produces many effects that might be described as negative and stressful, such as nausea, depression of the central nervous system, and impairment of cognitive and motor functioning. Alcohol's aversive properties have been well demonstrated in the conditioned taste-aversion paradigm. In this procedure, animals are given a novel-tasting solution followed by administration of alcohol. Following this training, animals avoid the novel-tasting solution, as if they had been poisoned (Cappell & LeBlanc, 1977).

Some researchers have argued that these aversive effects of alcohol argue against the TRH and, by implication, also call into question the broader TRT. Powers and Kutash (1985) argued against this broad-brush approach and recommended that more effort be put into identifying the conditions under which alcohol serves a stress-response dampening effect and how this multivariate approach might assist in formulating a more elaborate account of the development of alcohol abuse and dependence.

DEFINITION OF TERMS

Key Terms

A shift in terminology has taken place over the past decade in research into the TRT. Researchers more commonly refer to the independent variables they manipulate as stressors—stimuli that induce stress or tension (e.g., social stressors, physical stressors, cognitive disruption) and the dependent variables are now described generically as stress responses (e.g., heart rate changes, self-reported stress levels, catecholamine levels).

It was noted earlier that alcohol's effects on stress can be variable, sometimes reducing it, sometimes increasing it, or at other times producing no change at all. Because the SRD effect of alcohol is not always predictable, it satisfies the conditions for intermittent reinforcement, a more powerful reinforcement schedule than continuous reinforcement (Skinner, 1926). This schedule of reinforcement may be important in the development and maintenance of SRD effects (Powers & Kutash, 1985).

Independent and Dependent Variables

Two fundamental assumptions that underpin research into the SRD effects of alcohol require consideration: (1) Experimental manipulation of stress/tension is possible; and (2) stress responses can be measured. Studies of the SRD model have investigated stress responses in great detail examining the direct and indirect effects of alcohol. Important parameters of the stressor, such as its type (physical, social, self-evaluative), time of onset (e.g., whether stress is greater in anticipation of giving a public speech or when actually giving the speech; for a review, see Sayette, 1993b), duration, and controllability (e.g., being able or unable to escape an aversive noise; Noel, Lisman, Schare, & Maisto, 1992) have been manipulated, as have the conditions of alcohol consumption, including dose, time of ingestion (before or after stressor onset), and expectancies (whether subjects are told they will receive alcohol).

A variety of stress-induction procedures or stressors have been employed in tests of TRT. They have included such diverse procedures as experimental conflict paradigms, approach–avoidance conflict, cognitive dissonance, and fear procedures. In the experimental conflict procedure, the aim is to produce conflict between two behaviors and to measure the suppression of one by the other. In this paradigm, alcohol is thought to reduce the tension, stress, fear, or anxiety instilled by this conflict and thereby reduce the suppression on responding. Evidence of tension reduction could include faster approach in an approach–avoidance conflict (behavioral measure); reduced dissonance (cognitive measure) in a cognitive dissonance paradigm; reduced time (behavioral measure) to carry out an aversive task (e.g., handle a snake or a mouse); and reports of less fear, anxiety, or tension (self-report measure) under these conditions. Other stressors include physically noxious stimuli such as shock or loud noise, and social stressors such as being required to give a self-evaluative speech or to make a positive impression on a member of the opposite sex.

As diverse as this list of stressors, so too is the range of stress responses. Fear, anxiety, tension, stress, frustration, and anger have all been reported as dependent measures in studies of the tension-reducing or stress-response dampening effects of alcohol. The most commonly reported physiological measures of stress include cardiovascular effects such as heart rate (HR) (e.g., Keane & Lisman, 1980; Sayette, 1993b; Stasiewicz & Maisto, 1993), blood pressure (e.g., Vogel & Netter, 1989), and digital pulse volume amplitude (DPVA) (Stewart et al., 1992); electrodermal activity (Bond & Lader, 1991; Finn, Zeitouni, & Pihl, 1990); and catecholamine levels (e.g., adrenaline and noradrenaline) (Vogel & Netter, 1989). More recently, researchers have begun to use detailed examination of facial expression as an index of emotional responsiveness to stressors (Sayette, Smith, Breiner, & Wilson, 1992). Clearly, a wide range of physiological, behavioral, cognitive, and emotional states have been included under the labels stress or tension.

In the case of changes in HR, a commonly used indicator of stress response, Sayette (1993b) provides compelling evidence that many reported SRD effects using this measure may be an artifact of the timing of the measures. For example, if a stimulus elicits an initial increase in HR (e.g., a low dose of alcohol), this is typically followed by a return to baseline HR. The outcome and interpretation of a study will vary depending on when the baseline is taken and when, during the sequence of HR changes elicited by the stimulus, a supposed measure of SRD is observed. The time course of the effects of the stressor and alcohol alone must be well understood, before the interpretation of these stimuli in combination can be evaluated.

A range of correlational studies and explicit experimental tests of the assumptions of the TRT have been conducted using humans and other animals as subjects. A sampling of these studies conducted since 1987 are considered in the next sections.

CORRELATIONAL STUDIES

Comorbidity

Correlational research on the comorbidity of anxiety disorders and alcohol-related disorders provides indirect evidence of the relationship between alcohol use and tension reduction. To consider this evidence, we must extend the definition of tension to include anxiety and other forms of negative affect. These correlational studies demonstrate that increased anxiety and increased alcohol consumption often co-occur, but they cannot shed light on the causal linkages that may exist between these disorders. In the TRT of drinking and alcoholism, people who experience higher levels of anxiety may drink as a means of self-medication. They drink to relieve their distress. Comorbidity studies provide a cross-sectional snapshot of the co-occurrence of different disorders within particular populations. They do not typically provide longitudinal information regarding the primacy of one disorder over another. Therefore, it is not possible to establish the causal links between anxiety and alcohol consumption from these studies. Nevertheless, they provide interesting indirect evidence of the stress–alcohol nexus.

Measures of state–trait anxiety and negative affect have been found to be positively (Kalodner, Delucia, & Ursprung, 1989) and negatively (Green, Burke, Nix, Lambrecht, & Mason, 1995) correlated with increased alcohol consumption in males and females. Studies of clinical populations such as social phobics (Holle, Heimberg, Sweet, & Holt, 1995) and sufferers of posttraumatic stress disorder (PTSD) (Stewart, 1996) have found positive correlations with alcohol-related disorders. Interestingly, these links have been observed in populations as young as adolescents (Colder & Chassin, 1993; Hussong & Chassin, 1994). Oei and Loveday (1997) noted that anxiety disorders such as agoraphobia, PTSD, general anxiety disorder, and panic and social disorders are more prevalent in patients suffering from alcohol disorders than in the general community. In each case, the authors concerned interpreted the results of their studies as supportive of TRT: People drink alcohol to reduce tension or anxiety. Their results cannot, however, address that hypothesis. Contrary evidence exists that suggests anxiety is not the primary condition in such cases (Vaillant, 1983).

Studies of the comorbidity of alcohol and the various anxiety disorders reveal large inconsistencies in the observed co-occurrence rates. For example, the rate of comorbidity between panic disorder and alcohol-related disorders ranges from 1% to 20%. Similarly, the rate of co-occurrence of PTSD with alcohol related disorders is reported as ranging from 19% to 40%. A number of factors contribute to this variability, such as the use by different researchers of different criteria for the diagnosis of disorders, the use of different diagnostic instruments, and other qualities of the actual clinical sample studied.

When compared with the prevalence of anxiety disorders found in the general population from the Epidemiologic Catchment Area (ECA) study (Robins et al., 1984), alcohol-disordered groups, on average, reveal a higher rate of co-occurrence of many of these diagnoses. In particular, panic disorder, agoraphobia, social phobia, generalized anxiety disorder, and PTSD are found more commonly in people suffering from alcohol-related disorders. The co-occurrence of simple phobia and obsessive–compulsive disorder with alcohol-related problems appears to be less pronounced (for reviews, see Allan, 1995; Brady & Lydiard, 1993; Cowley, 1992; Stewart, 1996).

Studies of patients in treatment for anxiety disorders with co-occurring alcohol-related disorders show a similar pattern of results. The ECA study found alcohol abuse and/or dependence occurring in their community samples at a rate of 13.3% (Robins et al., 1984). It would seem that only patients with social phobia and agoraphobia (with and without panic) have coexisting alcohol disorders at greater rates than occur in the general community. However, the small number of studies examining generalized anxiety disorder, obsessive–compulsive disorder, and PTSD would lend caution to the interpretation that these disorders are less likely to coexist with alcohol abuse or dependence. A review of alcohol abuse and dependence in patients with PTSD found these occur at rates of between 41% and 85%, respectively (Keane & Wolfe, 1990; Stewart, 1996). Panic disorder (with and without agoraphobia) seems to be the only anxiety disorder unrelated to higher levels of alcohol problems, occurring at rates the same or lower than in the general community.

The ECA study, which surveyed some 20,000 people across five cities and towns in the United States in the early 1980s, found evidence of significant rates of co-occurring alcohol-related disorders and anxiety disorders. Nearly 25% of individuals with anxiety disorders had a substance abuse disorder (Regier, Farmer, & Rae, 1991). Those with lifetime diagnoses of alcoholism showed 2.4 times more risk for panic disorder, 2.1 times more risk for obsessive–compulsive disorder, and 1.4 times more risk for phobic disorder (Helzer & Pryzbeck, 1987).

Furthermore, the National Comorbidity Study (NCS), conducted in the United States between 1990 and 1992 using DSM-III-R criteria, examined the co-occurrence of anxiety disorders (panic disorder with and without agoraphobia, generalized anxiety disorder, simple phobia, social phobia, agoraphobia with and without panic, PTSD) and addictive disorders (alcohol abuse without dependence, alcohol dependence, drug abuse without dependence, other drug dependence) (Kessler et al., 1996). Comorbidity was examined using a sample of over 5,000 noninstitutionalized civilians who were diagnosed with one psychiatric or addictive disorder. All the anxiety disorders, except panic disorder, were significantly related to alcohol abuse and dependence. Social phobia was the only anxiety disorder significantly related to alcohol abuse without dependence. The lifetime co-occurrence data found all anxiety disorders were significantly related to alcohol abuse and dependence. PTSD was significantly related to both alcohol abuse without dependence, and alcohol abuse and dependence (Kessler et al., 1996). Overall, the results of these two epidemiological studies suggest that the association found in the clinical studies is not an artifact due to specific factors of the samples studied.

Levels of Alcohol Consumption and Stress

Indirect evidence for TRH is available through a large body of literature in which authors examine the relationship between some measure of stress (e.g., life-event stress, state–trait anxiety) and pattern of alcohol consumption (generally assessed through self-report measures). For example, O'Doherty (1991) found that alcoholic subjects reported fewer stressful life events (quantity and frequency) not directly related to drinking than matched controls. Similarly, subjects exhibiting high alcohol consumption in a study by Neff (1993) reported lower frequency of stressful life events; however, the effect was true for males only. In contrast, other studies have found no relationship between number of stressful life events and increased alcohol consumption (Glass, Prigerson, Kasl, & Mendes de Leon, 1995). In a study on the interaction between stress, alcohol, and depression in the elderly, Krause (1995) reported that alcohol reduced tension related to certain, less important stressful events, and increased tension resulting from more salient stressors. Orcutt and Harvey (1991) found that self-reported tension reduction after drinking occurred for men and women, but only on work days.

Causal Relationships: Mediation or Moderation?

In summary, although there appears to be general consensus in the theoretical literature about the tension-reducing role of alcohol, research has revealed mixed support for the TRH. On the whole, observational studies provide data that are consistent with the TRH, whereas the experimental evidence is less supportive.

Age and Gender

Most of the research conducted on TRT prior to 1987 used as subjects college students who were in late adolescence or early adulthood. Recent studies have begun to examine the tension-reduction theory of alcohol use as an explanation of drinking behavior in early and middle adolescence (e.g., Colder & Chassin, 1993; Hussong & Chassin, 1994; Johnson & Pandina, 1993). Some studies have found links between levels of stress or anxiety and alcohol consumption (e.g., Kalodner et al., 1989), while others have found little or no indication of such a relationship (e.g., Brook, Gordon, Whiteman, & Cohen, 1986). The research findings on TRT of alcohol consumption in this population tend to parallel those seen with adults. Some subgroups use alcohol in response to stress, while others do not. Individual differences in coping strategies, personality, and social support interact with stress to augment or attenuate stress-induced drinking. Emotional states such as anxiety and depression, and personality variables such as impulsivity, operate to mediate or moderate the influence of stress on alcohol intake (Hussong & Chassin, 1994).

Among adolescents, stressful life events combined with low family support were associated with higher levels of alcohol consumption and other problem behaviors when examined in a cross-sectional analysis (Windle, 1992). Prospective longitudinal analyses of similar data indicated that these factors best predicted problem behaviors in young women rather than young men. Some authors have suggested that this difference in response to stress may be due to differences in sex-role development, in which girls are more dependent on family support, whereas boys of a similar age are expected to be more independent. Alternatively, Isenhart (1993) noted that among an inpatient sample of male alcohol abusers, those who scored high on masculine gender-role stress (i.e., who felt stressed because they felt unable to live up to the male role expectation in certain circumstances) generally scored higher on alcohol abuse than those who scored low on this factor. The importance of role identity and social support were underlined in a study by Richman, Rospenda, and Kelley (1995), where they found that men and women reported increased distress and increased levels of alcohol consumption during the transition into parenthood. These changes seemed to be the result of deterioration of other social roles (e.g., that of spouse). This finding is in contrast with other research which indicated people tend to "mature-out" of earlier problem drinking as they grow older and take on the responsibilities of adulthood, such as parenting (e.g., Power & Estaugh, 1990). Yet the findings from this group of older, first-time parents suggest that some individuals may be at risk of slipping back into drinking problems as role changes lead to increased stress.

In these studies, stress and stressful life events are equated with the concept of tension as it is used in the TRT. Unlike the more specific definition of stress, as applied in the SRD experiments of Sher and others, stress in the present studies encompasses all those daily hassles and other more significant life events that can adversely affect our capacity to operate efficiently. It is presumed that increases in stress mediate the transition from lower to higher levels of alcohol consumption.

Gender differences in alcohol pharmacokinetics may also influence alcohol's impact as a tension reduction agent. Breslin, Hayword, and Baum (1994) noted that women showed greater bioavailability of alcohol, even after body composition was controlled, and a faster rate of alcohol elimination than men. There were no interactions between gender and stress in this study. Men and women exposed to stressors such as cold pressor and a distressing film showed reduced levels of intoxication and changes in the blood alcohol concentration (BAC) curve. The influence of stress on the psychopharmacological response to alcohol may, in part, account for the relationship between increased alcohol consumption and stress. If stress reduces alcohol's impact as a stress-reducing agent and also increases anxiety, then it may contribute to the motivation to consume alcohol in two ways. In other words, alcohol may be least effective in individuals who may desire to use it most for its SRD effects—in those who are most reactive to stress.

There is some indication that as people grow older, their tolerance to alcohol's effects may decrease, which may partially explain why people reduce alcohol consumption as they approach old age (e.g., Atkinson & Kofoed, 1982). Reports have been inconsistent regarding levels of drinking problems found among the elderly. It has been suggested that these differences may be attributable to different samples being used in different studies. Rates of alcohol consumption and alcohol-related problems tend to vary across clinical or hospitalized populations and community-based samples of the elderly (Glass et al., 1995; LaForge, Nirenberg, Lewis, & Murphy, 1993).

One factor noted as influencing whether exposure to stress increases alcohol consumption among the elderly is their baseline level of consumption. People who were abstainers or infrequent drinkers were less likely to resort to increased alcohol consumption in response to stress than those who were regular or heavy drinkers (Glass et al., 1995). These researchers also noted that the type of event experienced by the elderly person affected whether alcohol consumption was likely to occur and that this varied between genders. For example, events relating to one's spouse (e.g., illness or hospitalization) were more likely to increase drinking among elderly men than women. Changes of living circumstances and health status (which often co-occurred) also affected use of alcohol. Poor health or relocation to a nursing home or hospital tended to be associated with reduced alcohol intake, perhaps more due to limitations on access to opportunities to drink rather than a reduced motivation to drink. Although data from survey studies such as those gathered by Glass et al. provide indications of the kinds of variables that may influence people's reactions to stress, these results provide no clear evidence of any causal relationship between stress and alcohol intake. In this study, as in many others that monitor life events, the impact of these events was presumed to be stressful, but no measure of the level of stress experienced was collected. Prospective studies that examine the time course of stress and alcohol intake, and that control for alternative explanations of the consumption data, are needed to make causal links between these variables and adequately test TRT.

Gender and age influence responses to stress and to alcohol. These demographic variables combine in complex ways to affect the relationship between stress and alcohol intake. Gender and age differences in basic alcohol pharmacokinetics operate in combination with variations in psychological variables such as social roles and expectations to produce a plethora of effects. It should not be surprising, then, that no simple relationship can be predicted between alcohol and stress.

EXPERIMENTAL STUDIES

Following the distinction made by Cappell and Greeley (1987), the experimental studies are divided according to the principal tenets of the TRT: (1) Alcohol reduces tension, and (2) people and other animals consume alcohol for its tension-reducing properties. Research on animals other than humans is considered briefly, and then the more extensive developments in investigations into the TRH using humans as experimental subjects are considered in some detail.

Experiments with Animals: Does Alcohol Reduce Tension/Stress?

The studies considered measure physiological responses to stress induced by restraint or immobilization. The physiological measures include changes in levels of the catecholamines, epinephrine (E) and norepinephrine (NE), and certain amino acids in the plasma and brain in response to the stressor, before and after alcohol injection. Thus, the response to stress is operationally defined as changes in these physiological measures. Livezey, Balabkins, and Vogel (1987) reported a reduction and delay in the catecholamine response to immobilization stress in male and female rats after consumption of 1 g/kg of alcohol. Changes in NE and E were not as large in rats that had consumed alcohol before exposure to the stressor as that seen in control rats. The SRD effect was stronger for male rats. The authors also observed that there were large variations in the stress reactions and SRD effects of alcohol observed among the rats, which they attributed to genetic differences. Those rats displaying the greatest initial (prealcohol) stress reaction showed the greatest stress reduction in response to alcohol. This may indicate a specificity of the SRD effects of alcohol on animals who are more reactive to stress. Alternatively, it could also indicate a problem due to the law of initial values (i.e., those animals with the greatest initial response to stress have more room to change than those who showed a small initial response) and suggests that data from such studies should be interpreted with caution.

Milakofsky, Miller, and Vogel (1989) found that alcohol reduced the change in certain amino acid levels typically produced by immobilization. Rats injected with alcohol showed smaller increases in amino acid levels than control rats when exposed to an immobilization stressor.

Exposure to social stressors has proven popular in investigation of the tension-reducing effects of alcohol on rats. Generally, social stress for rats is operationally defined with respect to subordination or fight stress; that is, it is hypothesized that alcohol inhibits the reduction of fighting behavior normally observed in subordinate rats due to fear and anxiety (Blanchard, Flores, Magee, Weiss, & Blanchard, 1992). This is demonstrated by increased fighting among subordinate rats when under the influence of alcohol.

Experiments with Animals: Does Tension/Stress Increase Alcohol Consumption?

This hypothesis has been tested more extensively over the past decade. Roske, Baeger, Frenzel, and Oehme (1994) observed that male rats increased voluntary consumption of alcohol in response to social-isolation stress but not immobilization stress. In contrast, rats reduced alcohol intake when exposed to acute stress such as formaldehyde or saline injections (Champagne & Kirouac, 1989).

Using the social stressor of fight stress described earlier, it was hypothesized that, after alcohol consumption, if fight stress is reduced, then, in accordance with the second tenet of TRT, voluntary alcohol intake by subordinate rats should increase in response to exposure to fight stress.

While such observations appear to support TRT (Blanchard, Yudko, & Blanchard, 1993; Hilakivi-Clarke & Lister, 1992), it must be noted that studies of this nature do not demonstrate a causal relationship between alcohol consumption and tension reduction. The increased alcohol consumption observed in these studies could be caused by a number of factors other than the anticipation of stress reduction by the rats. For example, the rats may increase alcohol consumption as a behavioral alternative to fighting.

Thus, recent animal studies indicate through behavioral and physiological measures that TRT is a plausible explanation of the effects of alcohol on stress, particularly in socially stressful situations.

Experiments with Human Subjects: Does Alcohol Reduce Stress/Tension?

The experiments addressing this question typically involve oral administration of alcohol either before or after some stressor, and observation of behavioral, physiological, or self-report responses of subjects.

As reported by Young, Oei, and Knight (1990), there is much support from the correlational literature for the idea that the tension-reducing effects of alcohol are influenced by alcohol related expectancies. Indeed, alcohol expectancies are thought to be important mediators of alcohol consumption in their own right (e.g., Darkes & Goldman, 1993; Gustafson, 1991; Keane & Lisman, 1980; Oei & Baldwin, 1994; Vuchinich, Tucker, & Sobell, 1979; Young, Knight, & Oei, 1990). Hence, many studies of the TRH have addressed the issue of alcohol expectancies by including a placebo condition as part of the research design. By manipulating expected and actual beverage content, researchers have attempted to examine the influence of the expected effects of alcohol on SRD independently of the pharmacological effects of the drug.

An extensive search of the literature revealed 15 studies published after 1988 that have included placebo control groups in experiments that investigate the TRH that alcohol reduces tension. None of the studies reviewed provided unequivocal support for the TRH. Corcoran (1994) found no evidence of tension reduction while most studies provided partial support for the idea that alcohol reduces anxiety (Conrod, Pihl, & Ditto, 1995; Finn et al., 1990; Josephs & Steele, 1990; Netter & Vogel, 1990; Noel et al., 1992; Sayette, Breslin, & Wilson, 1994; Sayette & Wilson, 1991; Sayette et al., 1992; Steele & Josephs, 1988; Stewart, Finn, & Pihl, 1992; Stritzke, Patrick, & Lang, 1995; Vogel & Netter, 1989; Young, Oei, & Knight, 1990; Zeichner, Giancola, & Allen, 1995). Direct comparison of these studies is difficult due to the different methodologies and manipulations used (i.e., different stressors and measures of stress effects). In accordance with the recommendations for research into the SRD effects of alcohol developed by Levenson and colleagues (1980), most studies supplied subjects with moderate to high doses of alcohol (i.e., greater than 0.39 g/kg), alcohol was administered immediately before or shortly after exposure to the stressor, and all studies successfully elicited some stress response from subjects as validated through manipulation checks.

Expectancy effects were not evident in the placebo groups tested in these studies (i.e., when subjects expected alcohol but did not consume it, tension reduction effects of alcohol were not observed). Thus, on the basis of these data, it appears that when an alcohol-induced tension-reduction effect occurred, it was due to some property of the alcohol and not an interaction involving alcohol expectancies.

As Cappell and Greeley (1987) pointed out, manipulation of subjects' expectations of the type of beverage they have received is quite different from examining what subjects believe the effects of alcohol to be. If an individual does not have an expectation that alcohol reduces tension, then belief that he or she has consumed alcohol is likely to be irrelevant to self-reports of tension levels. In order to address this issue, it is necessary to examine specific alcohol expectancy beliefs (i.e., prior beliefs about the effects alcohol may induce). Young et al. (1990) posited that there are two possible methods to control for such preheld expectancy beliefs: (1) Manipulate alcohol expectancies in the experiment or (2) determine alcohol expectancies prior to the experiment. Of the experiments reviewed earlier, three attempted to control for expectancy beliefs by determining them prior to the experiment (Corcoran, 1994; Sayette et al., 1994; Young, Knight, & Oei, 1990). Preheld alcohol expectancy beliefs did not correlate with tension-reduction effects in any of these studies. This is consistent with previous research (e.g., Sher & Walitzer, 1986). However, in the Young, Knight, and Oei study (1990), independent and subjective measures of tension were lower after alcohol consumption, despite no reported change in alcohol expectancies by subjects (alcohol expectancies were measured before, during, and after drinking).

The results of studies examining the effects of alcohol on experimentally manipulated stressors are considered below according to the type of stressor used.

Physical Stress

Six studies employed physical stressors: Five used shock (Conrod et al., 1995; Finn & Pihl, 1987, 1988; Finn et al., 1990; Stewart et al., 1992), and one used aversive noise (Noel et al., 1992). The dependent measure of stress-response dampening in the study using aversive noise was latency to learn an escape response in a human shuttle-box apparatus (Noel et al., 1992). A learned helplessness paradigm was used by varying the controllability of the noise. Dose (placebo, 0.26 and 0.59 g/kg) and timing of alcohol delivery (before or after exposure to uncontrollable aversive noise) were also manipulated. The groups that received the moderate-dose of alcohol before exposure to uncontrollable noise showed less impairment of escape learning than those receiving the low dose or placebo indicating an SRD effect. The groups who consumed their respective beverages after exposure to uncontrollable noise showed a different pattern of results; the moderate dose group showed impairment of escape learning (i.e., longer escape latencies) relative to the low dose and placebo groups. Results from the control group suggested that it is possible that controllable noise facilitated learning. Therefore, it is also possible that the moderate dose of alcohol did likewise, rather than merely attenuate the learned helplessness effects produced by uncontrollable noise.

A series of studies by Pihl and associates investigated the role of risk for alcoholism as a moderating factor in the SRD effects of alcohol. Risk for alcoholism was assessed through family history targeting men with multigenerational family history positive for alcoholism as those at greatest risk. In the five studies employing shock as a stressor, multigenerational family history of alcoholism was measured. These studies found that men with multigenerational family histories positive (MFH+) for alcoholism showed greater cardiovascular reactivity to shock when sober than men who had no family history of alcoholism (FH–) (Conrod et al., 1995; Finn & Pihl, 1987, 1988; Finn et al., 1990; Stewart et al., 1992). In these studies, only men in the MFH+ group showed stress-response dampening effects of alcohol, and only at moderately high to high doses of alcohol (0.59, 0.79, and 1.04 g/kg). It was also noted that alcohol significantly raised baseline HR in the MFH+ group but, again, only at the higher doses. In the study by Conrod et al. (1995) an additional control group was added— men who were the sons of essential hypertensives (HT+). Like the MFH+ men, the HT+ group exhibited an elevated cardiovascular and muscular tension response to stress. Alcohol increased resting HR in all groups, but the greatest increase was seen in the MFH+ group. Likewise, this group showed the greatest increase in muscle tension in the left frontalis muscle of the forehead when given alcohol. When responsiveness to the shock stimulus was measured under the alcohol condition, again, only the MFH+ group showed a significant reduction in responsiveness on the HR and electromyographic (EMG) measures. Conrod et al. argued that the specificity of these effects to the MFH+ group provided evidence that different mechanisms control HR responsiveness to shock in HT+ and MFH+ men. The specificity of the SRD effect of alcohol also strengthened the claim that certain forms of alcoholism may be inherited and that SRD may be one of the mechanisms whereby alcohol's reinforcing effects are mediated.

These findings parallel those reported by Sher and Levenson (1982), in which they found that individuals identified as being at greater risk for developing alcoholism, as measured by personality inventories, were also those who showed greater responsiveness to the SRD effects of alcohol. The findings with the multigenerational familial history measure are more robust than those using measures of personality. This may be due to the greater reliability of the family history measure or because it is a better indicator of genetic influences on the effects experienced from alcohol consumption.

The failure to find an SRD effect among men with family histories of essential hypertension is reminiscent of the findings reported by Sher (1987) of early studies failing to find a greater SRD effect among anxious subjects. Different mechanisms may control different forms of anxiety, and perhaps only some of these are susceptible to the tension-reducing effects of alcohol.

Social Stress

Six of the studies that showed partial support for TRH employed a social stressor (usually comprising instructions to prepare and/or perform a brief speech about one's physical appearance; Josephs & Steele, 1990; Sayette et al., 1992, 1994; Sayette & Wilson, 1991; Steele & Josephs, 1988; Zeichner et al., 1995). Of these, alcohol significantly reduced physiological measures of stress reaction in the presence of a distracting task (Josephs & Steele, 1990; Steele & Josephs, 1988), in hostile men and not in nonhostile men (Zeichner et al., 1995), and when alcohol was consumed prior to, and not following, exposure to a stressor (Sayette & Wilson, 1991). In studies where stress or anxiety was measured via self-report, four studies reported a reduction in anxiety after alcohol consumption (Josephs & Steele, 1990; Sayette et al., 1994; Steele & Josephs, 1988; Vogel & Netter, 1989). Two studies conducted by Sayette and colleagues found an improvement in mood after alcohol consumption (Sayette et al., 1992, 1994). One study did not show this trend of reduced anxiety (Sayette & Wilson, 1991). It is possible that this is due to the fact that in this study, subjects were all men, whereas the subject samples in the majority of studies that showed positive effects on mood and anxiety consisted of men and women.

Cognitive Stress

Vogel and Netter (1989) conducted a study in which the stressor was an increasingly difficult math task. Physiological indicators of stress were unaffected by alcohol, but subjects reported less anxiety and aggression in the alcohol condition when performing this task. A reanalysis of these data by Netter and Vogel (1990), dividing the groups on the basis of their level of habitual alcohol consumption, revealed that those who were high habitual consumers showed attenuated SRD effects on NE and E levels, and on emotional stress compared with low habitual consumers. The reduced efficacy of alcohol as a stress-response dampening agent in high habitual consumers may reflect the development of tolerance to this effect of alcohol in this group.

Stritzke et al. (1995) conducted a study in which subjects were exposed to very pleasant and very unpleasant slides. They found that alcohol dampened emotional responding (in the form of the startle response) to both types of stimuli, indicating a general reduction in arousal by alcohol rather than an effect specific to negative emotional states. If alcohol dampens what might be perceived as positive emotional states as well as negative ones, how might this be incorporated into TRT?

Findings from these studies combined with those from earlier research indicate that there are important individual differences among subjects that may significantly influence the SRD effects of alcohol. These include such factors as family history for alcoholism and personality variables that are associated with increased risk for developing drinking problems. The largest SRD effects seem to appear in subjects who are at greater risk for developing alcoholism. If these findings are reliable, then they may well account for many of the inconsistencies in results from previous research on the TRH. They may also provide a mediating or moderating mechanism to account for the apparently greater reinforcing effects of alcohol experienced by some drinkers. If there is a heritable tendency to receive greater tension-reducing effects from alcohol, then this may explain the susceptibility of some and not other drinkers to develop problems controlling alcohol consumption.

Experiments with Human Subjects: Does Stress/Tension Increase Alcohol Consumption?

Corcoran and Parker (1991) manipulated stress by asking college students to prepare a brief essay on a favorite leisure activity (low-stress condition) or give a 10-minute speech on their most embarrassing body part (high stress). They hypothesized that subjects in the high-stress condition would drink more alcohol. No such relationship was observed. Samoluk and Stewart (1996) manipulated stress through the presentation of anxiety-relevant and anxiety-irrelevant questions. Subjects were exposed to one of the sets of questions and then asked to engage in a taste-rating task. Samoluk and Stewart also controlled for anxiety sensitivity. High-anxiety-sensitive subjects consumed more alcohol than their counterparts who scored low on the anxiety sensitivity scale, but only when answering anxiety-irrelevant questions. The anxiety manipulation in this study was not effective; therefore, it is difficult to interpret these results with respect to TRT. The contrived nature of both manipulations, like many used in previous research, has resulted in uninterpretable findings (Cappell & Greeley, 1987).

Although a number of early studies of the TRH showed the importance of considering individual differences in risk for alcoholism when attempting to explain seemingly contradictory experimental outcomes, no one has attempted to test this factor in studies involving alcohol consumption as the dependent variable. If alcohol is more effective as a tension-reducing agent in those at risk for alcoholism, then it should follow that these same individuals will be more likely to consume more alcohol when stressed. This hypothesis may, however, be difficult to test in the laboratory, where other factors come into play. For example, subjects may wish to look socially acceptable and inhibit drinking. The quantity of alcohol required to produce the desired effect may not be readily consumed in the typical "taste test" procedure. The level and kind of stress required to induce increased drinking may be difficult to achieve under the highly constrained conditions of the laboratory. Innovative strategies will have to be developed in order to provide an adequate test of this hypothesis.

INDIVIDUAL DIFFERENCES: GENETIC INFLUENCES AND PERSONALITY

A common factor considered in studies on the SRD effects of alcohol was multigenerational familial history of alcoholism (MFHA, where a subject's father, grandfather, and at least one other paternal relation is alcoholic). Three of four studies investigating this factor employed electric shock as the stressor (Conrod et al., 1995; Finn et al., 1990; Stewart et al., 1992). Collectively, these studies revealed physiological and behavioral tension-reducing effects of alcohol only in subjects positive for family history of alcoholism. The fourth study used a social stressor and found that the only differential effect attributable to family history of alcoholism was improved mood after alcohol (Sayette et al., 1994).

Personality traits that have been linked with increased alcohol use include self-defeating personality (Schill & Beyler, 1992), impulsivity (Hussong & Chassin, 1994), anxiety (Kushner, Sher, Wood, & Wood, 1994), hostility in men (Zeichner et al., 1995), and powerlessness (Seeman & Seeman, 1992). Also, men who score high on avoidant forms of emotion-focused coping tend to respond to stress with increased alcohol consumption (Cooper, Russell, Skinner, Frone, & Mudar, 1992). These studies demonstrate that there are many factors that act as moderators or mediators of alcohol as a SRD agent. The significant influence of these and other variables on alcohol's impact as a tension reducer underscores the view that a simple TRT or SRD model of alcohol consumption is inadequate to account for most problem-drinking behavior. Interactive models that incorporate the effects of individual differences on subjects' responsiveness to stress and on alcohol's impact on stress responses have supplanted the simpler, single-factor explanatory models such as TRT and SRD.

METHODOLOGICAL ISSUES

Appropriate Control Conditions

Placebo control groups have long been recognized as useful control conditions in studies of TRT. As the section on experimental studies indicated, a number of studies have demonstrated that expectancies can influence the

SRD effects of alcohol, but these effects tend to be the exception rather than the rule. The majority of studies employing a placebo control condition did not find any SRD effects when subjects were administered placebo beverages. In the majority of studies, changes induced by alcohol were apparently attributable to its pharmacological effects. However, without the placebo-control-condition confirmation, this explanation would be less convincing.

Sayette (1993b) cautions that the use of HR as an index of stress response in alcohol administration research is not ideal because potential confounds exist in the interpretation of these measures as SRD effects. Sayette presents a persuasive argument that many reports of SRD effects of alcohol may be artifacts of the normal homeostatic functioning of the cardiovascular system in response to various environmental events, such as consuming a beverage. Initially, consumption of a placebo beverage elicits a reduction in HR. Once this reduction in HR reaches peak, it returns to baseline. If the stress effect is measured during the period when HR is returning to preconsumption baseline in the control condition, then this could be interpreted as an enhanced stress response. Alternatively, consumption of a low dose of alcohol (the dosage range typically used in studies of SRD) produces an increase in HR. Once this response has reached peak, homeostatic mechanisms return it to baseline. Measurement of the stress response during this period when HR is decreasing could be construed as a SRD effect of alcohol. Sayette presents several tables that demonstrate the point at which the HR response to stress is measured greatly influences whether a SRD effect is observed. Unless the difference in HR observed between alcohol and nonalcohol prestress baselines is greater than 4 beats per minute, a SRD effect is unlikely to be observed. The studies by Finn, Pihl, and colleagues (Conrod et al., 1995; Finn & Pihl, 1987, 1988; Finn et al., 1990; Stewart et al., 1992) may be compromised by differential reactions to alcohol, independent of the stress response. Unless the time course of cardiovascular changes in response to alcohol are taken into consideration, the interpretation of results in studies of the SRD effects of alcohol should be carried out with caution.

The problem of baseline levels of activity and homeostatic regulatory properties of physiological systems is clearly one that must be examined for all measures of the stress response. Sayette's thorough review of HR data on the SRD effects of alcohol should be replicated with other physiological indices.

Design Issues

Another factor that has been identified as important in the assessment of SRD effects is the timing of the stressor. It is unclear in some studies precisely when the stressor is introduced. In studies using social stress, such as subjects being asked to deliver a self-disclosing speech, it is debatable at what point the stress occurs—at the time the instruction is given, during countdown to the speech, or at the point where the speech is given. Sayette et al. (1992) measured stress responses at all three points. In addition to the standard measures of self-reported anxiety and HR change, these researchers also examined facial expression as an index of the emotional response to a stressor. Three groups were tested: those given a 0.67 g/kg dose of vodka mixed with tonic (alcohol); those who were told they would be given alcohol but were actually given tonic (placebo); and those who were told they would be drinking tonic, and were given tonic (control). The alcohol group differed from the placebo and no-drink control groups by showing significantly less emotion during the initial 10 seconds of the instructions and throughout the full 30-second instruction period. HR changes mirrored the facial expression results but were not statistically significant at the conventional $p < .05$ level. No significant differences were observed at other periods.

OTHER DRUGS AS TENSION REDUCTION AGENTS

Although it is generally accepted that other drugs, such as the benzodiazepines, have a much better therapeutic index as stress-reducing agents than alcohol (see Cappell & Greeley, 1987), there has been less experimental work explicitly examining the SRD effects of other drugs. In the case of illicit drugs such as heroin, ethical considerations would reduce the likelihood of conducting laboratory experiments with this class of drugs. Correlational studies of the relationship between stress and other drug use are as inconclusive as those investigating the alcohol–stress interaction (e.g., O'Doherty, 1991). Confounding factors such as the stress-producing effects of drug use make it difficult to disentangle the causal direction of any relationship between stress and drug use. While stress may be associated with greater drug use, it may be possible that this is because drug use creates its own stressful situations. More prospective studies are needed to help clarify the causal pathways between factors.

SUMMARY AND CONCLUSIONS

A recent survey of 3,075 students in 10 U.K. universities indicated that alcohol and other drug consumption was on the rise (Webb, Ashton, & Kamali, 1996). The primary reason given for drug use was pleasure rather than social pressure or stress. Although high levels of anxiety were reported by this sample, anxiety was not related to drinking or drug taking. On the face of it, this survey would seem to call into question the value of a TRT of alcohol use. Nevertheless, much research provides some support for the TRT and SRD model of alcohol consumption, and cannot be ignored.

The take-home message from current literature (1987–1997) on the use of alcohol and other drugs to reduce stress has not changed greatly from that given in 1987—some individuals, for example, those who may be genetically predisposed to experience greater stress-buffering effects from alcohol (Sher, Bylund, Walitzer, Hartmann, & Ray-Prenger, 1994), who hold certain beliefs about alcohol (e.g., that alcohol produces positive mood-enhancing effects; Zarantonello, 1986), will, under certain circumstances (e.g., stressful situations in which the individual experiences powerlessness; Seeman & Seeman, 1992) consume alcohol for its stress-response dampening effects. However, these same individuals may also consume alcohol at other times for other reasons (e.g., to enhance a pleasurable experience). The literature has moved from a consideration of TRT or SRD as comprehensive explanations of alcohol or other drug use to considering these as minitheories of one aspect of drug use. There is now more interest in the mechanism(s) by which alcohol produces its SRD effects when they occur.

Alcohol problems are seen as one response to stressful life situations, along with other responses, such as emotional distress, anxiety and other psychological and physiological problems (e.g., Horwitz & Davies, 1994). There is a substantial body of evidence that indicates that alcohol and other drug use are often found in combination with other forms of psychopathology (e.g., depression, anxiety disorders, PTSD; see "Comorbidity" section of this chapter). Depending upon the populations sampled in studies of stress and alcohol consumption, more or less support for TRT can be found. Samples of dependent drinkers, depressed or anxious individuals, are more apt to show a positive relationship between life stresses and alcohol use (e.g., Kalodner et al., 1989). General population samples, however, are less consistent in their findings (e.g., Webb et al., 1996).

Another important factor in the mediation and/or moderation of the stress–alcohol consumption link is the individual's beliefs or expectancies regarding the effects that alcohol can produce. Those who hold stronger beliefs about alcohol's positive effects tend to drink more and, as some research has shown, may be more likely to drink in response to stressors (e.g., Cooper et al., 1992; McKirnan & Peterson, 1988).

FUTURE DIRECTIONS FOR RESEARCH

The caveats placed on interpretation of the TRT and SRD models of alcohol consumption have led numerous researchers to propose more complex interactive models of the relationship between stress and drug use. An approach that has been gathering momentum is the stress-vulnerability model of stress-induced drinking (e.g., Cooper et al., 1992). According to the stress-vulnerability approach, a number of factors that are known to moderate the impact of life stresses upon individuals come to influence whether alcohol consumption is likely to become a response to stress. Several factors have been identified that influence the individual's vulnerability to stress, and these include gender, alcohol expectancies, and coping style (Cooper et al., 1992). Using these factors, subgroups of individuals can be identified that appear vulnerable to developing alcohol use problems in response to stress. In the study conducted by Cooper and colleagues, men who relied on avoidant forms of emotion-focused coping and who held strong positive expectancies were more vulnerable to drinking in response to stress than women or men who held low expectancies and were low on avoidant coping style. The direction of causality operating among these factors could not be determined in this cross-sectional study. What is needed is larger-scale prospective studies that include appropriately selected control groups (see Lewinsohn, Gotlib, & Seeley, 1995) and measurement intervals (see Sher, Wood, Wood, & Raskin, 1996). These field studies should be complemented by well-controlled experimental investigations of the possible mediating mechanisms underlying alcohol's SRD potential in targeted vulnerable groups.

Recent research on TRT has shown increased sophistication in the manipulation and measurement of alcohol's tension-reducing effects. This improvement in methodology has been accompanied by an increase in the number of alternative accounts of the mechanisms underlying these phenomena. Since the 1980s, studies of TRT have been supplanted, to some extent, by studies on the stress-response dampening effects of alcohol (e.g., Sher, 1987; Sher & Levenson, 1982). Sher (1987) described the SRD model as "a narrower more molecular model which relies on fewer hypothetical constructs than the TRH," "a psychobiological minitheory which can be embedded in the context of a broader cognitive-social learning framework" (p. 258). The SRD model is more circumscribed in its predictions regarding alcohol's stress-response dampening effects. It acknowledges that alcohol can increase, as well as decrease, stress responses and that not all stressful situations will elicit drinking behavior. Individual differences (e.g., family history of alcoholism, prealcoholic personality characteristics, and comorbidity with anxiety and stress-related disorders) and stressful environmental circumstances (e.g., occupational stress, controllability of events, personal trauma) are recognized as important predisposing factors in the link between alcohol and SRD.

The proposed mechanisms through which these factors mediate the SRD effects of alcohol are reflected in several different theoretical viewpoints. These theories reflect different levels of analysis of the problem, ranging from physiological to emotional accounts of behavior.

PHYSIOLOGICAL ACCOUNTS

Reports on the direct pharmacological effects of alcohol on stress-response are variable (for reviews, see Sayette, 1993a; Sher, 1987) and change as a function of the dose of alcohol and individual differences in responsiveness of subjects to the stressor when sober (Stewart et al., 1992). Several pharmacological explanations of alcohol's stress-reducing properties have been posited. Based on an analysis of epidemiological evidence, Volpicelli (1987) suggested that alcohol consumption increases not in anticipation of stress but following stressful events. Indeed, a number of studies have shown that subjects tend to avoid drinking before engaging in an anticipated event which may require cognitive readiness and agility (e.g., Tucker, Vuchinich, Sobell, & Maisto, 1980). Also, many experimental models used to test the TRT first expose subjects to a stressor and then measure its impact on subsequent alcohol consumption (e.g., Corcoran & Parker, 1991; Samoluk & Stewart, 1996). According to Volpicelli, it is not during the experience of tension that drinking is most likely to occur, but during the period of tension relief, after the stressful event is over. Evidence indicates that during this period, there is a relative deficiency in endorphin activity, and Volpicelli suggests that alcohol consumption increases at this time to compensate for endorphin deficiency. Blum and colleagues (e.g., Blum, Hamilton, & Wallace, 1977; Vereby & Blum, 1979) have demonstrated that alcohol stimulates endorphin activity. Other lines of research indicate that there are links between the pharmacological effects of alcohol and the opioid drugs morphine and naloxone (Blum, Futterman, Wallace, & Schwetner, 1977; Blum, Wallace, Schwetner, & Eubanks, 1976).

On the other hand, Roske et al. (1994) observed an increase in alcohol consumption in rats during a stressor that apparently increased opioid activity. They observed different effects of two types of stress—social isolation and intermittent immobilization—on alcohol consumption. Only social isolation increased consumption of alcohol by rats. The two stressors also were found to have differing effects on the functional state of the endogenous opioid system. The social isolation condition was associated with activation of the peripheral endogenous opioid system, while immobilization was associated with a functionally insufficient opioid system.

Sher et al. (1994) observed that men with low platelet monoamine oxidase (MAO) activity showed stronger stress-response dampening on HR when administered a 0.625 g/kg dose of alcohol than did men with higher levels of this enzyme. Although it is not possible to relate these peripheral enzyme levels to central activity of the catecholamines and serotonin, links have been established between platelet MAO and behavior. Low platelet MAO levels were associated with antisociality, increased use of cigarettes, and increased level of drug use, but not alcohol use or abuse in this sample.

The pharmacological effects of alcohol on stress vary with the dose of alcohol ingested, the inherited physiological makeup of the individual, and the kind of stressor; therefore, it is difficult to pinpoint a single physiological mechanism that might account for this drug's potential as a pharmacological stress-reducing agent. The variety of physiological models that might account for alcohol's SRD properties has led some researchers to turn to other levels of analysis of the problem. Over the past decade of research on the TRT and the SRD model of alcohol use, cognitive explanations of these effects have taken a more prominent role. Several of the more successful cognitive models are considered in the next section.

Cognitive Models

Perhaps the earliest cognitive model of the SRD effects of alcohol is that provided by expectancy theory (e.g., Goldman, Brown, & Christiansen, 1987). In essence, this model predicts that a drinker's expectation that alcohol will reduce stress or relieve tension will influence whether this effect is observed. As long as subjects believe they have consumed alcohol and expect this tension-reducing effect, it will be experienced, irrespective of whether alcohol has been consumed.

Other researchers have attempted to incorporate other cognitive mediating factors to explain alcohol's SRD effect. Steele and Josephs (1988) posited an attention-allocation model, which holds that alcohol dampens stress responses through impairment of information processing coupled with a distracting activity. Alcohol impairment coupled with distraction prevents the allocation of attention to the stressor, thereby preventing or impairing its cognitive processing. If the stressor is processed less effectively, its ability to elicit a stress response will be dampened. If however, alcohol is consumed in the absence of a distracting stimulus, it is not expected to produce SRD and can possibly lead to increased focusing on the stressor and an elevated stress response. Although this model can account for much data that run contrary to simpler TRT and SRD explanations, it cannot explain instances in which, for example, SRD effects have been observed in the absence of an obvious distracting stimulus (e.g., Stewart et al., 1992).

Sayette (1993a) proposed an alternative cognitive account of SRD effects, which posits that alcohol's pharmacological action is to interfere with a person's ability to appraise stressful information. The appraisal-disruption model proposes that alcohol constrains the spread of activation of information that is associated with the stressful stimulus and stored in long-term memory, thereby preventing thorough processing of the stimulus and its accompanying stress response. For alcohol to be an effective stress-response dampener in this model, it should be administered *before* exposure to the stressor; it will be most effective when the stressor is both difficult to process and occurs in individuals who are particularly sensitive to alcohol's cognitive impairing effects (cf. Volpicelli, 1987). It also predicts that the SRD effect of alcohol should be most apparent immediately after the stressful information is presented. Responses to stressors that are processed before alcohol intake, or ones that are easily or more readily processed (e.g., ones that are extremely threatening or familiar) will be less likely to be affected by alcohol. For a review of the evidence for and against this model, see Sayette (1993a).

Behavioral Models

Traditional behavioral accounts of how alcohol's tension-reducing effects may be mediated include the notions of disinhibition and escape–avoidance learning. By releasing the individual from the inhibiting effects of tension on behavior, alcohol facilitates escape–avoidance learning. The two-factor avoidance model proposed by Stasiewicz and Maisto (1993) represents one of the more current behavioral accounts of TRT. It proposes that drinking is an instrumentally conditioned avoidance response (CAR) to a classically conditioned emotional response (CER). A negative affective state, such as a CER of fear or anxiety, can motivate alcohol consumption as a CAR. The model recommends that extinction of emotional as well as drug-related cues for drinking is required for better treatment outcomes.

In their 1987 review, Cappell and Greeley made the point that single-factor theories of alcohol consumption are, by definition, limited. While it may be reasonable to assume that some people sometimes drink to reduce stress or relieve tension, research shows that regular drinkers report positive (e.g., enhanced sexual responding, increased arousal) and negative (e.g., reduced tension, relief from withdrawal) reinforcing effects of alcohol as motives for drinking (Goldman et al., 1987). An overarching principle that can account for alcohol's influence as an incentive object is its capacity to affect emotions. When we talk about alcohol serving as a positive or negative reinforcer and motives for drinking, we are implicitly acknowledging alcohol's capacity to modify the emotional/motivational reaction to ongoing events. We need to know whether the effects of alcohol on emotions are specific or general. Is alcohol equally effective in modulating positive and negative emotional states?

Recent research into the measurement of emotional states reveals an interesting approach to the study of emotion that permits the researcher to assess more objectively not only the intensity of an emotional experience, but also its valence or direction (Stritzke et al., 1995). Previous research relied mainly upon self-report as the index of emotional valence. The more objective physiological indicators (e.g., autonomic measures) were used primarily as measures of emotional intensity or arousal. By using startle-probe methodology, researchers can detect the valence of an emotional state. This is based upon a synergistic match–antagonistic mismatch principle: When exposed to a startle stimulus such as a sudden loud burst of noise while experiencing an unpleasant or aversive emotional state, the magnitude of the startle response will be enhanced because of a synergistic match between the negative emotion and the startle response. Conversely, when experiencing a positive or appetitive emotion, the presentation of the startle stimulus results in an attenuated startle response because of an antagonistic mismatch between the aversive startle probe and the ongoing positive emotion.

Stritzke et al. (1995) conducted a study to examine the effect of alcohol on emotional intensity and valence using pleasant and unpleasant slides to induce emotion. Alcohol merely suppressed general arousability, without differentially affecting appetitive or aversive response mobilization (i.e., the startle response was attenuated during pleasant slide presentations and augmented during unpleasant slides, only less so under the influence of alcohol for both conditions). If alcohol simply produces a generalized reduction in arousal, unlike the benzodiazepines, which disrupt affective valence without dampening the startle response, then what are the implications for motivational accounts of alcohol consumption? Alcohol's effects on positive affect are as yet unclear. If, as the data presented here suggest, alcohol has a general suppressing effect on emotional intensity, what are the implications for the SRD model and TRT? Will suppression of positive emotional states also prove to rewarding? If so, then the notion of tension reduction, with alcohol functioning as a kind of negative reinforcer, may need to be reconsidered. Alcohol appears to attenuate both appetitive and aversive stimulation. Is this through some effect on attention or on the quality of the emotional experience?

Over the last 50 years, advances in identifying different forms of stress and their various effects have been important in gaining a more sophisticated understanding of how stress and alcohol might interact (Powers, 1987). This may be a fruitful direction in which to take TRT experiments.

REFERENCES

Adamson, R., & Black, R. (1959). Volitional drinking and avoidance learning in the white rat. *Journal of Comparative and Physiological Psychology*, *52*, 734–736.

Allan, C. A. (1995). Alcohol problems and anxiety disorders—A critical review. *Alcohol and Alcoholism*, *30*, 145–151.

Atkinson, R. M., & Kofoed, L. L. (1982). Alcohol and drug abuse in old age: A clinical perspective. *Substance Alcohol Actions—Misuse*, *3*, 353.

Blanchard, R. J., Flores, T., Magee, L., Weiss, S., & Blanchard, D. (1992). Pregrouping aggression and defense scores influences alcohol consumption for dominant and subordinate rats in visible burrow systems. *Aggressive Behavior*, *18*, 459–467.

Blanchard, R. J., Yudko, E. B., & Blanchard, D. (1993). Alcohol, aggression and the stress of subordination. *Journal of Studies on Alcohol* (Suppl. 11), 146s–155s.

Blum, K., Futterman, S., Wallace, J. E., & Schwetner, H. A. (1977). Naloxone-induced inhibition of alcohol dependence in mice. *Nature*, *265*, 49–51.

Blum, K., Hamilton, M. L., & Wallace, J. E. (1977). Alcohol and opiates: A review of common mechanisms. In K. Blum (Ed.), *Alcohol and opiates: Neurochemical and behavioral mechanisms* (pp. 203–236). New York: Academic Press.

Blum, K., Wallace, J. E., Schwetner, H. A., & Eubanks, J. D. (1976). Morphine suppression of ethanol withdrawal in mice. *Experimentia*, *32*, 79–82.

Bond, A., & Lader, M. (1991). Does alcohol modify responses to reward in a competitive task? *Alcohol and Alcoholism*, *26*, 61–69.

Brady, J. V. (1956). Assessment of drug effects on emotional behavior. *Science*, *123*, 1033–1034.

Brady, K. T., & Lydiard, R. B. (1993). The association of alcoholism and anxiety. *Psychiatric Quarterly*, *64*, 135–149.

Brook, J. S., Gordon, A. S., Whitemen, M., & Cohen, P. (1986). Dynamics of childhood and adolescent personality traits and adolescent drug use. *Developmental Psychology*, *22*, 403–414.

Brown, R. A., & Cutter, H. S. G. (1977). Alcohol, customary drinking behavior, and pain. *Journal of Abnormal Psychology*, *86*, 179–188.

Cappell, H. (1975). An evaluation of tension models of alcohol consumption. In R. J. Gibbins, Y. Israel, H. Kalant, R. E. Popham, W. Schmidt, & R. G. Smart (Eds.), *Research advances in alcohol and drug problems* (Vol. 2, pp. 177–210). New York: Wiley.

Cappell, H., & Greeley, J. (1987). Alcohol and tension reduction: An update on research and theory. In H. T. Blane & K. E. Leonard (Eds.), *Psychological theories of drinking and alcoholism* (pp. 15–54). New York: Guilford Press.

Cappell, H., & Herman, C. P. (1972). Alcohol and tension reduction: A review. *Journal of Studies on Alcohol*, *33*, 33–64.

Cappell, H., & LeBlanc, A. E. (1977). Gustatory avoidance conditioning by drugs of abuse: Relationships to general issues in research on drug dependence. In N. W. Milgram, L. Krames, & T. M. Alloway (Eds.), *Food aversion learning* (pp. 133–167). New York: Plenum.

Champagne, F., & Kirouac, G. (1989). The effects of formaldehyde on voluntary ethanol consumption in the laboratory rat: A comparison of two methods of determination of a single test solution. *Journal of General Psychology*, *116*, 91–101.

Colder, C. R., & Chassin, L. (1993). The stress and negative affect model of adolescent alcohol use and the moderating effects of behavioral undercontrol. *Journal of Studies on Alcohol*, *54*, 326–333.

Conger, J. J. (1951). The effect of alcohol on conflict behavior in the albino rat. *Quarterly Journal of Studies on Alcohol*, *12*, 1–49.

Conger, J. J. (1956). Alcoholism: Theory, problem and challenge: II. Reinforcement theory and the dynamics of alcoholism. *Quarterly Journal of Studies on Alcohol*, *13*, 296–305.

Conrod, P. J., Pihl, R. O., & Ditto, B. (1995). Autonomic reactivity and alcohol-induced dampening in men at risk for alcoholism and men at risk for hypertension. *Alcohol: Clinical and Experimental Research*, *19*, 482–489.

Cooper, M. L., Russell, M., Skinner, J., Frone, M. R., & Mudar, P. (1992). Stress and alcohol use: Moderating effects on gender, coping, and alcohol expectancies. *Journal of Abnormal Psychology*, *101*, 139–152.

Corcoran, K. J. (1994). Predicting reduction in tension following alcohol consumption in a stressful situation with the alcohol expectancy questionnaire. *Addictive Behaviors*, *19*, 57–62.

Corcoran, K. J., & Parker, P. S. (1991). Alcohol expectancy questionnaire tension reduction scale as a predictor of alcohol consumption in a stressful situation. *Addictive Behaviors*, *16*, 129–137.

Cowley, D. S. (1992). Alcohol abuse, substance abuse and panic disorder. *American Journal of Medicine, 92*(Suppl. 1A), 41s–48s.

Cutter, H. S. G., Maloof, B., Kurtz, N. R., & Jones, W. C. (1976). "Feeling no pain": Differential responses to pain by alcoholics and nonalcoholics before and after drinking. *Journal of Studies on Alcohol*, *37*, 273–277.

Darkes, J., & Goldman, M. S. (1993). Expectancy challenge and drinking reduction:

Experimental evidence for a mediational process. *Journal of Consulting and Clinical Psychology, 61,* 344–353.

Dengerink, H. A., & Fagan, N. J. (1978). Effects of alcohol on emotional responses to stress. *Journal of Studies on Alcohol, 39,* 525–539.

Ellis, F. W. (1966). Effects of ethanol on plasma corticosterone levels. *Journal of Pharmacology and Experimental Therapeutics, 153,* 121–127.

Estes, W., & Skinner, B. F. (1941). Some quantitative properties of anxiety. *Journal of Experimental Psychology, 29,* 390–400.

Finn, P. R., & Pihl, R. O. (1987). Men at risk for alcoholism: The effect of alcohol on cardiovascular response to unavoidable shock. *Journal of Abnormal Psychology, 96,* 230–236.

Finn, P. R., & Pihl, R. O. (1988). Risk for alcoholism: A comparison between two different groups of sons of alcoholics on cardiovascular reactivity and sensitivity to alcohol. *Alcoholism: Clinical and Experimental Research, 12,* 742–747.

Finn, P. R., Zeitouni, N. C., & Pihl, R. O. (1990). Effects of alcohol on psychophysiological hyperactivity to nonaversive and aversive stimuli in men at high risk for alcoholism. *Journal of Abnormal Psychology, 99,* 79–85.

Gabel, P. C., Noel, N. E., Keane, T. M., & Lisman, S. A. (1980). Effects of sexual versus fear arousal on alcohol consumption in college males. *Behaviour Research and Therapy, 18,* 519–526.

Geller, I., Croy, D. J., & Ryback, R. S. (1974). Effects of ethanol and sodium pentobarbital on conflict behavior of goldfish. *Pharmacology, Biochemistry and Behavior, 2,* 545–548.

Glass, T. A., Prigerson, H., Kasl, S. V., & Mendes de Leon, C. F. (1995). The effects of negative life events on alcohol consumption among older men and women. *Journal of Gerontology, 50B,* S205–S216.

Glowa, J. R., & Barrett, J. E. (1976). Effects of alcohol on punished and unpunished responding of squirrel monkeys. *Pharmacology, Biochemistry and Behavior, 4,* 169–174.

Goddard, P. J. (1958). Effect of alcohol on excretion of catecholamines in conditions giving rise to anxiety. *Journal of Applied Physiology, 13,* 118–120.

Goldman, M. S., Brown, S. A., & Christiansen, B. A. (1987). Expectancy theory: Thinking about drinking. In H. T. Blane & K. E. Leonard (Eds.), *Psychological theories of drinking and alcoholism* (pp. 181–226). New York: Guilford Press.

Goldman, P. S., & Doctor, R. F. (1966). Facilitation of bar pressing and "suppression" of conditioned suppression in cats as a function of alcohol. *Psychopharmacologia, 9,* 64–72.

Green, E. K., Burke, K. L., Nix, C. L., Lambrecht, K. W., & Mason, D. C. (1995). Psychological factors associated with alcohol use by high school athletes. *Journal of Sport Behavior, 18,* 195–208.

Gustafson, R. (1991). Is the strength and desirability of alcohol-related expectancies positively related? A test with an adult Swedish sample. *Drug and Alcohol Dependence, 28,* 145–150.

Helzer, J. E., & Pryzbeck, T. R. (1987). The co-occurrence of alcoholism with other psychiatric disorders in the general population and its impact on treatment. *Journal of Studies on Alcohol, 49,* 219–224.

Higgins, R. L., & Marlatt, G. A. (1973). Effects of anxiety arousal on the consumption of alcohol by alcoholics and social drinkers. *Journal of Consulting and Clinical Psychology, 41,* 426–433.

Higgins, R. L., & Marlatt, G. A. (1975). Fear of interpersonal evaluation as a determinant of alcohol consumption in male social drinkers. *Journal of Abnormal Psychology, 84,* 644–651.

Hilakivi-Clarke, L., & Lister, R. G. (1992). Social status and voluntary alcohol consumption in mice: Interaction with stress. *Psychopharmacology, 108,* 276–282.

Hodgson, R. J., Stockwell, T. R., & Rankin, H. J. (1979). Can alcohol reduce tension? *Behaviour Research and Therapy, 17,* 459–466.

Holle, C., Heimberg, R. G., Sweet, R. A., & Holt, C. S. (1995). Alcohol and caffeine use by social phobics: An initial inquiry into drinking patterns and behavior. *Behaviour Research and Therapy, 33,* 561–566.

Holroyd, K. A. (1978). Effects of social anxiety and social evaluation on beer consumption and social interaction. *Journal of Studies on Alcohol, 39,* 737–744.

Horwitz, A. V., & Davies, L. (1994). Are emotional distress and alcohol problems differential outcomes to stress?: An exploratory test. *Social Science Quarterly, 75,* 607–621.

Hull, C. L. (1943). *Principles of behavior.* New York: Appleton–Century–Crofts.

Hussong, A. M., & Chassin, L. (1994). The stress–negative affect model of adolescent alcohol use: Disaggregating negative affect. *Journal of Studies on Alcohol, 55,* 707–718.

Isenhart, C. E. (1993). Masculine gender role stress in an inpatient sample of alcohol abusers. *Psychology of Addictive Behaviors, 3,* 177–184.

Jellinek, E. M. (1945). The problem of alcohol. In Yale Studies on Alcohol, *Alcohol, science and society* (pp. 13–30). Westport, CT: Greenwood Press.

Johnson, V., & Pandina, R. J. (1993). A longitudinal examination of the relationships among stress, coping strategies, and problems associated with alcohol use. *Alcoholism: Clinical and Experimental Research, 17,* 696–702.

Josephs, R. A., & Steele, C. M. (1990). The two faces of alcohol myopia: Attentional mediation of psychological stress. *Journal of Abnormal Psychology, 99,* 115–126.

Kalodner, C. R., Delucia, J. L., & Ursprung, A. W. (1989). An examination of the tension reduction hypothesis: The relationship between anxiety and alcohol in college students. *Addictive Behaviors, 14,* 649–654.

Keane, T. M., & Lisman, S. A. (1980). Alcohol and social anxiety patterns in males: Behavioral, cognitive, and physiological effects. *Journal of Abnormal Psychology, 89,* 213–222.

Keane, T. M., & Wolfe, J. (1990). Comorbidity in post-traumatic stress disorder: An analysis of community and clinical samples. *Journal of Applied Social Psychology, 20,* 1776–1788.

Kessler, R. C., Nelson, C. B., McGonagle, K. A., Edlund, M. J., Frank, R. G., & Leaf, P. J. (1996). The epidemiology of co-occurring addictive and mental disorders. *American Journal of Orthopsychiatry, 66,* 17–31.

Kimble, G. A. (1961). *Hilgard and Marquis' conditioning and learning.* New York: Appleton–Century–Crofts.

Krause, N. (1995). Stress, alcohol use, and depressive symptoms in later life. *Gerontologist, 35,* 296–307.

Kushner, M. G., Sher, M. D., Wood, M. D., & Wood, P. K. (1994). Anxiety and drinking behavior: Moderating effects of tension-reduction alcohol outcome expectancies. *Alcoholism: Clinical and Experimental Research, 18,* 852–860.

LaForge, R. G., Nirenberg, T. D., Lewis, D. C., & Murphy, J. B. (1993). Problem drinking, gender, and stressful life events among hospitalized elderly drinkers. *Behavior, Health, and Aging, 3,* 129–138.

Levenson, R. W., Sher, K. J., Grossman, L. M., Newman, J., & Newlin, D. B. (1980). Alcohol and stress response dampening: Pharmacological effects, expectancy, and tension reduction. *Journal of Abnormal Psychology, 89,* 528–538.

Lewinsohn, P. M., Gotlib, I. H., & Seeley, J. R. (1995). Specificity of psychosocial risk factors for depression and substance abuse in older adolescents. *Journal of the American Academy of Child and Adolescent Psychiatry, 34,* 1221–1229.

Lienert, G. A., & Traxel, W. (1959). The effects of meprobamate and alcohol on galvanic skin response. *Journal of Psychology, 48,* 329–334.

Lindman, R. (Ed.). (1980). *Anxiety and alcohol: Limitations of tension reduction theory in nonalcoholics* (Monograph Suppl. 1). Abo, Finland: Abo Akademi, Department of Psychology.

Livezy, G. T., Balabkins, N., & Vogel, W. H. (1987). The effect of ethanol (alcohol) and stress on plasma catecholamine levels in individual female and male rats. *Neuropsychobiology, 17,* 193–198.

Logue, P. E., Gentry, W. D., Linnoila, M., & Erwin, C. W. (1978). Effects of alcohol consumption on state anxiety in male and female nonalcoholics. *American Journal of Psychiatry, 135,* 1079–1081.

Masserman, J. H., Jacques, M. G., & Nicholson, M. R. (1945). Alcohol as a preventive of experimental neuroses. *Quarterly Journal of Studies on Alcohol, 6,* 281–299.

Masserman, J. H., & Yum, K. S. (1946). The influence of alcohol on experimental neuroses in cats. *Psychosomatic Medicine, 8,* 36–52.

McKirnan, D. J., & Peterson, P. L. (1988). Stress, expectancies, and vulnerability to substance abuse: A test of a model among homosexual men. *Journal of Abnormal Psychology, 97,* 461–466.

Mello, N. K. (1968). Some aspects of the behavioral pharmacology of alcohol. In D. H. Efron et al. (Eds.), *Pharmacology: A review of progress, 1957–1967* (PHS Publication No. 1836). Washington, DC: U.S. Government Printing Office.

Milakofsky, L., Miller, J. M., & Vogel, W. H. (1989). Effect of ethanol on plasma amino acids and related compounds of stressed male rats. *Pharmacology, Biochemistry and Behavior, 32,* 1071–1074.

Miller, N. E. (1961). Some recent studies of conflict behavior and drugs. *American Psychology, 16,* 12–24.

Miller, P. M., Hersen, M., Eisler, R. M., & Hilsman, G. (1974). Effects of social stress on operant drinking of alcoholics and social drinkers. *Behaviour Research and Therapy, 12,* 67–72.

Neff, J. A. (1993). Life stressors, drinking patterns, and depressive symptomatology: Ethnicity and stress-buffer effects of alcohol. *Addictive Behaviors, 18,* 373–387.

Netter, P., & Vogel, W. H. (1990). The effect of drinking habit on catecholamine and behavioral responses to stress and ethanol. *Neuropsychobiology, 24,* 149–158.

Noel, N. E., Lisman, S. A., Schare, M. L., & Maisto, S. A. (1992). Effects of alcohol consumption on the prevention and alleviation of stress-reactions. *Addictive Behaviors, 17,* 567–577.

O'Doherty, F. (1991). Is drug use a response to stress? *Drug and Alcohol Dependence, 29,* 97–106.

Oei, T. P. S., & Baldwin, A. R. (1994). Expectancy theory: A two-process model of alcohol use and abuse. *Journal of Studies on Alcohol, 55,* 525–533.

Oei, T. P. S., & Loveday, W. A. L. (1997). Management of comorbid anxiety and alcohol disorders: Parallel treatment of disorders. *Drug and Alcohol Review, 16,* 261–273.

Orcutt, J. D., & Harvey, L. K. (1991). The temporal patterning of tension reduction: Stress and alcohol use on weekdays and weekends. *Journal of Studies on Alcohol, 52,* 415–424.

Pihl, R. O., & Yankofsky, L. (1979). Alcohol consumption in male social drinkers as a function of situationally induced depressive affect and anxiety. *Psychopharmacology, 65,* 251–257.

Polivy, J., Schueneman, A. L., & Carlson, K. (1976). Alcohol and tension reduction: Cognitive and physiological effects. *Journal of Abnormal Psychology, 85,* 595–600.

Power, L., & Estraugh, V. (1990). The role of family formation and dissolution in shaping drinking behaviour in early adulthood. *British Journal of Addiction, 85,* 521–530.

Powers, R. J. (1987). Stress as a factor in alcohol use and abuse. In E. Gottheil, K. A. Druley, S. Pashko, & S. P. Weinstein (Eds.), *Stress and addiction* (pp. 248–260). New York: Brunner/Mazel.

Powers, R. J., & Kutash, I. L. (1985). Stress and alcohol. *International Journal of the Addictions, 20,* 461–482.

Regier, D. A., Farmer, M. E., & Rae, D. S. (1990). Comorbidity of mental disorders with alcohol and other drug use: Results from the Epidemiologic Catchment Area (ECA) Study. *Journal of the American Medical Association, 264,* 2511–2518.

Reynolds, G. S., & van Sommers, P. (1960). Effects of ethyl alcohol on avoidance behavior. *Science, 132,* 42–43.

Richman, J. A., Rospenda, K. M., & Kelley, M. A. (1995). Gender roles and alcohol abuse across the transition to parenthood. *Journal of Studies on Alcohol, 56,* 553–557.

Rimm, D., Briddell, D., Zimmerman, M., & Caddy, G. (1981). The effects of alcohol and the expectancy of alcohol on snake fear. *Addictive Behavior, 6,* 47–51.

Robins, L., Helzer, J., Weissman, M. M., Orvaschel, H., Gruenberg, E., Burke, J. D. Jr., & Regier, D. A. (1984). Lifetime prevalence of specific psychiatric disorders in three sites. *Archives of General Psychiatry, 41,* 949–958.

Roske, I., Baeger, I., Frenzel, R., & Oehme, P. (1994). Does a relationship exist between the quality of stress and the motivation to ingest alcohol? *Alcohol, 11,* 113–124.

Samoluk, S. B., & Stewart, S. H. (1996). Anxiety sensitivity and anticipation of a self-disclosing interview as determinants of alcohol consumption. *Psychology of Addictive Behaviors, 10,* 45–54.

Sayette, M. A. (1993a). An appraisal–disruption model of alcohol's effects on stress responses in social drinkers. *Psychological Bulletin, 114,* 459–476.

Sayette, M. A. (1993b). Heart rate as an index of stress response in alcohol administration research: A critical review. *Alcoholism: Clinical and Experimental Research, 17,* 802–809.

Sayette, M. A., Breslin, F. C., & Wilson, G. T. (1994). Parental history of alcohol abuse and the effects of alcohol and expectations of intoxication on social stress. *Journal of Studies on Alcohol, 55,* 214–223.

Sayette, M. A., Smith, D. W., Breiner, M. J., & Wilson, G. T. (1992). The effect of alcohol on emotional response to a social stressor. *Journal of Studies on Alcohol,* *53,* 541–545.

Sayette, M. A., & Wilson, G. T. (1991). Intoxication and exposure to stress: Effects of temporal patterning. *Journal of Abnormal Psychology, 100,* 56–62.

Schill, T., & Beyler, J. (1992). Self-defeating personality and strategies for coping with stress. *Psychological Reports, 71,* 67–70.

Seeman, M., & Seeman, A. Z. (1992). Life strains, alienation, and drinking behavior. *Alcoholism: Clinical and Experimental Research, 16,* 199–205.

Seligman, M. E. P. (1968). Chronic fear produced by unpredictable shock. *Journal of Comparative and Physiological Psychology, 66,* 402–411.

Sher, K. J. (1987). Stress-response dampening. In H. T. Blane, & K. E. Leonard (Eds.), *Psychological theories of drinking and alcoholism* (pp. 227–271). New York: Guilford Press.

Sher, K. J., Bylund, D. B., Walitzer, K. S., Hartmann, J., & Ray-Prenger, C. (1994). Platelet monoamine oxidase (MAO) activity: Personality, substance use, and the stress-response dampening effect of alcohol. *Experimental and Clinical Psychopharmacology, 2,* 53–81.

Sher, K. J., & Levenson, R. W. (1982). Risk for alcoholism and individual differences in the stress-response-dampening effect of alcohol. *Journal of Abnormal Psychology, 91,* 350–367.

Sher, K. J., & Walitzer, K. S. (1986). Individual differences in the stress-response-dampening effect of alcohol: A dose-response study. *Journal of Abnormal Psychology, 95,* 150–167.

Sher, K. J., Wood, M. D., Wood, P. K., & Raskin, G. (1996). Alcohol outcome expectancies and alcohol use: A latent variable cross-lagged panel study. *Journal of Abnormal Psychology, 105,* 561–574.

Skinner, B. F. (1926). *The behavior of organisms.* New York: Appleton Century.

Stasiewicz, P. R., & Maisto, S. A. (1993). Two-factor avoidance theory: The role of affect in the maintenance of substance use and substance use disorder. *Behavior Therapy, 24,* 337–356.

Steele, C. M., & Josephs, R. A. (1988). Drinking your troubles away: II. An attention-allocation model of alcohol's effect on psychological stress. *Journal of Abnormal Psychology, 97,* 196–205.

Steele, C. M., Southwick, L. L., & Critchlow, B. (1981). Dissonance and alcohol: Drinking your troubles away. *Journal of Personality and Social Psychology, 41,* 831–846.

Stewart, S. (1996). Alcohol abuse in individuals exposed to trauma: A critical review. *Psychological Bulletin, 120,* 83–112.

Stewart, S. H., Finn, P. R., & Pihl, R. O. (1992). The effects of alcohol on the cardio-vascular stress response in men at high risk for alcoholism: A dose response study. *Journal of Studies on Alcohol, 53,* 499–506.

Stritzke, W. G. K., Patrick, C. J., & Lang, A. R. (1995). Alcohol and human emotion: A multidimensional analysis incorporating startle-probe methodology. *Journal of Abnormal Psychology, 104,* 114–122.

Tamerin, J. S., & Mendelson, J. H. (1969). The psychodynamics of chronic inebriation observations of alcoholics during the process of drinking in an experimental group setting. *American Journal of Psychiatry, 125,* 886–889.

Tucker, J., Vuchinich, R., Sobell, M., & Maisto, S. A. (1980). Normal drinkers' alcohol consumption as a function of conflicting motives induced by intellectual performance stress. *Addictive Behaviors, 5,* 171–178.

Vaillant, G. E. (1983). *The natural history of alcoholism.* Cambridge, MA: Harvard University Press.

Van Thiel, D. (1983). Adrenal response to ethanol: A stress response? In L. A. Poherecky & J. Brick (Eds.), *Stress and alcohol use* (pp. 23–27). New York: Elsevier.

Vereby, V., & Blum, K. (1979). Alcohol euphoria, possible mediation via endorphinergic mechanisms. *Journal of Psychedelic Drugs, 11,* 305–311.

Vogel, R. A., Frye, G. D., Wilson, J. H., Kuhn, C. M., Koepke, K. M., Mailman, R. B., Mueller, R. A., & Breese, G. R. (1980). Attenuation of the effects of punishment by ethanol: Comparisons with chlordiazepoxide. *Psychopharmacology, 71,* 123–129.

Vogel, W. H., & DeTurck, K. H. (1983). Effects of ethanol on plasma and brain catecholamine levels in stressed and unstressed rats. In L. A. Poherecky & J. Brick (Eds.), *Stress and alcohol use* (pp. 429–438). New York: Elsevier.

Vogel, W. H., & Netter, P. (1989). Effect of ethanol and stress on plasma catecholamines and their relation to changes in emotional state. *Alcoholism: Clinical and Experimental Research, 13,* 284–290.

Volpicelli, J. R. (1987). Uncontrollable events and alcohol drinking. *British Journal of Addiction, 82,* 381–392.

Vuchinich, R. E., Tucker, J. A., & Sobell, M. B. (1979). Alcohol, expectancy, cognitive labelling, and mirth. *Journal of Abnormal Psychology, 88,* 641–651.

Wallgren, H., & Savolainen, S. (1962). The effect of ethyl alcohol on a conditioned avoidance response in rats. *Acta Pharmacologia and Toxicologia, 19,* 59–67.

Webb, E., Ashton, C. H., & Kamali, F. (1996). Alcohol and drug use in UK university students. *Lancet, 348,* 922–925.

Williams, A. F. (1966). Social drinking, anxiety, and depression. *Journal of Personality and Social Psychology, 3,* 689–693.

Wilson, G. T., & Abrams, D. (1977). Effects of alcohol on social anxiety and physiological arousal: Cognitive versus pharmacological processes. *Cognitive Theory and Research, 1,* 195–210.

Windle, M. (1992). A longitudinal study of stress buffering for adolescent problem behaviors. *Developmental Psychology, 28,* 522–530.

Young, R. McD., Knight, R. G., & Oei, T. P. S. (1990). The stability of alcohol-related expectancies in social drinking situations. *Australian Journal of Psychology, 42,* 321–330.

Young, R. McD., Oei, T. P. S., & Knight, R. G. (1990). The tension reduction hypothesis revisited: An alcohol expectancy perspective. *British Journal of Addiction, 85,* 31–40.

Zarantonello, M. M. (1986). Expectations for reinforcement from alcohol use in a clinical sample. *Journal of Studies on Alcohol, 47,* 485–488.

Zeichner, A., Giancola, P. R., & Allen, J. D. (1995). Effects of hostility on alcohol stress-response-dampening. *Alcoholism: Clinical and Experimental Research, 19,* 977–983.

3

Personality and Alcoholism: Issues, Methods, and Etiological Processes

KENNETH J. SHER
TIMOTHY J. TRULL
BRUCE D. BARTHOLOW
ANGELA VIETH

INTRODUCTION

Alcoholism is among the most highly prevalent disorders in the United States (Grant et al., 1994; Kessler et al., 1994; Meyers et al., 1984; Robins et al., 1984) and many other modern societies (Helzer & Canino, 1992). The disorder poses a significant threat to affected individuals, their families, and the larger community. Understanding those variables that are involved in the etiology and maintenance of alcoholism is thus a high priority for both clinicians who treat alcoholics and public health workers attempting to prevent alcohol dependence and related problems. Although a number of biological, psychological, and social factors have been implicated in the etiology of alcoholism (e.g., National Institute on Alcohol Abuse and Alcoholism [NIAAA], 1997), the general belief that personality plays an important role in causing alcoholism has been a major theme for much of this century and remains so to this day.

Over the past 50 years, hundreds of studies have examined the personality correlates of alcoholics, many of these in search of a so-called "alcoholic personality" (e.g., see Sutherland, Schroeder, & Tordella, 1950) that was thought to underlie alcoholic behavior. In the first edition of the American Psychiatric Association's (APA) *Diagnostic and Statistical Manual of Mental Disorders* (DSM-I; American Psychiatric Association, 1952), alcoholism was considered a form of personality disorder, implying that disordered personality functioning is a core component of alcoholism. During the 1950s and 1960s, critical reviews of the literature began to cast serious doubt on the existence of a distinct "alcoholic personality" (e.g., Lisansky, 1960; Syme, 1957). In the 1960s, the behavioral movement in academic clinical psychology and influential critiques of the utility of personality for understanding behavior (e.g., Mischel, 1968) tended to diminish the influence of personological accounts of alcoholism. However, interest in personality-based explanations for alcoholism began to increase in the late 1960s and early 1970s with the publication of influential longitudinal studies documenting personality differences in individuals prior to the development of alcohol problems (Hoffman, Loper, & Kammeier, 1974; Jones, 1968, 1971).

By the 1980s, the alcohol research community generally came to recognize that, although there was no single constellation of personality traits that was unique to alcoholics, personality measures could be used to distinguish "clinical alcoholics" (i.e., individuals seeking treatment for alcoholism or individuals meeting diagnostic criteria for alcoholism) from various comparison groups. Perhaps more important was the realization (e.g., Barnes, 1983) that those traits that are most sensitive in differentiating clinical alcoholics from others are not necessarily the same as those that distinguish "prealcoholics" (i.e., nonalcoholic individuals who later become alcoholic) from their peers. By the mid-1980s, personality once again became a major focus of research on alcoholism and associated disabilities by major theorists (e.g., Cloninger, 1987a, 1987b). Although research continues to indicate that both clinical alcoholics and prealcoholics can be distinguished from relevant comparison groups on a number of different personality traits (e.g., Cox, 1985; Sher & Trull, 1994), there does not appear to be a distinctive personality organization that characterizes either prealcoholics or clinical alcoholics (e.g., Sher & Trull, 1994; Sutker & Allain, 1988). The major goal of this chapter is to highlight what we now know about the role of personality in the etiology and maintenance of alcoholism. We begin by providing some background regarding current conceptions of personality.

DEFINING PERSONALITY

A critical but often overlooked issue in the study of personality and alcoholism concerns the definition of personality employed. Although there is considerable variability in how different theorists define personality, most formal definitions note that personality is "internal, organized, and characteristic of an individual over time and situations . . . [and has] motivational and adaptive significance" (Watson, Clark, & Harkness, 1994, p. 18). Many individual-difference variables that have been related to alcoholism may or may not be considered in the personality–alcoholism relation, depending upon the definition of personality used. As we have pointed out elsewhere (Sher & Trull, 1994), relatively narrow, alcohol-specific traits (e.g., alcohol-outcome expectancies, drinking self-efficacy [Young, Oei, & Crook, 1991], and drinking-related locus of control [Donovan & O'Leary, 1978]) can be considered personality traits under some definitions of personality but not others. For example, individually held, alcohol-outcome expectancies have been shown to be relatively strong correlates of both nonpathological and pathological alcohol involvement (e.g., Goldman, 1994; Goldman, Brown, & Christiansen, 1987) and could be considered "internal, organized . . . [and to have] motivational and adaptive significance" (Watson et al., 1994, p. 18). However, despite being somewhat trait-like, expectancies are not as "characteristic of an individual over time and situations" as most commonly employed personality constructs (although a case could probably be made in support of this idea).

To make matters more complex, traits related to antisociality (e.g., history of childhood conduct problems) have been shown repeatedly to be robust predictors of alcoholism, and this finding has often been used to support the importance of personality in alcoholism. Leading theorists, however, debate the relevance of these findings relating antisociality to personality. At one end of the spectrum, Zucker and Gomberg (1986) claim that "antisocial behavior is part of personality and it plays a significant etiological role" (p. 785). At the other end of the spectrum are those (e.g., Nathan, 1988) who question whether these characteristics should be conceptualized as reflecting personality, because the adaptive and motivational components are unclear. Although, under some circumstances, certain antisocial behaviors could be considered indicators of specific personality traits (e.g., traits related to impulsivity or anger), it seems hazardous to equate heterogeneous aggregates of behaviors (e.g., antisociality) with strong evidence for the presence of a specific, motivationally important trait.

WHAT ARE THE BASIC DIMENSIONS
OF PERSONALITY?

Examining the relation between personality and alcoholism presupposes that clearly identified dimensions of personality exist and can be agreed upon; this is not necessarily the case. Numerous personality traits have been studied, and it is often unclear if the various traits represent unique, partially overlapping, or largely overlapping constructs. A brief overview of various models of personality is useful in providing order to the numerous personality traits that have been investigated over the years.

Several models of personality have been promoted as comprehensive accounts of the major dimensions underlying adult personality. The most widely accepted among these "general factor models" (Watson et al., 1994) focus on either three major dimensions (Big Three) or five major dimensions (Big Five). We briefly discuss the most widely utilized versions of each of these influential models.

Big Three Models

The late Hans Eysenck might be considered the father of the Big Three models. Half a century ago, Eysenck began a program of research that identified the three personality dimensions of Neuroticism (N) versus Emotional Stability, Extraversion (E) versus Introversion, and Psychoticism (P) versus Super-Ego Control. Secondary traits relevant to these three higher-order personality dimensions are assessed in the Eysenck Personality Questionnaire (Eysenck & Eysenck, 1975). A listing of the secondary traits for N, E, and P, respectively, appears in Table 3.1 (Eysenck, 1990).

Tellegen's (1985) model of personality in many ways resembles Eysenck's (see Table 3.1). The three higher-order personality dimensions include Negative Emotionality, Positive Emotionality, and Constraint. These roughly correspond to Eysenck's N, E, and P (reverse-scored), respectively. Scales designed to measure the components of Tellegen's model are included in the Multidimensional Personality Questionnaire (Tellegen, 1994; Tellegen & Waller, in press).

TABLE 3.1. Personality Traits Included in Eysenck's, Tellegen's, and Cloninger's Big Three Personality Models

Eysenck	Tellegen	Cloninger
Neuroticism	Negative Emotionality	Harm Avoidance
Anxious, Depressed, Guilt, Feelings, Low Self-Esteem, Tense, Irrational, Shy, Moody, Emotional	Aggression, Alienation, Stress Reaction	Cautious, Apprehensive, Fatigable, Inhibited
Extraversion	Positive Emotionality	Reward Dependence
Sociable, Lively, Active, Assertive, Sensation-Seeking, Carefree, Dominant, Surgent, Venturesome	Achievement, Social Potency, Well-Being, Social Closeness	Ambitious, Sympathetic, Warm, Industrious, Sentimental, Persistent, Moody
Psychoticism	Constraint	Novelty Seeking
Aggressive, Cold, Egocentric, Impersonal, Impulsive, Antisocial, Unempathic, Creative, Tough-minded	Traditionalism, Harm Avoidance, Control	Impulsive, Excitable, Exploratory, Quick Tempered, Fickle, Extravagant

A final Big Three model is noteworthy as well, because it has been frequently applied in the research literature on alcohol use disorders. Cloninger's (1987a) three-dimensional model of personality targets the higher-order temperamental constructs of Harm Avoidance, Reward Dependence, and Novelty Seeking (see Table 3.1). Component personality traits associated with these three dimensions are assessed by the Tridimensional Personality Questionnaire (TPQ; Cloninger, 1987b). In the most recent revision of his theory, Cloninger proposes Persistence (which was previously considered a subfactor of Reward Dependence) as a fourth major dimension of temperament, and adds three (nontemperamental) character traits (Self-Directedness, Cooperativeness, and Self-Transcendence), to yield a seven-factor theory of personality (e.g., Svrakic, Whitehead, Przybeck, & Cloninger, 1993). It should be noted that Cloninger's original three temperamental supertraits are not isomorphic with those of Eysenck and Tellegen (Sher, Wood, Crews, & Vandiver, 1995; Zuckerman & Cloninger, 1996), and concerns over the factor structure of the TPQ have been raised by some researchers (e.g., Cannon, Clark, Leeka, & Keefe, 1993; Earleywine, Finn, Peterson, & Pihl, 1992). However, other investigators find the factor structure proposed by Cloninger to be empirically reasonable (e.g., Bagby, Parker, & Joffe, 1992; Sher et al., 1995; Waller, Lilienfeld, Tellegen, & Lykken, 1991). Much of this controversy surrounding the validity of the proposed factor structure stems from the lack of a consistently accepted metric for evaluating model fit in factor-analytic studies.

Big Five Models

In recent years, the Five-Factor Model of personality (or Big Five) has gained prominence in the field. This model's roots are often traced to the work of Allport and Odbert (1936), who collected personality-relevant terms from an English dictionary in order to develop a taxonomy of traits or attributes. Cattell (1943), using a reduced list of these terms, applied several methods to form a set of synonym clusters and develop a set of 35 rating scales. Subsequently, a number of independent factor-analytic investigations using Cattell's scales or modified versions of these scales reported finding five higher-order factors that could adequately account for the variance in these personality traits. Similar findings emerged regardless of whether data were from self-reports or peer ratings; from men, women, or children; or from English, Dutch, German, or Japanese samples (for a review of the history of the Big Five, see John, 1990; Wiggins & Trapnell, 1997). Although several versions of the Big Five exist, we focus on only two of these versions: one that developed from the lexical tradition (Goldberg), and one that developed from the questionnaire tradition (Costa & McCrae).

Goldberg (1982, 1990) has played a prominent role in the movement to identify the orthogonal personality factors that best account for the wide variety of personality trait terms that exist in the natural language. Investigators within this lexical tradition have examined the interrelationships among personality trait descriptors in order to develop an empirically based, dimensional model of personality. Goldberg's work is especially noteworthy because of its comprehensiveness, and his model has proved to be robust to variations in factor extraction and factor rotation. Goldberg (1992) has provided the following labels for the five factors of his model: Surgency (Extraversion), Agreeableness, Conscientiousness, Emotional Stability (i.e., reverse-scored Neuroticism), and Intellect (see Table 3.2 for descriptors). Goldberg presents several versions (unipolar vs. bipolar markers) of Big Five instruments to assess traits related to these five higher-order dimensions (for a review, see Widiger & Trull, 1997).

Interestingly, when Costa and McCrae first began their research on major dimensions of personality, there was no consensus on the Big Five (Costa & McCrae, 1992). These investigators compared competing systems of personality structure and identified major dimensions that were common across models. Their subsequent work involved the identification and fur-

TABLE 3.2. Personality Traits Included in Goldberg's and Costa and McCrae's Big Five Personality Models

Goldberg	Costa and McCrae
Surgency	Extraversion
Extraverted, Energetic, Talkative, Enthusiastic, Bold, Active, Self-Confident, Forceful, Spontaneous, Sociable	Warmth, Gregariousness, Assertiveness, Activity, Excitement-Seeking, Positive Emotions
Agreeableness	Agreeableness
Warm, Kind, Cooperative, Unselfish, Polite, Agreeable, Trustful, Generous, Flexible, Fair	Trust, Straightforwardness, Altruism, Compliance, Modesty, Tender-Mindedness
Conscientiousness	Conscientiousness
Organized, Responsible, Reliable, Conscientious, Practical, Thorough, Hardworking, Thrifty, Cautious, Serious	Competence, Order, Dutifulness, Achievement Striving, Self-Discipline, Deliberation
Emotional Stability	Neuroticism
Calm, Relaxed, At Ease, Even-tempered, Good-natured, Not Envious, Stable, Contented, Secure, Unemotional	Anxiety, Angry Hostility, Depression, Self-Consciousness, Impulsiveness, Vulnerability
Intellect	Openness to Experience
Intelligent, Perceptive, Analytical, Reflective, Curious, Imaginative, Creative, Cultured, Refined, Sophisticated	Fantasy, Aesthetics, Feelings, Actions, Ideas, Values

ther elaboration of major personality dimensions that were not clearly represented in the previous models of Eysenck, Guilford, Cattell, and others. The five factors that comprise Costa and McCrae's Big Five model include Neuroticism (N), Extraversion (E), Openness to Experience (O), Agreeableness (A), and Conscientiousness (C). Their Revised NEO-Personality Inventory (NEO-PI-R; Costa & McCrae, 1992) is the most popular measure of the Big Five. One of its most important, distinguishing features is its assessment of a wide variety of personality facets or traits that comprise the five higher-order personality dimensions of N, E, O, A, and C (see Table 3.2).

Integration

Two recent investigations suggest that the Big Three and Big Five models share similarities beyond the obvious resemblance of N and E in both sets of models. Zuckerman, Kuhlman, and Camac (1988) conducted a series of factor analyses of scores from 46 scales from a variety of popular personality inventories (including measures of the Big Three and Big Five models) and examined the factor structure and construct validity of a variety of factor solutions. Zuckerman et al. argued that their three-factor solution was most useful to those investigators who wanted to make "broader" (regarding content) predictions, predictions over longer time frames, and to those who were interested in theory testing. Zuckerman et al.'s three-factor solution of Sociability, Impulsive–Unsocialized–Sensation-Seeking, and Emotionality as supertraits resembles Eysenck's dimensions of Extraversion, Psychoticism, and Neuroticism, respectively.

A second recent attempt to integrate these models was conducted by Watson et al. (1994), who administered two Big Three and two Big Five instruments to a large sample of undergraduates and identified five factors using exploratory factor-analytic techniques. However, no subscale from a Big Three measure loaded on the fifth factor, leading the authors to settle on a four-factor integrative model. The higher-order personality dimensions identified in this model were Neuroticism or Negative Emotionality, Extraversion or Positive Emotionality, Conscientiousness or Constraint; and Agreeableness. Furthermore, Watson et al. presented a catalog of lower-order personality traits that comprise each of these major dimensions.

Thus, currently, a substantial body of research points to a highly replicable structure of personality traits, and the Big Three and Big Five approaches can serve as useful structures both for organizing the vast literature on alcoholism and personality and for generating research hypotheses (see Martin & Sher, 1994; Sher & Trull, 1994).

Despite the widespread acceptance of three- and five-factor trait theories discussed earlier, this trait approach, typically assessed via self-report personality inventories, represents only one strategy for studying characteristics that some might consider aspects of personality. For example, over the years, a number of personality traits have been linked to alcoholism, including dispositional self-awareness (or self-consciousness; e.g., Hull, 1987), augmentation–reduction (e.g., Petrie, 1967), and field dependence (e.g., Witkin, Karp, & Goodenough, 1959), to name just a few. The relation among these personality dimensions and Big Three and Big Five traits is not at all clear.

GENERAL MODELS OF THE RELATION BETWEEN PERSONALITY AND ALCOHOLISM

There are a number of ways that personality and alcoholism can be related; some of these are substantively important, whereas others are artifactual. Here, we highlight several alternative models of this general relationship and focus on those that are etiologically relevant.

Causal versus Noncausal Relationships

It is always important to remember that correlations between personality variables and alcoholism can be obtained because of unrecognized confounds at the measurement or design level. At the measurement level, some personality scales contain items that directly reference substance use. As a case in point, the Disinhibition subscale of the Sensation-Seeking Scale— Version V (Zuckerman, Eysenck, & Eysenck, 1978) is a frequently employed self-report measure of sensation seeking and impulsivity containing two items that directly assess substance use ("I often like to get high [drinking liquor or smoking marijuana]," "I feel best after taking a couple of drinks"). Failure to address this confounding of item content inflates the magnitude of the correlation between disinhibition and alcohol consumption (Darkes, Greenbaum, & Goldman, 1998).

Also, it is possible that personality and alcoholism can be spuriously related because of "third variable" causation (see the top panel of Figure 3.1). For example, throughout the adult years, alcoholism is more prevalent among males than among females (Robins et al., 1984). However, many personality variables are related to gender (e.g., Costa & McCrae, 1992); thus, correlations between personality measures and alcoholism can spuriously result because both are associated with gender (Figure 3.1). Consequently, in studying personality/externalizing disorder relations, it is essential that plausible third variable explanations are evaluated and, when possible, ruled out.

Direction of Influence

Aside from artifactual and spurious relations, research on personality and alcoholism has suggested several models relating personality to alcohol use

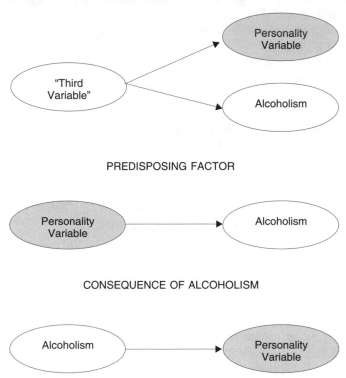

FIGURE 3.1. Three basic models of the relation between personality variables and alcoholism: (1) spurious ("third variable") relation, (2) etiological (predisposing variable) relation, and (3) consequential relation.

and abuse. First, there are those models that posit personality as a *predisposing* factor (middle panel of Figure 3.1). In these models, personality traits are thought to lead to alcoholism for any of a number of reasons. For example, as we discuss later, personality traits could provide the primary motivational basis for alcohol consumption (e.g., negative affect regulation, sensation seeking). Alternatively, personality traits could affect the likelihood that an individual who is already drinking is likely to continue drinking despite the fact that alcohol is interfering with his or her life (e.g., deficits in inhibitory control). Yet a third possibility is that personality traits contribute to the development of specific, alcohol-related consequences (e.g., alcohol-related aggression) in someone who has consumed alcohol (e.g., in individuals high in trait aggressiveness).

Second, there are models that view personality characteristics as a *consequence* of alcoholism (see bottom panel of Figure 3.1). Such models assume that the psychosocial (e.g., life stress, demoralization) and biological (e.g., ethanol toxicity, brain insult) consequences of alcoholism disorders result, either directly or indirectly, in personality changes. For example, there is considerable evidence that the cross-sectional correlates of clinical alcoholism differ from the prospective correlates of risk for alcoholism, leading to the previously mentioned distinction between *prealcoholic* and *clinical alcoholic* personalities (Barnes, 1983). Further support for the distinction between *prealcoholic* and *clinical alcoholic* traits comes from studies comparing changes in personality traits in alcoholics over an extended period of abstinence. Some "traits" appear stable (especially those related to psychopathic traits), whereas others appear to "normalize" (especially those related to anxiety and depression; see Barnes, 1983).

The Relation of Personality with Other Causal Variables

Presently, it is assumed that there is no single personality trait or constellation of traits that reliably predicts or diagnoses alcoholism. In addition, it is clear that multiple factors at varying levels of biopsychosocial organization, from genetic to broad social forces, contribute to the development of alcoholism. Often, theorists and researchers deal with the issue of multifactorial causation in one of two ways: (1) They ignore other domains of explanatory variables, or (2) they create atheoretical additive models that include both personality and other types of variables but do not specify ways in which they are related (e.g., Bry, McKeon, & Pandina, 1982). A number of models in the area of alcoholism, however, place personality variables into causal models incorporating other etiological constructs. In these models, personality variables are viewed in the context of mediating and moderating relationships (e.g., see Petraitis, Flay, & Miller, 1995).

With respect to *mediating relationships,* personality variables have been viewed in one of two ways. First, personality variables have been posited to mediate the effects of more distal variables, such as family history, on outcome (e.g., Cloninger, 1987a; Sher, 1991; Tarter, 1988; see top panel of Figure 3.2). Second, personality variables have been viewed as having only indirect effects on disorders; that is, their primary effects are mediated by other variables more proximal to outcome (see middle panel of Figure 3.2). To illustrate the notion of an indirect effect, it has been posited that individuals who are high on traits related to negative affectivity are more likely to experience subjective distress and consequently turn to alcohol for "self-medication" purposes (e.g., Sher, 1991). In this case, subjective distress would be considered the mediator of the effect of the personality-trait neuroticism. Additionally, personality variables can be thought to occupy the "middle" of multistage causal chains, both mediating the effects of more distal variables and exerting their effects through mediators more proximal to outcome (see bottom panel of Figure 3.2). For example, Sher, Walitzer, Wood, and Brent's (1991) data suggest that the effect of family history on offspring alcoholism could be mediated by such a

MEDIATING DISTAL VARIABLES

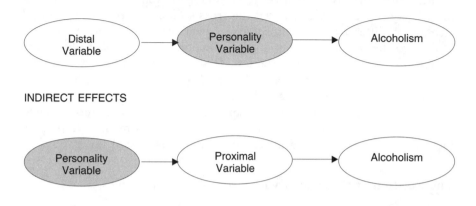

INDIRECT EFFECTS

MULTISTAGE CAUSAL CHAINS

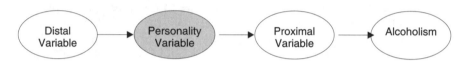

FIGURE 3.2. Three basic models in which personality plays "mediating" or "mediated" roles.

multistage chain where family history (a distal variable) is related to behavioral undercontrol (a personality variable), which in turn is related to alcohol-outcome expectancies (a proximal variable), which in turn is related to alcohol involvement (the outcome).

In addition to mediating-type relationships, there is ample evidence to suggest that personality can play a *moderating* role in alcohol use and alcoholism, interacting with various risk factors to exacerbate or attenuate the likelihood of consumption or disorder; that is, one's relative standing on a personality dimension can determine the strength of relation between a predictor variable and an alcohol-related outcome (see Figure 3.3). For example, the trait of dispositional self-awareness (a personality variable) has been shown to interact with life events (a predictor variable) in determining the likelihood of relapse (Hull, Young, & Jouriles, 1986). Similarly, self-awareness has been shown to interact with family history of alcoholism in predicting offspring alcohol problems (Rogosch, Chassin, & Sher, 1990) and appears to moderate the relationship between alcohol-outcome expectancies and alcohol use (Bartholow, Sher, & Strathman, 1998). Consideration of the interaction of personality variables with environmental variables has the potential to explain more variance in behavior than prediction

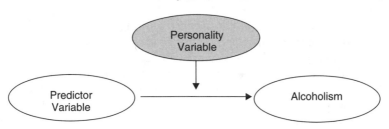

FIGURE 3.3. Personality as a moderator of other predictors of alcoholism.

based solely on main effects of personality and environmental variables (Magnusson & Endler, 1977).

Thus, independent of the content of specific relationships, the basic structure of personality–alcoholism relationships can vary across several domains, including the extent to which a variable is (1) artifactual/spurious or substantively meaningful, (2) causal or consequential, (3) mediating direct effects (i.e., transmitting the effects of more distal variables), (4) mediated by other variables and thus having only indirect effects (i.e., transmits its effect through its influence on a more proximal variable), and (5) moderating the effects of other variables. As discussed in a later section, we believe it is more useful from both basic and applied perspectives not only to search for personality correlates of alcoholism, but also to try to test specific models of how personality could be related to alcoholism.

GENERAL METHODOLOGICAL CONCERNS

There are numerous important methodological issues to consider in research on personality and alcoholism. Several of the most crucial issues that bear on the nature of the types of inferences that can be drawn from a given study are described here.

Diagnostic Subtypes

A critical methodological issue concerns the *heterogeneity* of membership within the diagnostic category of alcoholism. As reviewed by Babor (1996; Babor & Lauerman, 1986), clinicians and researchers have posited the presence of subtypes of alcoholism since at least the middle of the last century. These typologies have been derived using a variety of techniques, ranging from clinical description (e.g., Jellinek, 1960) to cluster analysis of psychometric data (e.g., Partington & Johnson, 1969). Numerous cluster-analytic investigations have been conducted in the past, and the number and type of clusters found by different investigators vary considerably (Morey & Blashfield, 1981). This is not surprising given the range of cluster-analytic techniques employed, the varying nature of the data bases subjected to clustering, and the diversity of subject samples studied. Nevertheless, there appears to be consistent evidence for at least two clusters that could broadly be termed a personality disorder cluster and a neurotic cluster (Morey & Blashfield, 1981). This general finding is compatible with the typology proposed more than 60 years ago by Knight (1937), and with more recent typologies that distinguish forms of alcoholism: (1) an earlier onset form marked by greater antisociality, and (2) a later onset form marked by greater negative emotionality (Babor et al., 1992; Cloninger, 1987b; Finn et al., 1997).

A key question confronting proponents of categorical subtypes is whether there is unique, configural information that is captured in a typology that is "missed" by solely considering basic, multiple dimensions of the phenomenon (Sher, 1994). However, typology researchers have not systematically attempted to demonstrate the validity of their derived categorical constructions against the (arguably) more parsimonious model that the phenotype is best described by a few underlying dimensions.

Although we are not yet convinced that subtyping alcoholics into discrete categories represents the most useful approach to investigating personality-based hypotheses regarding the causes and effects of alcoholism, failure to consider heterogeneity *could* conceivably obscure potentially important personality correlates. Cloninger's (1987a) theory of Type 1 and Type 2 alcoholism provides an interesting *hypothetical* example of this potential problem. Cloninger proposed that there are two *prototypical* types of alcoholics, one characterized by early and the other by late age of onset, and each with opposite patterns on primary dimensions of personality. Conceivably, a sample of alcoholics composed of equal numbers of each type would be expected to have a mean value near the general population mean on each of the three personality traits in Cloninger's model (see earlier discussion), and as such may not be distinguishable from a control group with respect to basic dimensions of personality. We note, however, that it is not necessary to adopt a subtyping approach in order to observe the types of associations Cloninger hypothesized. Indeed, for example, a corollary of Cloninger's hypothesis is that in a heterogeneous sample of alcoholics, certain traits should be nonlinearly related to alcoholism (e.g., by showing a quadratic relation). We have explicitly tested this hypothesis and failed to find such effects (Sher et al., 1995). Nevertheless, Cloninger's theory illustrates the potential pitfalls of failing to consider important sources of heterogeneity within a sample when studying personality correlates.

The issue of subtyping becomes more complex when subtypes are derived from personality data, and theorists have long proposed alcoholism subtypes based upon personality variables. For example, many of the cluster-analytic studies of alcoholics conducted to date have been based on personality scale data (e.g., Morey & Blashfield, 1981). Studies demonstrating personality differences among groups differentiated on the basis of personality data run the risk of becoming tautological, and care must be taken to avoid this pitfall by always validating personality-based subtypes with external criteria (Morey & Blashfield, 1981).

Comorbidity

For many years, it has been recognized that alcohol use disorders are highly comorbid with antisocial personality disorder (APD). Moreover, this generalization appears to be true in clinical (e.g., Hesselbrock, Meyer, & Keener, 1985), criminal (e.g., Lewis, Cloninger, & Pais, 1983), and general population samples (e.g., Helzer & Pryzbeck, 1988), and these associations persist even when overlap in diagnostic criteria is eliminated (Grande, Wolf, Schubert, Patterson, & Brocco, 1984; Lewis, 1984). As noted by Sher and Trull (1994) however, considerably less is known concerning comorbidity between alcoholism and other personality disorders.

Over the past 15 years, it has become clear that personality disorders other than APD frequently co-occur with alcoholism in both clinical samples and nonclinical samples (Alnaes & Torgersen, 1988; Drake & Vaillant, 1985; Mendelsohn, Barbor, Mello, & Pratt, 1986; Poldrugo & Forti, 1988; Widiger & Rogers, 1989). Table 3.3 presents studies in which alcohol use disorders and personality disorders have been examined. Taken together, the studies presented in Table 3.3 document that personality disorders often co-occur with alcohol use disorders, especially antisocial and borderline personality disorders. However, caution is appropriate when interpreting the findings of the clinical studies in that they are likely to overestimate comorbidity, because individuals with multiple disorders are more likely to seek treatment (e.g., Cohen & Cohen, 1984). Consequently, it is important to note that those few studies based on nonclinical samples also indicate extensive comorbidity (e.g., Drake, Adler, & Vaillant, 1988; Drake & Vaillant, 1985; Tousignant & Kovess, 1989; Zimmerman & Coryell, 1989).

In another recent study, Alterman et al. (1998) found that nonclinical participants at high familial risk for developing alcoholism reported significantly more drinking in the past 30 days and diagnosed with significantly more personality pathology (particularly APD) than a low-risk group. Furthermore, the greatest amount of personality pathology was found among high-risk participants with a greater density of familial alcoholism (defined as having an alcoholic biological father as well as significant additional familial alcoholism).

Given extensive (Axis I and Axis II) comorbidity, one critical implication concerns the ability to unambiguously attribute a personality characteristic to a specific disorder; that is, if alcoholics are found to differ from a control sample, is this difference specific to alcoholism per se or to a co-occurring condition (e.g., APD, borderline personality disorder, drug abuse, anxiety disorder)? Unfortunately, there is no simple way of disentangling comorbid disorders to arrive at specific correlates of a target disorder. It is tempting to think that a specificity design (Garber & Hollon, 1991)

TABLE 3.3. Comorbidity between Alcoholism and Personality Disorders in a Sample of Recent Studies

Study	Sample	% comorbid diagnosis
Alnaes & Torgersen (1988) (N = 38)	Outpatient	AvPD, DPD, OCD, P-A, BPD, NPD, HPD, APD = 92%
Casey & Tyrer (1990) (N = 41)	Presenting for Tx to GP	Unsp. = 67%
DeJong et al. (1993) (N = 178)	Inpatient	BPD = 17%
Derksen (1990) (N = 15)	Outpatient	BPD = 53%
Drake & Vaillant (1985) (N = 62)	Community	DPD, P-A, HPD, Unsp. = 37%
Drake et al. (1988) (N = 62)	Community	BPD = 3%
Haver & Dahlgren (1995) (N = 60)	Inpatient, outpatient	BPD = 12%, Unsp. = 12%
Jonsdottir-Baldurson & Horvath (1987) (N = 51)	Inpatient	BPD = 27%
Morgenstern et al. (1997) (N = 366)	Inpatient, outpatient	APD = 23%, BPD = 22%, NPD = 21%
Nace et al. (1986) (N = 74)	Inpatient	BPD = 18%
Nace et al. (1991) (N = 100)	Inpatient	BPD = 17%, PPD = 7%, HPD = 6%
Nurnberg et al. (1993) (N = 50)	Outpatient	PPD = 44%, APD = 20%, P-A = 18%, BPD = 16%
Poldrugo & Forti (1988) (N = 404)	Alcoholics presenting for Tx	APD = 9%, BPD = 4%
Stravynski et al. (1986) (N = 167)	Abstinent alcoholics presenting for Tx	AvPD = 20%
Tousignant & Kovess (1989) (N = 21)	Community	BPD = 19%
Vaglum & Vaglum (1985) (N = 64)	Inpatient	BPD = 66%, Unsp. = 22%
Zimmerman & Coryell (1989) (N = 145)	Community	APD = 14%, P-A = 10%, HPD = 8%, BPD = 7%, OCD = 5%

Note. PD, personality disorder; APD, antisocial PD; AvPD, avoidant PD; BPD, borderline PD; DPD, dependent PD; HPD, histrionic PD; NPD, Narcissistic PD; PPD, paranoid PD; OCD, obsessive–compulsive disorder; P-A, passive–aggressive PD; Unsp., personality disorder not otherwise specified; Tx, treatment; GP, general practitioner. Sample sizes (Ns) refer to numbers of participants in each study diagnosed with alcoholism, which does not necessarily equal the study N.

contrasting, say, groups of alcoholic subjects with and without comorbid diagnoses (and possibly other informative control groups) to shed light on the construct of "pure alcoholism." However, so-called "pure" cases of alcoholism could be highly atypical of alcoholism and do not clearly represent an optimal group from which to generalize. It is within this context of high comorbidity and diagnostic overlap that the question of personality and alcoholism needs to be viewed. Later, we describe a general statistical approach that can help address some of the complexities associated with diagnostic heterogeneity/subtypes.

An additional complexity to the comorbidity issue concerns the extent that alcoholism can be thought to be primary or secondary to a comorbid disorder (e.g., Schuckit, 1985). Primary and secondary alcoholism are typically distinguished on the basis of the temporal ordering of age of onset for alcoholism and comorbid diagnoses; alcoholism is considered *primary* if its onset precedes that of another diagnosis, or *secondary* if its onset succeeds that of another diagnosis. Although, in practice, it is often difficult to resolve the temporal ordering of alcoholism and a comorbid diagnosis, the primary–secondary distinction can be useful conceptually. As noted earlier, the idea that there are fundamentally different types of alcoholism has profound implications for the design and interpretation of studies on alcoholism.

Research Design

Although the implications of different research designs for studying the personality correlates of alcoholism are well known, they nonetheless warrant brief comment. First, *cross-sectional* designs, the most frequently employed research designs in personality and psychopathology research, fail to resolve the temporal relation between personality and diagnostic status; that is, correlations between diagnostic status and personality can reflect causal, consequential, or spurious associations. *Prospective* designs, although employed relatively infrequently, are much more useful in resolving temporal precedence. Despite the value of prospective designs, we emphasize that the establishment of a prospective relation between personality and alcoholism does not establish a causal relation, and "third-variable" alternative explanations need to be considered in evaluating this research. Furthermore, alcoholism can sometimes have a protracted and insidious onset with behavioral antecedents (e.g., oppositionality, conduct problems) appearing in childhood and/or adolescence; that is, what may be prodromal aspects of certain forms of alcoholism (at least those associated with antisociality) are evident early in development; ideally, prospective studies should evaluate whether various personality traits predict (i.e., account for additional variance) over and above these early behavioral manifestations of disorder. Failure of personality traits to increment prediction beyond childhood behavior problems does not necessarily negate the importance of personality but does raise interpretative questions.

Because of the limitations of cross-sectional studies, and the cost and difficulty of conducting prospective studies, there has been a dramatic increase in the use of cross-sectional *high-risk* designs in recent years. The basic rationale of the high-risk design was presented more than 30 years ago by Mednick and McNeil (1968), who argued that existing etiological research on schizophrenia was severely limited because schizophrenics were so affected by their illness that studying them told us more about the consequences of schizophrenia than its causes. They recommended the "longitudinal study of young children at high risk" (p. 687) in order to distinguish antecedents from consequences of disorder. They pointed out that the high-risk method had cross-sectional utility in that "differences between the high- and low-risk groups may relate to factors predisposing to mental illness" (p. 689). Because the high-risk method has the potential to discover "predisposing" factors prior to the ultimate development of the disorder, it frequently has been employed in the study of a range of psychopathological conditions. Over the last 10 years, numerous cross-sectional high-risk studies have been conducted in the area of alcoholism. However, high-risk versus low-risk differences on a variable do not establish etiological relevance, but merely reflect the "characteristics, correlates and/or consequences of the risk criterion" (McNeil & Kaij, 1979, p. 548). Thus, high-risk versus low-risk differences, by themselves, suggest, but do not establish, a trait as being etiologically relevant; demonstration of an etiologically relevant role involves both prospective prediction and elimination of artifactual, alternative explanations.

Sampling

Much of the personality research on alcoholism is conducted on samples ascertained on the basis of their status as patients in treatment facilities. Given that only some proportion of individuals with a given disorder are likely to receive treatment or become incarcerated, the generalizability of findings based on clinical and institutionalized samples is always an issue (see Cohen & Cohen, 1984). For example, alcoholics in treatment have been shown to have more comorbid psychopathology than those not in treatment (Woodruff, Guze, & Clayton, 1973), and, as noted earlier, comorbidity (including comorbidity not causally associated with the target disorder) increases the likelihood of entering treatment (Berkson, 1946). Also, as pointed out by Cohen and Cohen (1984), the most severe cases (i.e., persons who have the most frequent or lengthy treatments) are the most likely to be sampled in studies utilizing patients. Nonclinical samples are frequently employed in studies of alcohol use and sometimes in studies of alcohol use disorders. However, all too frequently, these nonclinical samples are based on convenience and/or are not systematically ascertained, thus limiting their generalizability to a known population.

Beyond the effects of sampling on sample composition, the setting from which subjects are selected might have important effects on the assessment of personality itself. For example, with respect to psychopathy, Eysenck and Gudjonsson (1989) have argued that incarceration status may affect personality scores. Specifically, these authors speculate that incarceration (and presumably, residential treatment of alcoholism) may lower the overall level of Extraversion scores due to restrictions placed on inmates' activities. On the other hand, Eysenck and Gudjonsson propose that incarceration may inflate Neuroticism scores because imprisonment (and possibly, inpatient treatment environments) may engender the development of fears and anxieties that otherwise would not be present. However, given the recent shift away from prolonged residential treatment of alcoholism and toward outpatient treatment, this potential concern is reduced.

"Control Groups" and the Problem of Specificity

The choice of control groups and control variables always involves numerous considerations and varies as a function of the basic research design employed. The issues involved in selecting controls for cross-sectional studies using clinical participants differ substantially from those using general population and/or high-risk prospective studies. A detailed consideration of these issues is beyond the scope of this chapter (but for a discussion of these issues, see Sher, 1991; Sher & Trull, 1996). Nevertheless, a major consideration of control groups in alcoholism research often involves the ability to show effects specific to alcoholism (i.e., as distinct from control groups with other behavior problems, as well as from "normal" control groups).

As we view it, the problem of comorbidity represents a significant challenge to thinking about control groups in the usual way; that is, it is possible that a given individual suffers from several conditions (e.g., drug use disorder, an anxiety disorder, a depressive disorder, and a personality disorder) in addition to his or her alcoholism. Attempting to develop discrete control groups (e.g., an anxiety disorder group, a depressive disorder group, an anxiety + depressive disorder group, a personality disorder group, a personality disorder + anxiety disorder group) is impractical, if not impossible. Consequently, we believe it is necessary to have nonalcoholic control subjects with psychopathology (especially those conditions most frequently comorbid with alcoholism) and without psychopathology (in order to model variance associated with all diagnostic variables, including alcoholism). However, because of comorbidity it is probably more useful to think in terms of diagnostic *control variables* (e.g., drug use disorder, APD, anxiety disorder, affective disorder) rather than control groups. We believe that, in general, it is useful always to consider two broad classes of control variables: (1) other forms of disinhibitory psychopathology (e.g., drug use disorders, APD), and (2) internalizing psychopathology (e.g., anxiety and depressive disorders).

Assessment of a broad range of psychopathology in a multivariate context permits a number of probing comparisons. For example, using factors to assess broadband domains of psychopathology permit an assessment of personality traits that characterize disinhibitory psychopathology as distinct from psychopathology more generally, and of the unique correlates of alcoholism over and above disinhibitory psychopathology. We illustrate this conceptual approach in Figure 3.4 using a structural equation model.

As can be seen in Figure 3.4, the structural path from the personality variable factor to the disinhibitory psychopathology factor (shown by the letter *a*) represents the effect of a personality variable on disinhibitory psychopathology. (Note that differences in the size of this effect can be compared with, say, the effect on internalizing psychopathology [indicated here by path *b*] by testing the reasonableness of the hypothesis that the two paths are equal. In an analogous way, the effects of the personality variable on other psychopathology factors, for example, "psychoses," also could be modeled and compared).

Perhaps more intriguing, the path (shown by the letter *c*) from the per-

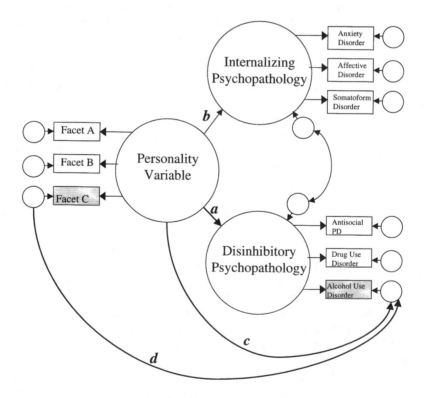

FIGURE 3.4. Structural equation model illustrating how it is possible to isolate progressively more specific personality correlates of alcoholism. See text for explanation of paths *a*, *b*, *c*, and *d*.

sonality factor to the unique variance of alcoholism (i.e., the residual) that is not a part of the disinhibitory factor can be thought to represent a unique personality correlate of alcoholism. Please note that such a unique effect is not necessarily the most important type of effect for understanding the alcoholism–personality relation; it is very possible that an effect on the "disinhibitory psychopathology" factor represents most of the important personality variation associated with alcoholism in a heterogeneous population. However, such unique effects can inform the question "How do individuals who suffer from alcohol use disorders differ from others who might have other forms of substance use disorders or antisociality?"

This general model is also capable of revealing highly specific effects between narrowband personality variables and alcohol use disorders. For example, under alternative Big Three and Big Five models of personality (see Tables 3.1 and 3.2), the superfactors are composed of more specific primary factors. Modeling of residual pathways (e.g., the path from the residual of Facet C to the residual of alcohol use disorder, path d) can be used to reveal unique effects of narrowband personality traits on alcohol use disorders above the more general associations between the personality superfactor and disinhibitory psychopathology. Recent papers by McArdle, Hamagami, and Hulick (1994) and Muthen (1994) give an overview of methodological developments, with particular emphasis on the application of these techniques to the study of alcohol consumption and alcoholism.

To date, we are not aware of any studies of personality and alcoholism that have used such designs. However, in a recent paper, we (Trull & Sher, 1994) used canonical correlation techniques to model both the general relation between psychopathology and personality, and a unique effect for substance use disorders and depression using a measure of the five-factor model of personality (the NEO-FFI). Certainly other analytic approaches are also possible. Our major point is that important sources of heterogeneity should be assessed and modeled in appropriate analyses in order to derive valid conclusions.

The general approach to modeling comorbidity also can be applied to modeling other sources of heterogeneity. For example, alcoholics have been subtyped on the basis of sex, family history, and age of onset of drinking problems (in addition to comorbid psychopathology). However, these subtyping dimensions tend to be intercorrelated (see Martin & Sher, 1994), and use of appropriate strategies for examining multivariate effects at varying levels of diagnostic specificity permits optimally informative analyses.

Assessing Personality

The overwhelming majority of research on personality in alcoholism has relied on the use of self-report questionnaires, which may be problematic. For example, Shedler, Mayman, and Manis (1993) presented evidence suggesting that many individuals who score low on measures of neuroticism appear to be defensively denying neurotic symptoms. Additionally, many studies have suggested that changes in mood states may markedly affect subjects' responses to self-report personality measures (Hirschfeld et al., 1983), and it is well known that clinical alcoholism is associated with transient affective disturbance that resolves over a period of abstinence (e.g., Schuckit, 1994). Thus, the biased reporting of personality characteristics may undermine the validity of self-report measures of personality traits.

To circumvent this potential threat to both reliability and validity, some investigators have employed informant ratings as primary measures of target subjects' personality traits. Informant ratings also have the advantage of applicability to very young samples. For example, in a study of the personality predictors of adolescent drug use, Block and his colleagues (Block, Block, & Keyes, 1988) obtained personality ratings on 3- and 4-year-olds. However, sole reliance on this latter method also runs the risk of potentially biasing assessments of personality. For example, the number of informants employed for each target is typically, though not always, small, the degree of familiarity between targets and informants is rarely quantified or controlled, and the possibility that informant reports (like self-reports) may be subject to bias is rarely considered (i.e., informants may be motivated to bias their reports).

Given these possible sources of subjectivity, it seems tempting to use observable, behavioral acts as "objective" indices of personality dispositions. For example, Buss and Craik (1980) have been strong proponents of the act-frequency approach to personality, in which frequencies of specified behaviors over a designated time period are considered indicative of an individual's personality traits or dispositions. However, the limitations of this seemingly "objective" personality assessment method must also be recognized (e.g., Block, 1989; Widiger & Trull, 1987). Although behaviors may be useful in inferring a personality trait, behaviors and traits are not equivalent concepts for a number of reasons: (1) Behavior can sometimes result primarily from environmental versus dispositional factors; (2) any individual behavior can be indicative of a variety of correlated or even uncorrelated traits; and (3) the base rates of certain behaviors that have been nominated as indicative of a particular personality trait are often so low in the general population as to provide little predictive power or utility.

These three limitations are especially important to research on personality and alcoholism, because the most robust predictor of alcoholism appears to be premorbid antisocial behavior (e.g., conduct problems). However, antisocial behavior (for example) can be indicative of a number of personality dispositions, as well as caused by a variety of environmental factors (e.g., poverty). Unfortunately, the motivational bases underlying antisociality are rarely assessed in prospective studies, and significance of personality per se is often obscure.

Another long-standing approach to assessing personality utilizes performance on behavioral tasks (e.g., using the Kinesthetic Figural After effect to assess augmentation–reduction and the Rod and Frame Test to assess field dependency), and these behavioral measures may not correlate highly with self-report measures. Currently, traits related to self-control or its absence (e.g., constraint, impulsivity, conscientiousness) are thought to be extremely important to the development of alcoholism, other substance abuse, and a range of externalizing behavior problems. However, it is clear that behavioral assessment of these traits using laboratory tasks are, at best, only weakly related to measures based on self-reports and informant ratings (e.g., White et al., 1994).

Despite the limitations of personality assessment, existing personality research has made significant progress toward understanding the psychological basis of alcoholism. Much of our improved understanding is based on a more sophisticated approach to the study of personality and alcoholism, and the various ways that personality variables can be related to alcoholism. In addition, given the limitations inherent in reliance on any single method of assessment, the importance of studies using multiple assessment methods (e.g., White et al., 1994) needs to be stressed. Such studies have the potential to resolve some of the assessment-related problems mentioned earlier.

Developmental and Gender Issues

The etiological relevance of various personality traits and associated processes is likely to vary across developmental stage. For example, antisocial alcoholism is associated with an early age of onset (Zucker, 1987), and some personality traits (e.g., those related to impulsivity/disinhibition) are particularly associated with this form of alcoholism (Sher & Trull, 1994). Alternatively, other personality traits (e.g., those related to neuroticism) may be more relevant to alcoholism appearing later in life. Thus, it is very possible that the personality correlates of alcoholism differ as a function of stage of life. Although no systematic program of research has examined this possibility in detail, several studies provide indirect evidence to support this distinction, at least in clinical samples. For example, Varma, Basu, Malhotra, Sharma, and Mattoo (1994) reported that alcoholic patients with an early age of onset were younger and displayed more novelty seeking and general disinhibition than did a later age-of-onset group. Also, Gomberg (1997) reported that younger problem drinkers with earlier onset show greater impulsivity and more antisociality, whereas older problem drinkers with later onset manifest more negative emotionality. These data and related theory suggest the need to consider age differences across samples (and age heterogeneity within samples) when interpreting the literature on alcoholism and personality.

Similarly, male alcoholics tend to be more psychopathic, aggressive, and impulsive than female alcoholics, and female alcoholics tend to be more affectively disturbed than male alcoholics (e.g., Hesselbrock, 1991).

However, it could be hazardous to assume that gender represents a subtyping variable delineating two different "species" of alcoholism. Most of the literature on gender and alcoholism is based on studies lacking normal controls, and the types of differences noted between female and male alcoholics could conceivably reflect pervasive gender differences in personality. For example, in one recent study, Martin and Sher (1994) demonstrated that the traditional personality differences between males and females diagnosed with alcohol use disorders were no greater in magnitude than those found between nonalcoholic males and females in an age-homogeneous sample. Data from the Epidemiologic Catchment Area (ECA) study indicate that although gender relates to the number of conduct problems experienced in childhood and adolescence, conduct problems predict substance use and abuse equally well in boys and girls (Robins & McEvoy, 1990). A recent longitudinal study of a large, representative sample of adolescents failed to show gender differences in the prospective relation between delinquency (assessed at ages 14–15) and various measures of alcohol involvement assessed 4 years later (Windle, 1990). It is quite possible that many of the putative differences between male and female alcoholism are an artifact of age of onset; female alcoholics typically have a later age of onset than males, although this trend appears to be changing (Reich, Cloninger, Van Eerdewegh, Rice, & Mullaney, 1988). As this brief discussion illustrates, and as recently suggested elsewhere (Hesselbrock & Hesselbrock, 1997), the issue of sex-specific etiological factors in alcoholism is far from resolved. Further investigation of specific patterns of sex-related comorbidity with alcoholism are needed before firm conclusions can be drawn.

THE RELEVANCE OF MAJOR PERSONALITY TRAITS TO ALCOHOLISM

Numerous reviews of empirical studies relating personality traits to alcoholism have been conducted over the past two decades (e.g., Barnes, 1979, 1983; Cox, 1979, 1985; Lang, 1983; Nathan, 1988; Sher & Trull, 1994; Sutker & Allain, 1998; Tarter, 1988; Tarter & Vanyukov, 1994) and only a brief overview of major findings is presented here. In order to organize the major findings, we adopt a Big Three approach that is suitable for describing the majority of studies relating alcoholism to personality traits and encompasses three broadband traits: (1) Neuroticism/Negative Emotionality, (2) Impulsivity/Disinhibition, and (3) Extraversion/Sociability. These dimensions are similar (but not identical) to the ones offered by Eysenck and Eysenck (1975), Tellegen (1985) and Zuckerman, Kuhlman, and Camac (1988).

At the outset, it is important to note that, to varying degrees, each of these three broadband dimensions have been found to correlate with risk for alcoholism (usually, as defined by family history), prealcoholism (as determined via prospective or follow-back longitudinal studies), or clinical alcoholism. In order to highlight what we consider to be the most important findings to emerge from this immense literature, we briefly summarize the conclusions from our earlier review (Sher & Trull, 1994). Although a number of more recent studies have been published by ourselves (e.g., Sher et al., 1995) and others (e.g., McGue, Slutske, Taylor, & Iacono, 1997), most new published data are consistent with the conclusions of the earlier review. We note, however, that one relevant, new prospective study (Schuckit & Smith, 1996) failed to find evidence of broadband personality traits predicting the onset of alcohol use disorders. However, the sampling frame and the inclusion–exclusion criteria employed in that study (which was designed to study ethanol sensitivity) clearly were not optimal for examining personality effects.

Neuroticism/Negative Emotionality

A number of lines of evidence suggest that neuroticism/negative emotionality is associated with clinical alcoholism. For example, alcoholism is associated with high rates of anxiety (e.g., Kessler et al., 1997; Kushner et al., 1996; Mullan, Gurling, Oppenheim, & Murray, 1986; see also Sher & Trull, 1994) and, to a somewhat lesser degree, mood disorder. In addition, clinical alcoholics typically score high on psychometric measures of neuroticism/negative emotionality (i.e., scales assessing neuroticism and harm avoidance) (e.g., Brooner, Templer, Svikis, Schmidt, & Monopolis, 1990; Kannapan & Cherian, 1989; Meszaros, Willinger, Fischer, Schonbeck, & Aschauer, 1996; Mullan et al., 1986). Furthermore, rates of alcoholism are particularly high among individuals with extremely elevated negative emotionality scores as measured by the Multidimensional Personality Questionnaire (McGue et al., 1997).

What is less clear is the extent to which neuroticism/negative emotionality is associated with future alcoholism. Researchers continue to debate whether high comorbidity with neurotic (i.e., anxiety and depressive disorders) disorders is a consequence or a cause of alcoholism. In one study, clinical alcoholics showed elevated scores on the Depression, Hysteria, and Psychasthenia scales of the Minnesota Multiphasic Personality Inventory, relative to scores obtained an average of 13 years earlier, suggesting that neurotic symptoms increased with the clinical manifestation of alcoholism (Kammeier, Hoffman, & Loper, 1973). Furthermore, in their study of alcoholic twin pairs, Mullan and colleagues (1986) suggested that both clinically diagnosed neurotic illness and high neuroticism scale scores are more likely to be a consequence than a cause of alcoholism.

Findings from several major longitudinal studies do not suggest a strong causal role for neuroticism/negative emotionality (e.g., Jones, 1968; Robins, Bates, & O'Neal, 1962; Vaillant & Milofsky, 1982). In contrast, other prospective studies do implicate negative emotionality as predictive of later alcohol involvement (Caspi et al., 1997; Chassin, Curran, Hussong, & Colder, 1996; Cloninger, Sigvardsson, & Bohman, 1988; Labouvie, Pandina, White, & Johnson, 1990; Sieber, 1981). However, it should be noted that Cloninger et al. (1988) specify that *low* negative affectivity (characterized by low scores on the Harm Avoidance scale of the TPQ) is most relevant to the development of early-onset alcoholism, whereas people high in negative affect are susceptible to alcohol dependence occurring later in life.

This divergent pattern of findings indicates that our understanding of the role played by neuroticism/negative emotionality in alcohol abuse is far from complete, particularly given that the existing data base of informative prospective studies remains relatively sparse. Furthermore, the issue may be best resolved by considering moderating variables influencing the relationship between negative emotionality and alcohol use. For example, there is some evidence (e.g., Jones, 1971) that this dimension might be more etiologically relevant for women than for men.

Impulsivity/Disinhibition

The broad personality dimension that appears to be most relevant to alcoholism is that of impulsivity/disinhibition. This dimension incorporates traits such as sensation seeking, aggressiveness, impulsivity, and psychoticism. The high rates of comorbidity between alcohol use disorders and both antisocial and borderline personality disorder (see "Comorbidity" section) provide support for the idea that clinical alcoholics tend to be impulsive (e.g., Rieger et al., 1990), and alcoholics tend to score high on psychometric measures assessing this dimension (e.g., Bergman & Brismar, 1994; Plutchik & Plutchik, 1988). Moreover, alcoholics with comorbid APD experience a more severe and chronic course of alcoholism, and engage in more drug use, compared to those without this comorbid diagnosis (e.g., Holdcraft, Iacono, & McGue, 1998).

Additionally, cross-sectional high-risk studies (e.g., Alterman et al., 1998; Sher, 1991) demonstrate that traits reflecting impulsivity/disinhibition are elevated in the offspring of alcoholics. Most importantly, prospective studies consistently indicate that impulsive/disinhibited individuals are at elevated risk for the development of alcohol-related problems (e.g., Bates & Labouvie, 1995; Caspi et al., 1997; Cloninger et al., 1988; Hawkins, Catalano, & Miller, 1992; Pederson, 1991; Schuckit, 1998; Zucker, Fitzgerald, & Moses, 1995; Zucker & Gomberg, 1986). For example, Cloninger et al. (1988) reported that children assessed at age 11 who were thought to be high in novelty seeking were at elevated risk to develop early-onset alcohol abuse by age 27. The importance of impulsivity/disinhibition as an early predictor of later alcohol problems has been outlined in detail by Zucker et al. (1995). These authors hypothesize that the prospective relation between childhood impulsivity/disinhibition (or childhood conduct disorder) and later drinking problems marks an etiological process whereby these traits lead to poor school performance and relational problems. These troubles in turn may lead such individuals to associate with similar peers, who are likely to begin using alcohol and other drugs early in adolescence. Moreover, conduct disorder and alcohol dependence have been linked to the influence of genes that increase the risk for both disorders (Slutske et al., 1998).

However, as noted in an earlier section ("Defining Personality"), there is some debate surrounding whether antisocial and impulsive behaviors are best thought of as indexing an underlying personality dimension (i.e., the personality perspective) or as representing early signs of a developmental disorder that ultimately manifests itself in the form of alcoholism (i.e., the developmental disorder perspective). Clearly, interpretation of these data is driven by the characteristics used to define personality.

To help resolve this issue, studies demonstrating that personality variables can statistically explain the relation between antisocial behavior and alcoholism can be of theoretical relevance. In one such study, Earleywine and Finn (1991) demonstrated that the cross-sectional relation between alcohol use and a scale that heavily samples antisocial behavior can be statistically explained by the effect of sensation seeking on both variables. Although alcohol use, not alcoholism per se, was investigated in this study, this type of statistical modeling could be extended to clinically more relevant outcomes and used to identify the most critical etiological variables, and thereby advance the antisociality–alcoholism debate considerably.

In summary, our reading of the literature suggests that, to some extent, both the personality perspective and the developmental disorder perspective have some validity, but that a personality-based interpretation is clearly defensible because some assessments do not directly index antisocial and aggressive behavior. Given the recent research attention directed at this issue, our understanding of these relationships should be more clear within the next few years.

Extraversion/Sociability

The evidence concerning the relationship between extraversion/sociability and alcoholism can best be described as mixed. Most reviews of the clinical literature (e.g., Barnes, 1983; Cox, 1985) do not suggest that, as a group, alcoholics differ from controls on the dimension of extraversion/sociability, although as dependence becomes severe, levels of extraversion/sociability may decrease (Rankin, Stockwell, & Hodgson, 1982). Moreover, high-risk, cross-sectional studies do not typically indicate that children of alcoholics differ from controls on this trait (Sher, 1991), although one recent study found that sociability predicted substance use for adolescent children of alcoholics but not for controls (Molina, Chassin, & Curran, 1994). On the other hand, at least one other, recent cross-sectional study using a non-clinical sample did not find a significant relationship between extraversion and either alcohol use frequency or alcohol problems (Stacy & Newcomb, 1998). However, prospective studies have noted the possibility that extraversion/sociability may be etiologically relevant to the development of drinking problems. For example, Jones (1968) reported that prealcoholics were rated as being high in expressiveness and gregariousness. Also, sociability has been found prospectively to predict frequency of intoxication (Sieber, 1981). Another, more recent prospective study found that higher extraversion scores predicted emergent, current alcohol dependence among young adults over a 3.5-year interval (Kilbey, Downey, & Breslau, 1998).

From the previous discussion, the findings in this literature may appear to be inconsistent: Some studies find that alcoholics do not differ from controls on extraversion/sociability; others indicate that this trait may relate to the development of alcohol problems. However, it seems possible that extraversion/sociability is a risk factor for the *development* of drinking problems, and that this trait becomes increasingly "masked" in those whose levels of dependence increase over time (i.e., alcoholics). Another possibility is that another, third variable may play a role in determining the influence of extraversion on alcohol misuse. For example, some recent evidence suggests a gender difference, wherein high extraversion scores may be more relevant for predicting alcohol problems in women than in men (e.g., Heath et al., 1997; Prescott, Neale, Corey, & Kendler, 1997). Furthermore, it is currently unclear whether these "outgoing" characteristics most accurately reflect true sociability or (misattributed) disinhibition (Tarter, 1988). In our view, the literature would benefit greatly from additional systematic investigations of this association with prospective data, including consideration of other potential moderating and mediating processes.

MODELS OF THE RELATION BETWEEN ALCOHOLISM AND PERSONALITY: MOVING THE FIELD FORWARD

Most of the previous discussion has focused on issues important in determining a relation between specific personality traits and alcoholism. As we have argued elsewhere (Sher & Trull, 1994), we strongly believe that personality variables are most useful when conceptualized in the nexus of other causal variables in etiological models and not simply as static trait descriptions. In addition, we have described several ways that personality could be related to the development of alcoholism (Sher & Trull, 1994). More specifically, we conjectured that personality variables appear to be relevant for understanding three major models of alcoholism etiology: (1) pharmacological vulnerability (i.e., that some individuals are pharmacologically predisposed to experience the effects of alcohol in a way that makes them vulnerable to excessive consumption or to pronounced difficulties from alcohol), (2) affect regulation (i.e., some individuals are motivated to drink in order to "self-medicate" transient or chronic negative affective states or to seek altered states of consciousness), and (3) deviance proneness (i.e., that some individuals are differently socialized and excessive consumption represents the outcome of this socialization).

Pharmacological Vulnerability

It has long been believed that certain individuals have difficulty "holding their liquor." In the late 19th century, Fere (1899) asserted that "all subjects do not offer the same susceptibility to the action of medicaments and poisons" and noted that "Lasegue has specially insisted upon the differences of aptitude for intoxication . . . [and has labeled these individuals] *alcoholizable.*" Risk for alcoholism (as determined by family history) appears to be related to both greater *and* lesser sensitivity to the acute effects of alcohol (Newlin & Thomson, 1990). Although prospective confirmation of vulnerability attributable to greater sensitivity awaits further study, a recent prospective study showed decreased sensitivity to alcohol is associated with onset of alcohol use disorders (Schuckit & Smith, 1996) in a sample not evidencing alcohol dependence in their early 20s.

But who are the alcoholizables? Seventy years ago, the noted social psychologist William McDougall (1929) speculated that "the markedly extraverted personality is very susceptible to the influence of alcohol" (p. 301), because such a person has lower levels of baseline cortical inhibition. Ten years later, the influential psychiatric theorist, Hervey Cleckley (1941), posited that individuals with psychopathic personalities were prone to "fantastic and uninviting behavior after drink" (p. 184). Although clinical and anecdotal evidence suggest that some individuals are exquisitely sensitive to disinhibition by alcohol, empirical evidence for personality-based individual differences in such effects is sparse (Urschell & Woody, 1994).

Over the past 50 years, there has been persistent interest in the hypothesis that personality traits can influence sensitivity to drug effects. For example, Eysenck (1957) and his colleagues (e.g., Claridge, 1970; Claridge, Canter, & Hume, 1973; Franks, 1964) have examined the effects of alcohol and other drugs on sedation thresholds and behavioral performance in efforts to test hypotheses concerning the relation between arousal and personality. Recent interest in the neuropharmacological bases of personality variation (e.g., Cloninger, 1987a; Zuckerman, 1991, 1995) has provided further rationale for the study of personality-based individual differences in alcohol sensitivity by refining and providing an empirical basis for the speculations of earlier theorists such as McDougall and Eysenck; that is, if alcohol affects the major neurotransmitter (e.g., dopamine, norepinephrine, serotonin) and hormonal (e.g., testosterone) systems thought to underlie variation in temperament and personality, individual differences in personality could reflect variation in the baseline functioning of these neurotransmitter systems (see Fromme & D'Amico, Chapter 11, this volume).[1] This baseline functioning could determine, in part, the nature and extent of alcohol's effects on these systems. (An alternative conceptualization of the relation between personality and drug effects is that personality dimensions represent basic patterns of reacting to biologically meaningful stimuli. From this perspective, individual differences in reactivity to alcohol could reflect characteristic patterns of response to other drugs.)

Perhaps the most intriguing findings to date are those showing that individuals who are high on the trait of impulsivity/disinhibition appear to be more sensitive to the stress-reducing properties of alcohol, especially on cardiovascular measures (Levenson, Oyama, & Meek, 1987; Sher, Bylund, Walitzer, Hartmann, & Ray-Prenger, 1994; Sher & Levenson, 1982). For example, in one study, Sher and Levenson (1982) reasoned that individuals who show higher levels of the stress-response dampening effects of alcohol may be those for whom alcohol's effects are most reinforcing. These authors found that highly impulsive and uninhibited participants (as measured by the MacAndrew Alcoholism scale of the MMPI) showed an increased stress-response dampening effect from alcohol on cardiovascular measures. In another, more recent study, Sher et al. (1994) reported that individuals with the lowest activity levels of platelet monoamine oxidase (MAO, an enzyme important in the catabolism of the catecholamines and serotonin; see Note 2) had elevated scores on a measure of antisociality and showed stronger stress-response dampening on heart rate, as compared to those with high MAO activity.

Somewhat analogous findings have been noted with respect to coronary prone (i.e., Type A) personalities, who tend to show attenuated cardiovascular reactivity after consuming alcohol (Zeichner, Edwards, & Cohen, 1985). Similarly, those high in trait hostility appear to show pronounced alcohol-related dampening of cardiovascular responses (Zeichner, Giancola, & Allen, 1995). In other studies (e.g., Nagoshi, Wilson, & Rodriguez, 1991); traits related to impulsivity/disinhibition have been found to relate (negatively) to alcohol effects on motor performance. Although these findings are provocative, they have been difficult to replicate on a consistent basis (Niaura, Wilson, & Westrick, 1988; Sher & Walitzer, 1986). To date, the literature relating basic dimensions of personality to alcohol effects must be considered promising but inconclusive. It is not surprising that a clear pattern of findings have yet to emerge given the (1) relatively small samples that characterize much of this literature, (2) variability with respect to the measures used to assess personality, (3) variability in the experimental protocols used to study alcohol effects, and (4) modest reliability of many of the effects under investigation. Because accumulating evidence suggests that individual differences in alcohol effects can prospectively predict the development of alcohol problems (Schuckit & Smith, 1996; Volavka et al., 1996), further evaluation of the relation between personality and alcohol effects is clearly warranted.

Although most researchers and theorists believe that the mechanisms underlying personality-based individual differences in alcohol effects are attributable to common neuropharmacological substrates for personality and alcohol effects, Hammersley, Finnigan, and Millar (1994) suggest an alternative indirect mechanism. These investigators posit that effects are indirect and mediated by personality-based differences in baseline consumption levels; that is, individuals high on certain personality traits are likely to drink more (for reasons other than personality-based individual differences in alcohol effects), and those who drink more are likely to experience alcohol differently due to differential experience (e.g., sensitization, tolerance, expectancy). Although this perspective represents an important alternative hypothesis that always needs to be considered, it does not appear capable of explaining some of the most intriguing findings to date.

Affect Regulation

For many years, it has been recognized that individuals consume alcoholic beverages for a variety of reasons. For example, in population-based surveys, drinkers frequently report drinking to socialize, to conform, and to alter their mental state, and these motives are strongly related to drinking status (e.g., Cahalan, Cisin, & Crossley, 1969). Similarly, individuals hold a number of beliefs concerning the anticipated effects of alcohol consumption (e.g., Goldman et al., 1987). Taken together, research on alcohol outcome expectancies and on self-reported reasons for drinking has identified a number of motives underlying alcohol use.[2] In recent years, personality variables have been shown to relate to these motives and, indeed, to have much of their effects mediated by these motives. Mediation of personality effects via drinking motives represents, perhaps, the most intuitively plausible mechanism of personality effects; that is, if personality traits contribute to the motivation of behavior in general, one would expect them to relate to specific alcohol-related motivations.

Drinking to regulate one's emotional state represents one major class of motives. Research on reasons for drinking and alcohol-outcome expectancies indicates that emotional regulation represents an important class of motives, and that these motives are related to basic dimensions of personality. Although the diversity of measures for assessing personality, reasons for drinking, and alcohol expectancies make it difficult to make highly specific statements, a number of studies have documented consistent statistical associations between personality variables and alcohol motivational variables. Traits related to impulsivity/disinhibition, to neuroticism/negative emotionality, and to extraversion/sociability have been consistently related to alcohol expectancies and motives (Brown & Munson, 1987; Cooper, Frone, Russell, & Mudar, 1995; Earleywine, 1994; Galen, Hendersen, &

Whitman, 1997; Galizio, Gerstenhaber, & Friedensen, 1985; Henderson, Goldman, Coovert, & Carnevalla, 1994; Leonard & Blane, 1988; Mann, Chassin, & Sher, 1987; Sher et al., 1991), as well as alcohol abuse (see previous section on the relevance of personality traits to alcoholism). In some of these studies (e.g., Henderson et al., 1994; Sher et al., 1991) clear evidence was found for the general hypothesis that some of the effect of personality (especially traits related to impulsivity/disinhibition) is mediated via alcohol expectancies.

A recent study by Cooper et al. (1995) provides a well-integrated formulation of the relation between personality and drinking motives. These researchers found that traits related to impulsivity/disinhibition are most strongly associated with drinking for "enhancement" (i.e., to enhance positive emotions) and that traits related to neuroticism/negative emotionality are most strongly associated with drinking to "cope" (i.e., to dampen negative emotions). Of greatest interest, enhancement motives appeared to mediate the effects of impulsivity/disinhibition on drinking; coping motives appeared to mediate the effects of neuroticism/negative emotionality. In other words, there was a relatively high degree of specificity between personality traits and drinking motives. Moreover, specific motives appeared to mediate the effects of specific personality traits on drinking behavior.

Although Cooper et al.'s (1995) findings are both provocative and compelling, existing research suggests that personality traits do not account for an overwhelming proportion of variance in drinking motives. Additionally, in several studies, direct effects of personality variables on drinking behavior remain after controlling for the mediating effects of drinking motives (e.g., Henderson et al., 1994; Sher et al., 1991). Thus, although there appears to be quite a bit of validity for the hypothesis that personality variables exert their effects via drinking motives (especially those motives involved in affect regulation), there are undoubtedly additional mechanisms relating personality to drinking.

Although the preceding discussion focused on correlational data derived from self-report measures of alcohol expectancies and reasons for drinking, further support for the mediating role of affect regulation (on personality–alcohol relations) comes from both correlational and experimental data assembled in the evaluation of the self-awareness model of alcohol (Hull, 1987). This model is based upon the proposition that many painful affective states (such as depression over a failure experience) are mediated by a state of self-awareness, and alcohol can reduce this distress by interfering with psychological mechanisms subserving self-awareness. Individuals high in private self-consciousness (i.e., the trait counterpart of the state of self-awareness) are particularly vulnerable to experience negative affect when confronted with negative information about the self and are also very likely to obtain relief from alcohol when experiencing negative affect mediated via self-awareness processes. A detailed description of the self-awareness model of alcohol use and abuse and empirical support for the model is beyond the scope of the current review. The review by Hull (1987) remains the best overview of this topic at this time (but also see Sayette, Chapter 7, this volume).

Other evidence for the affect regulation model is indirect and based on the high comorbidity between alcohol use disorders and the anxiety and mood disorders (see earlier discussion). Neuroticism/negative emotionality is a vulnerability factor for both anxiety disorders and mood disorders, and low extraversion/sociability may be a vulnerability factor for depression (Clark, Watson, & Mineka, 1994). To the extent that anxiety and mood disorders put an individual at risk for alcoholism, personality traits predictive of anxiety and depression become implicated in the prediction of comorbid alcohol disorders via an affect regulation pathway. It is important to emphasize that not all individuals are likely to increase their alcohol consumption when anxious or depressed and that the association between affective disturbance and drinking appears to be moderated by expectancies (Kushner, Sher, Wood, & Wood, 1994); that is, only those individuals who believe alcohol is helpful in coping with psychological distress are likely to drink when distressed.

Deviance Proneness

As we have noted elsewhere, although "the major explanatory concept in the deviance-proneness model is deficient socialization . . . personality variables probably play an important role" in this model (Sher & Trull, 1994, p. 96). The essence of the model can be summarized in the following way: Temperamental traits in childhood related to impulsivity/disinhibition[3] in transaction (see Sameroff & Chandler, 1974) with ineffective parental control (e.g., Dishion, Patterson, & Reid, 1988) can lead to deficits in socialization. These socialization deficits are associated with a range of problem behaviors including poor academic performance and school failure, delinquent behavior, association with deviant peers, and substance use and abuse (Sher, 1991). Theories differ in the extent that these various problem behaviors are viewed as indicators of a general syndrome of problem behavior or are causally related to each other (e.g., Jessor & Jessor, 1977; Kaplan, 1975; Oetting & Beauvais, 1986; also see Windle & Davies, Chapter 5, this volume). Among those who believe that these behavior problems are causally related to each other, there are clear differences in the extent that state-like intrapersonal variables (e.g., self-esteem) are posited to mediate the functional relations between specific problem behaviors.[4] Regardless of the theoretical perspective adopted, there is considerable evidence for linkages among personality variables and indices of deficits in socialization (e.g., decreased attachments to family, school, religious institutions; involvement with deviant peer groups) (see Petraitis et al., 1995).

Within the general class of models that we would refer to as deviance proneness, personality variables are typically viewed as considerably upstream (i.e., very distal) from alcohol involvement (e.g., for examples, see Petraitis et al., 1995); that is, they are thought to influence behavior by affecting long-term socialization processes brought about by parents, schools, and other institutions in the community. However, as suggested by Caspi et al. (1997), it is also possible that a "risky" personality style is associated with a style of decision making that is quite proximal to alcohol use episodes (Beyth-Marom, Austin, Fischoff, Palmgran, & Jacobs-Quadrel, 1993). We do not view these two models as incompatible and believe that personality and social deviance can be associated because of the effect of personality on the development of socialization and on impulsive decision making. In the former case, personality is quite distal to proximal variables such as the norms of deviant peer groups, which are viewed as having a large effect on alcohol (and other drug) involvement. In the latter case, personality is thought to represent a vulnerability to making "risky" decisions, and personality effects—although still mediated (by decision making) and thus still indirect—are nonetheless more proximal in a causal sense.

Other Comments

The above three classes of models should not be viewed as exhaustive of all possible models of the effect of personality on alcoholism. Equally important, these models are not mutually exclusive. As we have noted elsewhere, "Individuals (especially those who are high on traits related to impulsivity and disinhibition) may develop pathological alcohol involvement because they are particularly sensitive to the pharmacological effects of alcohol, because they are motivated to get high or otherwise seek . . . reinforcement from alcohol, and because their socialization experiences put them on a trajectory for social deviance" (Sher & Trull, 1994, p. 96). From the perspectives outlined here, personality variables represent important sources of influence on alcoholism etiology via multiple pathways. Consequently, understanding the role of personality in alcoholism is akin to understanding many aspects of the multiple causes of alcoholism.

However, in all of these models, the effects of personality are largely indirect and mediated by variables more proximal to drinking. Thus, consideration of personality variables would not necessarily improve short-term prediction of drinking problems over and above the prediction afforded by proximal influences. However, the situation changes considerably when we are interested in predicting over the longer term; that is, in contrast to most proximal sources of influence that are typically situational (e.g., peer groups) or state-like (e.g., distress, drinking motives), personality is, by definition, trait-like. Consequently, the practical utility of studying personality variables may be in the identification of those at future risk of developing problems and those likely to develop chronic or life-course persistent problems. Because individual differences in personality variables are moderately to highly stable over the life course (especially after young adulthood; Costa & McCrae, 1994), preventive and treatment interventions are probably best targeted at the mediators of these traits and not the traits themselves.

Are the Personality Correlates of Alcohol Use Disorders Specific or Characteristic of Broadband Diagnostic Distinctions?

Before concluding, it is important to discuss whether the findings relating personality characteristics to alcoholism are specific to a narrow class of disorders (i.e., alcohol use disorders) or are generalizable to broader classes of disorders (e.g., substance use disorders, externalizing disorders, or even psychopathology in general) (see Sher & Trull, 1996). This issue is rarely systematically studied, and when it is studied, the issues are often addressed in a problematic way. We discussed the issue of problems of specificity from a methodological standpoint earlier in this chapter (General Methodological Concerns: "Control groups" and the problem of specificity), but feel that the evidence surrounding this matter is deserving of more comment.

In general, it seems likely that the personality correlates (and, presumably, associated mediational processes) of alcoholism share important similarities across other specific substance use disorders, other health-related problems, and psychological disorders in general. For example, comorbidity studies of drug abusers (most typically, cocaine or opioid dependent individuals) generally reported rates (40–70%) and types (primarily antisocial and borderline) of disorders similar to those found in samples of alcoholics (Ball, Tennen, Poling, Kranzler, & Rounsaville, 1997; Barber et al., 1996; Grilo et al., 1997; Kosten, Kosten, & Rounsaville, 1989; Kranzler, Satel, & Apter, 1994; Malow, West, Williams, & Sutker, 1989; Marlowe, Husband, Bonieskie, Kirby, & Platt, 1997; Miller, Belkin, & Gibbons, 1994; Oldham et al., 1995; Rousar, Brooner, Regier, & Bigelow, 1994; Zimmerman & Coryell, 1989). This general pattern of comorbidity between (nonalcohol) substance use disorders and personality disorders implicates high levels of impulsivity/disinhibition and neuroticism/negative emotionality personality traits and is generally similar to the pattern found for alcohol use disorders. In our own research with nonclinical young adults, we found that DSM-III and DSM-III-R alcohol use disorder, drug use disorder, and tobacco dependence showed similar patterns of personality correlates using both Cloninger's three-factor model and Costa and McCrae's five-factor model (Sher et al., 1995; Trull & Sher, 1994). Nevertheless, given extensive comorbidity, it is possible that these broad diagnostic groupings obscure substance-specific associations with various personality traits.

Researchers and clinicians have long posited that there is an association between personality traits and drugs-of-choice among addicts. For example, Khantzian (1990) asserts, "Each class of drugs-of-abuse interacts with painful affect states and related personality factors to make an individual's preferred drug appealing and compelling. . . . Addiction-prone individuals discover which drug suits them best through the unique qualities of their affect experience, and these choices are what distinguish addicts and alcoholics from each other" (p. 268). However, as recently noted by O'Connor, Berry, Morrison, and Brown (1995), there is little in the way of replicable findings relating choice-of-drug to personality traits and other individual difference variables, and numerous methodological problems characterize much of the research in this area (e.g., acute, chronic, and withdrawal effects of different drugs). Additionally, cohort, regional, cultural, and social-class factors that influence exposure and availability of different substances (Heath, 1990) might greatly overshadow subtle but theoretically meaningful personality-based effects. Thus, although it is certainly possible that there are theoretically important differences in the personality correlates of specific substance dependencies (e.g., see O'Connor et al., 1995), at present, the similarities appear much greater than these possible differences.

Not only are there important similarities in the personality correlates of individuals who abuse or become dependent upon different substances, but there also appear to be important similarities in the personality correlates of various health-risk behaviors more generally. This is not surprising in that a variety of behaviors that could be considered "risky" tend to cluster in a "syndrome of problem behavior" (Donovan, Jessor, & Costa, 1988). For example, Caspi et al. (1997) found that four distinct (though arguably related) health behaviors showed a similar pattern of personality correlates. More specifically, unsafe sexual behavior, dangerous driving habits, violence conviction, and alcohol dependence were all associated with both high negative emotionality and low constraint (i.e., high impulsivity/disinhibition). Moreover, Caspi et al. found a monotonic relationship between the number of health-risk behaviors encountered and negative emotionality and constraint. Although the supertrait of positive emotionality was not related to these health-risk behaviors, one facet of positive emotionality, social closeness, was. Specifically, social closeness was found to correlate negatively with involvement in health-risk behaviors. We note this latter finding because it demonstrates that facets of higher-order personality traits can be meaningfully related to a disorder even when the higher-order trait is not.

Trull and Sher (1994) found, using Costa and McCrae's (1992) NEO-FFI (a brief Big Five measure), that the personality pattern of high Neuroticism, high Openness to Experience, low Extraversion, low Agreeableness, and low Conscientiousness was associated with a wide range of Axis I disorders in young adults (including substance use disorders, anxiety disorders, and mood disorders). Although quantitative deviations from this general pattern were associated with individual diagnoses, the general pattern was quite consistent across a range of diagnoses. Findings from a recent study by Krueger, Caspi, Moffitt, Silva, and McGee (1996) are generally consistent with Trull and Sher's (1994) findings. However, noncomorbid cases of each disorder appeared to show a less extreme and less consistent profile.[5] It is therefore not surprising that McGue et al. (1997) found that more severe alcohol use disorders were associated with higher levels of impulsivity/disinhibition and negative emotionality than less severe disorders; more severe cases tended to be more comorbid (with other externalizing, and with depressive, symptomatology).

As noted throughout the chapter, we believe that personality variables are most informative when they help us to elucidate basic etiological processes. To this extent, it is important to note that researchers studying other drugs of abuse have adopted models similar to the types of models advocated here. For example, Gilbert and Gilbert (1995) described a number of ways that traits such as extraversion, neuroticism, and psychoticism (impulivity/disinhibition) potentially subserve mechanisms that could be described as reflecting pharmacological vulnerability and affect regulation. Stacy, Newcomb, and Bentler (1995) explored the extent to which the effect of personality variables on cocaine use are mediated by motives for use and find some support for this notion. Clearly, research on the specificity of personality traits (and their mediation) in substance use disorder is still in its infancy. Methodological complexities such as unmeasured third variables (associated with both personality traits and with exposure to and availability of different substances), coupled with the high comorbidity among various forms of substance use disorders, have typically not been addressed. Studies that attempt to address the inherent complexity of examining specificity issues are most likely to be successful in isolating unique effects when they exist. As discussed earlier, higher-order factor models and residual techniques offer a potentially powerful approach for delineating those effects that are common to the various forms of substance use disorder and those that are specific to alcohol use disorder (see Sher, 1996).

THE FUTURE OF RESEARCH ON ALCOHOLISM AND PERSONALITY

Over 30 years ago, Mischel (1968) noted that personality variables by themselves probably explain only a small proportion of most behavioral outcomes, and the area of alcoholism is no exception (Sher & Trull, 1994). Although we know that the observed correlation between personality and various criteria can be increased by extending observation periods and aggregating criterion behaviors over time (Epstein, 1979), existing evidence does not suggest that personality variation alone will ever provide a complete accounting of who does and who does not develop an alcohol use disorder.

This is not to say, however, that personality does not represent a critical domain for understanding the genesis and maintenance of alcohol problems. Existing data suggest that personality variables play an important etiological role in the genesis of drinking problems, and a comprehensive understanding of vulnerability to alcoholism will need to take personality processes into account. However, elucidation of these processes involves considerably more than simply indexing trait differences between alcohol-dependent groups (or subgroups) and various control groups—the dominant research strategy employed. Rather, personality research on alcoholism must be integrated into investigations of genetic transmission, stress and coping, ethanol reactivity, and social-psychological and developmental processes. It is only in the context of meaningfully elaborated etiological models that we can begin to assess the importance of personality for understanding alcoholism and related phenomena.

The importance of personality as an explanatory concept with respect to alcohol involvement has moved in and out of favor for many years. As we stand on the cusp of the 21st century, it seems fair to say that the etiological significance of personality variables has never been stronger. As research on the etiology of alcoholism becomes increasingly informed by research on behavior genetics, social development, decision making, stress and coping, and behavioral pharmacology, personality variables can be viewed as the nexus of these distinct etiological influences. To a large extent, further elucidation of the role of personality variables may lie in the hands of investigators who are exploring the mediation of genetic influences, stress and coping processes, psychiatric comorbidity, and individual differences in the "prized and punishing effects" (Steele & Josephs, 1990) of alcohol.

At present, there are a number of important questions regarding the role of personality in alcohol use disorders that have not yet been comprehensively addressed. In addition to the potential mechanisms discussed earlier, several additional research questions need to be considered. These are briefly described as follows:

  • *The changing role of personality in the development of alcohol involvement.* Not all individuals who ever drink alcohol go on to become regular drinkers; not all regular drinkers go on to drink heavily or with problems; and not all heavy or problem drinkers develop chronic drinking problems. Although some variables, particularly those related to impulsivity/disinhibition, appear to be relevant to alcohol involvement at all stages of drinking careers (Sher, Gotham, Watson, & Meier, 1998), the general issue of differential correlates of personality over the lifetime course of drinking has not been well mapped.
  • *The role of personality in predicting continuity versus discontinuity in drinking across major life transitions.* The period of late adolescence and early adulthood is associated with the highest prevalences of heavy alcohol use and alcohol use disorders (Grant et al., 1994; Johnston, O'Malley, &

Bachman, 1996; Kessler et al., 1997). The large declines in these prevalences that occur in the mid- to late 20s is often termed "maturing out" and is associated with the adoption of various adult roles (Sher & Gotham, 1998). For example, prospective examination of drinking patterns with these role transitions indicates (sometimes large) decreases in the prevalence of heavy drinking as a function of marriage, pregnancy (for both women and, to a lesser degree, their spouses), and full-time employment and homemaker status (e.g., Bachman, Wadsworth, O'Malley, Johnston, & Schulenberg, 1997). However, some individuals do not appear to "mature out," and personality traits represent an important class of variables that can moderate the effect of these "normalizing" influences (Gotham, Sher, & Wood, 1997). Research on the role of personality within this developmental context is only just beginning and holds promise for understanding the relation between personality and the larger social-developmental context.

Additionally, the likelihood and timing of various role transitions can be affected by alcohol involvement (e.g., role selection; Mensch & Kandel, 1988), and these changes in role statuses can affect alcohol involvement (e.g., role socialization; Yamaguchi, 1990). It is not yet known to what extent these role-selection effects are determined, in part, by personality. However, the critical influence of these role transitions, and the finding that these are often "selected" by the individual, suggests that we need to understand how ostensibly "environmental" effects might be distally "caused" by personality.

• *The role of personality in alcohol-related comorbidity.* It is reasonable to hypothesize that various forms of comorbidity between alcohol use disorders and other forms of psychopathology are mediated via common personality diatheses. For example, Cloninger (1987a, 1987b) hypothesizes the same personality correlates for APD and a subtype (Type 2) of alcoholism. Although data directly bearing on this hypothesis are sparse, the general notion is supported by recent cross-sectional findings that note the similarity of the personality correlates of alcohol use disorders and other Axis I disorders (Krueger et al., 1996; Trull & Sher, 1994). Because the overwhelming majority of comorbidity studies rely on cross-sectional data, it has not yet been possible to examine potential mechanisms of comorbidity and clearly establish personality traits as "causes" of comorbidity. However, prospective data capable of distinguishing alternative models of comorbidity causation are becoming increasingly available and should be able to inform this hypothesis in the near future.

• *The extent to which personality traits mediate genetic influences on the development of alcoholism.* Although the notion that personality might mediate the genetics of alcoholism has been a major hypothesis for some time (e.g., Cloninger, 1987a), to date critical data are scarce. Slutske et al.'s (1998) finding that symptoms of conduct disorder explain a major part of the genetic risk for alcoholism is clearly consistent with this idea. However, as noted earlier, there are hazards associated with equating antisocial symptoms with personality, and replication and extension of these findings with "purer" personality measures are clearly needed. It is important to highlight, however, that if personality variables are found to mediate genetic risk for alcoholism, then not only is personality identified as a key etiological factor, but also causal mechanisms (i.e., affect regulation, deviance proneness, and pharmacological vulnerability) associated with the personality variable are potentially implicated.

Clearly, the most recent period of research on personality and alcoholism has moved us from a simple "trait description" phase to one in which psychological processes and the associated role of personality in these processes are emphasized. In the next period, we hope to see these processes elaborated, understood in the context of adolescent and adult development, and extended to understand related psychopathology.

ACKNOWLEDGMENTS

Preparation of this chapter was supported, in part, by National Institute on Alcohol Abuse and Alcoholism Grant No. R01 AA7231 to Kenneth J. Sher. We gratefully acknowledge Wendy Slutske for her assistance in previewing an earlier version of this chapter.

NOTES

1. In a recent study, we (Sher, Bylund, Walitzer, Hartmann, & Ray-Prenger, 1994) examined the relation between a presumed indicator of a neuropharmacological substrate of personality and alcohol effects. More specifically, we assessed the extent that individual differences in platelet monoamine oxidase (MAO) activity correlated with alcohol effects. (MAO is an enzyme that plays an important role in the breakdown of norepinephrine, dopamine, and serotonin, and has been correlated with personality traits and psychiatric conditions associated with impulsivity; e.g., Zuckerman, 1991.) Low platelet MAO activity was associated with decreased cardiovascular responding after alcohol consumption, a finding consistent with those reported by Levenson et al. (1987) and Sher and Levenson (1982). However, the finding did not generalize to other alcohol effects, and MAO activity was unrelated to alcohol consumption in this particular sample.

2. Although alcohol-outcome expectancies and reasons for drinking represent constructs that are conceptually and empirically distinct (Cooper et al., 1995), both can be viewed as indexing motivational processes. Our own view of the relationship is that expectancies are exogenous to reasons for drinking, which, in turn, are more proximal predictors of alcohol use.

3. As Caspi and Silva (1995) have shown, individuals characterized as "undercontrolled" at age 3 are those most likely to be high on negative emotionality and impulsivity/disinhibition in late adolescence.

4. Although emphasizing what they term "experimental substance use," Petraitis et al. (1995) describe a number of specific theories that we would consider to fit under the broad rubric of deviance proneness.

5. Note that in the Krueger et al. (1996) study, so-called "pure" (i.e., noncomorbid) cases of each disorder were clearly in the minority.

REFERENCES

Allport, G. W., & Odbert, H. S. (1936). Trait-names: A psycho-lexical study. *Psychological Monographs, 47* (Whole No. 211).

Alnaes, R., & Torgersen, S. (1988). The relationship between DSM-III symptom disorders (Axis I) and personality disorders (Axis II) in an outpatient population. *Acta Psychiatrica Scandinavica, 78,* 485–492.

Alterman, A. I., Bedrick, J., Cacciola, J. S., Rutherford, M. J., Searles, J. S., McKay, J. R., & Cook, T. G. (1998). Personality pathology and drinking in young men at high and low familial risk for alcoholism. *Journal of Studies on Alcohol, 59,* 495–502.

American Psychiatric Association. (1952). *Diagnostic and statistical manual of mental disorders.* Washington, DC: Author.

Babor, T. F. (1996). The classification of alcoholics: Typology theories from the 19th century to the present. *Alcohol Health and Research World, 20,* 6–14.

Babor, T. F., Hofmann, M., DelBoca, F. K., Hesselbrock, V., Meyer, R. E., Dolinsky, Z. S., & Rounsaville, B. (1992). Types of alcoholics: I. Evidence for an empirically derived typology based on indicators of vulnerability and severity. *Archives of General Psychiatry, 49,* 599–608.

Babor, T. F., & Lauerman, R. (1986). Classification and forms of inebriety: Historical antecedents of alcohol typologies. In M. Galanter (Ed.), *Recent developments in alcoholism* (Vol. 5, pp. 113–144). New York: Plenum.

Bachman, J. G., Wadsworth, K. N., O'Malley, P. M., Johnston, L. D., & Schulenberg, J. E. (1997). *Smoking, drinking, and drug use in young adulthood.* Mahwah, NJ: Erlbaum.

Bagby, R. M., Parker, J. D. A., & Joffe, R. T. (1992). Confirmatory factor analysis of the Tridimensional Personality Questionnaire. *Personality and Individual Differences, 13,* 1245–1246.

Ball, S. A., Tennen, H., Poling, J. C., Kranzler, H. R., & Rounsaville, B. J. (1997). Personality, temperament, and character dimensions and the DSM-IV personality disorders in substance abusers. *Journal of Abnormal Psychology, 106,* 545–553.

Barber, J. P., Frank, A., Weiss, R. D., Blaine, J., Siqueland, L., Moras, K., Calvo, N., Chittams, J., Mercer, D., & Salloum, I. M. (1996). Prevalence and correlates of personality disorder diagnoses among cocaine dependent outpatients. *Journal of Personality Disorders, 10,* 297–311.

Barnes, G. E. (1979). The alcoholic personality: A reanalysis of the literature. *Journal of Studies on Alcohol, 40,* 571–633.

Barnes, G. E. (1983). Clinical and personality characteristics. In B. Kissin & H. Begleiter (Eds.), *The pathogenesis of alcoholism: Psychosocial factors* (Vol. 6, pp. 113–196). New York: Plenum.

Bartholow, B. D., Sher, K. J., & Strathman, A. (1998). *Individual differences in pri-*

vate self-consciousness moderate the expectancy—alcohol use relation: Data from a longitudinal study. Manuscript submitted for publication.

Bates, M. E., & Labouvie, E. W. (1995). Personality–environment constellations and alcohol use: A process-oriented study of intraindividual change during adolescence. *Psychology of Addictive Behaviors, 9,* 23–35.

Bergman, B., & Brismar, B. (1994). Hormone levels and personality traits in abusive and suicidal male alcoholics. *Alcoholism: Clinical and Experimental Research, 18,* 311–316.

Berkson, J. (1946). Limitations of the application of fourfold table analysis to hospital data. *Biometrics Bulletin, 2,* 47–53.

Beyth-Marom, R., Austin, L., Fischoff, B., Palmgran, C., & Jacobs-Quadrel, M. (1993). Perceived consequences of risky behaviors: Adults and adolescents. *Developmental Psychology, 29,* 549–563.

Block, J. (1989). Critique of the act frequency approach to personality. *Journal of Personality and Social Psychology, 56,* 234–245.

Block, J., Block, J. H., & Keyes, S. (1988). Longitudinally foretelling drug usage in adolescence: Early childhood personality and environmental precursors. *Child Development, 59,* 336–355.

Brooner, R. K., Templer, D., Svikis, D. S., Schmidt, C., & Monopolis, S. (1990). Dimensions of alcoholism: A multivariate analysis. *Journal of Studies on Alcohol, 51,* 77–81.

Brown, S. A., & Munson, E. (1987). Extroversion, anxiety and the perceived effects of alcohol. *Journal of Studies on Alcohol, 48,* 272–276.

Bry, B. H., McKeon, P., & Pandina, R. J. (1982). Extent of drug use as a function of the number of risk factors. *Journal of Abnormal Psychology, 91,* 273–279.

Buss, D. M., & Craik, K. H. (1980). The frequency concept of disposition: Dominance and prototypically dominant acts. *Journal of Personality, 43,* 379–392.

Cahalan, D., Cisin, I. H., & Crossley, H. M. (1969). *American drinking practices: A national survey of behavior and attitude* (Monograph No. 6). New Brunswick, NJ: Rutgers Center of Alcohol Studies.

Cannon, D. S., Clark, L. A., Leeka, J. K., & Keefe, C. K. (1993). A reanalysis of the Tridimensional Personality Questionnaire (TPQ) and its relations to Cloninger's Type 2 alcoholism. *Psychological Assessment, 5,* 62–66.

Casey, P. R., & Tyrer, P. (1990). Personality disorder and psychiatric illness in general practice. *British Journal of Psychiatry, 156,* 261–265.

Caspi, A., Begg, D., Dickson, N., Harrington, H.-L., Langley, J., Moffitt, T. E., & Silva, P. A. (1997). Personality differences predict health-risk behaviors in adulthood: Evidence from a longitudinal study. *Journal of Personality and Social Psychology, 73,* 1052–1063.

Caspi, A., & Silva, P. A. (1995). Temperamental qualities at age 3 predict personality traits in young adulthood: Longitudinal evidence from a birth cohort. *Child Development, 66,* 486–498.

Cattell, R. B. (1943). The description of personality: Basic traits resolved into clusters. *Journal of Abnormal and Social Psychology, 38,* 476–506.

Chassin, L., Curran, P. J., Hussong, A. M., & Colder, C. R. (1996). The relation of parent alcoholism to adolescent substance use: A longitudinal follow-up study. *Journal of Abnormal Psychology, 105,* 70–80.

Claridge, G. (1970). *Drugs and human behavior.* London: Praeger.

Claridge, G., Canter, S., & Hume, W. (1973). *Personality differences and biological variations: A study of twins.* New York: Pergamon.

Clark, L. A., Watson, D., & Mineka, S. (1994). Temperament, personality and the mood and anxiety disorders. *Journal of Abnormal Psychology, 103,* 103–116.

Cleckley, H. M. (1941). *The mask of sanity.* St. Louis: Mosby.

Cloninger, C. R. (1987a). Neurogenetic adaptive mechanisms in alcoholism. *Science, 236,* 410–416.

Cloninger, C. R. (1987b). A systematic method for clinical description and classification of personality variants. *Archives of General Psychiatry, 44,* 573–588.

Cloninger, C. R., Sigvardsson, S., & Bohman, M. (1988). Childhood personality predicts alcohol abuse in young adults. *Alcoholism, Clinical and Experimental Research, 12,* 494–505.

Cohen, P., & Cohen, J. (1984). The clinician's illusion. *Archives of General Psychiatry, 41,* 1178–1182.

Cooper, M. L., Frone, M. R., Russell, M., & Mudar, P. (1995). Drinking to regulate positive and negative emotions: A motivational model of alcohol use. *Journal of Personality and Social Psychology, 69,* 990–1005.

Costa, P. T., Jr., & McCrae, R. R. (1992). *Revised NEO Personality Inventory (NEO-PI-R) and NEO Five-Factor Inventory (NEO-FFI) professional manual.* Odessa, FL: Psychological Assessment Resources.

Costa, P. T., Jr., & McCrae, R. R. (1994). Set like plaster? Evidence for the stability of adult personality. In T. F. Heatherton & J. L. Weinberger (Eds.), *Can personality change?* (pp. 21–40). Washington, DC: American Psychological Association Press.

Cox, W. M. (1979). The alcoholic personality: A review of the evidence. In B. A. Major (Ed.), *Progress in experimental personality research* (Vol. 9, pp. 89–148). San Diego, CA: Academic Press.

Cox, W. M. (1985). Personality correlates of substance abuse. In M. Galizio & S. A. Maisto (Eds.), *Determinants of substance abuse* (pp. 209–246). New York: Plenum.

Darkes, J., Greenbaum, P. E., & Goldman, M. S. (1998). Sensation seeking–disinhibition and alcohol use: Exploring issues of criterion contamination. *Psychological Assessment, 10,* 71–76.

De Jong, C. A. J., van den Brink, W., Harteveld, F. M., & van der Wielen, G. M. (1993). Personality disorders in alcoholics and drug addicts. *Comprehensive Psychiatry, 34,* 87–94.

Derksen, J. (1990). An exploratory study of borderline personality disorder in women with eating disorders and psychoactive substance dependent patients. *Journal of Personality Disorders, 4,* 372–380.

Dishion, T. J., Patterson, G. R., & Reid, J. R. (1988). Parent and peer factors associated with drug sampling in early adolescence: Implications for treatment. In E. R. Rahdert & J. Grabowski (Eds.), *NIDA Research Monograph 77, Adolescent drug abuse: Analyses of treatment research* (pp. 69–93). Rockville, MD: National Institute on Drug Abuse.

Donovan, D. M., & O'Leary, M. R. (1978). The drinking-related locus of control scale: Reliability, factor structure and validity. *Journal of Studies on Alcohol, 39,* 759–784.

Donovan, J., Jessor, R., & Costa, F. M. (1988). Syndrome of problem behavior in adolescence: A replication. *Journal of Consulting and Clinical Psychology, 56,* 762–765.

Drake, R. E., Adler, D. A., & Vaillant, G. E. (1988). Antecedents of personality disorders in a community sample of men. *Journal of Personality Disorders, 2,* 60–68.

Drake, R. E., & Vaillant, G. E. (1985). A validity study of axis II of DSM-III. *American Journal of Psychiatry, 142*, 553–558.

Earleywine, M. (1994). Personality risk for alcoholism and alcohol expectancies. *Addictive Behaviors, 19*, 577–582.

Earleywine, M., & Finn, P. R. (1991). Sensation seeking explains the relation between behavioral disinhibition and alcohol consumption. *Addictive Behaviors, 16*, 123–128.

Earleywine, M., Finn, P. R., Peterson, J. B., & Pihl, R. O. (1992). Factor structure and correlates of the Tridimensional Personality Questionnaire. *Journal of Studies on Alcohol, 53*, 1–6.

Epstein, S. (1979). The stability of behavior: I. On predicting most of the people much of the time. *Journal of Personality and Social Psychology, 37*, 1097–1126.

Eysenck, H. J. (1957). Drugs and personality: I. Theory and methodology. *Journal of Mental Science, 103*, 119–131.

Eysenck, H. J. (1990). Biological dimensions of personality. In L. A. Pervin (Ed.), *Handbook of personality theory and research* (pp. 244–276). New York: Guilford Press.

Eysenck, H. J., & Eysenck, S. B. G. (1975). *Manual for the Eysenck Personality Questionnaire*. San Diego: Educational and Industrial Testing Service.

Eysenck, H. J., & Gudjonsson, G. H. (1989). *The cause and cures of criminality*. New York: Plenum.

Fere, C. (1899). *The pathology of emotions* (English ed., trans. R. Park). London: University Press.

Finn, P. R., Sharkansky, E. J., Viken, R., West, T. L., Sandy, J., & Bufferd, G. M. (1997). Heterogeneity in the families of sons of alcoholics: The impact of familial vulnerability type on offspring characteristics. *Journal of Abnormal Psychology, 106*, 26–36.

Franks, C. M. (1964). The use of alcohol in the investigation of drug-personality postulates. In R. Fox (Ed.), *Alcoholism: Behavioral research, therapeutic approaches*. New York: Springer.

Galen, L. W., Hendersen, M. J., & Whitman, R. D. (1997). The utility of novelty seeking, harm avoidance, and expectancy in the prediction of drinking. *Addictive Behaviors, 22*, 93–106.

Galizio, M., Gerstenhaber, L., & Friedensen, F. (1985). Correlates of sensation seeking in alcoholics. *International Journal of the Addictions, 20*, 1479–1493.

Garber, J., & Hollon, S. D. (1991). What can specificity designs say about causality in psychopathology research? *Psychological Bulletin, 110*, 129–136.

Gilbert, D. G., & Gilbert, B. O. (1995). Personality, psychopathology, and nicotine response as mediators of the genetics of smoking [Special Issue: Genetic, environmental, and situational factors mediating the effects of nicotine]. *Behavior Genetics, 25*, 133–147.

Goldberg, L. R. (1982). From ace to zombie: Some explorations in the language of personality. In C. D. Spielberger & J. N. Butcher (Eds.), *Advances in personality assessment* (Vol. 1, pp. 203–234). Hillsdale, NJ: Erlbaum.

Goldberg, L. R. (1990). An alternative "description of personality": The Big-Five factor structure. *Journal of Personality and Social Psychology, 59*, 1216–1229.

Goldberg, L. R. (1992). The development of markers for the Big-Five factor structure. *Psychological Assessment, 4*, 26–42.

Goldman, M. S. (1994). The alcohol expectancy concept: Applications to assessment, prevention, and treatment of alcohol abuse. *Applied and Preventive Psychology, 3,* 131–144.

Goldman, M. S., Brown, S. A., & Christiansen, B. A. (1987). Expectancy theory: Thinking about drinking. In H. Blane & K. E. Leonard (Eds.), *Psychological theories of drinking and alcoholism* (pp. 181–226). New York: Guilford Press.

Gomberg, E. S. L. (1997). Alcohol abuse: Age and gender differences. In R. W. Wilsnack & S. C. Wilsnack (Eds.), *Gender and alcohol: Individual and social perspectives.* New Brunswick, NJ: Rutgers Center of Alcohol Studies.

Gotham, H. J., Sher, K. J., & Wood, P. K. (1997). Predicting stability and change in frequency of intoxication from the college years to beyond: Individual-difference and role transition variables. *Journal of Abnormal Psychology, 106,* 619–629.

Grande, T. P., Wolf, A. W., Schubert, D. S. P., Patterson, M. B., & Brocco, K. (1984). Associations among alcoholism, drug abuse, and antisocial personality: A review of the literature. *Psychological Reports, 55,* 455–474.

Grant, B. F., Harford, T. C., Dawson, D. A., Chou, P., Dufor, M., & Pickering, R. (1994). Prevalence of DSM-IV alcohol abuse and dependence: United States, 1992. Special Focus: Women and alcohol. *Alcohol Health and Research World, 18,* 243–248.

Grilo, C. M., Martino, S., Walker, M. L., Becker, D. F., Edell, W. S., & McGlashan, T. H. (1997). Controlled study of psychiatric comorbidity in psychiatrically hospitalized young adults with substance use disorders. *American Journal of Psychiatry, 154,* 1305–1307.

Hammersley, R., Finnigan, F., & Millar, K. (1994). Individual differences in the acute response to alcohol. *Personality and Individual Differences, 17,* 497–510.

Haver, B., & Dahlgren, L. (1995). Early treatment of women with alcohol addiction (EWA): A comprehensive evaluation and outcome study: I. Patterns of psychiatric comorbidity at intake. *Addiction, 90,* 101–109.

Hawkins, J. D., Catalano, R. F., & Miller, Y. (1992). Risk and protective factors for alcohol and other drug problems in adolescence and early adulthood: Implications for substance abuse prevention. *Psychological Bulletin, 112,* 64–105.

Heath, A. C., Bucholz, K. K., Madden, P. A. F., Dinwiddie, S. H., Slutske, W. S., Bierut, L. J., Statham, D. J., Dunne, M. P., Whitfield, J., & Martin, N. G. (1997). Genetic and environmental contributions to alcohol dependence risk in a national twin sample: Consistency of findings in women and men. *Psychological Medicine, 8,* 1381–1396.

Heath, D. (1990). Cultural factors in the choice of drugs. In M. Galanter (Ed.), *Recent developments in alcoholism: Vol. 8. Combined alcohol and other drug dependence* (pp. 245–254). New York: Plenum.

Helzer, J. E., & Canino, G. J. (1992). Comparative analysis of alcoholism in ten cultural regions. In J. E. Helzer & G. J. Canino (Eds.), *Alcoholism in North America, Europe, and Asia* (pp. 289–308). New York: Oxford University Press.

Helzer, J. E., & Pryzbeck, T. R. (1988). The co-occurrence of alcoholism with other psychiatric disorders in the general population and its impact on treatment. *Journal of Studies on Alcohol, 49,* 219–224.

Henderson, M. J., Goldman, M. S., Coovert, M. D., & Carnevalla, N. (1994). Covariance structure models of expectancy. *Journal of Studies on Alcohol, 55,* 315–326.

Hesselbrock, M. N. (1991). Gender comparison of antisocial personality disorder and depression in alcoholism. *Journal of Substance Abuse, 3,* 205–220.

Hesselbrock, M. N., & Hesselbrock, V. M. (1997). Gender, alcoholism, and psychiatric comorbidity. In R. W. Wilsnack & S. C. Wilsnack (Eds.), *Gender and alcohol: Individual and social perspectives.* New Brunswick, NJ: Rutgers Center of Alcohol Studies.

Hesselbrock, M. N., Meyer, R. E., & Keener, J. J. (1985). Psychopathology in hospitalized alcoholics. *Archives of General Psychiatry, 42,* 1050–1055.

Hirschfeld, R., Klerman, G., Clayton, P., Keller, M., McDonald-Scott, P., & Larkin, B. (1983). Assessing personality: Effects of the depressive state on trait measurement. *American Journal of Psychiatry, 140,* 695–699.

Hoffman, H., Loper, R., & Kammeier, M. (1974). Identifying future alcoholics with the MMPI alcoholism scales. *Quarterly Journal of Studies on Alcohol, 35,* 490–498.

Holdcraft, L. C., Iacono, W. G., & McGue, M. K. (1998). Antisocial personality disorder and depression in relation to alcoholism: A community-based sample. *Journal of Studies on Alcohol, 59,* 222–226.

Hull, J. G. (1987). Self-awareness model. In H. T. Blane & K. E. Leonard (Eds.), *Psychological theories of drinking and alcoholism* (pp. 272–304). New York: Guilford Press.

Hull, J. G., Young, R. D., & Jouriles, E. (1986). Applications of the self-awareness model of alcohol consumption: Predicting patterns of use and abuse. *Journal of Personality and Social Psychology, 51,* 790–796.

Jellinek, E. M. (1960). *The disease concept of alcoholism.* New Haven, CT: Hillhouse.

Jessor, R., & Jessor, S. L. (1977). *Problem behavior and psychosocial development: A longitudinal study of youth.* San Diego: Academic Press.

John, O. P. (1990). The "Big-Five" factor taxonomy: Dimensions of personality in the natural language and in questionnaires. In L. A. Pervin (Ed.), *Handbook of personality: Theory and research* (pp. 66–100). New York: Guilford Press.

Johnston, L. D., O'Malley, P. M., & Bachman, J. G. (1996). *National survey results on drug use from the Monitoring the Future Study, 1975–1994: Volume II. College students and young adults.* Rockville, MD: National Institute on Drug Abuse.

Jones, M. C. (1968). Personality correlates and antecedents of drinking patterns in adult males. *Journal of Consulting and Clinical Psychology, 32,* 2–12.

Jones, M. C. (1971). Personality antecedents and correlates of drinking patterns in women. *Journal of Consulting and Clinical Psychology, 36,* 61–69.

Jonsdottir-Baldursson, T., & Horvath, P. (1987). Borderline personality-disordered alcoholics in Iceland: Descriptions on demographic, clinical, and MMPI variables. *Journal of Consulting and Clinical Psychology, 55,* 738–741.

Kammeier, M. L., Hoffman, H., & Loper, R. G. (1973). Personality characteristics of alcoholics as college freshmen and at time of treatment. *Quarterly Journal of Studies on Alcohol, 34,* 390–399.

Kannappan, R., & Cherian, R. R. (1989). Personality factors and alcoholism. *Journal of Personality and Clinical Studies, 5,* 43–46.

Kaplan, H. B. (1975). Increase in self-rejection as an antecedent of deviant responses. *Journal of Youth and Adolescence, 4,* 281–292.

Kessler, R. C., Crum, R. M., Warner, L. A., Nelson, C. B., Schulenberg, J., & Anthony, J. C. (1997). Lifetime co-occurrence of DSM-III-R alcohol abuse and dependence with other psychiatric disorders in the national comorbidity survey. *Archives of General Psychiatry, 54,* 313–321.

Kessler, R. C., McGonagle, K. A., Zhao, S., Nelson, C. B., Hughes, M., Eshleman, S., Wittchen, H., & Kendler, K. S. (1994). lifetime and 12-month prevalence of DSM-III-R Psychiatric disorders in the United States: Results from the national comorbidity survey. *Archives of General Psychiatry, 51,* 8–19.

Khantzian, E. J. (1990). Self-regulation and self-medication factors in alcoholism and the addictions. In M. Galanter (Ed.), *Recent developments in alcoholism: Vol. 8. Combined alcohol and other drug dependence* (pp. 255–271). New York: Plenum.

Kilbey, M. M., Downey, K., & Breslau, N. (1998). Predicting the emergence and persistence of alcohol dependence in young adults: The role of expectancy and other risk factors. *Experimental and Clinical Psychopathology, 6,* 149–156.

Knight, R. P. (1937). The dynamics and treatment of chronic alcohol addiction. *Bulletin of the Menninger Clinic, 1,* 233–250.

Kosten, T. A., Kosten, T. R., & Rounsaville, B. J. (1989). Personality disorders in opiate addicts show prognostic specificity. *Journal of Substance Abuse Treatment, 6,* 163–168.

Kranzler, H. R., Satel, S., & Apter, A. (1994). Personality disorders and associated features in cocaine-dependent inpatients. *Comprehensive Psychiatry, 35,* 335–340.

Krueger, R. F., Caspi, A., Moffitt, T. E., Silva, P. A., & McGee, R. (1996). Personality traits are differentially linked to mental disorders: A multitrait–multidiagnosis study of an adolescent birth cohort. *Journal of Abnormal Psychology, 105,* 299–312.

Kushner, M. G., Mackenzie, T. B., Fiszdon, J., Valentiner, D. P., Foa, E., Anderson, N., & Wangensteen, D. (1996). The effects of alcohol consumption on laboratory-induced panic and state anxiety. *Archives of General Psychiatry, 53,* 264–270.

Kushner, M. G., Sher, K. J., Wood, M., & Wood, P. K. (1994). Anxiety and drinking behavior: Moderating effects of tension-reduction expectancies. *Alcoholism: Clinical and Experimental Research, 18,* 852–860.

Lang, A. R. (1983). Addictive personality: A viable construct? In P. K. Levison, D. R. Gerstein, & D. R. Maloff (Eds.), *Commonalities in substance abuse and habitual behavior* (pp. 157–235). Lexington, MA: Lexington Books.

Leonard, K. E., & Blane, H. T. (1988). Alcohol expectancies and personality characteristics in young men. *Addictive Behaviors, 13,* 353–357.

Levenson, R. W., Oyama, O. N., & Meek, P. S. (1987). Greater reinforcement from alcohol for those at risk: Parental risk, personality risk, and gender. *Journal of Abnormal Psychology, 96,* 242–253.

Lewis, C. E. (1984). Alcoholism, antisocial personality, narcotic addition: An integrative approach. *Psychiatric Developments, 3,* 223–235.

Lewis, C. E., Cloninger, C. R., & Pais, J. (1983). Alcoholism, antisocial personality and drug use in a criminal population. *Alcohol and Alcoholism, 18,* 53–60.

Lisansky, E. S. (1960). The etiology of alcoholism: The role of psychological predisposition. *Quarterly Journal of Studies on Alcohol, 21,* 314–343.

Magnusson, D., & Endler, N. (1977). *Personality at the crossroads: Current issues in interactional psychology.* Hillsdale, NJ: Erlbaum.

Malow, R. M., West, J. A., Williams, J. L., & Sutker, P. B. (1989). Personality disorders classification and symptoms in cocaine and opioid addicts. *Journal of Consulting and Clinical Psychology, 57,* 765–767.

Mann, L. M., Chassin, L., & Sher, K. J. (1987). Alcohol expectancies and the risk for alcoholism. *Journal of Consulting and Clinical Psychology, 55,* 411–417.

Marlowe, D. B., Husband, S. D., Bonieskie, L. M., Kirby, K. C., & Platt, J. J. (1997). Structured interview versus self-report test vantages for the assessment of personality pathology in cocaine dependence. *Journal of Personality Disorders, 11,* 177–190.

Martin, E. D., & Sher, K. J. (1994). Family history of alcoholism, alcohol use disorders, and the five factor model of personality. *Journal of Studies on Alcohol, 55,* 81–90.

McArdle, J. J., Hamagami, F., & Hulick, P. (1994). Latent variable path models in alcohol use research. In R. Zucker, G. Boyd, & J. Howard (Eds.), *The development of alcohol problems: Exploring the biopsychosocial matrix of risk.* NIAAA Research Monograph No. 26 (pp. 341–386). Rockville, MD: Department of Health and Human Services.

McDougall, W. (1929). The chemical theory of temperament applied to introversion and extroversion. *Journal of Abnormal and Social Psychology, 24,* 293–309.

McGue, M., Slutske, W., Taylor, J., & Iacono, W. G. (1997). Personality and substance use disorders: I. Effects of gender and alcoholism subtype. *Alcoholism: Clinical and Experimental Research, 21,* 513–520.

McNeil, T. F., & Kaij, L. (1979). Etiological relevance of comparisons of high-risk and low-risk groups. *Acta Psychiatrica Scandinavia, 59,* 545–560.

Mednick, S. A., & McNeil, T. F. (1968). Current methodology in research on the etiology of schizophrenia: Serious difficulties which suggest the use of the high-risk group method. *Psychological Bulletin, 70,* 681–693.

Mendelsohn, J. H., Barbor, T. F., Mello, N. K., & Pratt, H. (1986). Alcoholism and prevalence of medical and psychiatric disorders. *Journal of Studies on Alcohol, 47,* 361–366.

Mensch, B. S., & Kandel, D. B. (1988). Dropping out of high school and drug involvement. *Sociology of Education, 61,* 95–113.

Meszaros, K., Willinger, U., Fischer, G., Schonbeck, G., & Aschauer, H. N. (1996). The tridimensional personality model: Influencing variables in a sample of detoxified alcohol dependents. *Comprehensive Psychiatry, 37,* 109–114.

Meyers, J. K., Weissman, M. M., Tischler, G. L., Holzer, C. E., Leaf, P., Orvaschel, H., Anthony, J. C., Boyd, J. H., Burke, J. D., Kramer, M., & Stoltzman, R. (1984). Six-month prevalence of psychiatric disorders in three communities: 1980–1982. *Archives of General Psychiatry, 41,* 959–967.

Miller, N. S., Belkin, B. M., & Gibbons, R. (1994). Clinical diagnosis of substance use disorders in private psychiatric populations. *Journal of Substance Abuse Treatment, 11,* 387–392.

Mischel, M. (1968). *Personality and assessment.* New York: Wiley.

Molina, B. S. G., Chassin, L., & Curran, P. (1994). A comparison of mechanisms underlying substance use for early adolescent children of alcoholics and controls. *Journal of Studies on Alcohol, 55,* 269–275.

Morey, L. C., & Blashfield, R. K. (1981). Empirical classifications of alcoholism: A review. *Journal of Studies on Alcohol, 42,* 925–937.

Morgenstern, J., Langenbucher, J., Labouvie, E., & Miller, K. J. (1997). The comorbidity of alcoholism and personality disorders in a clinical population: Prevalence rates and relation to alcohol typology variables. *Journal of Abnormal Psychology, 106,* 74–84.

Mullan, M. J., Gurling, H. M., Oppenheim, B. E., & Murray, R. M. (1986). The relationship between alcoholism and neurosis: Evidence from a twin study. *British Journal of Psychiatry, 148,* 435–441.

Muthen, B. (1994). *Psychometric modeling in epidemiology with an emphasis on longitudinal analysis of alcohol use* (ABMRF Monograph No. 1). Baltimore: Alcoholic Beverage Medical Research Foundation.

Nace, E. P., Davis, C. W., & Gaspari, J. P. (1991). Axis II comorbidity in substance abusers. *American Journal of Psychiatry, 148,* 118–120.

Nace, E. P., Saxon, J. J., & Shore, N. (1986). Borderline personality disorder and alcoholism treatment: A one-year follow-up study. *Journal of Studies on Alcohol, 47,* 196–200.

Nagoshi, C. T., Wilson, J. R., & Rodriguez, L. A. (1991). Impulsivity, sensation seeking, and behavioral and emotional responses to alcohol. *Alcoholism: Clinical and Experimental Research, 15,* 661–667.

Nathan, P. E. (1988). The addictive personality is the behavior of the addict. *Journal of Consulting and Clinical Psychology, 56,* 183–188.

National Institute on Alcohol Abuse and Alcoholism. (1987). *Ninth special report to the U.S. Congress on alcohol and health* (NIH Publication No. 97-4017). Washington, DC: U.S. Government Printing Office.

Newlin, D. B., & Thomson, J. B. (1990). Alcohol challenge with sons of alcoholics: A critical review and analysis. *Psychological Bulletin, 108,* 383–402.

Niaura, R., Wilson, G. T., & Westrick, E. (1988). Self-awareness, alcohol consumption, and reduced cardiovascular reactivity. *Psychosomatic Medicine, 50,* 360–380.

Nurnberg, H. G., Rifkin, A., & Doddi, S. (1993). A systematic assessment of the comorbidity of DSM-III-R personality disorders in alcoholic outpatients. *Comprehensive Psychiatry, 34,* 447–454.

O'Connor, L. E., Berry, J. W., Morrison, A., & Brown, S. (1995). The drug-of-choice phenomenon: Psychological differences among drug users who preferred different drugs. *International Journal of the Addictions, 30,* 541–555.

Oetting, E. R., & Beauvais, F. (1986). Peer cluster theory: Drugs and the adolescent. *Journal of Counseling and Development, 65,* 17–22.

Oldham, J. M., Skodol, A. E., Kellman, H. D., Hyler, S. E., Doidge, N., Rosnick, L., & Gallaher, P. E. (1995). Comorbidity of Axis I and Axis II disorders. *American Journal of Psychiatry, 152,* 571–578.

Partington, J. T., & Johnson, F. G. (1969). Personality types among alcoholics. *Quarterly Journal of Studies on Alcohol, 30,* 21–34.

Pederson, W. (1991). Mental health, sensation seeking, and drug use patterns: A longitudinal study. *British Journal of Addiction, 86,* 195–204.

Petraitis, J., Flay, B. R., & Miller, T. Q. (1995). Reviewing theories of adolescent substance use: Organizing pieces in the puzzle. *Psychological Bulletin, 117,* 67–86.

Petrie, A. (1967). *Individuality in pain and suffering,* Chicago: University of Chicago Press.

Plutchik, A., & Plutchik, R. (1988). Psychosocial correlates of alcoholism. *Integrative Psychiatry, 6,* 205–210.

Poldrugo, F., & Forti, B. (1988). Personality disorders and alcoholism treatment outcome. *Drug and Alcohol Dependence, 21,* 171–176.

Prescott, C. A., Neale, M. C., Corey, L. A., & Kendler, K. S. (1997). Predictors of problem drinking and alcohol dependence in a population-based sample of female twins. *Journal of Studies on Alcohol, 58*, 167–181.

Rankin, H., Stockwell, T., & Hodgson, R. (1982). Personality and alcohol dependence. *Personality and Individual Differences, 3*, 145–151.

Regier, D. A., Farmer, M. E., Rae, D. S., Locke, B. Z., Keith, S. J., Judd, L. L., & Goodwin, F. K. (1990). Comorbidity of mental disorders with alcohol and other drug abuse. *Journal of the American Medical Association, 264*, 2511–2518.

Reich, T. R., Cloninger, C. R., Van Eerdewegh, P., Rice, J. P., & Mullaney, J. (1988). Secular trends in the familial transmission of alcoholism. *Alcoholism: Clinical and Experimental Research, 12*, 458–464.

Robins, L. N., Bates, W., & O'Neal, P. (1962). Adult drinking patterns of former problem children. In D. Pittman & C. R. Snyder (Eds.), *Society, culture, and drinking patterns* (pp. 395–412). New York: Wiley.

Robins, L. N., Helzer, J. E., Weissman, M. M., Orvaschel, H., Gruenberg, E., Burke, J. D., Jr., & Regier, D. A. (1984). Lifetime prevalence of specific psychiatric disorders in three sites. *Archives of General Psychiatry, 41*, 949–958.

Robins, L. N., & McEvoy, L. (1990). Conduct problems as predictors of substance abuse. In L. Robins & M. Rutter (Eds.), *Straight and devious pathways from childhood to adulthood* (pp. 182–204). Cambridge, UK: Cambridge University Press.

Rogosch, F., Chassin, L., & Sher, K. J. (1990). Personality variables as mediators and moderators of family history risk for alcoholism: Conceptual and methodological issues. *Journal of Studies on Alcohol, 51*, 310–318.

Rousar, E., Brooner, R. K., Regier, M. W., & Bigelow, G. E. (1994). Psychiatric distress in antisocial drug abusers: Relation to other personality disorders. *Drug and Alcohol Dependence, 34*, 149–154.

Sameroff, A., & Chandler, M. (1974). Reproductive risk and the continuum of caretaking casualty. In F. D. Horowitz, M. Hetherington, S. Scarr-Salapatek, & G. Siegel (Eds.), *Review of child development research* (Vol. 4, pp. 187–244). Chicago: University of Chicago Press.

Schuckit, M. A. (1985). The clinical implications of primary diagnostic groups among alcoholics. *Archives of General Psychiatry, 42*, 1043–1049.

Schuckit, M. A. (1994). Alcohol and depression: A clinical perspective. Yrjo Jahnsson Foundation VIII Medical Symposium: Depression: Preventive and risk factors (1992, Porvoo, Finland). *Acta Psychiatrica Scandinavica, 89*(Suppl. 377), 28–32.

Schuckit, M. A. (1998). Biological, psychological, and environmental predictors of the alcoholism risk: A longitudinal study. *Journal of Studies on Alcohol, 59*, 485–494.

Schuckit, M. A., & Smith, T. L. (1996). An 8-year follow-up of 450 sons of alcoholic and control subjects. *Archives of General Psychiatry, 53*, 202–210.

Shedler, J., Mayman, M., & Manis, M. (1993). The illusion of mental health. *American Psychologist, 48*, 1117–1131.

Sher, K. J. (1991). *Children of alcoholics: A critical appraisal of theory and research.* Chicago: University of Chicago Press.

Sher, K. J. (1994). There are two types of alcoholism researchers, those who believe in two types of alcoholism and those who don't. *Addiction, 89*, 1061–1064.

Sher, K. J. (1996, June). *The course of alcohol problems in adolescence and young adulthood: Perspectives from a high-risk, prospective study.* Plenary address at the annual meeting of the Research Society on Alcoholism, Washington, DC.

Sher, K. J., Bylund, D. B., Walitzer, K. S., Hartmann, J., & Ray-Prenger, C. (1994). Platelet MAO activity: Personality, substance use, and the stress-response-dampening effect of alcohol. *Experimental and Clinical Psychopharmacology*, 2, 53–81.

Sher, K. J., & Gotham, H. J. (1998). *A developmental psychopathology perspective on alcohol use disorders in young adulthood.* Unpublished manuscript.

Sher, K. J., Gotham, H. J., Watson, A., & Meier, M. (1998). *Baseline and dynamic predictors of the course of alcohol use disorders in young adulthood.* Unpublished manuscript.

Sher, K. J., & Levenson, R. W. (1982). Risk for alcoholism and individual differences in the stress-response-dampening effect of alcohol. *Journal of Abnormal Psychology*, 91, 350–368.

Sher, K. J., & Trull, T. J. (1994). Personality and disinhibitory psychopathology: Alcoholism and antisocial personality. *Journal of Abnormal Psychology*, 103, 92–102.

Sher, K. J., & Trull, T. J. (1996). Methodological issues in psychopathology research. *Annual Review of Psychology*, 47, 371–400.

Sher, K. J., Walitzer, K. S. (1986). Individual differences in the stress-response dampening effect of alcohol: A dose-response study. *Journal of Abnormal Psychology*, 95, 159–167.

Sher, K. J., Walitzer, K. S., Wood, P. K., & Brent, E. E. (1991). Characteristics of children of alcoholics: Putative risk factors, substance use and abuse, and psychopathology. *Journal of Abnormal Psychology*, 100, 427–448.

Sher, K. J., Wood, M., Crews, T., & Vandiver, T. A. (1995). The Tridimensional Personality Questionnaire: Reliability and validity studies and derivation of a short form. *Psychological Assessment*, 7, 195–208.

Sieber, M. F. (1981). Personality scores and licit and illicit substance use. *Personality and Individual Differences*, 2, 235–241.

Slutske, W. S., Heath, A. C., Dinwiddie, S. H., Madden, P. A. F., Bucholz, K. K., Dunne, M. P., Statham, D. J., & Martin, N. G. (1998). Common genetic risk factors for conduct disorder and alcohol dependence. *Journal of Abnormal Psychology*, 107, 363–374.

Stacy, A. W., & Newcomb, M. D. (1998). Memory association and personality as predictors of alcohol use: Mediation and moderator effects. *Experimental and Clinical Psychopharmacology*, 6, 280–291.

Stacy, A. W., Newcomb, M. D., & Bentler, P. M. (1995). Expectancy in mediational models of cocaine use. *Personality and Individual Differences*, 19, 655–667.

Steele, C. M., & Josephs, R. A. (1990). Alcohol myopia: Its prized and dangerous effects. *American Psychologist*, 45, 921–933.

Stravynski, A., Lamontagne, Y., & Lavallee, Y. (1986). Clinical phobias and avoidant personality disorder among alcoholics admitted to an alcoholism rehabilitation setting. *Canadian Journal of Psychiatry*, 31, 714–719.

Sutherland, E. H., Schroeder, H. G., & Tordella, C. L. (1950). Personality traits and the alcoholic. *Quarterly Journal of Studies on Alcohol*, 11, 547–561.

Sutker, P. B., & Allain, A. N. (1988). Issues in personality conceptualizations of addictive behaviors. *Journal of Consulting and Clinical Psychology*, 56, 172–182.

Svrakic, D., Whitehead, C., Przybeck, T. R., & Cloninger, C. R. (1993). Differential diagnosis of personality disorders by the seven-factor model of temperament and character. *Archives of General Psychiatry*, 50, 991–999.

Syme, L. (1957). Personality characteristics of the alcoholic: A critique of current studies. *Quarterly Journal of Studies on Alcohol, 18,* 288–301.

Tarter, R. E. (1988). Are there inherited behavioral traits that predispose to substance abuse? *Journal of Consulting and Clinical Psychology, 56,* 189–196.

Tarter, R. E., & Vanyukov, M. (1994). Alcoholism: A developmental disorder. *Journal of Consulting and Clinical Psychology, 62,* 1096–1107.

Tausignant, M., & Kovess, V. (1989). Borderline traits among community alcoholics and problem drinkers: Rural–urban differences. *Canadian Journal of Psychiatry, 34,* 796–799.

Tellegen, A. (1985). Structures of mood and personality and their relevance to assessing anxiety, with an emphasis on self-report. In A. H. Tuma & J. D. Maser (Eds.), *Anxiety and the anxiety disorders* (pp. 681–716). Hillsdale, NJ: Erlbaum.

Tellegen, A. (1994). *Multidimensional Personality Questionnaire.* Minneapolis: University of Minnesota Press.

Tellegen, A., & Waller, N. G. (in press). Exploring personality through test construction: Development of the Multidimensional Personality Questionnaire. In S. R. Briggs & J. M. Cheek (Eds.), *Personality measures: Development and evaluation* (Vol. 1). Greenwich, CT: JAI Press.

Trull, T. J., & Sher, K. J. (1994). Relationship between the five-factor model of personality and Axis I disorders in a nonclinical sample. *Journal of Abnormal Psychology, 103,* 350–360.

Urschell, H. C., & Woody, G. E. (1994). Alcohol idiosyncratic intoxication: A review of the data supporting its evidence. In T. A. Widiger, A. J. Frances, H. A. Pincus, M. B. First, R. Ross, & W. Davis (Eds.), *DSM-IV sourcebook* (Vol. 1, pp. 117–128). Washington, DC: American Psychiatric Association Press.

Vaglum, S., & Vaglum, P. (1985). Borderline and other mental disorders in alcoholic female psychiatric patients: A case control study. *Psychopathology, 18,* 50–60.

Vaillant, G. E., & Milofsky, E. S. (1982). The etiology of alcoholism: A prospective viewpoint. *American Psychologist, 37,* 494–503.

Varma, V. K., Basu, D., Malhotra, A., Sharma, A., & Mattoo, S. K. (1994). Correlates of early- and late-onset alcohol dependence. *Addictive Behaviors, 19,* 609–619.

Volavka, J., Czobor, P., Goodwin, D. W., Gabrielli, W. F., Jr., Penick, E. C., Sarnoff, A. M., Jensen, P., Knop, J., & Schulsinger, F. (1996). The electroencephalogram after alcohol administration in high-risk men and the development of alcohol use disorders 10 years later: Preliminary findings. *Archives of General Psychiatry, 53,* 258–263.

Waller, N. G., Lilienfeld, S. O., Tellegen, A., & Lykken, D. T. (1991). The Tridimensional Personality Questionnaire: Structural validity and comparison with the Multidimensional Personality Questionnaire. *Multivariate Behavioral Research, 26,* 1–23.

Watson, D., Clark, L. A., & Harkness, A. R. (1994). Structures of personality and their relevance to psychopathology. *Journal of Abnormal Psychology, 103,* 18–31.

White, J. L., Moffitt, T. E., Caspi, A., Bartusch, D. J., Needles, D. J., & Stouthamer-Loeber, M. (1994). Measuring impulsivity and examining its relationship to delinquency. *Journal of Abnormal Psychology, 103,* 192–205.

Widiger, T. A., & Rogers, J. H. (1989). Prevalence and comorbidity of personality disorders. *Psychiatric Annals, 19,* 132–136.

Widiger, T. A., & Trull, T. J. (1987). Behavioral indicators, hypothetical constructs, and personality disorders. *Journal of Personality Disorders, 1,* 82–87.

Wiggins, J. S., & Trapnell, P. D. (1997). Personality structure: The return of the Big Five. In R. Hogan, J. Johnson, & S. Briggs (Eds.), *Handbook of personality psychology* (pp. 737–765). New York: Academic Press.

Windle, M. (1990). A longitudinal study of antisocial behaviors in early adolescence as predictors of late adolescent substance use: Gender and ethnic group differences. *Journal of Abnormal Psychology, 99,* 86–91.

Witkin, H. A., Karp, S. A., & Goodenough, D. R. (1959). Dependence in alcoholics. *Quarterly Journal of Studies on Alcohol, 20,* 493–504.

Woodruff, R. A., Guze, S. B., & Clayton, P. J. (1973). Alcoholics who see a psychiatrist compared to those who do not. *Quarterly Journal of Studies on Alcoholism, 34,* 1162–1171.

Yamaguchi, K. (1990). Drug use and its social covariates from the period of adolescence to young adulthood: Some implications from longitudinal studies. In M. Galanter (Ed.), *Recent developments in alcoholism: Vol. 8. Combined alcohol and other drug dependence* (pp. 125–143). New York: Plenum.

Young, R. M., Oei, T. P., & Crook, G. M. (1991). Development of a drinking self-efficacy questionnaire. *Journal of Psychopathology and Behavioral Assessment, 13,* 1–15.

Zeichner, A., Edwards, P. W., & Cohen, E. (1985). Acute effects of alcohol on cardiovascular reactivity to stress in college-age Type A (coronary prone) individuals. *Journal of Psychopathology and Behavioral Assessment, 7,* 75–89.

Zeichner, A., Giancola, P. R., & Allen, J. D. (1995). Effects of hostility on alcohol stress-response-dampening. *Alcoholism, Clinical and Experimental Research, 19,* 977–983.

Zimmerman, M., & Coryell, W. (1989). DSM-III personality disorder diagnoses in a nonpatient sample: Demographic correlates and comorbidity. *Archives of General Psychiatry, 46,* 682–689.

Zucker, R. A. (1987). The four alcoholisms: A developmental account of the etiologic process. In P. C. Rivers (Ed.), *Nebraska Symposium on Motivation, 1986: Alcohol and addictive behavior* (pp. 27–83). Lincoln: University of Nebraska Press.

Zucker, R. A., Fitzgerald, H. E., & Moses, H. D. (1995). Emergence of alcohol problems and the several alcoholisms: A developmental perspective on etiologic theory and life course trajectory. In D. Cicchetti & D. J. Cohen (Eds.), *Developmental psychopathology: Vol. 2. Risk, disorder, and adaptation* (pp. 677–711). New York: Wiley.

Zucker, R. A., & Gomberg, E. S. L. (1986). Etiology of alcoholism reconsidered: The case for a biopsychosocial process. *American Psychologist, 41,* 783.

Zuckerman, M. (1991). *Psychobiology of personality.* Cambridge, UK: Cambridge University Press.

Zuckerman, M. (1995). Good and bad humors: Biochemical bases of personality and its disorders. *Psychological Science, 6,* 325–332.

Zuckerman, M., & Cloninger, C. R. (1996). Relationships between Cloninger's, Zuckerman's, and Eysenck's dimensions of personality. *Personality and Individual Differences, 21,* 283–285.

Zuckerman, M., Eysenck, S., & Eysenck, H. J. (1978). Sensation seeking in England and America: Cross-cultural, age, and sex comparisons. *Journal of Consulting and Clinical Psychology, 46,* 139–149.

Zuckerman, M., Kuhlman, D. M., & Camac, C. (1988). What lies beyond E and N? Factor analyses of scales believed to measure basic dimensions of personality. *Journal of Personality and Social Psychology, 54,* 96–107.

4

Social Learning Theory

STEPHEN A. MAISTO
KATE B. CAREY
CLARA M. BRADIZZA

INTRODUCTION

The purpose of this chapter is to provide a review of theoretical and empirical advances in social learning theory (SLT) of alcohol, other drug use, and the substance use disorders[1,2] since publication of the first edition of this book in 1987. It is important to define at the outset a few major terms that are of central interest in this chapter. As we discuss later, different "social learning" theories have been published. However, these theories have in common emphases on learning from the social environment that is both direct (by personal experience of differential reinforcement) and indirect (by modeling of others), and on cognition as major determinants of behavior (e.g., Petraitis, Flay, & Miller, 1995). "Drinking" has been used to refer to a number of variables. Typically, it denotes quantity and frequency of alcohol consumption and is viewed as existing on a continuum. The low point of this continuum is abstinence from alcohol. One implication of this viewpoint is that the same principles may be used to enhance understanding of alcohol use at any point along the quantity–frequency continuum. In addition, drinking-related behavior or consequences may or may not meet DSM-IV (fourth edition of the *Diagnostic and Statistical Manual of Mental Disorders*; American Psychiatric Association, 1994) criteria for an alcohol use disorder.[3] Similarly, "drug use" usually has referred to the frequency and, less often, to the quantity of use of illicit psychoactive substances. In addition, drug-related behavior or consequences may not necessarily meet the DSM criteria for substance use disorder.

Consistent with the chapter on SLT in the first edition of this book (Abrams & Niaura, 1987), we begin this chapter by tracing the main principles and constructs of SLT as a general theory of behavior as they have been articulated over the last 30 years. In this regard, Bandura's (1969, 1977, 1986) work will be the focus, as it has been the most influential SLT approach in alcohol research. Then, we describe how SLT's major constructs have been applied to enhance understanding of alcohol use and the alcohol use disorders. This theoretical overview is the basis of a selective review of empirical literature that has appeared since 1987 on SLT variables in the alcohol (and other drugs) research area. This review concentrates on the most recent work that is available. Furthermore, the review of empirical literature primarily concerns topics that are relevant to SLT but that are not covered entirely by other chapters in this book. Therefore, we emphasize social-environmental variables, coping/social skills, cognitive variables, and relapse. After the literature review, we discuss methodological and substantive advances that the field has made since 1987, as well as the major theoretical and empirical questions to address in future research.

SOCIAL LEARNING AS A GENERAL THEORY OF BEHAVIOR

Social learning theory represents a general theory of behavior. As such, it is one approach to understanding human behavior, and its major constructs and principles are far-reaching and expressed in broad terms. The name "social learning" theory has been given to theories of human behavior that have been proposed by several prominent psychologists (Bandura, 1969, 1977, 1986; Dollard & Miller, 1950; Mischel, 1973; Rotter, 1954) and sociologists (Akers, 1977; Akers, Krohn, Lanza-Kaduce, & Radosevich, 1979; Burgess & Akers, 1966). Social learning theory may be defined as an approach that synthesizes principles of learning with those of cognitive psychology. It is a systematic effort to explain how the social and personal competencies that are often referred to as "personality" develop from the social context in which such learning occurs (Hilgard & Bower, 1975, p. 599).

As mentioned earlier, Bandura (1969, 1977, 1986) probably was the most influential contributor to the development of SLT. Furthermore, his ideas have formed the foundation for the work of psychologists who claim to take a SLT approach to the investigation of alcohol and other drug use and disorders. Therefore, we proceed with this section of the chapter by summarizing primary principles and constructs as they have been developed in Bandura's major publications on SLT. It should be noted that, for the most part, the principles and constructs that are included in the summary have a substantial amount of empirical support. This supporting evidence is reviewed in the three books by Bandura (1969, 1977, 1986) that are cited.

Social Learning Theory's View of Human Nature

One reason that Bandura's 1969 book was so important is that it presented an integrated statement about human nature that departed in major ways from the psychoanalytic and associative conditioning–learning views that dominated American psychology in the 1950s and 1960s. SLT did not view humans as impelled from within by psychological (e.g., traits, unconscious drives) or biological drives. Similarly, behavior was not viewed as controlled only by the external environment. Instead, according to SLT, "human functioning . . . involves interrelated control systems in which behavior is determined by external stimulus events, by internal processing systems and regulatory codes, and by reinforcing response–feedback systems" (Bandura, 1969, p. 19). This fundamental conception of human behavior has not changed in the decades that have passed since Bandura's book was published.

Bandura's (1969) SLT included four major principles or constructs that have been essential to the theory over the years and that in some cases have undergone some elaboration as a result of empirical findings. In our view, these four SLT elements are *differential reinforcement, vicarious learning, cognitive processes, and reciprocal determinism.* In the next sections, we describe each of these elements and identify any changes in thinking about them that have occurred over the years.

Differential Reinforcement

Differential reinforcement refers to the application of consequences for a behavior dependent on stimulus conditions. "Stimulus conditions" broadly make up the "setting." In SLT, the principle of differential reinforcement is used to help to explain variability in the same person's behavior in different settings; this principle has not been modified in versions of SLT that have appeared since 1969.

Positive or negative reinforcement, or punishment, or withdrawal of these three events, often occur directly from the external environment. Table 4.1 provides an illustration of differential reinforcement. In Table 4.1, the contrast of possible consequences for the behavior of moderate alcohol use is presented. If the individual drinks moderately in a setting such as a party, where hosts typically sanction alcohol use for adults, he or she will tend to experience positive outcomes. Examples of these outcomes listed in Table 4.1 include feeling relaxed, and experiencing pleasant social exchanges and social approval. However, in most places of employment, the same moderate alcohol use would tend to result in mostly punishing consequences. The individ-

TABLE 4.1. Example of Differential Consequences for a Behavior
in Different Settings

Setting	Behavior	Consequences
Social gathering, such as a party	Moderate alcohol use (e.g., two beers)	Relaxation Enjoyable social exchanges Social approval
Place of employment	Moderate alcohol use	Relaxation Disapproval of supervisors and peers Possible employment termination

ual may feel more relaxed upon drinking, but if that drinking is detected, then he or she likely would meet peers' and supervisors' disapproval, along with possible termination of employment. As a result of these differential consequences for moderate drinking in the two settings, it occurs more frequently at parties than at work. Note that differential consequences for a behavior also may occur vicariously, or may be implemented by the individual him- or herself. The self-administration of consequences for a behavior would be called self-reinforcement, or self-punishment, for example.

Vicarious Learning

In 1969, Bandura presented a considerable amount of evidence to support the idea that humans may acquire new behaviors through observation of others, or through communication by symbolic means such as spoken or written language. This process is called *vicarious learning*, or *modeling*. SLT posits that observation of a model being reinforced for a given behavior can increase the likelihood of that behavior in the observer. Similarly, observation of behavior that results in punishment may cause the observer to avoid similar behavior. In Bandura's subsequent presentations of SLT (1977, 1986), vicarious learning assumed a more prominent place. For example, by 1986, Bandura argued that virtually all that can be learned from direct experience can be acquired by vicarious learning. In this regard, vicarious learning allows a far more efficient way to acquire and regulate behavioral patterns than does learning by trial and error (direct experience).

Cognitive Processes

Bandura (1969) viewed cognitions as mediating environmental events and behavior, as indicated in the earlier section on SLT's view of human nature. Cognitive processes such as encoding, organizing, and retrieving information regulate behavior. In this view, environmental events provide the individual with information that is cognitively processed, and the results of that processing determine the overt behavior that will follow. A major piece of information that individuals glean from the environment is the probable consequences for enacting a behavior in a given setting. Accordingly, the *expectancies* of behavioral outcomes that are acquired play an important part in guiding later behavior, as individuals typically behave to access sources of reinforcement in the environment.

In 1977 and 1986, Bandura argued for the increasing importance of the individual and less of a role for the external environment as determinants of human behavior. Much of this shift in position was due to the greater emphasis on cognitive processes. In 1977, Bandura discussed the importance of humans' ability to use symbols as an extremely effective way to cope with their environment. For example, every day, individuals must cope with stress, which may be viewed as environmental events that present challenges to, or make demands on, individuals. As will be seen throughout this chapter, SLT emphasizes stress from the social environment. Cognitive processes help individuals cope with stress because they can use verbal and imaginal stimuli to process and retain representations of their experiences. These cognitive representations then guide later behavior. *Self-regulatory* functions also were emphasized. Individuals are capable of arranging environmental incentives, producing cognitive supports, and generating consequences for their own actions. As a result, people are able to exert a degree of control over their own behavior. Self-regulatory functions are acquired through interaction with the social environment and can be maintained by the external environment. However, once behaviors are acquired, self-regulation plays a role in which ones are enacted.

The proposition that behavior can be self-regulated sets the stage for the construct of *self-efficacy*. In its typical application, self-efficacy concerns the individual's beliefs regarding the likelihood that he or she can enact behavior at a level required to result in desired outcomes. Self-efficacy expectancies are distinguished from outcome expectancies in that the latter refer to beliefs about behavior–consequence probabilities, independent of whether the individual believes that he or she can enact the relevant behavior.

As implied by the definition of self-efficacy, it is hypothesized to be situation-specific. Moreover, as with outcome expectancies, self-efficacy is hypothesized to mediate environmental or cognitive events and behavior. Bandura (1977) argued that there are four sources of self-efficacy expectancies: performance accomplishments, vicarious experience, verbal persuasion, and emotional arousal.

In 1986, Bandura further emphasized cognitive processes in his discussions of *forethought capability* and *self-reflective capability*. Forethought capability means that most of human behavior is planned. Forethought is viewed as product of reflection and not of mechanical mediation between an environmental event and behavior. Self-reflective capability means that individuals can have thoughts about their own thoughts. Through self-reflection, individuals can monitor their own ideas, make predictions from them, and change their ideas based on evaluations of their adequacy or accuracy. A crucial concept that is included here is the notion of judgments of self-efficacy.

Reciprocal Determinism

Bandura introduced the idea of *reciprocal determinism* into SLT in his 1969 book. At that time, reciprocal determinism meant that behavior may be controlled by the environment, but that behavior may also alter (control) the environment. In this context, *reciprocal* means mutual action between factors that are seen as causal, and *determinism* means the production of effects by certain factors (Bandura, 1986). To give an example of reciprocal determinism, the heavy drinker may claim that he or she drinks excessively in reaction to the feelings that go along with social rejection that is the result of heavy drinking.

In 1977, Bandura introduced the "person" as a factor in the reciprocal determinism model. Therefore, in this view, the person, the environment, and behavior are seen as "interlocking" (Bandura, 1977, pp. 9–10) determinants of each other, as illustrated in Figure 4.1. The amount of influence that each of these three interrelated sets of factors exerts varies according to the setting and to the behavior in question. The person variables that were emphasized in this model were the cognitive processes that were discussed earlier. Bandura maintained this model in 1986, except that he changed the label reciprocal determinism to *triadic reciprocality*.

Summary

Our presentation of Bandura's thinking about four major elements of SLT shows an approach that sees much of human behavior as learned from the social environment. Traditional concepts of learning are enhanced by principles of vicarious learning, and together provide mechanisms for the transmission of information from the environment that the individual processes

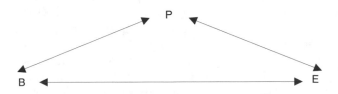

FIGURE 4.1. Interplay among the person (P), his or her behavior (B), and the environment (E) as an illustration of reciprocal determinism.

cognitively. This cognitive processing in turn results in the formulation of hypotheses about environmental consequences that direct the individual's actions in a given situation. As a behavior becomes established, it becomes increasingly under the control of internal standards and self-evaluation, relative to control by the external environment. Moreover, the person (primarily cognitions), the environment, and behavior are interdependent and influence each other ("triadic reciprocality") in the course of acquisition and maintenance of behavior.

Although Bandura (1986) considers SLT a "multivariate" theory that acknowledges the need to incorporate knowledge from multiple disciplines in order to understand human behavior, his emphasis is on situational and cognitive factors as determinants of behavior. Therefore, more distal environmental factors such as cultural variables, and intrapersonal factors such as personality characteristics, are given relatively little attention, although their importance is acknowledged. Finally, SLT encompasses a broad range of constructs but does not specify well how these constructs may combine, or how they may mediate or moderate each other to determine the development and maintenance of behavior. Indeed, Bandura acknowledged this in his 1986 book, and saw SLT at that time as focusing on the relationships between specific factors and their mechanisms of action. Nevertheless, SLT has served over the years as an excellent heuristic by stimulating a large volume of research, and by providing a way to integrate the findings that emerge. This has been true both for behavioral research in general, and for research on alcohol and other drug use in particular.

SOCIAL LEARNING THEORY OF ALCOHOL USE

As a general theory of behavior, SLT may be applied to enhance understanding of the development and maintenance of drinking and alcohol use disorders. Indeed, Bandura presented such an application in his 1969 book. (He did not include a similar discussion in his 1977 and 1986 books.) In Bandura's application of SLT to drinking behavior, he emphasized stress reduction as a major pharmacological action of alcohol and, therefore, as a major agent of negative reinforcement.

According to Bandura (1969), cultural and subcultural norms define whether alcohol use will be encouraged at all and, if so, in what quantities and under what conditions. These group norms are learned by observation of socializing agents, such as the drinking behavior of adults and the presentation of alcohol use in the media. Bandura argued that drinking behavior typically is begun by youth under nonstressful conditions as part of a more general socialization process, but in the course of experimenting with alcohol, the individual will experience the negative reinforcement of stress reduction through drinking alcohol on a number of occasions. If alcohol use is intermittently reinforced by stress reduction, it will tend to be used on future occasions when the individual experiences stress. If these stressful occasions of use become frequent enough and begin to interfere with the individual's life, then it becomes likely that an alcohol use disorder will develop. Bandura argued that this pattern is most likely to occur in families with one or more alcoholic parents, because in such a context, children are most likely to observe heavy drinking as a dominant response to stressful conditions. Moreover, once a pattern of habitual drinking is acquired, it may be maintained by the need to forestall alcohol withdrawal in individuals who have become physically dependent on alcohol. In other words, an abrupt drop in blood alcohol level is likely to lead to the painful experience of the alcohol withdrawal syndrome; avoidance of this state can motivate continued drinking.

From this description, Bandura's (1969) analysis sounds essentially like a simple tension reduction model of alcoholism (see Cappell & Greeley, 1987; Conger, 1956). However, Bandura included other features in his analysis that frequently are not discussed and that could be viewed as the bases of later applications of SLT to alcohol use, as will be evident later in this chapter. In this regard, Bandura's model is a coping deficits model, in that the use of alcohol under conditions of stress is seen as occurring in high frequency when alternative coping behaviors are not available to the individual. Often, this would occur if the individual had not acquired adequate social skills to enact behaviors that are healthier than excessive alcohol use in a given situation. Indeed, Bandura (1969) suggested that, for a large proportion of individuals with alcohol use disorder, skills training would be one component of a preferred treatment. The assumption here is that healthier ways of coping with stress are likely to result in access to more reinforcement from the social environment and, therefore, would be more likely to be acquired and displace alcohol use. This idea of sober behavior eliciting a greater amount of social reinforcement than drunken behavior also was the basis of Bandura's recommendation for what he called "multiform" therapy. This was the notion that treatment typically must include more than one component in order to give the alcoholic sufficient competencies and resources to gain access to social reinforcement for sober behavior. If sobriety does receive such reinforcement, then it is likely to be learned and maintained. Bandura argued that often alcoholics are individuals who have lost much of their access to social reinforcement, in large part due to their chronic, heavy drinking patterns. Therefore, a major task of treatment is to restore these sources of reinforcement for the individual. It is important to point out here that a SLT premise of multiform treatment is the idea of reciprocal determinism; it is believed that as the individual changes his or her behavior, the environment changes in response to it, which in turn affects the individual's future behavior.

To summarize, Bandura's (1969) analysis of drinking behavior emphasizes modeling as a major source of the acquisition of drinking patterns and ascribes an important role to negative reinforcement of alcohol use through stress reduction as an etiologic agent of alcoholism. However, the analysis is much broader, in that it argues for the influence of coping skills and social resources as major determinants of whether problem drinking patterns are changed, and if these changes are maintained. This early emphasis on coping skills and resources reflected Bandura's view that alcohol use, especially at the higher end of the continuum, in large part is an individual's effort to handle challenges in the social environment that may result in "stress." This viewpoint has been influential through the years in SLT-based research on substance use, as is evident in later sections of this chapter. Finally, Bandura recognized that, in addition to stress reduction, alcohol may have reinforcing properties that could influence an individual's pattern of drinking and whether it becomes a problem. However, his discussion gave these other reinforcing properties of alcohol relatively little attention.

Later Applications of Social Learning Theory to Alcohol Use

Since Bandura's (1969) SLT analysis of alcohol use and alcohol use disorders, no single attempt to explain these phenomena has claimed to be "social learning theory" (e.g., Cooper, Russell, & George, 1988). The framework that probably has come closest to a SLT of drinking behavior is the cognitive-behavioral approach, which indeed has been heavily influenced by Bandura's SLT. However, the cognitive-behavioral approach also incorporates other elements, such as social psychology. Several discussions of the cognitive-behavioral approach have been published (Dimeff & Marlatt, 1995; George & Marlatt, 1983; Marlatt & Gordon, 1985; Monti, Rohsenow, Abrams, & Binkoff, 1988), besides the SLT chapter by Abrams and Niaura (1987) that appeared in the first edition of this book. Marlatt and Gordon's (1985) cognitive-behavioral perspective on the development and maintenance of drinking patterns may be viewed, based on its content and clinicians' and researchers' perceptions, as best representing Bandura's SLT. Marlatt and Gordon's discussion (1985, pp. 9–10) was presented as applicable to "addictive behaviors" in general and has a number of central points:

• Addictive behaviors represent a category of "bad habits" (or learned maladaptive behaviors). Biological factors may contribute to predisposing an individual to alcohol problems, but specific patterns of use are learned.
• Addictive behaviors occur on a continuum of use; that is, behavior such as alcohol abuse is not seen in a categorical way (e.g., present or absent), but rather exists on continua of quantity and frequency of occurrence.
• All points along the continuum of addictive behavior are influenced by the same principles of learning. Therefore, the same mechanisms that may be applied to explain alcohol use can be invoked to explain alcohol use disorder.

• Addictive behaviors are learned habits that can be analyzed in the same way as any other habit.

• The determinants of addictive behaviors are situational and environmental factors, beliefs and expectations, and the person's family history and prior learning experiences with the substance or activity. Emphasis also is placed on the consequences of addictive behavior, to understand its reinforcement and punishing features.

• Besides the effects of alcohol (or other substance or activity in question), it also is important to discern the social and interpersonal reactions that the individual experiences before, during, and after engaging in the addictive behavior. Social factors are important both in the acquisition and later performance of the addictive behavior.

• Frequently, addictive behaviors are exhibited under conditions that are perceived as stressful. To that degree, they represent maladaptive coping behaviors.

• Addictive behaviors are strongly affected by the individual's expectations of achieving desired effects of engaging in the addictive behavior. Furthermore, self-efficacy expectancies (i.e., expectations of being able to use behavioral skills to cope with a situation without engaging in the addictive behavior) are important. If self-efficacy in a situation is low, and the individual believes (expects) that engaging in the addictive behavior would help to cope with it, then the likelihood of engaging in the behavior increases.

• The acquisition of new skills and cognitive strategies in a self-management program can result in changes in addictive behavior to new, more adaptive behaviors that come under control of cognitive processes of awareness and decision making. Accordingly, the individual can assume and accept a greater degree of responsibility for changing the addictive behavior.

From this summary of Marlatt and Gordon (1985), the influence of Bandura's SLT is apparent. Alcohol and other drug use patterns are primarily learned behaviors in which the social environment plays a prominent role. Patterns of use may become a problem for the individual if alcohol and other drugs are used frequently to cope with stress or other unpleasant feelings, which is most likely to happen when the individual does not possess an adequate degree of social or affect management skills to handle the situation effectively. Cognitions, both outcome and efficacy expectancies, play an important mediating role in patterns of alcohol use, so that their development and maintenance are key questions. Cognitive processes also are critical in the regulation of alcohol use, as well as in changing it.

This summary of SLT as a general theory of behavior and explanation of alcohol and other drug use provides the foundation for a review of the empirical support for the major constructs of SLT, and for their interplay in the hypothesized process of the development and maintenance of alcohol (and other drug) use patterns. Therefore, this chapter emphasizes constructs or phenomena critical to SLT that are not covered entirely in other chapters of this book.

The chapter proceeds with a review of empirical literature relevant to the constructs of social-environmental variables (including situational variables and modeling), coping skills, and cognitive variables (including self-efficacy and outcome expectancies), respectively. It should be noted that the literature on each topic is presented as if it stands alone, outside of a general conceptual framework. Our earlier review of Bandura's SLT shows that this is not the case, but that it is the most common way that each of the topics has been studied in the alcohol and drug area. On the other hand, our review of empirical work also shows recent attempts to evaluate SLT as an integrated theory of alcohol and other drug use. The review of the empirical literature is selective and emphasizes work published since 1987.

Following presentation of the first three topics, empirical studies that address reciprocal relationships between a SLT variable and substance use are discussed. Then, two studies that include multiple SLT determinants in specific efforts to evaluate the SLT approach to substance use are presented. The chapter's final empirical section concerns the problem of relapse. Relapse is included in this chapter because SLT has contributed to major clinical and research advances in the study of relapse. The last section of the chapter provides an overall summary and conclusions, and points to directions for future research on SLT and substance use.

We have noted that SLT views substance use as existing on a continuum, and that similar principles apply to understanding such use across the spectrum of quantity and frequency of consumption. However, empirical work on different SLT constructs has not always sampled research participants across the substance use continuum. (Because relapse, by definition, applies specifically to clinical populations, this consideration is not relevant.) For example, as will be seen later, research on coping skills has emphasized clinical populations, while research on cognitive variables reflects the sampling of a wider array of research participants. The problem of the representativeness of empirical work on SLT is discussed further in the last section of this chapter.

THREE SOCIAL LEARNING THEORY CONSTRUCTS

Social-Environmental Variables

Situation Factors

The situation surrounding a behavior plays a major part in its prediction by SLT and other learning theories. Here, *situation* typically refers to the external stimulus environment in which the behavior in question occurs. This immediate environment is distinguished from environmental variables that are more distal from the occurrence of behavior, such as cultural and legal factors. SLT is explicit in stating the part that the immediate environment plays in behavior and, by extension, in alcohol and other drug use. (It is important to note here that SLT actually emphasizes the reciprocal relationship between the individual and the situation, but in this section, we emphasize situation variables.) In research on substance use, the immediate context or situation has been defined as "the physical and social context of drug use and includes (a) the physical setting (e.g., room, location, space); (b) the setting's attributes (e.g., light, temperature, furniture, paraphernalia); (c) companions; and (d) the interaction among these elements" (McCarty, 1985, p. 248). Along these lines, fundamental questions are whether there is empirical evidence that elements of the immediate environment are associated with the use and effects of alcohol and other drugs.

There is a substantial amount of correlational and experimental data demonstrating a relationship between substance use and immediate environment factors in a range of user populations and for different substances. For example, Holyfield, Ducharme, and Martin (1994) analyzed data on drinking contexts obtained in a 1984 national survey of drinking practices among adults in the United States. These authors found in a multivariate analysis that the frequency of drinking at home, while socializing, and while drinking away from home each contributed significantly to variance in reports of current frequency of consuming alcohol. Frequency of drinking at home was the strongest predictor of the three drinking contexts evaluated. Setting variables also seem to affect drinking among adolescents. Beck and Treiman (1996) surveyed over 1,300 Washington, DC, area high school students and classified them as low, moderate, or high intensity drinkers. A discriminant function analysis showed that three social context variables of social facilitation, school defiance, and stress control loaded heavily on the primary discriminant function, which accounted for 86% of the variance.

The relationship between situation and substance use also is supported by experimental evidence, much of which concerns alcohol use. These data were published primarily in the 1970s and early 1980s, and were summarized nicely by McCarty (1985). His review of the data showed the following: A major contextual variable is the number of social companions. In this regard, the individual's drinking tends to be heavier when he or she is part of a group compared to when with one other person, or when alone. In experimental studies, the number of companions seems to have a greater effect on women than on men, perhaps because men's drinking tends to be greater at a baseline level than women's; therefore, it is more difficult for an environmental variable to affect men's drinking. The effect of number of companions on amount of alcohol consumption has been replicated in a variety of settings. Another situational variable that affects quantity of alcohol consumed on an occasion is social norms, which refer here to behavioral standards and expectations that are shared by group members and typically are observed as regularities in the behavior of group members (McCarty, 1985, p. 262). In the group situation, if the norm is heavier alcohol consumption, then group members will tend to conform to it. Heavy drinking at fraternity parties, or at weddings, illustrates this conformity to elevated drinking norms. Conversely, norms for tempered or zero alcohol use also will tend to be followed by group members. For example, few people allow themselves to drink heavily at job interviews, because normative expectations prohibit such behavior. Finally, attributes of the tavern or bar setting, such as cost of drinks, physical design and lighting, presence of entertainment, and staff characteristics have been shown to influence quantity of alcohol consumption in a situation. Although there is little experimental evidence, qualitative data have supported the effects of situational factors on consumption of drugs other than alcohol (Lenson, 1995; Weil, 1993; Zinberg, 1984).

The data are consistent in their support of the general proposition that situational factors affect substance use. Experimental data show that situational factors can alter the effects an individual experiences when under the influence of either alcohol or marijuana. In a frequently cited experiment by Pliner and Cappell (1974), men and women consumed moderate amounts of alcohol when alone or with others. When the research participants drank alone, they reported experiencing physical changes such as fuzzy thinking, sleepiness, and dizziness. However, participants who drank the same amount of alcohol, but with others, reported mood changes of feeling friendly and more pleasant. Subjects who drank a placebo beverage did not report any mood changes. It would appear from this experiment that the number of people with whom the individual drinks affects how he or she interprets alcohol-induced internal changes.

In summary, experimental, correlational, and qualitative data generally support the finding that situational factors affect both the consumption of alcohol and other drugs, and the effects that are experienced when those substances are consumed. Discovering the mechanisms that might explain these data is an important research task. Although several explanations are possible, from a SLT view, processes of classical, operant, and vicarious conditioning (learning) are of major importance. (Because learning factors in substance use is the subject of Chapter 8 by Vogel-Sprott and Fillmore, only highlights of learning processes relevant to situation effects are presented here.) In an analysis of learning mechanisms underlying the influence of situational variables on substance use and effects, the primary phenomenon of interest is *stimulus discrimination*. Bickel and Kelly (1988) noted that a "discriminative stimulus refers to a class of stimuli whose presence alters the probability of a class of responses previously reinforced in the presence of the stimulus class" (p. 122).

Modeling

Modeling may be thought of as a specific type of situational factor, that of the influence of others, who may be part of a situation, on one's own behavior. More specifically, modeling refers to a social influence process whereby observation of another performing a behavior influences the likelihood of a person engaging in that behavior. SLT states that models provide vicarious learning experiences with regard to the initiation of behavior. Modeling influences come into play before a person takes his or her first drink, because parents, siblings, peers, and the media are the first sources of information about drinking for most young people. Models can also provide normative information regarding previously acquired behavior. Hence, drinkers may look to other drinkers around them to learn how to use alcohol in a manner acceptable to their social group. The influence of modeling has been studied using both experimental and nonexperimental methods.

Experimental Studies. Early laboratory research established that modeling can be a proximal determinant of drinking (Abrams & Niaura, 1987). When college students had the opportunity to drink alcohol with another person, the students drank more in the presence of the heavy drinking confederate than in the presence of the light drinking confederate (Caudill & Marlatt, 1975; Hendricks, Sobell, & Cooper, 1978). Characteristics of the observer influence the modeling process in that the modeling effect is strongest for heavy versus light drinkers (Lied & Marlatt, 1979). The effects of modeling also seem to be pronounced for individuals with a positive family history of alcoholism. For example, in one study, the amount consumed with a heavy drinking model was greater in the positive family history group than the negative family history group; the family history positive group also consumed less than the family history negative group with a light drinking model (Chipperfield & Vogel-Sprott, 1988).

Characteristics of the model have been studied with mixed results. Neither model race (Watson & Sobell, 1982) nor social status (Collins, Parks, & Marlatt, 1985) have been found to interact with the primary effect of the model's consumption level. Model gender interacts with observer gender in that the modeling effect is strongest when males observe a heavy drinking male model (Cooper, Waterhouse, & Sobell, 1979). The warmth and sociability of the model are key to the modeling effect; drinkers tend not to match their drinking behavior to either heavy or light drinking models when the models behave in an indifferent or "cold" manner (Collins et al., 1985; Reid, 1978).

Nonexperimental Studies. Few laboratory studies of proximal modeling effects have been reported in the last decade. Instead, exploration of social influence on drinking behavior has used nonexperimental methods, employing structural equation modeling and hierarchical regression methods to study naturally occurring influences on behavior. Furthermore, modeling is often conceptualized as alcohol use by parents, peers, or siblings. For example, Webb and Baer (1995) tested a multivariate model of adolescent alcohol use that incorporated parental alcohol use (modeling), family disharmony, social skills, and self-efficacy in a sample of 805 seventh graders. Although they originally hypothesized that the adolescent's social skills would mediate the parental and family influences, a direct effect of parental alcohol use on adolescent alcohol use was observed and cross-validated. Webb and Baer concluded that both direct modeling of alcohol use by parents and general family environment are important influences on adolescent drinking, but the relationship between the two could not be determined with cross-sectional data. Ary, Tildesley, Hops, and Andrews (1993) addressed the influence of parental, sibling, and peer modeling on adolescent alcohol use in a prospective study of 173 families. All families had a target adolescent between the ages of 11 and 17, and at least one sibling 11 years of age or older. Parent modeling, defined as the frequency of parent alcohol use at Time 1, did not predict their children's use of alcohol at Time 1. Peer alcohol use did concurrently predict adolescents' drinking at Time 1, as did sibling alcohol use, somewhat more weakly. However, parent alcohol use did predict change in their adolescents' alcohol use at Time 2, 1 year later. Peer and sibling alcohol use predicted adolescents' Time 2 alcohol use only indirectly through prior drinking.

Hypothesized social influence factors have been divided into active influence (direct offers of alcohol) and passive influence (friends' drinking behavior and perceptions of friends' drinking). Graham, Marks, and Hansen (1991) tested the ability of these forms of social influence (assessed at Time 1) to predict adolescent drinking 6–12 months later (Time 2). In a sample of 526 seventh-grade students, all three of the factors making up active and passive influence helped to predict Time 2 drinking above and beyond Time 1 drinking. The pattern of findings did not differ between boys and girls. This study suggests that the drinking behavior modeled by one's three best friends does have an influence separate from the direct social pressure to drink.

Apparently the drinking behavior of parents does influence the drinking behavior of their children. Although the studies just reviewed show that parental modeling has an effect on future drinking by adolescents, the mechanism of this influence is unclear. Similarly, adolescent drinking resembles peer and sibling drinking at a given point in time. However, the causal relationships cannot be established. Perhaps the social influence occurs in a manner suggested by the laboratory studies: The presence of heavy drinking models in one's social group causes a matching of drinking styles. Alternatively, both adolescent alcohol use and peer/sibling alcohol use may share a common set of determinants.

Coping Skills

As reviewed earlier in this chapter, in 1969, Bandura hypothesized that alcohol problems resulted at least in part because of deficits in skills to manage (cope with) stressful events without the use of alcohol. According to this analysis, therefore, individuals who engage in regular, heavy drinking are using alcohol as a generalized coping response. This fundamental hypothesis received early experimental support in research on the effects of provocation (to aggression), opportunity to retaliate, and alcohol consumption in nonalcoholic men (Marlatt, Kosturn, & Lang, 1975). In this study, research participants were provoked by the experimenter's confederate. The findings showed that participants drank more alcohol in a "taste test" that served as an unobtrusive measure of ad lib alcohol consumption when they were not provided an opportunity to retaliate to the provocation compared to when they were. Furthermore, the coping skills hypothesis was carried forward to Marlatt and Gordon's (1985) influential outline of their SLT-based cognitive-behavioral model of addiction, presented earlier, and still is prominent (Monti, Rohsenow, Colby, & Abrams, 1995). Given the content of the coping skills model of substance use, most of the research relevant to it has concerned individuals with alcohol use disorders, although the hypothesis clearly has implications for the development of substance use disorder as well.

A few earlier studies concerning assessment of coping skills in clinical populations support the essential hypothesis that individuals with alcohol use disorder show a lower level of coping skills than do individuals in relevant comparison groups. Hamilton and Maisto (1979) compared individuals with or without alcohol use disorder on measures of assertiveness skill and discomfort. They found no differences between the groups on assertiveness; however, individuals with alcohol use disorder reported significantly more subjective discomfort in situations requiring the use of assertion skills. A study by Twentyman et al. (1982) compared problem and social drinkers on role-play tests involving general social skills and some alcohol-specific skills. The groups did not differ on their responses to general social skills, but problem drinkers gave less effective responses to situations involving drink-refusal skills. More recently, a study by Abrams et al. (1991) found that when alcoholic and nonproblem drinkers were compared on their role-play responses to general social situations, few differences were found. However, alcoholics were rated as less skillful and more anxious in their responses to alcohol-specific situations. Overall, these studies suggest there are few differences between individuals with alcohol use disorder and social drinkers in their level of general social skills. In contrast, alcoholics have consistently demonstrated less skillful responses in alcohol-specific situations.

The empirical literature on addiction-coping skills has emphasized the effectiveness of coping skills training interventions in the treatment of alcohol use disorders, and then in the treatment of other substance use disorders relative to other psychosocial treatments. In addition, coping skills training has been studied with regard to matching skills training to patient characteristics as well as to the effectiveness of coping skills training in combination with other treatments. To a lesser extent, coping skills assessment has been applied to special populations of alcohol abusers and to persons with other substance use disorders. A discussion of research on these topics follows.

Comparison of Coping Skills Treatment of Alcohol Use Disorders with Psychosocial Treatments

During the last decade, studies have compared coping skills treatments to other available psychosocial treatments. One such study sought to compare a group alcohol coping skills intervention to a process-oriented, inter-actional group therapy in a sample of female and male alcoholics recruited from an existing inpatient substance abuse unit (Kadden, Cooney, Getter, & Litt, 1989). The coping skills training focused on teaching relapse-prevention skills, while the interactional therapy was intended to foster insight and healthier interpersonal functioning by encouraging self-disclosure. Both the coping skills and interactional treatments were equally effective in reducing heavy drinking days at posttreatment. Similarly, the results at 2-year follow-up (Cooney, Kadden, Litt, & Getter, 1991) indicated no significant overall advantage of the coping skills intervention on the frequency of heavy drinking days.

At least one study compared a coping skills intervention with a second, behavioral treatment. Monti et al. (1990) administered a coping skills approach they labeled Communication Skills Training (CST) to two groups. In Group 1, CST was administered individually, and in Group 2, CST was administered in the presence of a significant other. The CST intervention was compared with an individually administered cognitive-behavioral treatment that included relaxation training and mood management components, termed Cognitive-Behavioral Mood Management Training (CBMMT). Participants in these standardized, 12-hour group treatments were 69 male alcoholics recruited from an inpatient unit of a VA Medical Center. In order to determine whether skills changed over the course of treatment, participants completed both the Simulated Social Interaction Test (SSIT; Monti, Wallander, Ahern, Abrams, & Munroe, 1984), which assesses general social skills, and the Alcohol-Specific Role-Play Test (ASRPT; Monti et al., 1993), both pre- and posttreatment. Alcoholics who received the individual CST treatment demonstrated greater improvement in the effectiveness of their alcohol-specific skills as compared with the other two groups. In addition, both CST groups consumed significantly less alcohol per drinking day during the 6-month posttreatment period as compared with alcoholics who received the CBMMT treatment. Effectiveness of coping responses in the ASRPT alcohol-related situations, but not in the SSIT general social situations, predicted number of abstinent days. The results of this study indicate that a communication-based coping skills intervention can result in better drinking outcomes relative to a more cognitively oriented behavioral treatment.

The Kadden et al. (1989) and Monti et al. (1990) studies suggest that coping skill interventions have not consistently resulted in better overall treatment outcomes for unselected samples of individuals assigned to these treatments. In an effort to isolate whether individuals with certain attributes are more likely to benefit from coping skills interventions, greater attention has been devoted to examining the relationship of patient characteristics to treatment outcome.

Patient–Treatment Matching Studies Involving Coping Skills Treatment

Kadden, Litt, Cooney, and Busher (1992) examined the data collected in their study comparing coping skills and interactional therapies to determine whether particular responses on a pretreatment alcohol role-play test interacted with type of treatment to predict outcome. These authors found that alcoholics who were rated as having better skills or less anxiety, or who reported lower levels of urge to drink during the role play, were more likely to be abstinent at the end of treatment if they had been assigned to the interactional group treatment. In contrast, alcoholics who were rated by an observer as having poorer skills or more anxiety were more likely to report abstinence if they received the coping skills treatment. This finding is consistent with the patient–treatment matching philosophy that skills remediation should be most effective for individuals with skills deficits.

These authors also examined whether patients could be matched to specific treatments based on pretreatment psychological variables. Consistent with Kadden et al.'s (1992) hypotheses, analyses of drinking outcomes indicated that at posttreatment, the coping skills intervention was more effective for individuals who were higher in sociopathy or psychopathology, and the interactional therapy was more effective for those individuals demonstrating lower levels of sociopathy and, to some extent, for individuals experiencing lower levels of psychopathology. However, contrary to predictions, individuals higher in neuropsychological impairment experienced fewer alcohol-related problems at posttreatment when assigned to the interactional treatment, while nonimpaired subjects experienced fewer problems in the coping skills treatment. Two-year follow-up data confirmed these initial findings (Cooney et al., 1991). In combination, the results of these studies indicate that individuals presenting with poorer initial coping skills, greater sociopathy, higher levels of psychopathology, or greater anxiety are good candidates for a coping skills intervention.

However, not all studies have found significant patient–treatment matching variables with coping skills interventions. Rohsenow and her colleagues (1991) analyzed data from a study comparing a coping skills intervention (CST) and a cognitive-behavioral treatment (CBMMT), discussed earlier in this section (Monti et al., 1990). They found that although individuals with higher levels of anxiety and urges during the alcohol-specific role plays had worse treatment outcomes in CBMMT, no significant inter-

actions were found between any of the pretreatment participant characteristics and CST. Therefore, in contrast to the studies by Kadden and his
colleagues (1992), this study failed to find evidence that coping skills interventions are better suited for certain individuals. The discrepancies between
these findings may be attributed to differences in the coping skills assessment administered at pretreatment, and to the fact that Rohsenow et al.
(1991) administered two behaviorally oriented treatments that resembled
each other more than did the coping skills and interactional interventions
in the Kadden et al. (1992) studies.

Adding Components to Coping Skills Treatment

Several studies have combined a coping skills intervention with either a second psychosocial intervention or with a pharmacological intervention.
Monti et al. (1993) administered a combination of cue exposure treatment
and urge coping skills training (CET) to 22 male alcoholics and compared
them to 18 male alcoholics in a contact-only control condition (CC) on
drinking outcome variables. At both 3- and 6-month follow-up, participants were asked to describe strategies they had used to cope with urges to
drink, including self-instruction, imagining negative consequences of returning to drinking, imagining positive consequences of sobriety, using imagery to reduce urges (e.g., slashing them with a sword), and substituting
alternative activities or consumption. At the 6-month follow-up, the CET
participants drank significantly less, were continuously abstinent longer,
had a higher percentage of abstinent days, and reported consuming fewer
drinks as compared with the CC group. In addition, the CET group reported greater use of coping strategies involving thinking about negative
consequences of drinking and the positive consequences of sobriety. These
strategies were significantly related to better drinking outcomes in both
groups. The results suggest that coping skills interventions can be effectively combined with other psychosocial interventions.

   Coping skills treatments have also been combined with a pharmacological intervention. O'Malley et al. (1996) investigated the separate and
combined effects of psychotherapy and pharmacotherapy on 6-month
drinking outcomes. The psychotherapy condition involved participation in
either coping skills training or supportive therapy, while the pharmacotherapy condition involved administration of naltrexone or placebo.
The results showed that among individuals receiving naltrexone, both the
coping skills and the supportive therapy groups resulted in similar rates of
drinking over the follow-up period. In contrast, among those individuals
receiving placebo, the coping skills group demonstrated significant decreases in drinking during the follow-up, while the supportive therapy
group showed a small increase in drinking. At the end of the 6-month follow-up, the two naltrexone groups and the placebo/coping skills groups
had similar rates of heavy drinking. The greater improvement of the coping

skills/placebo group in drinking outcomes over the follow-up period was attributed to a delayed emergence of the benefits associated with coping skills therapy. This study suggests that, in contrast to pharmacological interventions, coping skills treatments may not demonstrate improved outcomes at posttreatment but may take somewhat longer to emerge. Longer follow-up periods are needed to determine whether individuals receiving coping skills treatments continue to improve 1 or 2 years following the end of active treatment.

Coping Skills Assessment and Treatment in Special Populations

Little research has been done in applying coping skills assessment and treatment to special populations. Brown, Stetson, and Beatty (1989) assessed the self-report of coping responses in high-risk alcohol use situations among three samples of adolescents: alcohol abusing adolescents recruited from an inpatient treatment setting, nonabusing adolescents with a family history of alcohol abuse, and nonabusing adolescents without a family history of alcohol abuse. All three groups were asked about the cognitive and behavioral strategies used to cope in recent high-risk drinking situations. A comparison of cognitive coping responses indicated that in high-risk situations, alcohol abusers tended to focus on the potentially negative social repercussions from authority figures, whereas both groups of nonabusers tended to adopt an attitude of viewing themselves as nondrinkers. With respect to behavioral coping, more nonabusing adolescents reported avoiding or leaving a situation and declaring publicly they were not drinking as compared with abusing adolescents. Although correlational, this study suggests that examining differences in the types of coping strategies used by abusers and nonabusers to cope with high-risk drinking situations may be a useful initial step in assessing the viability of coping skills interventions with an adolescent population.

Coping Skills Interventions with Drug Users

Stephens, Roffman, and Simpson (1994) compared a relapse prevention treatment that included coping skills training with a social support intervention administered to men and women presenting for treatment of marijuana use. Posttreatment results indicated no significant differences between the treatment groups on drug-use outcome measures. However, men in the relapse prevention condition were more likely than those in the social support condition to report a reduced level of drug use, with no problems at the 3-month follow-up. Other gender differences did emerge, although they did not consistently indicate a better overall outcome for either gender. A limitation of this study is that it did not include the administration of a coping skills assessment pre- and posttreatment in order to determine if there were any differential changes in skills levels between groups over the course of treatment.

An earlier study by Hawkins and his colleagues (Hawkins, Catalano, Gillmore, & Wells, 1989; Wells, Catalano, Plotnick, Hawkins, & Brattesani, 1989) did include the administration of a coping skills role-play assessment before and after treatment. In this study, individuals received either the coping skills intervention or a control treatment. The results indicated that, contrary to predictions, the coping skills intervention did not result in better overall drug-use outcomes at 12-month follow-up. However, better performance on drug-specific coping skill role plays conducted at the end of treatment were predictive of less drug use and a greater number of weeks of abstinence in the first 6 months after treatment. However, responses to general social skills did not significantly predict posttreatment drug use.

The Relationship of Coping Skills to Substance Use in Community Samples

Several studies have examined the relationship of coping styles to alcohol use in samples of adolescents and adults recruited from the community. These studies have used the concepts of active, problem-focused coping and avoidant, emotion-focused coping. Problem-focused coping refers to cognitive or behavioral strategies intended to alter the source of the problem, whereas emotion-focused coping describes cognitive or behavioral strategies for managing the emotional distress, without any real efforts made to modify the stressor itself (Folkman & Lazarus, 1980). Studies have generally found that active, problem-focused coping is adaptive, and that avoidant, emotion-focused coping is maladaptive.

Cooper, Russell, Skinner, Frone, and Mudar (1992) examined the stress moderating effects of several variables, including demographics, alcohol expectancies, and coping style on alcohol use and related problems in a random community sample of black and white adults. They used several different measures to assess avoidant, emotion-focused coping and active, problem-focused coping. Relying on avoidant forms of coping predicted the frequency of alcohol-related problems, while engaging in active coping styles predicted decreased frequency of drinking to cope with problems. Furthermore, there was an interaction with gender such that men high in avoidance coping reported more alcohol problems than men low in avoidance coping; however, this relationship did not extend to women in the study. This study suggests that a maladaptive, avoidant, emotion-focused coping style may be an important component contributing to the development of problematic alcohol use.

These results are supported by a study conducted by Evans and Dunn (1995), in which they assessed the relationship of coping styles to alcohol use and alcohol-related problems in college students. This study is discussed later in this chapter in the section on concurrent evaluation of SLT constructs. Finally, not all studies have found a relationship between coping style and alcohol use or alcohol problems. Wagner (1993) examined the relationship of substance use involvement and several variables, including delay of gratification, impulsivity, peer substance use, stress, and coping style in a sample of high school students. Although initial multiple regression analyses supported the prediction that emotion-focused coping would predict greater substance use involvement, this relationship was weak when the proposed stress–coping model was evaluated using structural equation modeling. Peer substance use and perceived stress were far more powerful predictors of substance use involvement than was coping style.

Summary and Conclusions

This review suggests that coping skills interventions are not consistently more effective in the treatment of alcohol abuse when compared with other psychosocial interventions. Furthermore, although coping theory proposes a relationship between both general coping skills and alcohol-specific coping skills and substance use, the studies reviewed here suggest little relationship between responses to general social situations and alcohol treatment outcome. On the other hand, responses to alcohol and drug-specific situations have consistently predicted substance use following treatment. The data also provide some evidence that individuals with poorer coping skills and more psychopathology are more likely to benefit from coping skills treatment. Overall, these findings suggest that SLT needs to become more precise about the conditions that modify the relationship between coping skills and substance use. This conclusion also is consistent with the literature on relapse, which is reviewed later.

In addition to examining the effects of coping skills interventions alone, there is a need for more research on the effects of combining coping interventions with other psychosocial and pharmacological treatments. Moreover, few studies have assessed the application of coping skills interventions to special populations. For example, studies are needed to determine whether adolescents will tolerate the demands of a coping skills assessment, and whether coping skills interventions are effective with this population. Most coping skills studies have recruited only males or such small proportions of females that any effects of this treatment that are unique to women cannot be evaluated. In addition to women, it is not clear that the promising results of coping skills interventions will generalize to other racial or ethnic minority groups, and individuals with a co-occurring mental disorder. Given that coping skills interventions have been used primarily with white male patients, more effort should be made to recruit these subgroups in order to assess not only the effectiveness of these interventions, but also to determine whether coping skills interventions are viewed as acceptable treatments by these individuals.

A common difficulty among many of the studies reviewed is the duration of follow-up once active treatment has ended. Often, follow-up periods are only 6–12 months, which is too brief to determine the long-term outcomes of the coping skills interventions. A second common shortcoming among the studies reviewed has been the absence of procedures to determine the integrity of coping skills treatment. Therefore, it is impossible to judge whether the coping skill intervention is discernibly different from the comparison treatment.

Finally, although recent studies provide some support for the importance of coping styles in predicting negative alcohol outcomes in community samples, support for this idea is not universal. It may be that the importance of coping style as a vulnerability factor in substance abuse is dependent on the population being studied. Different factors may serve as risk factors for adults, as opposed to young adolescents. Whereas the Cooper et al. (1992) and Evans and Dunn (1995) studies were conducted with adults and young adults, the Wagner study involved adolescents. It is possible that among adolescents, other factors, such as peer influence, may play a more important role in the initiation of problematic substance use.

Cognitive Factors

SLT recognizes the role of cognitive mediational factors in alcohol and drug use behaviors. These include self-efficacy expectations (belief that one can enact a given behavior to achieve desired outcomes) and outcome expectancies (beliefs about behavior–consequences probabilities). We begin this section with a discussion of self-efficacy.

Self-Efficacy

Self-efficacy has been a focus in research on the development of alcohol use patterns as well as the process of recovery from problematic drinking. Much progress has been made regarding measurement of self-efficacy, but review of the recent literature indicates that some definitional inconsistencies persist. Specifically, some researchers have operationalized self-efficacy as confidence regarding one's ability not to drink heavily in a given set of situations (Annis & Davis, 1988), while others define self-efficacy as confidence in one's ability to abstain across situations (DiClemente, Carbonari, Montgomery, & Hughes, 1994; Young, Oei, & Crook, 1991). Ellickson and Hays (1991; Hays & Ellickson, 1990) introduced the construct of resistance self-efficacy, referring to the ability of adolescents to resist the pressure to drink in party or date situations. Although these definitions may be more similar than different, the slight variations in emphasis may differentially predict various measures of consumption. Despite the inconsistency in definition, literature published since the last review (Abrams & Niaura, 1987) affirms efficacy expectations as a key person variable linked to drinking behavior. However, its status as a mediator between situational and participant history variables and alcohol consumption remains to be established.

Psychometric Studies. The psychometric sophistication of self-efficacy assessment has developed substantially in the last decade. Several self-efficacy instruments with solid psychometric properties now are available. Annis's (1982) Situational Confidence Questionnaire (SCQ) evaluates confidence in the ability to resist drinking heavily. The original version contains 100 items representing high-risk situations derived from Marlatt and Gordon's (1985) typology: negative emotional states, negative physical states, positive emotional states, testing personal control, urges and temptations, interpersonal conflict, social pressure to drink, and positive emotional states. Thus, the SCQ yields eight scale scores as well as a general efficacy score. Several versions of the SCQ have been used, ranging from 39 items (Annis, 1987) to 15 items (Sitharthan & Kavanagh, 1990). Evidence exists for its factorial validity (Burling et al., 1989), known-groups validity (Miller, Ross, Emerson, & Todt, 1989), and predictive validity (Annis & Davis, 1988).

Two other self-efficacy scales measure abstinence efficacy, which denotes one's confidence for not drinking at all in a variety of situations. The Alcohol Abstinence Self-Efficacy Scale (AASE; DiClemente et al., 1994) consists of 20 items and yields two sets of scores: temptations to drink and confidence for not drinking in each situation. The temptation and efficacy scores are internally consistent and negatively correlated ($r = -.65$). Each separates into four factors representing high-risk situations: negative affect, social/positive, physical and other concerns, and withdrawal and urges. The factor structure of the AASE is invariant across gender, and no gender differences have been found in mean scores (DiClemente et al., 1994). The pattern of relationships among the subscales of the AASE and the Alcohol Use Inventory (AUI; Wanberg, Horn, & Foster, 1977) provide evidence of convergent and discriminant validity. The more problems reported on the AUI, the lower the self-efficacy score. Notably, the AASE scales were not related to daily drinking in this sample presenting for alcohol treatment.

Young, Oei, and Crook (1991) developed the 31-item Drinking Self-Efficacy Questionnaire (DSEQ). The DSEQ produces three factor scores (social pressure, opportunistic drinking, emotional relief), with good test–retest correlations (.84–.93) and alpha coefficients (.87–.94). Evidence for the validity of the DSEQ scales includes their ability to discriminate between problem and nonproblem drinkers, and to predict alcohol consumption in both student and community samples (Young et al., 1991). Additional research suggests a gender difference: In a sample of college students, females had higher opportunistic self-efficacy than males (Baldwin, Oei, & Young, 1993).

Since the previous review of SLT (Abrams & Niaura, 1987), enthusiasm for the study of self-efficacy and drinking behavior has been manifested in psychometric development of additional instruments to permit the reliable and valid assessment of this construct. The data suggest that the multiple dimensions of self-efficacy assessed by these scales may relate differentially to drinking patterns and problems. In addition to the psychometric studies, other recent research provides substantial evidence for the validity of the self-efficacy construct with regard to alcohol use. This evidence comes from diverse samples from nonclinical and clinical settings, including adolescents and adults, in Australia, Canada, and Norway, as well as the United States. First, we summarize evidence for construct and predictive validity derived from nonclinical samples and then describe and interpret the pattern of findings emerging from clinical samples of problem drinkers seeking treatment.

Nonclinical Samples. Self-efficacy has often been negatively related to alcohol consumption in nonclinical samples. For example, Young et al. (1991) reported that low self-efficacy significantly predicted concurrent alcohol consumption in both college student and community samples. Prospective studies also support the association between self-efficacy and consumption. In a sample of 241 women with recently confirmed pregnancies, those who started with higher abstinence self-efficacy drank less while they were pregnant than those with lower abstinence self-efficacy (Moore, Turner, Park, & Adler, 1996). Ellickson and Hays (1991) evaluated self-efficacy to resist drinking in two situations (at a party and on a date) in a longitudinal study of 1,138 eighth graders. These students were reassessed 9 months later on measures of alcohol and other drug use. Among the nonusers at Time 1, low-resistance self-efficacy predicted future alcohol use, demonstrating a direct effect in the structural model. Among the users at Time 1, low-resistance self-efficacy also predicted later alcohol use, but self-efficacy was mediated by expectations of use. This indirect effect indicates that self-efficacy influences adolescents' expectations of future alcohol use, which in turn predict alcohol use.

Additional research has addressed other aspects of construct validity, namely the relationship of self-efficacy to other variables known to be associated with alcohol use. Hays and Ellickson (1990) explored the relationships among self-efficacy for alcohol, marijuana, and cigarettes in the same large sample of eighth and ninth graders. They found that self-efficacy generalized across drugs, suggesting that a "generic" sense of self-efficacy may exist with regard to resisting use of these common drugs. Furthermore, self-efficacy for resisting alcohol during a date and at a party were distinct but correlated constructs. Similarly, resistance self-efficacy and degree of pressure to use were seen as related but distinct; thus, students did separate the perceived pressure to use from their ability to resist. Notably, the negative correlation between self-efficacy and pressure to use was strongest for alcohol and weakest for marijuana; this suggests that students felt less confident that they could resist drinking if pressured to do so, compared to resisting marijuana when pressured to use. The relation between self-efficacy and social skills in adolescents was explored by Webb and Baer (1995). Confidence in one's ability to control alcohol use was positively associated with level of social skills; in fact, association between poor social skills and use of alcohol was mediated by self-efficacy. These two studies suggest that self-efficacy may represent the ability of adolescents to enact the interpersonal skills necessary to resist social pressure to drink, a SLT-based hypothesis that often has been applied clinically.

Clinical Samples. The study of self-efficacy and treatment outcomes in clinical samples has produced a heterogeneous set of findings. Abstinence self-efficacy does differentiate individuals at various stages of recovery. Strom and Barone (1993) compared active abusers, recently detoxed abusers, and abstainers who had been sober for at least a year, and found that long-term abstainers reported higher levels of self-efficacy than either the active abusers or recently detoxed groups. A parallel finding was reported by Miller et al. (1989); these authors modified the SCQ to assess abstinence self-efficacy. Individuals who were sober for more than a year reported significantly stronger self-efficacy on seven of the eight SCQ scales than did individuals who were just admitted into alcohol treatment. Of course, self-efficacy differences found between groups who differ in recovery status may be explained by preexisting differences or by the experience of successful recovery. Thus, the studies just reviewed cannot address the predictive validity of self-efficacy in recovery from alcohol problems.

Several recent studies have explored the extent to which self-efficacy can predict outcome of alcohol treatment. When self-efficacy is assessed at pretreatment, it generally is not related to posttreatment outcomes (e.g., Langenbucher, Sulesund, Chung, & Morgenstern, 1996; Solomon & Annis, 1990). However, among clients who were drinking at follow-up, pretreatment self-efficacy did predict average daily consumption, even after controlling for intake drinking (Solomon & Annis, 1990). It should be noted that this finding was based on self-efficacy assessed by the SCQ, which measures confidence in not drinking heavily across a wide range of situations. Although not a sensitive predictor of abstinence, it appears related to exactly what it assessed—ability to control quantity of drinking if one does drink.

Completing treatment for an alcohol use disorder appears to enhance self-efficacy. Mean levels of self-efficacy for controlling heavy drinking increased from pretreatment to posttreatment to follow-up for both male and female participants in a controlled drinking program (Sitharthan & Kavanagh, 1990). In contrast to pretreatment self-efficacy, posttreatment self-efficacy has been shown to be a significant predictor of treatment outcome even at long-term follow-up. For example, Sitharthan and Kavanagh demonstrated that posttreatment self-efficacy predicted alcohol consumption 6 months later, even after controlling for demographic, alcohol history, and dependence variables, as well as consumption during treatment. However, in the same study, posttreatment self-efficacy for controlling heavy drinking was not predictive of number of abstinent days at follow-up. The differential prediction of drinking level versus abstinence is consistent with the findings of Solomon and Annis (1990).

McKay, Maisto, and O'Farrell (1993) provide further support for the ability of posttreatment self-efficacy to predict 12-month treatment outcome. Their findings differed from those of Sitharthan and Kavanagh (1990) in two important ways. First, high levels of posttreatment self-efficacy predicted more percent days abstinent and fewer percent days of heavy drinking, even after controlling for the corresponding consumption variable during treatment. Second, the relation of self-efficacy to outcome held only in the condition that did not receive any aftercare. Among the clients who did continue to participate in aftercare during follow-up, posttreatment self-efficacy did not predict any outcome variable. This study identifies continued contact with treatment as a moderator that alters the relationship between self-efficacy and outcome.

In summary, because self-efficacy appears to be modified by treatment experiences, posttreatment self-efficacy tends to be a better predictor of outcome. However, it appears that matching the type of self-efficacy assessed (abstinence vs. avoiding heavy drinking) with outcome variables (abstinent days vs. alcohol consumption) may be important. Furthermore, involvement with aftercare appears to eliminate the association between posttreatment self-efficacy and drinking outcomes. Thus, to maximize the predictive validity of self-efficacy, it should be assessed in a way that is parallel to the outcome it predicts, and it should be assessed at the point of last treatment contact.

Information from Other Drugs. The construct of self-efficacy has also been evaluated in the context of other drugs. In a laboratory study, cocaine-dependent patients were presented with cocaine-related cues (Avants, Margolin, Kosten, & Cooney, 1995). Those who did not respond to the cocaine cues with either increased cravings or decreased aversion to cocaine were identified as nonresponders. The nonresponders (n = 21) were compared to the responders (n = 48) on several variables, including abstinence self-efficacy. Nonresponders reported significantly higher self-efficacy for mood states than did responders. In contrast, the groups did not differ on self-efficacy for social pressure/cues or for stressful situations. The results of this study suggest that lack of a strong craving or approach response to cocaine cues is linked to confidence in one's ability to resist using cocaine when experiencing strong mood states. This interpretation is consistent with Bandura's (1977) suggestion that a key source of efficacy information is physiological responses to relevant situations.

Stephens and colleagues (Stephens, Wertz, & Roffman, 1993, 1995) explored the relationship of self-efficacy to resist marijuana use to marijuana treatment outcome. Contrary to SLT predictions, these authors found that self-efficacy did not mediate the effects of other variable groups (demographics, psychological distress, and drug use) on marijuana use or related problem outcomes; each predictor group, including self-efficacy, made a separate and independent contribution to the accounted for variance (Stephens et al., 1993). A follow-up set of analyses addressed hypothesized sources of self-efficacy for avoiding marijuana use (Stephens et al., 1995). These hypothesized sources (use behavior, temptation ratings, availability of coping responses, perceived stress, and contact with users) all significantly predicted self-efficacy. However, self-efficacy only partially mediated the effect of the source variable on posttreatment outcomes; that is, the predictive power of the source variables was reduced, but not eliminated, when self-efficacy entered the regression equation first, suggesting that the ability of the source variables to predict later marijuana use was not entirely accounted for by their contributions to self-efficacy. Similar studies testing predictions from SLT regarding alcohol self-efficacy are needed.

Summary. The construct of self-efficacy has generated a substantial amount of research in the alcohol field. Measurement and basic-construct-validity problems have been addressed. The relationship of self-efficacy to drinking behavior has cross-cultural validity and, when evaluated, no gender effects have emerged. Nonetheless, several questions remain. The first question concerns the significance of the distinction between abstinence self-efficacy and self-efficacy to resist drinking heavily. Existing data suggest that sometimes these differentially predict corresponding outcomes. Such conceptual and definitional heterogeneity with regard to self-efficacy has emerged with regard to other behaviors (Forsyth & Carey, 1998), and poses problems for interpretation of research data. The second question concerns the need to consider factors that moderate the influence of self-efficacy on drinking behavior; one such factor already identified is aftercare participation. The issue of moderators should also be considered in nonclinical samples. Finally, the sources of alcohol self-efficacy still are not well understood; although treatment participation does enhance self-efficacy, it is not clear what features of treatment account for this increase. If sources of alcohol self-efficacy could reliably be identified, then it might be possible to enhance individuals' resistance to problematic drinking.

Alcohol-Outcome Expectancies

Several measures have been developed to assess alcohol-outcome expectancies (e.g., Brown, Goldman, Inn, & Anderson, 1980; Fromme, Stroot, & Kaplan, 1993; Leigh & Stacy, 1991; Southwick, Steele, Marlatt, & Lindell, 1981; Young & Knight, 1989). These vary with regard to item structure, response options, and number of factors extracted. The two expectancy scales that have received the greatest psychometric attention are described to illustrate important measurement and conceptual issues.

The Alcohol Expectancy Questionnaire (AEQ; Brown et al., 1980) is the most commonly used instrument; it has a version suitable for use with adolescents, the AEQ-Adolescent (AEQ-A; Christiansen, Goldman, & Inn, 1982). Respondents indicate agreement or disagreement with 90 items reflecting reinforcement from alcohol (e.g., "Alcohol decreases my hostilities"). The AEQ yields six scales: global positive change, sexual enhancement, physical and social pleasure, social assertiveness, relaxation and tension reduction, arousal and aggression. The AEQ-A yields seven slightly different scales: global positive change, social facilitation, improved cognitive–motor abilities, sexual enhancement, cognitive–motor impairment, increased arousal, relaxation and tension reduction. Brown, Christiansen, and Goldman (1987) summarized supporting psychometric data. Subsequent research demonstrated that the strength of a person's belief in each expectancy item can be differentiated from simple endorsement of each item (Collins, Lapp, Emmons, & Isaac, 1990); thus, high scores on the AEQ scales may best be interpreted as breadth of endorsement rather than strength of expectancies.

The Effects of Drinking Alcohol scale (EDA; Leigh & Stacy (1991) consists of 34 items representing both positive and negative effects of alcohol (e.g., feel sleepy, get aggressive). A 6-point Likert-type scale indicates how likely–unlikely it is that alcohol would have each effect. Exploratory and confirmatory factor analyses support four positive expectancy factors (social facilitation, sex, fun, negative reinforcement) and four negative expectancy factors (negative emotions, negative social, negative physical, cognitive/performance). These factors are weakly correlated, suggesting that they are independent components of expectancy. Although both positive and negative expectancies predict drinking behavior, negative outcome expectancies have less influence on alcohol use than positive outcome expectancies (Leigh & Stacy, 1993; Stacy, Widaman, & Marlatt, 1990). Accumulated research suggests that negative expectancies differentiate nondrinkers from drinkers, but positive expectancies account for more variance in patterns of alcohol use among drinkers (Brown, 1993).

Independent confirmatory factor analysis on these expectancy measures calls into question the discriminative validity of subscales; that is, each identified subscale may not represent separate and distinct expectancy dimensions (Leigh, 1989). Rather, the scales may best be interpreted as correlated dimensions related to a general alcohol expectancy that nonetheless has predictive validity with regard to drinking behavior.

Outcome Expectancies and Drinking Behavior. A large body of literature supports the association between outcome expectancies and alcohol use and problems. These relationships hold across several instruments used to operationalize outcome expectancies, and across populations (e.g., adolescents, adults, and adults in treatment for alcohol use disorders), and cultures. Specifically, expectancies are positively associated with level of alcohol consumption in both adolescents and adults, and discriminate between problem and nonproblem drinkers (Brown, Christiansen, & Gold-man, 1987). In prospective studies, outcome expectancies predict alcohol use (Stacy, Newcomb, & Bentler, 1991) and high-risk drinking (Carey, 1995), even after accounting for the influence of previous drinking behavior. Among persons in treatment for alcoholism, greater expectancies were associated with more negative treatment outcome (Brown, 1985); that is, the more positive reinforcement from alcohol expected by participants before treatment, the less likely they were to be abstinent or drinking in a nonproblem way 1-year posttreatment. Some preliminary evidence indicates that experimental manipulation of expectancies may successfully lower expectancies and decrease drinking (Darkes & Goldman, 1993). These findings suggest that direct "expectancy challenge" could become a component of interventions for problem use.

Recent research sheds light on the developmental aspects of the expectancy–drinking behavior relationship. Evidence suggests that expectancies develop before the onset of drinking, and that late childhood and early adolescence may be the key period for expectancy development (Miller, Smith, & Goldman, 1990). Parental drinking patterns appear to contribute to the development of alcohol reinforcement expectancies; adolescents with alcoholic parents endorse expectancies with a greater degree of strength than adolescents with nonalcoholic parents (Brown, Creamer, & Stetson, 1987). In a sample of high school students, risk for developing drinking problems, as defined by personality variables, was positively associated with endorsement of alcohol expectancies (Mann, Chassin, & Sher, 1987). Furthermore, the relationship between personality risk and expectancies was strongest in students who reported a positive family history of alcoholism. These early representations of the likely outcomes of drinking alcohol influence the onset and course of one's drinking career. Vicariously developed expectancies predict the start of drinking and the development of drinking problems in adolescents (Christiansen, Smith, Roehling, & Goldman, 1989). Specifically, adolescents who expect social enhancement and improved cognitive and motor functioning are more likely to become involved with alcohol.

Questions have been raised about the nature of the relationship between expectancies and subsequent drinking behavior. If outcome expectancies predict later drinking behavior, does drinking influence the development of expectancies? This question is discussed later in this chapter in the section on empirical evidence for reciprocal determinism.

Distinction between Efficacy and Outcome Expectancies

SLT predicts that efficacy and outcome expectancies are distinct constructs that independently contribute to the prediction of behavior. This hypothesis has been evaluated in empirical studies of alcohol use. Burke and Stephens (1997) found consistently negative correlations between tension-reduction expectancies and self-efficacy for Positive Situations, Negative Situations, and Socially Anxious Situations. A similar pattern of negative correlations was found between self-efficacy and outcome expectancies in a study conducted in Australia (Baldwin et al., 1993). Thus, as beliefs in the positive effects of alcohol get stronger, self-efficacy for limiting or refusing opportunities to drink decreases. Despite consistent negative relationships, these constructs retain independent predictive power. Aas, Klepp, Laberg, and Aaro (1995) demonstrated that self-efficacy has a weaker relationship to drinking intentions than do outcome expectancies among Norwegian adolescents; however, self-efficacy did significantly predict intentions to drink, even after controlling for the influence of alcohol expectancies.

The unique predictive ability of self-efficacy and outcome expectancies generalizes to differential prediction of drinking indices. For example, high opportunistic and social-pressure self-efficacy were associated with less frequent drinking, whereas high expectancies for positive effects of alcohol were associated with more quantity consumed per occasion in Australian college students (Baldwin et al., 1993). Another study from this research group revealed slightly different findings with drinkers recruited from the community. Self-efficacy predicted usual frequency and maximum quantity consumed per occasion; outcome expectancies also predicted usual frequency and maximum frequency (Lee & Oei, 1993). These findings indicate that self-efficacy and outcome expectancies may be related to different aspects of drinking behavior. Additional study of these relationships appears warranted.

In summary, the empirical evidence supports the view that alcohol outcome expectancies mediate the effects of environmental, social, and psychological antecedents on drinking events. Thus, a person will drink alcohol in a social context (e.g., a party) if he or she holds outcome expectancies about the social-facilitation effects of alcohol. However, a person will not drink alcohol in another social context (e.g., in a job interview) if he or she holds outcome expectancies regarding the negative cognitive effects of alcohol. Given the existence of individual differences in outcome expectancies, exploration into the sources of specific expectancies is warranted. In addition, early evidence justifies further investigation of methods for modifying outcome expectancies when they have become maladaptive.

TWO SPECIAL TOPICS: RECIPROCAL DETERMINISM AND CONCURRENT EVALUATION OF SOCIAL LEARNING THEORY CONSTRUCTS

In this section we review empirical literature on two topics important to the evaluation of SLT. The first of these is reciprocal determinism, which was earlier defined as bidirectional causality between two variables. Therefore, one variable can both influence and be influenced by another variable. The second topic, concurrent evaluation, refers to how the literature on SLT and alcohol use has evolved. In this regard, the literature on SLT and alcohol use has consisted primarily of the evaluation of SLT constructs in isolation from one another and has paid little attention to their concurrent evaluation in *an evaluation of theoretically derived predictions*. This feature of the literature was reflected in the organization of our review of empirical research relevant to SLT in the preceding sections of this chapter. Evaluation of a construct by itself is an important step in advancing knowledge about the validity of a theory of which it is a part. However, it is essential for any multivariate theory such as SLT to move beyond this point to consider its multiple constructs concurrently for at least two reasons. First, evaluation of constructs in isolation does not allow an appreciation of SLT as a dynamic theory of alcohol use. Second, from a methodological view, it does not allow an appraisal of the independent contribution that the multiple constructs of SLT make to drinking behavior (Evans & Dunn, 1995). We begin this section with a discussion of empirical studies relevant to the concept of reciprocal determinism.

Reciprocal Determinism

As reviewed earlier, reciprocal determinism is a major feature of SLT that distinguishes it from more traditional learning theories. (In his 1986 book, Bandura extended this idea to triadic reciprocality.) In fact, this idea has been viewed as an essential feature of social behavior for some time (e.g., Rogosa, 1979), but until recently, it has received little systematic empirical attention because of a lack or inaccessibility of statistical methods needed for scientific study of reciprocal relationships between variables. Fortunately, this no longer is true because of advances that have been made in structural equation modeling (SEM) techniques (Hoyle, 1994), and in their accessibility to the research community. The application of SEM to longitudinal data provides one method of investigating reciprocal relationships between variables.

Several recently published studies involved the use of SEM to study reciprocal relationships between SLT-relevant constructs. Three of the articles concern the relationship between alcohol-related expectancies and alcohol (or other drug) use, and two of the articles concern the relationship between the individual's alcohol use and that of his or her peers. The latter two studies are relevant to the question of the effects of modeling on an individual's drinking behavior.

Expectancies and Alcohol Use

Stacy, Newcomb, and Bentler (1991) compared three models of the alcohol-expectancy relationship, including expectancy theory, self-perception/behavioral choice theory, and reciprocal determinism. Briefly, expectancy theory would predict that the primary causal path is from expectancy to alcohol consumption; that is, expectancy is viewed as being a causal mediator of alcohol consumption, so that expectancy would be predicted to influence alcohol consumption. However, expectancy theory says little about the effects of alcohol consumption on expectancy. According to self-perrception/behavioral choice theories, alcohol consumption is the primary determinant of expectancies. The latter are viewed as epiphenomena of drinking behavior and as not causing it. Finally, reciprocal determinism argues that expectancies affect drinking, which in turn may modify expectancies.

Stacy et al. (1991) used a two-wave longitudinal survey design to evaluate the relative validity of these three perspectives. The subjects were 584 men and women, who were selected from a larger study of drug use etiology and consequences. The mean age of subjects at the first interview was 17.95 years, and at the second interview 9 years later, their mean age was 26.95 years. In this study, four constructs were included in the models evaluated: frequency of alcohol and other drug use, quantity of alcohol and other drug use, alcohol and other drug problems, and the expectancy construct of cognitive motivation, which was measured separately for alcohol and marijuana.

The crux of the Stacy et al. (1991) research consisted of the application of SEM methods to evaluate which of three models (each representing one of the three theories described earlier) best fit the data. The results of such analyses showed the strongest and most consistent support for the expectancy theory model, and only weak and inconsistent support for the reciprocal determinism model. Specifically, support for expectancy theory was indicated by significant paths between alcohol or marijuana motivation at Wave 1 and drug use constructs at Wave 2. Inconsistent with the other two perspectives, paths between drug use constructs at Wave 1 were not expected to predict alcohol or marijuana motivation at Wave 2.

Smith, Goldman, Greenbaum, and Christiansen (1995) also designed a study to evaluate the reciprocal relationship between alcohol use and expectancies, and to determine whether expectancies predicted individual differences in changes in alcohol consumption over time. This longitudinal survey study differed from that of Stacy et al. (1991) in several ways. First, three waves of data collection were included, and an attempt was made to capture the time period in which adolescents tend to become regular drinkers. In this regard, the participants were public school students aged 12–14 at the first assessment, and the three assessments were 1 year apart. Another facet of this study was the use of latent-growth-modeling statistical methods to complement the use of SEM techniques. SEM methods evaluate average changes over time but do not emphasize individual differences in change (i.e., deviations from the average). Latent growth methods, however, focus on such deviations and provide information on individual differences in growth or change in a phenomenon over time. Such methods, therefore, are especially applicable to the study of drinking in adolescents.

The sample in this study included 461 boys (46%) and girls at the first assessment, and the 3-year sample did not differ appreciably from the original sample. The major constructs measured in this study were alcohol expectancies (regarding social facilitation) and drinking style. The results of evaluation of statistical models showed, first, that participants' drinking did increase over the course of the 3-year study period, and that there was significant variability in such change. As predicted, expectancies about alcohol's effects on social facilitation predicted growth in drinking: The stronger the social expectancy, the greater the increase in drinking over time. In addition, SEM techniques found support for the reciprocal determinism model for alcohol expectancy and drinking over time, relative to a model incorporating only autoregressive (correlation of a variable with itself, such as drinking at Time 1 with drinking at Time 2, over time) and cross-sectional (regarding variables measured at the same time point, in Time 2) relationships between drinking and expectancies. Importantly, analyses also showed that the relationship between social expectancy and changes in alcohol use applied to both boys and girls, and that the reciprocal relationship between alcohol use and expectancy over time also applied to participants of both sexes.

Sher, Wood, Wood, and Raskin (1996) reported a study that addresses questions raised in both the Stacy et al. (1991) and the Smith et al. (1995) studies. In this regard, Sher et al. tested the three models representing relationships between alcohol use and expectancies cited earlier (expectancy theory, self-perception/behavioral choice, and reciprocal determinism). They also evaluated the validity of the models with older participants than those in the Smith et al. study, as well as with different time lags of assessment in a four-wave longitudinal survey design. At the first assessments, participants were 489 male and female freshman at a large state university; data from 465 of these individuals were available for the longitudinal analyses. A total of 109 of the participants were male children of alcoholics, 127 were female children of alcoholics; 111 were male children of nonalcoholics, and 118 were female children of nonalcoholics. Each of the four waves of data collection were separated by 1 year.

Expectancies and alcohol consumption were the major constructs of interest in this study. The model evaluation for the four-wave data showed that the reciprocal determinism model provided a good fit to the data, after the autoregressive and cross-sectional relationships between expectancies and alcohol use were taken into account. Further analyses evaluated the three models using only two waves of data, the first and last years of the study. The results of these analyses did not support the reciprocal determinism model, but like Stacy et al. (1991) supported the expectancy theory model. The pattern of findings for the two- and four-wave data seemed to be consistent for both participant sexes and for both family histories (of alcoholism).

To summarize, these three studies of the relationship between alcohol use and expectancies lead to several conclusions. First, advances in statistical methods now make possible systematic evaluation of one of SLT's major principles, that of reciprocal determinism. Reciprocal determinism does seem to characterize the relationship between alcohol use and expectancies over time, especially in younger adolescents over shorter time periods. However, the data do not support such a relationship for older adolescents and young adults, and when assessment intervals are farther apart in time (Sher et al., 1996; Stacy et al., 1991). Sher et al.'s speculation about possible reasons for this pattern of findings, which centers on differences between adolescents and young adults in both alcohol use and expectancies, needs evaluation in future research. In conclusion, besides having heuristic value, the three studies cited here provide a base for a more refined statement about the expectancy–alcohol use relationship, especially regarding the conditions under which reciprocal determinism may hold.

Peer Influences on Individuals' Alcohol Use

Farrell (1994) reported a study designed to evaluate three hypotheses about the relationship between the individual's alcohol use and that of his or her peers. Peer cluster theory predicts that peer models and anger have direct effects on alcohol (and other drug) use, and that anger has an indirect effect through (i.e., is mediated by peer models). SEM techniques were used to compare the fit of this model to the data with the fit of a hypothesis that alcohol use in adolescents causes peers' use, and of a reciprocal determinism model. The participants in this three-wave longitudinal study were 1,122 boys (39%) and girls (61%) who were beginning the seventh grade at the first assessment, at the end of the seventh grade at the second assessment, and at the end of the eighth grade by the third assessment. A total of 91.9% of the sample were African American, 52% were from lower income families, and 57% were from single-parent households.

The major findings of model evaluation showed that the best fit for the data was the model in which the individual's alcohol use predicts peer use. However, the pattern of findings was different for boys and girls. For boys, the individual's alcohol use at Time 1 predicted peer use at Time 2. However, for girls, alcohol use at Time 2 significantly predicted peer alcohol use at Time 3. Despite these differences, the structure of the model was similar for boys and girls.

A study by Curran, Stice, and Chassin (1997) applied SEM and latent growth modeling to evaluate the peer–individual alcohol use relationship, and to evaluate individual differences in changes regarding individuals' and peers' alcohol use over time in a sample of adolescents. In this three-wave longitudinal study, the participants at Time 1 were 454 adolescents aged 10.5–15.5 years and their parents. This sample consisted of 246 children of alcoholics and 208 children of nonalcoholics. Assessments were spaced 1 year apart. The analyses reported in this study included participants who reported at least some alcohol use by themselves and by their peers, a total of 363 families. For this latter sample, the average age at Time 1 was 12.9 years, 56% were children of alcoholics, 48% were female, 25% were Hispanic, and 75% were white.

The results of the latent growth and SEM modeling were as follows. Although peer alcohol use increased for the entire group of participants over time, participants who reported lower alcohol use at Time 1 tended to increase in peer alcohol use at a steeper rate compared to adolescents who used more alcohol at Time 1. In addition, although the entire group showed increasing alcohol use over time, adolescents who reported higher peer alcohol use at Time 1 showed a steeper increase in their own alcohol use compared to adolescents who reported lower peer alcohol use. These trends in growth did not seem to vary as a function of participant sex and were not related to a measure of the adolescent's rebelliousness, which previously had been found to be related to adolescent drinking. Finally, application of SEM techniques showed that individuals with higher levels of alcohol use at one time period tended to report higher peer alcohol use at the next time period, and vice versa. Therefore, the reciprocal determinism model provided a good fit to the data compared to alternatives, which is not consistent with Farrell's (1994) data. Curran et al. (1997) suggest that the difference in results may be due to differences in the characteristics of the research participants. In this regard, Farrell's sample was predominantly African American adolescents, whose alcohol consumption has not been shown to be as strongly influenced by peers as is the drinking of white and Hispanic adolescents.

In summary, peer alcohol use has been shown consistently to be highly correlated with drinking in adolescents. This finding is relevant specifically to a SLT perspective of alcohol use, because the association between an individual's alcohol use and that of his or her peers has been assumed to reflect the action of modeling processes, as well as direct differential reinforcement, on the individual's drinking. The studies reviewed here suggest that the relationship between peer and adolescent alcohol use may be bidirectional, at least for white and Hispanic individuals. However, reciprocal determinism may not characterize the association between these two variables among African American adolescents.

To conclude this section, recent research using SEM techniques and longitudinal designs to evaluate the hypothesis of reciprocal determinism represent a significant advance in the application of SLT to substance use. Such research gives systematic empirical attention to a feature of social behavior long acknowledged but not investigated quantitatively. Therefore, the recent trend of combining SEM and related techniques along with longitudinal designs would advance this field. Moreover, the studies that have been done suggest that any such future research address moderators of reciprocal relationships among variables.

Concurrent Evaluation Studies

Cooper et al. (1988) presented a model that combined the SLT constructs of general coping skills, positive expectancies about alcohol's effects, the use of alcohol to cope with stress, and heavy alcohol use in prediction of the outcomes of alcohol abuse/alcohol dependence. It is important to note that, as reviewed in the section on the coping skills model, the construct of drinking to cope with stress focuses on alcohol-specific coping skills, in contrast to general coping skills. Cooper et al.'s use of their model to make predictions about the relationships among these constructs is consistent with the SLT and alcohol use literature up to 1988.

The subjects in this one-time survey study were 119 adults who met formal diagnostic criteria for current alcohol abuse or dependence and a comparison sample of 948 individuals who drank in the last year but had no history of alcohol use disorder. The mean age of the participants was 40 years; 57% of them were female, and 51% of them were African American. Measures of the major constructs all involved the use of established instruments. A series of multiple regression analyses were conducted in a way that is analogous to the use of path analysis in evaluation of the SLT-based model. In these analyses, both participant sex and age were included as control factors. The first set of analyses involved prediction of drinking to cope. As hypothesized, the results showed that individuals who scored higher on avoidance as a general way of coping, and who scored higher on expectancies, tended to score highest on using alcohol to cope. Similarly, individuals who scored lower on active, problem-focused general coping tended to use alcohol to cope if they also scored higher on expectancies. Therefore, expectancies moderated the relationship between general coping skills and using alcohol to cope. The second set of analyses concerned the prediction of alcohol consumption and also strongly supported the model. Individuals who were higher on expectancies, had fewer active general coping skills, and used alcohol to cope, tended to have the highest levels of alcohol consumption. Finally, the third set of analyses showed that individuals who reported using alcohol to cope, and who scored higher on expectancies, were most likely to have a diagnosis of alcohol use disorder. When the results of these three sets of parallel analyses were combined in an evaluation of the entire path model, the findings strongly supported the model's validity.

Evans and Dunn (1995) reported a survey study designed to replicate and extend Cooper et al.'s (1988) research. Evans and Dunn collected data from 157 college students (68% female) with a mean age of 19 years. The participants were asked to respond to measures of coping styles, positive alcohol expectancies, alcohol use in the last 30 days, and alcohol problems. This study added a measure of another construct central to SLT, that of self-efficacy. Therefore, Evans and Dunn's study was similar in aims to that of Cooper et al., and it measured most of the same constructs.

Multiple regression analyses showed that being male and scoring higher on the expectancy measure and lower on self-efficacy all predicted a higher level of alcohol consumption. The effects of coping style and coping style × expectancies interaction were not significant. This latter finding may have been due to Evans and Dunn's use of a coping measure that was made alcohol-specific, rather than the general coping skills measure used by Cooper et al. In the prediction of alcohol problems, participant gender, expectancies, alcohol consumption, avoidant coping style, and self-efficacy all were statistically significant. Males who scored higher on expectancies, who drank more, who used an avoidant coping style, and who were lower on self-efficacy were more likely to report more alcohol problems. Again, the coping × expectancy terms in the regression model were not significant. The pattern of findings from these two sets of analyses were interpreted as being consistent with those of Cooper et al. and of SLT.

In summary, two studies have been published with the explicit aim of simultaneous evaluation of constructs central to SLT in the prediction of alcohol use and problems. Despite considerable differences in the samples and data-analytic procedures used in the two studies, their results generally may be viewed as consistent with SLT. The studies also suggest that avoidant coping may be a strong predictor of alcohol problems, which is in contrast to the more important role typically given to active coping by social learning theorists. The Cooper at al. (1988) and Evans and Dunn (1995) research stands out because of their evaluation of hypotheses that specifically follow from SLT, as well as their methodological sophistication. Throughout the literature on the etiology and modification of substance use patterns, it is possible to find research that uses multivariate analyses in the evaluation of two or more constructs that are relevant to SLT. However, few of these studies have been designed to evaluate the validity of SLT-based predictions. The Cooper et al. and Evans and Dunn studies achieved that end. On the other hand, it also is important to note that the findings of both of these studies would be bolstered by replication and extension through the use of longitudinal designs and more robust statistical modeling techniques, such as SEM. Furthermore, neither of the two studies included a comparison of the SLT model to other possible models. A comparative evaluation of models is essential to an appraisal of their worth.

RELAPSE

The previous sections of this chapter have emphasized what typically have been thought of as SLT-based independent variables or determinants of alcohol or other drug use. (This traditional way of thinking about these variables does not follow the idea of reciprocal determinism, which suggests that a given variable can serve as both an independent and dependent variable in the same causal sequence, due to feedback relationships among variables.) In this section, however, we review research on the topic of relapse, which usually is viewed as a dependent variable. More specifically, relapse is one type of outcome that most often is studied in the context of alcohol or other drug treatment. The term relapse is borrowed from the treatment of physical diseases and generally refers to the recurrence of a disease state after some period of remission.

When applied to phenomena that have behavioral, psychological, and social components, such as the substance use disorders, scientists hold mixed views about the utility of the term "relapse" (Miller, 1996). Nevertheless, research designed to advance understanding of the problem of relapse has been a fundamentally important part of addictions research for the last 20 years. Despite the importance of this topic, no consensus has emerged on a definition of relapse. In practice, relapse most often has meant a return to alcohol or other drug use after some time period of voluntary, committed abstinence from those substances by individuals with substance use disorder. Because relapse research is concerned with the topic of maintenance of behavior change, it is considered to be among the most important clinical research areas in the addictions (Allen, Lowman, & Miller, 1996; Rounsaville, 1986).

Marlatt and Gordon's (1985) Social Learning Theory Model of the Relapse Process

Marlatt and Gordon's (1985) model of the relapse process is the most representative and influential of the SLT-based models, although others have applied SLT principles to make major contributions to the study of relapse (Annis, 1986; Litman, 1986). Marlatt and Gordon's model depicts a two-stage process of relapse. Initial use of a substance following abstinence is called a lapse, which results from the individual's exposure to a high-risk situation, the lack of availability or use of coping skills to handle that situation without consuming a substance, low levels of self-efficacy expectancies to cope with the situation without resorting to substance use, and expectancies that use of a substance will help to cope with the situation effectively. (It is worth mentioning again that, although initial use following a period of abstinence is called a lapse in this and other models, the empirical literature often does not distinguish between a lapse and a relapse.) A lapse may extend to further use of a substance, called a relapse, primarily as a result of cognitive and affective processes. Specifically, if an individual attributes the lapse to global, internal (personal) qualities that are enduring, a lapse is most likely to proceed to a relapse. An example of such an attribution is "I don't have enough willpower." Movement into a relapse may be the result of two processes. First, such global, stable, and internal attributions may give the individual a perception of loss of control over his or her substance use, which could result in abandoning any attempts to control it once a lapse has occurred. Second, additional substance use may be an effort to alleviate the negative affect that tends to be generated with such attributions, so that a cycle of use → negative affect → further use is generated. The cognitions and negative affect hypothesized to follow from a lapse are called the abstinence violation effect (AVE).

A component of the Marlatt and Gordon (1985) model that has received a lot of attention from researchers is the taxonomy of high-risk situations. The most commonly used version of the taxonomy consists of two general categories, called intrapersonal and interpersonal determinants. The basis of this taxonomy was a study that Marlatt and his colleagues conducted in the early 1970s and consisted of a 3-month follow-up interview of a sample of males following completion of an episode of aversion therapy for alcoholism. A subsequent series of studies resulted in the current version of the high-risk situation taxonomy and the current model of the relapse process (see Marlatt, 1996).

It should be noted that there have been questions about the generalizability and accuracy of Marlatt and Gordon's (1985) model of relapse, principally because of the method of data collection and the characteristics of the sample from which the data in Marlatt's initial study of relapse precipitants were obtained. These methodological questions pertain primarily to the development of the taxonomy of high-risk situations. In this regard, because the taxonomy was derived from a content analysis of responses to an open-ended interview conducted at varying lengths of time after the event (first drink) in question, it may be that problems inherent in retrospective self-report data may have seriously biased the accuracy of the data and, therefore, the inferences that were made from them (Hammersley, 1994). However, recent studies of individuals with alcohol use disorder (Hodgins, el-Guebaly, & Armstrong, 1995) and with cocaine use disorder (McKay, Rutherford, & Alterman, 1996) suggest that any retrospective bias in reports of relapse determinants is not a major problem. The objection that the model is based on data from a small sample of male alcoholics and is therefore likely not to be representative has been addressed by years of research on the taxonomy and other components of the relapse model with a variety of populations of alcohol and other drug abusers (as well as smokers, compulsive gamblers, and obese individuals). This latter research has supported the relevance of the general model to these different populations.

Evidence for the Marlatt and Gordon Model

As with SLT in general, evidence for the Marlatt and Gordon (1985) model of relapse may be evaluated by examining its individual components and their simultaneous appraisal. The individual components considered here include high-risk situations (the taxonomy), coping skills, self-efficacy, and the AVE.

High-Risk Situations

In the relapse literature, situations that are identified as "high-risk" are those contexts in which a lapse or a relapse is more likely to occur because of the unavailability of, or the lack of self-efficacy to use, coping mechanisms that do not involve the use of alcohol or other drugs (Myers, Martin, Rohsenow, & Monti, 1996). Research on high-risk situations generally has followed Marlatt's original methods, and the results overall have supported the taxonomy as a way to describe individuals' attributions for what caused a lapse or a relapse to occur. In particular, among adult alcohol and other drug abusers, negative emotional states, whether related to situations involving other people or not, are the most frequently cited reasons given for a return to substance use following a period of intentional abstinence (Allen et al., 1996; Hodgins et al., 1995; Kadden, 1996; McKay, Rutherford, Alterman, & Cacciola, 1996; Zywiak, Connors, Maisto, & Westerberg, 1996). On the other hand, for adolescents, the little research that has been done suggests that situations involving social pressure to use alcohol or other drugs are more powerful determinants of a return to substance use than negative emotional states (Brown, Vik, & Creamer, 1989; Brown, Myers, Mott, & Vik, 1994). The evidence regarding sex differences is mixed. For alcohol use, men and women have similar distributions of reported relapse precipitants (Hodgins et al., 1995; Rubin, Stout, & Longabaugh, 1996). However, for individuals with cocaine use disorder, women more frequently reported unpleasant affect and interpersonal problems on the day of relapse, prior to their use, than men did, and men reported positive experiences more often (McKay, Rutherford, Cacciola, Kabasakalian-McKay, & Alterman, 1996).

Although the Marlatt taxonomy of high-risk situations has been supported on a descriptive level, recent data suggest that the taxonomy, as a measurement of high-risk situations, may have some difficulties in meeting standards of reliability (Longabaugh, Rubin, Stout, Zywiak, & Lowman, 1996) and validity (Maisto, Connors, & Zywiak, 1996; Stout, Longabaugh, & Rubin, 1996). It is possible that the taxonomy's failure to meet psychometric standards may be due to procedural and methodological problems. Because the Marlatt classifications are made by raters' content analysis of qualitative information, it may be that ambiguities in the coding system itself impose limits on the level of interrater agreement that can be achieved. These limits also could be due to the procedural requirement that raters assign a relapse precipitant to only one category. However, sometimes high-risk situations are complex and may contain more than one type of determinant, which would lead to disagreements among raters (e.g., Saunders & Houghton, 1996). Therefore, the operationalization of high-risk situations could affect the quality of measurement. Questionnaires based on the Marlatt taxonomy have been developed to allow identification of more than one precipitant in a high-risk situation (Inventory of

Drinking Situations and Reasons for Drinking Questionnaire; Annis, 1982; Heather, Stallard, & Tebbutt, 1991, respectively). These questionnaires have achieved scientifically acceptable levels of both reliability and validity. A conclusion that may be reached from this research is that the Marlatt taxonomy has clinical utility, but the evidence for its scientific value is not strong. More quantitative methods of measuring high-risk situations for relapse suggest that, consistent with SLT, the construct of high-risk situation has heuristic value in efforts to increase knowledge about relapse.

Coping Skills

Consistent with information reviewed earlier, coping skills is a construct central to SLT models of relapse. The importance of this variable has received empirical support in studies of adult and adolescent alcohol and other drug abusers (Donovan, 1996; Myers & Brown, 1996). Moreover, the clinical trials and survey research that examined social skills variables in the context of other SLT constructs reviewed in earlier sections provide some empirical evidence that is consistent with the global prediction that the availability and use of coping skills are related to patterns of substance use, including relapse. It would seem that for knowledge to advance about the relationship between coping skills and relapse, it would be necessary to specify further the conditions under which the stress–coping skills–substance use relationship holds.

One distinction that seems important is *type of stressor*. For example, Brown et al. (1990) evaluated male alcoholics 3 months after they completed an inpatient alcohol treatment program. Individuals who relapsed (defined as any alcohol or other drug use during the 3-month period) reported the same number of total stressors as did nonrelapsers. However, the relapsers said they had experienced a greater number of severe, ongoing, stressors independent of alcohol than did the nonrelapsers. This finding suggests that it may be important to specify whether or not stressors are related to substance use, as well as to their chronicity and severity.

Type of coping response also is important. The literature shows that several classifications of coping strategies or responses have been developed. One classification system includes active behavioral, active cognitive, and emotional coping (see, e.g., Finney & Moos, 1991). Behavioral coping strategies typically attempt to alter the stressor directly, or they involve taking action to avoid the source of stress in question. Cognitive coping typically refers to thinking of the negative consequences of using substances in the past and the benefits derived from staying away from them. Finally, emotional coping refers to ways to alleviate negative emotions (Donovan, 1996; Myers, Brown, & Mott, 1993). Another distinction that has been made is ways to cope with general life stressors ["substance independent," as in the Brown et al. (1990) study described earlier], and temptation coping, which concerns ways to avoid substance use (Myers et al., 1993). In adults with alcohol use disorders, the utility of different types of coping strategies seems to depend on the time in the change process in question. In this regard, early in the change process, behavioral strategies tend to be most effective (Annis, Schober, & Kelly, 1996), but as maintenance of change proceeds in time, cognitive strategies seem to be more effective (Donovan, 1996). However, behavioral, problem-focused coping tends to be the most effective strategy in adolescents (Brown et al., 1994). Overall, this pattern of findings suggests that the relationship between stress and the effective use of coping behaviors is a dynamic one, and that it is important to specify parameters of both the "stressor" and coping strategies in question. Related to this point, and as noted earlier, the literature has shown that individuals who evidence the most resilience to relapsing are those who have a variety of coping strategies available and implement them according to situational demands (Brown, Vik, Patterson, & Grant, 1995; Donovan, 1996; Litman, 1986).

In closing this section, it is important to try to explain the discrepancies in findings from the three areas of social skills research reviewed in this chapter (coping skills and relapse, coping skills intervention trials, and evaluation of social skills variables in the context of other SLT constructs in survey studies). Essentially, the clinical trials literature suggests that temptation (alcohol-specific) coping is critical to drinking outcomes but shows little contribution of general coping skills to those outcomes. In contrast, the relapse and survey research suggests that general and temptation coping skills both contribute to drinking behavior. In trying to understand this set of findings, first, it is important to recognize that a global comparison of the outcomes of treatment groups that constitute a randomized clinical trial does not alone provide an evaluation of a specific construct. Rather, any treatment group differences that are observed could be attributed to factors other than the specific construct that an intervention is purported to represent (in this case, general or temptation coping skills). A second possibility is that the clinical trials and the relapse research both concern clinical populations, but the outcomes that the two bodies of research emphasize differ. It may be that the outcomes measured in the relapse literature are more sensitive to the effects of general coping skills variables; however, given the categorical nature of many of the relapse definitions that have been used, this possibility seems unlikely.

A third possibility is that the intervention literature has tended to pit general versus temptation coping skills against each other in horse race style, and their *relative* effects on drinking outcomes have been measured. The relapse and survey studies, however, essentially have been correlational, sometimes multivariate investigations of the relationship between existing (in research participants) levels of different types of coping skills and measures of relapse or of drinking behavior and related problems. The latter two types of designs would seem to offer a more sensitive context in which to evaluate the contributions of the different types of coping skills to substance use, and the conditions under which they hold. For example, analyses of intervention group differences would not be sensitive to degrees of coping skills that participants may have. Clinical trials also have tended not to evaluate situational moderators of coping skills effects, which provide a more sensitive design for any effects of coping skills to emerge. In conclusion, it would appear that knowledge about coping skills and substance use would be best advanced if clinical trials and other types of research considered the range of coping skills possibilities, situational and temporal factors that may moderate their effects, and their mechanisms of action.

Self-Efficacy

As reviewed earlier, according to SLT, one determinant of whether an individual implements a coping strategy in a situation is the expectation that he or she can enact the strategy effectively. The lower such self-efficacy expectancies are, the less likely a coping strategy will be used. This hypothesis suggests that increasing self-efficacy to cope with high-risk situations (without use of undesired levels of alcohol or other drugs) would be a major goal of SLT-based interventions for substance use disorders. Accordingly, our earlier review of the self-efficacy construct showed that level of self-efficacy should increase during treatment, and that there should be a positive relationship between end-of-treatment levels of self-efficacy and treatment outcomes (including relapse). Additional data suggest that the effectiveness of "aftercare" treatment for individuals with substance use disorder may be related to the utility of such treatment in enhancing the self-efficacy of individuals who are relatively low in such expectations at the completion of an initial treatment episode (McKay et al., 1993).

Although clinical research has provided correlational evidence that is consistent with SLT's prediction of a relationship between self-efficacy and relapse, it has not provided evidence about what mechanism underlies the relationship. This gap in the research is the same as that identified earlier in review of research on self-efficacy and substance use in nonclinical samples. Theoretically, improvements in self-efficacy enhance treatment outcomes, because individuals have a greater degree of belief that they can enact any coping skills available to them when they encounter situations posing risk for heavy substance use. With a higher level of self-efficacy, the individual is more likely to implement coping skills when they are needed. However, there is no direct evidence from clinical research that this process underlies the self-efficacy treatment outcome relationship.

Abstinence Violation Effect

The AVE has received little research attention in studies of lapse and relapse among individuals with alcohol or other drug problems relative to its influence on smoking research. In the last few years, however, several studies concerning the AVE and alcohol and other drug use have been published. Birke, Edelmann, and Davis (1990) studied a small sample (n = 30, although only 23 participants appeared for their interviews) of illicit drug users referred to a community clinic in the United Kingdom. Evaluations of the participants' attributions for their relapses did not provide evidence for the AVE. However, the small sample size, self-selection bias, and other methodological problems make these findings difficult to interpret. A much stronger study by Stephens, Curtin, Simpson, and Roffman (1994) does provide support for the AVE. In this study, individuals participating in a controlled clinical trial of interventions for marijuana abuse were followed up for 1 year after the intervention had ended. Individuals who resumed regular marijuana use after an initial lapse made a greater degree of internal, global, and stable attributions for their lapses, and they experienced a greater degree of loss of control (over marijuana use), than did individuals who lapsed but who did not return to regular use. However, there were no differences between lapsers and relapsers in the amount of guilt reported following the lapse. Additional analyses supplemented the retrospective data by showing that attributions for earlier lapses predicted future frequency of marijuana use; that is, individuals who made more internal and global attributions for their lapses at an earlier follow-up period reported more frequent marijuana use 2–3 and 5–6 months after the lapse assessment. These prospective data help to rule out the possibility that attribution differences between lapsers and relapsers were due to the biasing effects of one group of participants relapsing to regular marijuana use.

A study by Walton, Castro, and Barrington (1994) provided additional support for the AVE construct. These authors evaluated a treatment sample of stimulant abusers and found that individuals classified as relapsers following treatment tended to make more global and stable attributions for their substance use than did individuals classified as lapsers. An interesting feature of this study was that the attributions of abstainers for their success were also assessed. These data showed that abstainers tended to make internal, stable, and global attributions for not using substances following treatment. Therefore, the same attribution style characterizes both successful abstainers and relapsers, with considerably different outcomes. In another study that supports the AVE construct, McKay, Rutherford, Alterman, and Cacciola (1996) found that individuals who relapsed following treatment for cocaine dependence tended to believe more strongly than did lapsers that an initial lapse dooms a person to a full-blown relapse. Therefore, relapsers appeared to experience a loss of control over their cocaine use following their initial use.

Simultaneous Evaluation of the Marlatt and Gordon Model Constructs

Only one study (Miller, Westerberg, Harris, & Tonigan, 1996) has been reported that was designed to evaluate the full Marlatt and Gordon (1985) relapse process model. This study involved the prediction of relapse among individuals admitted for alcohol treatment. Data collected 4 months following treatment entry were used to predict relapse status 2 months later. The predictor variables measured consisted of the major constructs of the Marlatt and Gordon model, including high-risk situations, coping responses (in situations where individuals might be at risk to start drinking again, after they have reached a goal of stopping), self-efficacy, positive alcohol-outcome expectancies, and the AVE. The results of a multivariate analysis that evaluated the independent contribution of each of these constructs to relapse status showed that coping responses and AVE were significant predictors. Use of positive thinking was negatively related, and use of avoidance coping was positively related to the likelihood that the individual had relapsed. In addition, stronger beliefs in the disease model of alcoholism (e.g., a belief that alcoholics cannot control their drinking) increased the probability of relapse. None of the other variables made significant contributions to predicting relapse status.

Conclusions about Social Learning Theory Approaches to Relapse

Several conclusions emerge from this discussion of empirical research on SLT approaches (Marlatt & Gordon, 1985) to relapse. The concept of high-risk situation generally seems to be useful for research and clinical purposes. However, the Marlatt and Gordon taxonomy of high-risk situations has some problems as a method to measure high-risk situations for research purposes and seems to have its greatest utility in the clinical setting. Quantitative methods of measuring high-risk situations, which allow for simultaneous consideration of multiple dimensions in defining high risk, do possess adequate levels of reliability and validity for use in research. It also is notable that research on high-risk situations for alcohol or other drug use would be advanced further with the introduction of near *real time* measurement of lapse–relapse antecedents, as has appeared in the smoking literature (e.g., Shiffman et al., 1997). In this regard, the available research has been based solely on retrospective reports of lapses and relapses. Although it was found in one study cited earlier (Hodgins et al., 1995) that retrospective reports of relapses do not seem to introduce serious biases in conclusions about them, it would appear that the ability to record information about an event closer in time to its occurrence would enhance the sensitivity of studies because of the decreased burden on memory.

Research on coping skills and relapse show findings that are consistent with the global SLT prediction that skill in coping with stressors is associated with substance use patterns. Furthermore, it is important to specify stressors and coping skills in order to advance knowledge about the coping skills–substance use relationship. The data also suggest that changes in patterns of substance use are maintained best over the long term by individuals who have a variety of coping skills at their disposal and apply them to meet situational demands. Findings on the construct of self-efficacy also have been consistent with SLT predictions, as they show that a greater degree of self-efficacy before or at the end of treatment for substance use disorders is correlated with the individual's substance use following treatment. However, the relapse literature has not provided direct evidence on what mechanism underlies this correlation. Research on the last single component of Marlatt and Gordon's model reviewed, the AVE, generally has supported the validity of this construct. Finally, the simultaneous evaluation of the major constructs in Marlatt and Gordon by Miller (1996) suggests that the most important components of the model are coping skills and the AVE.

Despite the general level of empirical support for Marlatt and Gordon's (1985) model, it has been subjected to some criticism (e.g., Saunders & Houghton, 1996). One is that the Marlatt and Gordon model gives little attention to macroenvironmental factors such as availability of substances and subcultural norms regarding their use, which may contribute to the prediction of relapse (see, e.g., Shiffman, 1989; Donovan, 1996). Indeed, Marlatt (1996) has noted the importance of macroenvironmental variables in understanding relapse. Although it is true that the Marlatt and Gordon model does not include such factors, their absence is not surprising. The model is a psychological one that focuses on the immediate relapse situation. Accordingly, it emphasizes the setting in which actual substance use occurs and the psychological variables that may influence the individual's decision to use substances in that situation. Because there are not nearly enough data available to underlie a model that covers all aspects of the complex problem of relapse with any precision, it would seem that no model should be expected to do so.

GENERAL SUMMARY AND CONCLUSIONS

This chapter has provided an outline of SLT as a general theory of behavior and as an approach to the understanding of the development and maintenance of substance use patterns. The chapter then provided a critical review of empirical literature evaluating selected SLT constructs in studies of alcohol and other drug use in both clinical and nonclinical populations, with an emphasis on research published since 1987. Overall, the essential and frequently global propositions of SLT regarding substance use patterns were found to be consistent with the data. Furthermore, in the last 10 years, the areas of research covered by this review have developed by their increased precision in hypotheses about relationships between variables, the mechanisms that underlie them, and the conditions under which they hold. That said, the review also has pointed out ways that research addressing specific subareas of SLT of substance use can improve and advance knowledge. In the concluding paragraphs of this chapter, we discuss general directions for future research on SLT approaches to understanding substance use patterns that apply across the subareas defined in the chapter.

Methodology

The quality of the methodology of the research covered was good in general. Naturally, there were several exceptions that were noted in the review, but the quality and replicability of the data, as evidenced by the degree of consistency of findings across areas, have been high enough to solidify support for the SLT approach to substance use. Two additional major points regarding methodology emerge from this review. The first is that recent research has included application of sophisticated, multivariate correlational techniques such as structural equation modeling. These techniques allow the systematic, quantitative investigation of hypotheses central to SLT that previously had been difficult to test. Examples included in this review are evaluations of the validity of SLT-derived multivariate models and reciprocal determinism. Although use of SEM and related methods such as path analysis *do not* allow inferences about causal relationships among variables, they have excellent heuristic value in helping to generate hypotheses about causal relationships.

The second methodological point is the importance of methods allowing causal inferences. In the 1970s and early 1980s, there was a considerable amount of *experimental* research published that was driven by application of SLT principles to substance use, particularly alcohol use. The consistency of the experimental data that emerged with selected propositions of SLT lends substantial credibility to this theoretical approach. Unfortunately, the frequency of experimental research has decreased in recent years in the SLT–substance use area, with some notable exceptions. Although the array of research methods that have been used to investigate a SLT approach to substance use are a strength, true experiments are needed to establish clear cause–effect relationships between variables. Therefore, a reemergence of experimental work would be a boost to the field.

Populations of Research Participants

In the last 10 years, SLT-relevant research increasingly has included female as well as male participants and drugs other than alcohol. Some of the subareas reviewed show more evidence of this trend than others. For example, the area of coping skills interventions has lagged behind others in involvement of female research participants and in evaluation of drug use other than alcohol. Despite the increase in the number of studies that include women, research that involves ethnic or racial groups other than whites, adolescents, or the elderly still is too infrequent. However, again, there have been some notable exceptions, such as Sandra Brown and her colleagues' studies of relapse in adolescents, and studies of African American and Hispanic populations (Farrell, 1994; Walton et al., 1994). Importantly, inclusion of different ethnic or racial groups permits the identification of differences between subgroups, such as the case of the reciprocal relationship between peer models and the individual's alcohol use (Curran et al., 1997; Farrell, 1994).

The need to expand the representativeness of SLT research also applies to alcohol (and other drug) use as an individual characteristic. The empirical literature that was reviewed showed discrepancies among different subareas of SLT research in the degree to which the alcohol use continuum was sampled in recruiting research participants. Because SLT is a theoretical approach that is hypothesized to be relevant to the explanation of the development and maintenance of the full spectrum of substance use, empirical work designed to evaluate SLT should reflect that hypothesis.

In conclusion, this selective review of research on SLT approaches to substance use shows significant advances in recent work and knowledge, with promising directions for future research. Continuing this trend will enhance SLT by making it more precise, with resulting greater predictive value. Such an evolution of the SLT approach will only increase the utility of the prevention, clinical methods, and programs behind which it stands.

NOTES

1. Technically, it is redundant to refer to "alcohol and other drug use," because alcohol is a drug. However, this terminology reflects how the clinical and research literature have been organized, with most of the research by far focusing on alcohol, and other literature emphasizing other drugs. In this chapter, "other drugs" refers to psychoactive substances other than nicotine or caffeine that are used in illicit or in nonprescriptive ways.

2. The term "substance" covers both alcohol and other drugs, and its use is in keeping with the research and clinical literature, and with conventions of the fourth edition of the *Diagnostic and Statistical Manual of Mental Disorders* (DSM-IV) published in 1994 by the American Psychiatric Association.

3. Particularly in older literature, but still currently, the "alcohol use disorder" of DSM-IV is referred to as alcoholism, alcohol addiction, and other terms. We may use the terms "alcoholism," "alcoholic," or "alcohol abuser" occasionally if they are consistent with what was written in the source cited, or to reduce awkwardness in language.

4. It is important to recognize that SEM methods may be applied to correlational data, such as in the Stacy et al. (1991) study, to evaluate the plausibility of different explanatory models. Although the results of using SEM techniques with correlational data provide information about a model's utility, they cannot be the bases of inferences about causal relationships among variables. Such inferences require data obtained from true experiments.

REFERENCES

Aas, H., Klepp, K.-I., Laberg, J. C., & Aaro, L. E. (1995). Predicting adolescents' intentions to drink alcohol: Outcome expectancies and self-efficacy. *Journal of Studies on Alcohol, 56*, 293–299.

Abrams, D. B., Binkoff, J. A., Zwick, W. R., Liepman, M. R., Nirenberg, T. D., Munroe, S. M., & Monti, P. M. (1991). Alcohol abusers' and social drinkers' responses to alcohol-relevant and general situations. *Journal of Studies on Alcohol, 52*, 409–414.

Abrams, D. B., & Niaura, R. S. (1987). Social learning theory. In H. T. Blane & K. E. Leonard (Eds.), *Psychological theories of drinking and alcoholism* (pp. 131–178). New York: Guilford Press.

Akers, R. L. (1977). *Deviant behavior: A social learning approach* (2nd ed.). Belmont, CA: Wadsworth.

Akers, R. L., Krohn, M. D., Lanzer-Kaduce, L., & Radosevich, M. (1979). Social learning and deviant behavior: A specific text of a general theory. *American Sociological Review, 44*, 636–655.

Allen, J., Lowman, C., & Miller, W. R. (1996). Perspectives on precipitants of relapse. *Addiction, 91*(Suppl.), S3–S4.

American Psychiatric Association. (1994). *Diagnostic and statistical manual of mental disorders* (4th ed.). Washington, DC: Author.

Annis, H. M. (1982). *Situational Confidence Questionnaire.* Toronto, Ontario: Addiciation Research Foundation.

Annis, H. M. (1986). A relapse prevention model for treatment of alcoholics. In W. R. Miller & N. Heather (Eds.), *Treating addictive behaviors: Processes of change*, (pp. 407–433). New York: Plenum.

Annis, H. M. (1987). *The Situational Confidence Questionnaire (SCQ-39).* Toronto, Ontario: Addiction Research Foundation.

Annis, H. M., & Davis, C. S. (1988). Assessment of expectancies. In D. Donovan & G. Marlatt (Eds.), *Assessment of addictive behaviors* (pp. 84–111). New York: Guilford Press.

Annis, H. M., Schober, R., & Kelly, E. (1996). Matching addiction outpatient counseling to client readiness to change: The role of structured relapse prevention counseling. *Experimental and Clinical Psychopharmacology, 4*, 37–45.

Ary, D. V., Tildesley, E., Hops, H., & Andrews, J. (1993). The influence of parent, sibling, and peer modeling and attitudes on adolescent use of alcohol. *International Journal of the Addictions, 28*(9), 853–880.

Avants, S. K., Margolin, A., Kosten, T. R., & Cooney, N. L. (1995). Differences between responders and nonresponders to cocaine cues in the laboratory. *Addictive Behaviors, 20*, 215–224.

Baldwin, A. R., Oei, T. P. S., & Young, R. (1993). To drink or not to drink: The differential role of alcohol expectancies and drinking refusal self-efficacy in quantity and frequency of alcohol consumption. *Cognitive Therapy and Research, 17*, 511–530.

Bandura, A. (1969). *Principles of behavior modification.* New York: Holt, Rinehart & Winston.

Bandura, A. (1977). *Social learning theory.* Englewood Cliffs, NJ: Prentice-Hall.

Bandura, A. (1986). *Social foundations of thought and action: A social cognitive theory.* Englewood Cliffs, NJ: Prentice-Hall.

Beck, K. H., & Treimman, K. A. (1996). The relationship of social context of drinking, perceived social norms, and parental influence to various drinking patterns of adolescents. *Addictive Behaviors, 21,* 633–644.

Bickel, W. K., & Kelly, T. H. (1988). The relationship of stimulus control to the treatment of substance abuse. In B. A. Ray (Ed.), *Learning factors in substance abuse* (pp. 122–140). Rockville, MD: Department of Health and Human Services.

Birke, S. A., Edelmann, R. J., & Davis, P. E. (1990). An analysis of the abstinence violation effect in a sample of illicit drug users. *British Journal of Addiction, 85,* 1299–1307.

Brown, S. A. (1985). Reinforcement expectancies and alcoholism treatment outcome after a one-year follow-up. *Journal of Studies on Alcohol, 46,* 304–308.

Brown, S. A. (1993). Drug effect expectancies and addictive behavior change. *Experimental and Clinical Psychopharmacology, 1,* 55–67.

Brown, S. A., Christiansen, B. A., & Goldman, M. S. (1987). The Alcohol Expectancy Questionnaire: An instrument for the assessment of adolescent and adult alcohol expectancies. *Journal of Studies on Alcohol, 48,* 483–491.

Brown, S. A., Creamer, V. A., & Stetson, B. A. (1987). Adolescent alcohol expectancies in relation to personal and parental drinking patterns. *Journal of Abnormal Psychology, 96,* 117–121.

Brown, S. A., Goldman, M. S., Inn, A., & Anderson, L. R. (1980). Expectations of reinforcement from alcohol: Their domain and relation to drinking patterns. *Journal of Consulting and Clinical Psychology, 48,* 419–426.

Brown, S. A., Myers, M. G., Mott, M. A., & Vik, P. W. (1994). Correlates of success following treatment for adolescent substance abuse. *Applied and Preventive Psychology, 3,* 61–73.

Brown, S. A., Stetson, B. A., & Beatty, P. A. (1989). Cognitive and behavioral features of adolescent coping in high-risk drinking situations. *Addictive Behaviors, 14,* 43–52.

Brown, S. A., Vik, P. W., & Creamer, V. A. (1989). Characteristics of relapse following adolescent substance abuse treatment. *Addictive Behaviors, 14,* 291–300.

Brown, S. A., Vik, P. W., McQuaid, J. R., Patterson, T. L., Irwin, M. R., & Grant, I. (1990). Severity of psychosocial stress and outcome of alcoholism treatment. *Journal of Abnormal Psychology, 99,* 344–348.

Brown, S. A., Vik, P. W., Patterson, T. L., & Grant, I. (1995). Stress, vulnerability, and adult alcohol relapse. *Journal of Studies on Alcohol, 56,* 538–545.

Burgess, R. L., & Akers, R. L. (1966). A differential association reinforcement theory of criminal behavior. *Social Problems, 14,* 128–147.

Burke, R. S., & Stephens, R. S. (1997). Effect of anxious affect on drinking self-efficacy in college students. *Psychology of Addictive Behaviors, 11,* 65–75.

Burling, T. A., Reilly, P. M., Moltzen, J. O., & Ziff, D. C. (1989). Self-efficacy and relapse among inpatient drug and alcohol abusers: A predictor of outcome. *Journal of Studies on Alcohol, 50,* 354–360.

Capell, H., & Greeley, J. (1987). Alcohol and tension reduction: An update on research and theory. In H. T. Blane & K. E. Leonard (Eds.), *Psychological theories of drinking and alcoholism* (pp. 15–54). New York: Guilford Press.

Carey, K. B. (1995). Alcohol-related expectancies predict quantity and frequency of heavy drinking among college students. *Psychology of Addictive Behaviors, 9,* 236–241.

Caudill, B. D., & Marlatt, G. A. (1975). Modeling influences in social drinking: An experimental analogue. *Journal of Consulting and Clinical Psychology, 43,* 405–415.

Chipperfield, B., & Vogel-Sprott, M. (1988). Family history of problem drinking among young male social drinkers: Modeling effects on alcohol consumption. *Journal of Abnormal Psychology, 97,* 423–428.

Christansen, B. A., Goldman, M. S., & Inn, A. (1982). The development of alcohol-related expectancies in adolescents: Separating pharmacological from social learning influences. *Journal of Consulting and Clinical Psychology, 50,* 336–344.

Christansen, B. A., Smith, G. T., Roehling, P. V., & Goldman, M. S. (1989). Using alcohol expectancies to predict adolescent drinking behavior after one year. *Journal of Consulting and Clinical Psychology, 57,* 93–99.

Collins, R. L., Lapp, W. M., Emmons, K. M., & Isaac, L. M. (1990). Endorsement and strength of alcohol expectancies. *Journal of Studies on Alcohol, 51,* 336–342.

Collins, R. L., Parks, G. A., & Marlatt, G. A. (1985). Social determinants of alcohol consumption: The effects of social interaction and model status on the self-administration of alcohol. *Journal of Consulting and Clinical Psychology, 53,* 189–200.

Conger, J. J. (1956). Alcoholism: Theory, problem, and challenge: II. Reinforcement theory and the dynamics of alcoholism. *Quarterly Journal of Studies on Alcohol, 13,* 296–305.

Cooney, N. L., Kadden, R. M., Litt, M. D., & Getter, H. (1991). Matching alcoholics to coping skills or interactional therapies: Two-year follow-up results. *Journal of Consulting and Clinical Psychology, 59,* 598–601.

Cooper, A. M., Waterhouse, G. J., & Sobell, M. B. (1979). Influence of gender on drinking in a modeling situation. *Journal of Studies on Alcohol, 40,* 562–570.

Cooper, M. L., Russell, M., & George, W. H. (1988). Coping, expectancies, and alcohol use: A test of social learning formulations. *Journal of Abnormal Psychology, 97,* 218–230.

Cooper, M. L., Russell, M., Skinner, J. B., Frone, M. R., & Mudar, P. (1992). Stress and alcohol use: Moderating effects of gender, coping, and alcohol expectancies. *Journal of Abnormal Psychology, 101,* 139–152.

Curran, P. J., Stice, E., & Chassin, L. (1997). The relation between adolescent alcohol use and peer alcohol use: A longitudinal random coefficients model. *Journal of Consulting and Clinical Psychology, 65,* 130–140.

Darkes, J., & Goldman, M. S. (1993). Expectancy challenge and drinking reduction: Experimental evidence for a mediational process. *Journal of Consulting and Clinical Psychology, 61,* 344–353.

DiClemente, C. C., Carbonari, J. P., Montgomery, R. P. G., & Hughes, S. O. (1994). The alcohol abstinence self-efficacy scale. *Journal of Studies on Alcohol, 55,* 141–148.

Dimeff, L. A., & Marlatt, G. A. (1995). Relapse prevention. In R. H. Hester & W. R. Miller (Eds.), *Handbook of alcoholism treatment approaches* (2nd ed., pp. 176–194). Needham Heights, MA: Allyn & Bacon.

Dollard, J., & Miller, N. E. (1950). *Personality and psychotherapy.* New York: McGraw-Hill.

Donovan, D. M. (1996). Assessment issues and domains in the prediction of relapse. *Addiction, 91*(Suppl.), S29–S38.

Ellickson, P. L., & Hays, R. D. (1991). Beliefs about resistance self-efficacy and drug prevalence: Do they really affect drug use? *International Journal of the Addictions, 25*, 1353–1378.

Evans, D. M., & Dunn, N. J. (1995). Alcohol expectancies, coping responses, and self-efficacy judgments: A replication and extension of Cooper et al.'s 1988 study in a college sample. *Journal of Studies on Alcohol, 56*, 186–193.

Farrell, A. D. (1994). Structural equations modeling with longitudinal data: Strategies for examining group differences and reciprocal relationships. *Journal of Consulting and Clinical Psychology, 62*, 477–487.

Finney, J. W., & Moos, R. H. (1991). The long-term course of treated alcoholism: I. Mortality, relapse, and remission rates comparison with community controls. *Journal of Studies on Alcohol, 52*, 44–54.

Folkman, S., & Lazarus, R. S. (1980). An analysis of coping in a middle-aged community couple. *Journal of Health and Social Behavior, 21*, 219–239.

Forsyth, A. D., & Carey, M. P. (1998). Measuring self-efficacy in the context of HIV-risk-reduction: Research challenges and recommendations. *Health Psychology, 17*, 559–568.

Fromme, K., Stroot, E., & Kaplan, D. (1993). The comprehensive effects of alcohol: Development and psychometric assessment of a new expectancy questionnaire. *Psychological Assessment, 5*, 19–26.

George, W. H., & Marlatt, G. A. (1983). Alcoholism: The evolution of a behavioral perspective. *Recent Developments in Alcoholism, 1*, 105–138.

Graham, J. W., Marks, G., & Hansen, W. B. (1991). Social influence processes affecting adolescent substance use. *Journal of Applied Psychology, 76*, 291–298.

Hamilton, F., & Maisto, S. (1979). Assertive behavior and perceived discomfort of alcoholics in assertion-required situations. *Journal of Consulting and Clinical Psychology, 47*, 196–197.

Hammersley, R. (1994). A digest of memory phenomena for addiction research. *Addiction, 89*, 283–293.

Hawkins, J. D., Catalano, R. F., Gillmore, M. R., & Wells, E. A. (1989). Skills training for drug abusers: Generalization, maintenance, and effects on drug use. *Journal of Consulting and Clinical Psychology, 57*, 559–563.

Hays, R. D., & Ellickson, P. L. (1990). How generalizable are adolescents' beliefs about pro-drug pressures and resistance self-efficacy? *Journal of Applied Social Psychology, 20*, 321–340.

Heather, N., Stallard, A., & Tebbutt, J. (1991). Importance of substance cues in relapse among heroin users: Comparison of two methods of investigation. *Addictive Behaviors, 16*, 41–49.

Hendricks, R. D., Sobell, M. B., & Cooper, A. M. (1978). Social influences on human ethanol consumption in an analogue situation. *Addictive Behaviors, 3*, 253–259.

Hilgard, E. R., & Bower, G. H. (1975). *Theories of learning* (4th ed.). Englewood Cliffs NJ: Prentice-Hall.

Hodgins, D. C., el-Guebaly, N., & Armstrong, S. (1995). Prospective and retrospective reports of mod states before relapse to substance use. *Journal of Consulting and Clinical Psychology, 63*, 400–407.

Holyfield, L., Ducharme, L. J., & Martin, J. K. (1994). *Drinking context, alcohol be-*

liefs, and patterns of alcohol consumption: Evidence for a comprehensive model of problem drinking. Unpublished manuscript, University of Georgia.

Hoyle, R. H. (1994). Introduction to the special section: Structural equation modeling in clinical research. *Journal of Consulting and Clinical Psychology, 62,* 427–428.

Kadden, R. M. (1996). Is Marlatt's relapse taxonomy reliable or valid? *Addiction, 91*(Suppl.), S139–S146.

Kadden, R. M., Cooney, N. L., Getter, H., & Litt, M. D. (1989). Matching alcoholics to coping skills or interactional therapies: Posttreatment results. *Journal of Consulting and Clinical Psychology, 57,* 698–704.

Kadden, R. M., Litt, M. D., Cooney, N. L., & Busher, D. A. (1992). Relationship between role-play measures of coping skills and alcoholism treatment outcomes. *Addictive Behaviors, 17,* 425–437.

Langenbucher, J., Sulesund, D., Chung, T., & Morgenstern, J. (1996). Illness severity and self-efficacy as course predictors of DSM-IV alcohol dependence in a multisite clinical sample. *Addictive Behaviors, 21,* 543–553.

Lee, N. K., & Oei, T. P. S. (1993). The importance of alcohol expectancies and drinking refusal self-efficacy in the quantity and frequency of alcohol consumption. *Journal of Substance Abuse, 5,* 379–390.

Leigh, B. C. (1989). Confirmatory factor analysis of alcohol expectancy scales. *Journal of Studies on Alcohol, 50,* 268–277.

Leigh, B. C., & Stacy, A. W. (1991). On the scope of alcohol expectancy research: Remaining issues of measurement and meaning. *Psychological Assessment, 5,* 216–229.

Lenson, D. (1995). *On drugs.* Minneapolis: University of Minnesota Press.

Lied, E. R., & Marlatt, G. A. (1979). Modeling as a determinant of alcohol consumption: Effect of subject sex and prior drinking history. *Addictive Behaviors, 4,* 47–54.

Litman, G. K. (1986). Alcoholism survival: The prevention of relapse. In W. R. Miller & N. Heather (Eds.), *Treating addictive behaviors* (pp. 391–405). New York: Plenum.

Longabaugh, R., Rubin, A., Stout, R. L., Zywiak, W. H., & Lowman, C. (1996). The reliability of Marlatt's taxonomy for classifying relapses. *Addiction, 91*(Suppl.), S73–S88.

Maisto, S. A., Connors, G. J., & Zywiak, W. H. (1996). Construct validation analyses on the Marlatt typology of relapse precipitants. *Addiction, 91*(Suppl.), S89–S98.

Mann, L. M., Chassin, L., & Sher, K. J. (1987). Alcohol expectancies and the risk for alcoholism. *Journal of Consulting and Clinical Psychology, 55,* 411–417.

Marlatt, G. A. (1996). Taxonomy of high-risk situations for alcohol relapse: Evolution and development of a cognitive behavioral model. *Addiction, 91*(Suppl.), S37–S49.

Marlatt, G. A., & Gordon, J. R. (Eds.). (1985). *Relapse prevention.* New York: Guilford Press.

Marlatt, G. A., Kosturn, C. F., & Lang, A. R. (1975). Provocation to anger and opportunity for retaliation as determinants of alcohol consumption in heavy drinkers. *Journal of Abnormal Psychology, 84,* 652–659.

McCarty, D. (1985). Environmental factors in substance abuse: The microsetting. In M. Galizio & S. A. Maisto (Eds.), *Determinants of substance abuse* (pp. 247–282). New York: Guilford Press.

McKay, J. R., Maisto, S. A., & O'Farrell, T. J. (1993). End-of-treatment self-efficacy, aftercare, and drinking outcomes of alcoholic men. *Alcoholism: Clinical and Experimental Research, 17,* 1078–1083.

McKay, J. R., Rutherford, M. J., & Alterman, A. I. (1996). An investigation of potential time effects in retrospective reports of cocaine relapses. *Addictive Behaviors, 21,* 37–46.

McKay, J. R., Rutherford, M. J., Alterman, A. I., & Cacciola, J. S. (1996). Development of the Cocaine Relapse Interview: An initial report. *Addiction, 91,* 535–548.

McKay, J. R., Rutherford, M. J., Cacciola, J. S., Kabasakalian-McKay, R., & Alterman, A. I. (1996). Gender differences in relapse experiences of cocaine patients. *Journal of Nervous and Mental Disease, 184,* 616–622.

Miller, P. J., Ross, S. M., Emmerson, R. Y., & Todt, E. H. (1989). Self-efficacy in alcoholics: Clinical validation of the situational confidence questionnaire. *Addictive Behaviors, 14,* 217–224.

Miller, P. M., Smith, G. T., & Goldman, M. S. (1990). Emergence of alcohol expectancies in childhood: A possible critical period. *Journal of Studies on Alcohol, 51,* 343–349.

Miller, W. R. (1996). What is relapse? Fifty ways to leave the wagon. *Addiction, 91*(Suppl.), S15–S28.

Miller, W. R., Westerberg, V. S., Harris, R. J., & Tonigan, J. S. (1996). What predicts relapse? Prospective testing of antecedent models. *Addiction, 91*(Suppl.), S155–S172.

Mischel, W. (1973). Toward a cognitive social learning reconceptualization of personality. *Psychological Review, 80,* 252–283.

Monti, P. M., Abrams, D. B., Binkoff, J. A., Zwick, W., Liepman, M. R., Nirenberg, T. D., & Rohsenow, D. J. (1990). Communication skills training, communications skills training with family, and cognitive behavioral mood management training for alcoholics. *Journal of Studies on Alcohol, 51,* 263–270.

Monti, P. M., Rohsenow, D. J., Abrams, D. B., & Binkoff, J. A. (1988). Social learning approaches to alcohol relapse: Selected illustrations and implications. In B. A. Ray (Ed.), *Learning factors in substance abuse* (pp. 141–160). Rockville, MD: Department of Health and Human Services.

Monti, P. M., Rohsenow, D. J., Colby, S. M., & Abrams, D. B. (1995). Coping and social skills training. In R. K. Hester & W. R. Miller (Eds.), *Handbook of alcoholism treatment approaches: Effective alternative* (2nd ed., pp. 221–241). Boston: Allyn & Bacon.

Monti, P. M., Rohsenow, D. J., Rubonis, A. V., Niaura, R. S., Sirota, A. D., Colby, S. M., Goddard, P., & Abrams, D. B. (1993). Cue exposure with coping skills treatment for male alcoholics: A preliminary investigation. *Journal of Consulting and Clinical Psychology, 61,* 1011–1019.

Monti, P. M., Wallander, J. L., Ahern, D. K., Abrams, D. B., & Munroe, S. M. (1984). Multi-modal measurement of anxiety and social skills in a behavioral role-play test: Generalizability and discriminant validity. *Behavioral Assessment, 6,* 15–25.

Monti, P. M., Rohsenow, D. J., Abrams, D. B., Zwick, W. R., Binkoff, J. A., Munroe, S. M., Fingeret, A. L., Nirenberg, T. D., Liepman, M. R., Pedraza, M., Kadden, R. M., & Cooney, N. L. (1993). Development of a behavior-analytically derived alcohol-specific role-play assessment instrument. *Journal of Studies on Alcohol, 54,* 710–721.

Moore, P. J., Turner, R., Park, C. L., & Adler, N. E. (1996). The impact of behavior and addiction on psychological models of cigarette and alcohol use during pregnancy. *Addictive Behaviors, 21,* 645–658.

Myers, M. G., & Brown, S. A. (1996). The Adolescent Relapse Coping Questionnaire. *Journal of Studies on Alcohol, 457,* 40–46.

Myers, M. G., Brown, S. A., & Mott, M. A. (1993). Coping as a predictor of adolescent substance abuse treatment outcome. *Journal of Substance Abuse, 5,* 15–29.

Myers, M. G., Martin, R. A., Rohsenow, D. J., & Monti, P. M. (1996). The Relapse Situation Appraisal Questionnaire: Initial psychometric characteristics and evaluation. *Psychology of Addictive Behaviors, 10,* 237–247.

O'Malley, S. S., Jaffe, A. J., Chang, G., Rode, S., Schottenfeld, R., Meyer, R. E., & Rounsaville, B. (1996). Six-month follow-up of naltrexone and psychotherapy for alcohol dependence. *Archives of General Psychiatry, 53,* 217–224.

Petraitis, J., Flay, B. R., & Miller, T. Q. (1995). Reviewing theories of adolescent substance use: Organizing pieces in the puzzle. *Psychological Bulletin, 117,* 67–86.

Pliner, P., & Cappell, H. (1974). Modification of affective consequences of alcohol: A comparison of social and solitary drinking. *Journal of Abnormal Psychology, 83,* 418–425.

Reid, J. B. (1978). Study of drinking in natural settings. In G. A. Marlatt & P. E. Nathan (Eds.), *Behavioral approaches to alcoholism* (pp. 58–74). New Brunswick, NJ: Rutgers Center for Alcohol Studies.

Rogosa, D. (1979). Causal models in longitudinal research: Rationale, formulation, and interpretation. In J. R. Nesselroade & P. B. Baltes (Eds.), *Longitudinal research in the study of behavior and development* (pp. 263–302). New York: Academic Press.

Rohsenow, D. J., Monti, P. M., Binkoff, J. A., Liepman, M. R., Nirenberg, T. D., & Abrams, D. B. (1991). Patient–treatment matching for alcoholic men in communication skills versus cognitive-behavioral mood management training. *Addictive Behaviors, 16,* 63–69.

Rotter, J. B. (1954). *Social learning theory and clinical psychology.* Englewood Cliffs, NJ: Prentice-Hall.

Rounsaville, B. J. (1986). Clinical implications of relapse research. In F. M. Tims & C. G. Lenkefeld (Eds.), *Relapse and recovery in drug abuse* (pp. 172–184). Rockville, MD: Department of Health and Human Services.

Rubin, A., Stout, R. L., & Longabaugh, R. (1996). Gender differences in relapse situations. *Addiction, 91*(Suppl.), S111–S120.

Saunders, B., & Houghton, M. (1996). Relapse revisited: A critique of current concepts and clinical practice in the management of alcohol problems. *Addictive Behaviors, 21,* 843–855.

Sher, K. J., Wood, M. O., Wood, P. K., & Raskin, G. (1996). Alcohol outcome expectancies and alcohol use: A latent variable cross-lagged panel study. *Journal of Abnormal Psychology, 105,* 561–574.

Shiffman, S. (1989). Conceptual issues in the study of relapse. In M. Gossop (Ed.), *Relapse and addictive behavior* (pp. 149–179). London: Tavistock/Routledge.

Shiffman, S., Enberg, J. B., Puty, J. A., Perz, W. G., Guys, M., Kassel, J. D., & Hickcox, M. (1997). A day at a time: Predicting smoking lapse from daily urge. *Journal of Abnormal Psychology, 106,* 104–116.

Sitharthan, T., & Kavanagh, D. J. (1990). Role of self-efficacy in predicting outcomes from a programme for controlled drinking. *Drug and Alcohol Dependence, 27,* 87–94.

Smith, G. T., Goldman, M. S., Greenbaum, P. E., & Christiansen, B. A. (1995). Expectancy for social facilitation from drinking: The divergent paths of high-expectancy and low-expectancy adolescents. *Journal of Abnormal Psychology, 104,* 32–40.

Solomon, K. E., & Annis, H. M. (1990). Outcome and efficacy expectancy in the prediction of post-treatment drinking behaviour. *British Journal of Addiction, 85,* 659–665.

Southwick, L., Steele, C., Marlatt, G. A., & Lindell, M. (1981). Alcohol-related expectancies: Defined by phase of intoxication and drinking experience. *Journal of Consulting and Clinical Psychology, 49,* 713–721.

Stacy, A. W., Newcomb, M. D., & Bentler, P. M. (1991). Cognitive motivation and drug use: A 9-year longitudinal study. *Journal of Abnormal Psychology, 100,* 502–515.

Stacy, A. W., Widaman, K. F., & Marlatt, G. A. (1990). Expectancy models of alcohol use. *Journal of Personality and Social Psychology, 58,* 918–928.

Stephens, R. S., Curtin, L., Simpson, E. E., & Roffman, R. A. (1994). Testing the abstinence violation effect construct with marijuana cessation. *Addictive Behaviors, 19,* 23–32.

Stephens, R. S., Roffman, R. A., & Simpson, E. E. (1994). Treating adult marijuana dependence: A test of the relapse prevention model. *Journal of Consulting and Clinical Psychology, 62,* 92–99.

Stephens, R. S., Wertz, J. S., & Roffman, R. A. (1993). Predictors of marijuana treatment outcomes: The role of self-efficacy. *Journal of Substance Abuse, 5,* 341–353.

Stephens, R. S., Wertz, J. S., & Roffman, R. A. (1995). Self-efficacy and marijuana cessation: A construct validity analysis. *Journal of Consulting and Clinical Psychology, 63,* 1022–1031.

Stout, R. L., Longabaugh, R., & Rubin, A. (1996). Predictive validity of Marlatt's relapse taxonomy versus a more general relapse code. *Addiction, 91*(Suppl.), S99–S110.

Strom, J., & Barone, D. F. (1993). Self-deception, self-esteem, and control over drinking at different stages of alcohol involvement. *Journal of Drug Issues, 23,* 705–714.

Twentyman, G. T., Greenwald, D. P., Greenwald, M. A., Kloss, J. D., Kovaleski, M. E., & Zibung-Hoffman, P. (1982). An assessment of social skill deficits in alcoholics. *Behavioral Assessment, 4,* 317–326.

Wagner, E. F. (1993). Delay of gratification, coping with stress, and substance use in adolescents. *Experimental and Clinical Psychopharmacology, 1,* 27–43.

Walton, M. A., Castro, F. G., & Barrington, E. H. (1994). The role of attributions in abstinence, lapse, and relapse following substance abuse treatment. *Addictive Behaviors, 19,* 319–331.

Wanberg, K. W., Horn, J. L., & Foster, F. M. (1977). A differential assessment model for alcoholism: The scales of the Alcohol Use Inventory. *Journal of Studies on Alcohol, 38,* 512–543.

Watson, D. B., & Sobell, M. B. (1982). Social influences on alcohol consumption by black and white males. *Addictive behaviors, 7,* 87–91.

Webb, J. A., & Baer, P. E. (1995). Influence of family disharmony and parental alcohol use on adolescent social skills, self-efficacy, and alcohol use. *Addictive Behaviors, 20,* 127–135.

Weil, A. (1993). *From chocolate to morphine: Everything you need to know about mind altering drugs.* Boston: Houghton Mifflin.

Wells, E. A., Catalano, R. F., Plotnick, R., Hawkins, J. D., & Brattesani, K. A. (1989). General versus drug-specific coping skills and posttreatment drug use among adults. *Psychology of Addictive Behaviors, 3,* 8–21.

Young, R. M., & Knight, R. G. (1989). The Drinking Expectancy Questionnaire: A revised measure of alcohol related beliefs. *Journal of Psychopathology and Behavioral Assessment, 11,* 99–112.

Young, R. M., Oei, T. P. S., & Crook, G. M. (1991). Development of a drinking self-efficacy questionnaire. *Journal of Psychopathology and Behavioral Assessment, 13,* 1–15.

Zinberg, N. E. (1984). *Drug, set, and setting.* New Haven, CT: Yale University Press.

Zywiak, W. H., Connors, G. J., Maisto, S. A., & Westerberg, V. S. (1996). Relapse research and the Reasons for Drinking Questionnaire: A factor analysis of Marlatt's relapse taxonomy. *Addiction, 91*(Suppl.), S121–S130.

5

Developmental Theory and Research

MICHAEL WINDLE
PATRICK T. DAVIES

INTRODUCTION

Major changes in the conceptualization and measurement of alcohol disorders and alcohol-related behaviors have emerged in recent years, culminating theoretically in the fostering of a biopsychosocial developmental paradigm (e.g., Donovan, 1988; Windle & Searles, 1990; Zucker, 1989; Zucker, Fitzgerald, & Moses, 1995). This biopsychosocial developmental paradigm, presented subsequently, may be most sharply contrasted with a narrow-range version of the medical disease model that emphasizes singularity with regard to factor prominence (e.g., the "alcoholic gene," the "alcoholic personality"), reductionism to the biological level with regard to necessary and sufficient conditions to infer causality, and "hard" determinism (i.e., inevitability) with regard to ultimate disease manifestation or outcome. The biopsychosocial developmental paradigm, by contrast, emphasizes multiple-factor influences on substance-related behaviors, the conjoint influence of variables from different levels of analysis (e.g., biochemical, cognitive, social variables), and dynamic, probabilistic behavior–outcome relations (i.e., the occurrence as well as the nature of expression of alcohol-related behaviors depend on a range of emerging, interactive factors that may vary across individuals and across time). A further characteristic of the biopsychosocial paradigm is the integral role of temporal factors related to lifespan development and to the timing of factors (e.g., pubertal onset, onset and duration of drinking) that may influence alternative life-course trajectories among individuals.

In the first edition of this volume (Blane & Leonard, 1987), Sadava (1987) reviewed the significance of evolving perspectives of interactionism to account for the complex relations among person and structural (or environmental) variables and alcohol-related outcome variables. Sadava contrasted extant theoretical perspectives and research programs (e.g., Huba & Bentler, 1982; Jessor & Jessor, 1977) that emphasized the potential significance of multiplicative interactive effects rather than simple additive effects. Interaction effects refer to conditional relationships, whereby the effect of a given independent variable (e.g., paternal alcoholism) on a dependent variable (e.g., offspring alcohol problems) is contingent on the level of a second independent variable (e.g., maternal support/protectiveness). This conditional relationship among independent variables is not constant across the levels of the two independent variables; hence, the functional relationship is conditional, or contingent, for these variables. For illustrative purposes, Figure 5.1 provides a simulated representation of an interactive effect among the three variables mentioned previously (i.e., paternal alcoholism, maternal support, offspring alcohol problems). For family history–negative (FHN) children, the number of alcohol problems among offspring is relatively constant across the levels of maternal support. However, for family history–positive (FHP) children, the number of alcohol problems among offspring varies contingent (or conditional) on the level of maternal support; lower maternal support is associated with more alcohol problems, whereas higher maternal support is associated with fewer alcohol problems.

Conceptually, this example of a single interaction effect demonstrates that the nature of interrelationships among variables is often much more

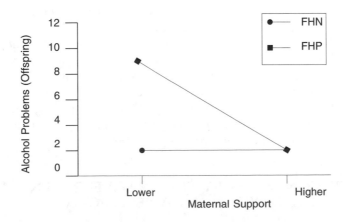

FIGURE 5.1. Simulated interactive relationship between family history of alcoholism, maternal support, and offspring alcohol problems.

complex than conceptual (and statistical) model implementations assume. That is, one cannot simply "add together" a constant influence of two (or more) factors (e.g., family history status and maternal support) and optimally predict outcomes (e.g., alcohol problems among offspring); rather, the impact of these factors varies, conditional on the values of the variables involved and the organized system of interrelations regulating these behaviors. Historically, this revision in conceptual approaches to substance use studies from more linear, additive models to interactive (multiplicative) models has corresponded to theoretical perspectives in developmental and personality psychology originating in the mid-1970s and early 1980s (e.g., Bronfenbrenner, 1977; Endler & Magnusson, 1976; Lerner, 1978; Magnusson, 1988). Sadava (1987) provided a useful review of some major substance use research programs (e.g., Huba & Bentler, 1982; Jessor & Jessor, 1977; Zucker & Noll, 1982) that have adopted (or were consistent with) the interactionist approach. Because of the substantive significance of these research programs and of the interactionist approach, findings from these studies are included in the materials subsequently reviewed.

However, a primary objective of this chapter is to extend the general conceptualization of interactionism to a broader lifespan developmental psychopathology perspective so as to coherently integrate extant findings and to provide a framework for subsequent research that is compatible with this perspective. We view the lifespan developmental psychopathology perspective as one that incorporates the general tenets of interactionism but involves major elaborations with regard to both conceptual and methodological features described subsequently, and which is consistent with the biopsychosocial paradigm. In the following pages, we first address the basic tenets and fundamental concepts of a lifespan developmental perspective. We then turn to a selective review of alcohol use studies across different portions of the lifespan (e.g., childhood, adolescence, young adulthood); studies were selected to help illuminate concepts relevant to the lifespan developmental psychopathology perspective rather than to comprehensively review the literature. After this selective review, we highlight and discuss two recent methodological advances (e.g., in research design and statistical modeling); these methodological advances are important because they facilitate the statistical testing of complex hypothesized relations generated by the developmental psychopathology perspective. Finally, we provide a brief summary of the material presented in this chapter.

BASIC CONCEPTS OF LIFESPAN DEVELOPMENTAL PSYCHOPATHOLOGY PERSPECTIVE

There are several concepts associated with a developmental psychopathology perspective that differ from many other theoretical orientations. These concepts are discussed now in relation to the dynamic diathesis–

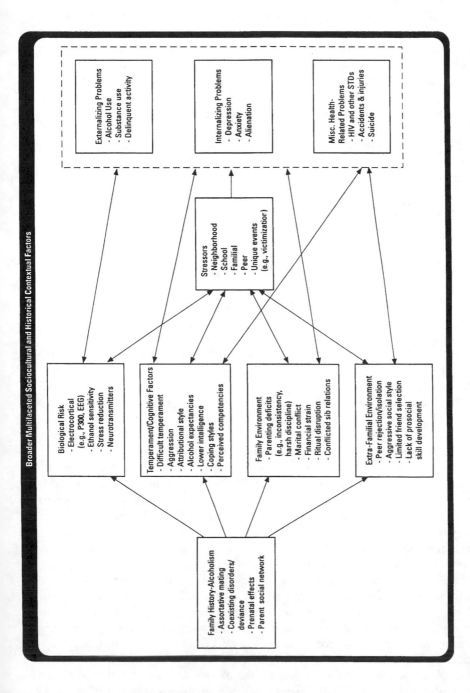

FIGURE 5.2. Dynamic diathesis–stress model of developmental psychopathology: An application to children of alcoholics (COAs).

stress model provided in Figure 5.2, which provides a representation of the major factors contributing to the expression of alcohol disorders and other forms of psychopathology and maladjustment among children of alcoholics (COAs). Parenthetically, the model presented here is not limited to COAs but may be used to represent putative causal factors for other disorders (e.g., major depressive disorder) by selecting those domain-specific risk factors identified as most relevant for the particular disorder (e.g., depressive attributional style as a psychological risk factor for depressive disorder). However, the *domains* identified in Figure 5.2 appear to have varying levels of support as potential putative factors across a wide range of psychiatric and substance abuse disorders, and features of maladjustment (e.g., dropping out of school, criminality).

The model in Figure 5.2 identifies and classifies risk factors for the expression of emotional and behavioral problems among COAs into several broad categories that correspond to different levels of analysis (e.g., biological, psychological, social). For example, a family history of alcoholism may pose increased risk for the expression of emotional and behavioral problems among offspring for several reasons, including increased genetic risk associated with assortative mating (i.e., alcoholic women marrying alcoholic men) (e.g., Hall, Hesselbrock, & Stabenau, 1983; Windle, 1997a), or from prenatal neurotoxic assaults associated with heavy alcohol consumption by mothers during pregnancy (e.g., Streissguth, Bookstein, Sampson, & Barr, 1995). Similarly, a reduction in the amplitude of the P300 electrocortical response has been associated with an increased risk for alcoholism (e.g., Begleiter, Porjesz, Bihari, & Kissin, 1984), as have individual differences in sensitivity to alcohol (e.g., Schuckit, 1994).

The model provided in Figure 5.2 seeks not only to identify and categorize major risk factors for emotional and behavioral problems among COAs, but also to highlight their intrinsic dynamic, interactive nature; that is, from a developmental process model orientation, it is important to attempt to map the ways in which constellations of factors coalesce into meaningful patterns (or organized behavioral regularities) across time to yield given outcomes (e.g., the expression of an alcohol disorder or coexisting alcohol and depressive disorders). Thus, a child with two alcoholic parents may be at genetic risk via both parental lineages, at risk prenatally due to mother's drinking, and at risk socially because of disrupted parenting (e.g., inconsistency of discipline), family financial strain, and marital conflict among the two alcoholic parents. This constellation of risk factors will likely increase the number of stressors within the family, and contingent on a range of other mediating and moderating sociocultural (e.g., socioeconomic status) and resource factors (e.g., level of social and community support), will result in either the nonoccurrence of any disorder (via protective factor influences), or the manifestation of one or more of the problems identified in Figure 5.2 (e.g., externalizing problems, internalizing problems, physical health problems).

For the illustrative case of COAs, findings from adoptee research designs have indicated at least a fourfold risk for an alcohol disorder among male offspring (e.g., for a review, see Russell, 1990). Despite the substantial increased risk for an alcohol disorder among COAs, it is important to recognize that the majority of COAs will *not* develop an alcohol disorder; rather, some will develop other expressions of psychopathology (e.g., major depressive disorder) or maladjustment, and still others will develop into well-adjusted adults. Hence, outcomes based solely on initial (COA) status are inadequate to account for the diverse manifestations observed. In order to "make sense" of the diversity, or heterogeneity, of outcomes among COAs, it is necessary to recognize that multiple risk and protective factors are involved in the ultimate expression of drinking-related behaviors and other forms of maladjustment, and that factors such as those summarized in Figure 5.2 need to be considered simultaneously. Furthermore, these factors must be studied prospectively (i.e., longitudinally) to understand how the timing of certain events (e.g., early-onset problem drinking, childhood proactive aggression) may contribute to negative regulatory cycles that may foster undesirable outcomes (e.g., alcohol disorder), and to identify other coevolving risk-associated behaviors (e.g., affiliation with deviant peers) that may propel individuals toward an entrenched unhealthy lifestyle.

A longitudinal focus on the organizational features of these coevolving and coadaptational processes across levels of analysis and across time characterizes a *transactional approach* to developmental psychopathology (e.g., Cicchetti, 1984; Sameroff, 1983; Sroufe & Rutter, 1984). By transaction, reference is made to the exchange of material and information across open systems that contributes to the stability and change in forms of behavior. Thus, this perspective emphasizes bidirectional (e.g., parent-to-child *and* child-to-parent influences) rather than unidirectional influences (e.g., parent-to-child only), continuity *and* discontinuity in behavior across time, and the multilevel multiplicity of influential factors (i.e., multivariate cross-level influences) on selected behaviors. As noted in the introduction to this chapter, this approach differs substantially from one that suggests a single-factor cause to account for a given outcome such as alcoholism. Furthermore, it extends beyond the statistical concept of interaction associated with the analysis of variance model to suggest "real-world," ongoing exchange processes among organisms and their environments in the organization and regulation (and dysregulation) of human behavior.

The concepts of equifinality and multifinality, adopted from general systems theory (e.g., von Bertalanffy, 1968), are commonly used in developmental psychopathology frameworks (e.g., Cicchetti & Rogosch, 1996; Sroufe & Rutter, 1984). *Equifinality* refers to the same end state being achieved from alternative initial conditions and through alternative processes. Thus, referring to Figure 5.2, an alcohol disorder (same end state) may occur via different initial conditions (e.g., parental assortative mating for alcoholism vs. prenatal effects on the central nervous system of the fetus) and/or alternative ongoing processes (e.g., disruptive parenting and financial strain vs. a more difficult temperament and peer rejection). *Multifinality* refers to the notion that any single component, or factor, may vary in terms of its influence (both in terms of valence and magnitude) contingent on the values (or functioning) of other components of the system operating as a whole. Hence, a risk factor such as family history of alcoholism will not always (inevitably) result in an alcohol disorder; rather, its impact will be moderated by the values of other factors. A positive, socially outgoing temperamental style, in conjunction with community-support agents, may yield a developmental pathway toward positive mental health among the offspring of alcoholics (e.g., Werner & Smith, 1982). In other circumstances, a family history of alcoholism may impact levels of marital conflict and financial strain that increase the probability of depression in offspring, but not necessarily alcoholism. Equifinality and multifinality are important concepts to a developmental psychopathology perspective because they relate to the heterogeneity and multiplicity of both putative causal influences and "outcomes" that characterize the behaviors under investigation.

Two other concepts of importance to the developmental psychopathology perspective (and to interactional approaches) are moderators and mediators, which assist in the description and statistical testing of the presumed causal dynamics involved in characterizing interrelationships among variables (e.g., Baron & Kenny, 1986). A *moderator variable* attenuates or exacerbates the relationship between a second independent variable (the moderator variable being the first) and an outcome variable. For example, in the earlier example portrayed in Figure 5.1, maternal support moderated the influence of family history of alcoholism on alcohol problems among offspring. In this instance, higher maternal support attenuated the impact of paternal alcoholism on offspring functioning. Other moderator relationships may be characterized by an exacerbation or synergy, whereby two (independent) variables interact to produce an effect on a dependent variable that is greater than their two independent additive effects. For example, levels of difficult temperament among fathers and their sons may be such that higher levels by both parties may result in greatly heightened levels of interpersonal conflict and violence (e.g., Blackson, Tarter, Martin, & Moss, 1994). Such moderator variable relationships are of importance in describing the nonlinear relationships that are sometimes found in alcohol studies and that may better describe the functional form of interrelationships among variables.

A *mediator variable* provides the proposed intervening process or mechanism used to explain the relationship between a variable (or variables) and an outcome (or outcomes). For example, Figure 5.3 provides an illustration of a single mediator model in which the influence of family history of alcoholism is posited to influence the expression of an alcohol disorder through the mediating mechanism of conduct disorder; that is, this model postulates a process or mechanism whereby the risk for familial al-

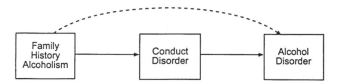

FIGURE 5.3. Mediator and partial mediator model of family history of alcoholism, childhood conduct disorder, and adult alcohol disorder.

coholism influences the expression of conduct disorder among offspring in childhood, which, in turn, influences the expression of an alcohol disorder in adulthood. Hence, this "full mediation" model suggests that the complete influence of familial alcoholism on offspring alcohol-disorder status in adulthood occurs via childhood conduct disorder. If this influence is only partial, that is, if other factors associated with familial alcoholism (e.g., sensitivity to alcohol) also influence alcohol disorder outcomes in adulthood, then this would be described as a "partial mediational" model and would be indicated by the inclusion of the dotted line in Figure 5.3, in addition to the bold lines.

Mediational models (full and partial) may be extended to multiple intervening, mediational variables, as exemplified in Figure 5.4. According to the fully mediated model portrayed in Figure 5.4, the influences of familial alcoholism on alcohol disorder status and school difficulties are fully medi-

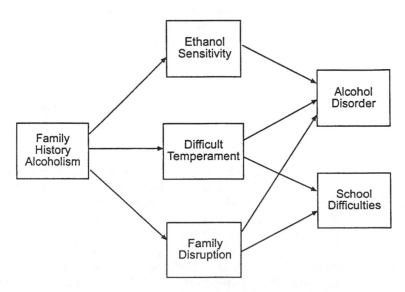

FIGURE 5.4. Multiple mediator model of the influence of family history of alcoholism on alcohol-disorder status and school difficulties.

ated by three factors: ethanol sensitivity, difficult temperament, and family disruption. However, this specified model further postulates that all three factors are involved in the mediational process for alcohol-disorder status, but that only difficult temperament and family disruption are involved in the mediational process for school difficulties. The use of these two figures (i.e., Figures 5.3 and 5.4) illustrates the nature of the kinds of questions that may be posed from a developmental psychopathology perspective with regard to the multiplicity of influences, the multiplicity of outcomes, and the specification of theoretically driven intervening processes. Such models may be extended to time-ordered, prospective data and to the inclusion of bidirectional influence models. In addition, as discussed later in this chapter, there have been significant methodological changes in methods of data collection and data analyses (i.e., alternative longitudinal statistical models) that enable the specification, testing, and evaluation of complex hypothesized relations that are consistent with those discussed in this chapter (e.g., Bryant, Windle, & West, 1997).

The concept of *developmental pathways* has often been used to identify a subset of the most prominent and distinctive patterns characterizing trajectories toward given end states, such as an alcohol disorder. For example, the alcohol subtype literature (e.g., Cloninger, Bohman, & Sigvardsson, 1981; Zucker, 1987) may be viewed as an attempt to identify distinctive, time-ordered, etiological pathways for alcohol disorders; that is, an antisocial alcoholic subtype has been identified that is characterized by higher rates of childhood conduct problems and an early age of onset for alcohol use and alcohol-related problems, whereas a second alcoholic subtype has been characterized by low rates of childhood conduct problems and a substantially later onset of alcohol-related problems. As a second example, Schulenberg, Wadsworth, O'Malley, Bachman, and Johnston (1996) used four-wave prospective data to identify distinctive pathways related to binge drinking in the transition from adolescence to young adulthood. For one of their comparisons, Chronic versus Decreased subgroups were similar in their levels of binge drinking in their senior year of high school (both averaging approximately four binge episodes in the preceding 2 weeks); however, across time, the Chronic group persisted in high levels of binge drinking, whereas the Decreased group members significantly reduced their levels of binge drinking. It is of importance to note that in their senior year, members of these two groups also did not differ on a number of other variables (e.g., antisociality, rebelliousness, grade point average, time spent with friends) that may have accounted for the different binge-drinking trajectories. The findings of the study indicated that being female, having higher self-efficacy and work readiness, less drinking to get drunk, and greater loneliness significantly differentiated those youth who decreased their binge drinking relative to those who persisted in their binge drinking. In this application, different pathways were indicated for those who began at the same initial state (i.e., as heavy binge drinkers) but diverged across the transition from adolescence to young adulthood in distinctive ways that were associated with a given set of precursor variables (e.g., higher self-efficacy).

The incorporation of concepts such as developmental pathways, equifinality, and multifinality in alcohol studies may be of value to "tease out" the multiplicity of influences on the range of variables of interest to alcohol researchers, and to entertain notions of distinctive patterns (or subtypes) that may more adequately account for the heterogeneity observed in most domains under investigation. Alcohol researchers have interests in a broad range of outcome variables, including alcohol use onset, frequency and quantity of use, adverse social consequences, dependency symptoms, binge drinking, and so on. These outcome variables typically manifest highly significant bivariate associations (e.g., Pearson correlations >.4), but they certainly are not identical phenotypes. Furthermore, it is highly unlikely that the range of risk and protective factors that have been identified in alcohol studies generalizes across all of these phenotypes; the generality and specificity of interrelations between risk and protective factors, and these phenotypes are not currently known.

In studying alcohol-related behaviors and time-course issues (e.g., initiation, escalation), researchers have often focused on the period of adolescence. A developmental perspective, however, underscores the fact that the impact of alcohol contexts on individuals' subsequent alcohol use and mental health may begin much earlier in the life course; that is, alcohol problems are often viewed as a manifestation of a developmental history of adaptational failures in key developmental tasks (e.g., emotional regulation, establishment of a personal identity). These prior failures are potentially malleable in the sense that success in coping with subsequent developmental challenges may affect movement toward more healthy developmental pathways (e.g., abstinence, modest levels of alcohol consumption) (Sroufe, 1997). In the following section, we selectively review research studies to illustrate how adherence to developmental principles may elucidate the study of the precursors, time course, and sequelae of alcohol and substance use.

Infancy and Toddlerhood

The constitutional risk posed by parental alcoholism to offspring is evident very early in the lifespan. Newborns of mothers who consume even moderate levels of alcohol during pregnancy exhibit greater irritability, tremulousness, information-processing impairments (e.g., delays in habituating to novel stimuli), and low activity (e.g., Streissguth, Barr, & Martin, 1983). Infants and young children of alcoholics (whether or not exposed to alcohol prenatally) are also at risk for manifesting defining features of difficult temperament, including high levels of emotional reactivity, negative affect, distractability, and impulsivity (Streissguth, 1986; Windle, 1990). A teratogenic model of alcohol effects for prenatally exposed infants has been useful in illustrating one possible source underlying this diathesis. In support of a teratogenic pathway of alcohol effects, dose–response relationships have been found between maternal alcohol consumption during pregnancy and offspring vulnerability. Thus, although high levels of prenatal exposure to alcohol appear to have highly adverse and even fatal effects on offspring, even moderate levels of maternal alcohol consumption increase risk for developmental impairments indicative of subtle, but persistent, neuropsychological deficits (e.g., poor attention span, poor spatial organization, and poor short-term memory). These findings are robust even after statistically controlling for extraneous prenatal (e.g., diet) and environmental variables (e.g., parental education, family stress) (Streissguth, Barr, & Sampson, 1990; Streissguth et al., 1983).

Although the significance of research on prenatal alcohol exposure cannot be understated, narrowly focusing on diathesis at the earliest part of the lifespan necessitates integrating a teratogenic model within a larger developmental diathesis–stress model. Alcoholism, even in one parent (e.g., fathers), may increase risk for diathesis through the mediating influences of an inherited genetic substrate. Genetic vulnerability models, for example, have proposed that the neurobiological mechanisms underlying parental alcoholism are inherited by offspring and are phenotypically manifested in the form of difficult temperament styles in infancy and toddlerhood (e.g., Tarter, Alterman, & Edwards, 1985). Assortative mating processes, whereby partners with significant histories of alcoholism, substance use, and psychopathology pair up (e.g., Hall et al., 1983; for a review, also see McGue, Chapter 10, this volume), may additively or multiplicatively increase the biological vulnerability of these young children. To account for behavioral outcomes among COAs exposed prenatally to alcohol, the teratogenic and genetic pathways to diathesis must be considered in the context of a complex constellation of comorbid risk factors in the prenatal (e.g., poor diet, lack of prenatal care), perinatal (e.g., obstetric problems), and early postnatal (e.g., poverty, impoverished caregiving environment) periods of development (e.g., Rodning, Beckwith, & Howard, 1989; Streissguth et al., 1990).

Biological risk processes alone, however, cannot fully account for the developmental impairments of offspring whose mothers consumed alcohol prenatally, or of COAs. The higher than normal prevalence of insecure attachments among infants of mothers who consumed large amounts of alcohol prenatally are not easily explained by an exclusive focus on biological processes (O'Connor, Sigman, & Brill, 1987). Furthermore, developmental pathways rooted in any context of early risk, including early alcohol effects, become increasingly differentiated and diverse over time (Sroufe, 1997). For example, some sources of biological risk (e.g., prenatal alcohol exposure) become progressively diluted over time (Windle & Tubman, in press), as many infants who initially show maladaptive patterns of functioning are able to make successive adaptations toward healthy developmental trajectories, and still other infants who initially showed constitutional integrity may respond in maladaptive ways to developmental challenges.

By subsuming the study of biological risk within transactional, developmental conceptualizations of the interplay between diathesis and stress, developmental psychopathology frameworks have begun to address this complexity. Such frameworks specify that understanding the ways in which young COAs (or children exposed prenatally via maternal drinking) negotiate stage-salient or developmental tasks may help unravel the multivariate complexities underlying the effects of family alcoholism. Particularly salient challenges faced by children approaching late infancy include the establishment of (1) ways of modulating arousal and negative affect; (2) harmonious, synchronous interactions with caregivers; (3) secure attachment bonds with caregivers; and (4) interpersonal trust. Successfully negotiating these tasks has been hypothesized to probabilistically increase children's success in adaptively coping with subsequent tasks and pursuing healthy developmental trajectories. Failure to successfully resolve these issues, however, has been hypothesized to probabilistically increase children's risk for subsequent maladaptive functioning over the course of development (Cicchetti, 1993; Sroufe, 1990).

The utility of this approach is exemplified in a series of studies by O'Connor and colleagues (e.g., O'Connor, Sigman, & Kasari, 1992, 1993). Illustrating the transactional interplay between developmental tasks, their hypothesis was that impairments in modulating negative affect among infants prenatally exposed to alcohol would increase the risk for mother–child interactive disturbances (developmental task 2) by virtue of escalating cycles of negative interactions between heavy drinking, distressed mothers and their difficult infants. These interactive disturbances, in turn, were hypothesized to increase the probability of insecure parent–child relationships (developmental task 3) and accompanying internal representations of attachment figures as untrustworthy (developmental task 4). Consistent with these hypotheses, analyses with structural equation models supported a multichain pathway whereby (1) maternal alcohol consumption during pregnancy predicted infant negative affect at 1 year of age; (2) negative affect, in turn, was linked with parenting styles indicative of a lack of synchrony (e.g., maternal intrusiveness, rejection); and (3) parental interactive disturbances were associated with insecure parent–child attachment patterns (O'Connor et al., 1992).

In a separate study, Eiden and Leonard (1996) reported that heavy paternal alcohol use was associated with a significantly higher prevalence of insecurely attached infants; almost two-thirds of the infants in the paternal heavy drinking group were so classified. Also, heavier paternal drinking was significantly associated with both higher maternal depression and lower maternal marital satisfaction. There was also a synergistic relationship between heavy paternal alcohol use and maternal depression that increased the prediction of insecure infant attachments. These findings exemplify how heavy paternal alcohol use may influence the resolution of important challenges in infancy (e.g., developing a secure attachment) via the disruptions of mother–child and family relationships.

Although many of the tasks faced in infancy remain salient across development, the transition from infancy to toddlerhood is also accompanied by a new series of developmental tasks, including the awareness of the self as distinct, the exploration of social and object worlds, self-control, emotion regulation, and understanding the emotional states of others (Rodning et al., 1989; Sroufe, 1990). Since these tasks are already challenging in themselves, their resolution may be highly sensitive to the deleterious effects of family alcoholism relative to other domains of functioning. A focus on the emergence of these domains of functioning and skills may be a rich source of hypotheses regarding the specific aspects of the dynamic diathesis–stress matrix that may be most salient in understanding toddler development. For example, an emerging understanding of the emotional states of others in conjunction with the salience of developing adaptive emotion-regulation strategies in toddlerhood may result in greater sensitivity to deleterious aspects of the emotional climate in the alcoholic family system. As such, interparental discord may emerge as an increasingly powerful mediator of the effects of parental alcohol problems during the toddler years (El-Sheikh & Cummings, 1997). In comparison to non-COAs, COAs are exposed to higher levels of interparental conflict, violence, and emotional instability (e.g., Heyman, O'Leary, & Jouriles, 1995; Leonard & Senchak, 1993). Accumulating evidence suggests that marital conflict, in itself, increases children's vulnerability to psychopathology directly through emotional channels (e.g., Cummings & Davies, 1996).

Even in the context of the multiple risks commonly experienced by toddlers of alcoholic parents within both stress and diathesis components of the model, it is important not to "overpathologize" toddlers or their developmental contexts; most of these young COAs develop along more or less adaptive developmental trajectories (Windle & Tubman, in press). Thus, prioritizing the search for protective factors (i.e., moderators) is an essential step in understanding multifinality in young COAs' developmental pathways and outcomes. Toward this end, personality variables such as high ego integration and low levels of impulsivity and sensation seeking have been shown to ameliorate the risk of children of substance-using parents (Brooks, Whiteman, Shapiro, & Cohen, 1996). A critical task of future research involves identifying the mediating processes through which the moderating nature of personality factors, spousal substance use, and so forth, ultimately have their influence on children.

Childhood

As children progress into and through the childhood years, maturational growth and developmental tasks are likely to result in a number of changes in the nature and magnitude of relations among variables in the dynamic diathesis–stress model. Maturational growth and the increasing differentiation of domains of functioning in the preschool years are specifically theorized to generate a number of qualitatively different pathways through which parental alcohol problems may pose their risk. For example, dramatic increases in cognitive development (e.g., constructing, accessing, and recalling symbolic representations of social experiences) allow young children, beginning in the preschool years, to increasingly employ schemas as guides to their behavior across time and contexts. An implication is that the repeated exposure of children to socialization agents who are alcoholics or regular drinkers provides greater access to acquisition of knowledge concerning the defining features of alcoholic beverages, norms of alcohol consumption, and the psychological precursors and sequelae of alcohol consumption (Gaines, Brooks, Maisto, Dietrich, & Shagena, 1988). These schemas, in turn, may provide early motivational and instructional scripts for the subsequent development of more refined alcohol expectancies, motives for drinking, and heavy alcohol consumption in adolescence and adulthood (e.g., Zucker, Kincaid, Fitzgerald, & Bingham, 1995).

Although researchers have yet to test explicitly the mediating role of evolving alcohol schemas during childhood in the intergenerational linkage of alcohol consumption, initial evidence is supportive, as linkages have been demonstrated between (1) early experiences with parental alcohol use and children's identification of, knowledge about, and intentions to drink as early as the preschool and elementary school years (Gaines et al., 1988; Noll, Zucker, & Greenberg, 1990; Zucker et al., 1995); and (2) alcohol expectancies, theorized to be a developmental derivative of early alcohol schemas, which predict subsequent alcohol involvement during early adolescence (e.g., Christiansen, Smith, Roehling, & Goldman, 1989). Prospectively tracing the pathways between living with a socialization agent who is a heavy drinker and the developmental differentiation and integration of alcohol schemas from early childhood through adolescence and subsequent alcohol consumption remain critical tasks for future research.

The increasing ability to take another's social and emotional perspective (i.e., decline in egocentrism) during early to middle childhood constitutes another maturational change that may provide important conceptual tools for tracking the multiple trajectories toward risk for psychopathology among COAs. Declines in egocentrism are specifically accompanied by increased concerns and worries among young children about the psychological and physical welfare of family members (Cicchetti, Cummings, Greenberg, & Marvin, 1990). Features of the larger family climate that serve as indicators of the psychological and emotional well-being of family members (e.g., family cohesion, interparental conflict) may thus assume even greater salience as mediators in the transmission of disturbance from alcoholic parents to their offspring. This is significant for COAs given the empirical findings of the high prevalence of family discord in alcoholic families (El-Sheikh & Cummings, 1997). Recent data support the hypothesis that the general emotional tenor of the family plays a more significant role in the development of children's worries about drinking than parental drinking per se (e.g., Shell, Groppenbacher, Roosa, & Gensheimer, 1992). High levels of involvement in family problems may, in turn, increase children's vulnerability to psychological problems, especially with regard to internalizing symptoms (e.g., depression, anxiety) (Cummings, Davies, & Simpson, 1994; Grych, Seid, & Fincham, 1992). Thus, developmental advances in social-perspective-taking skills during childhood may pave the way for stronger mediational pathways between parental alcoholism, family discord, and child psychological problems.

In spite of these early demonstrations of the importance of the alcoholic family system to children's development (e.g., parent–child relations, marital and family conflict), much remains to be known about the mediating and moderating role of family processes and children's personality and coping styles (El-Sheikh & Cummings, 1997; Whipple, Fitzgerald, & Zucker, 1995). A noteworthy exception is Zucker's (1994) model of gender-specific developmental trajectories to alcoholism. Zucker has hypothesized that risk and vulnerability for antisocial trajectories to alcoholism begin early in childhood, with boys being especially prone to following this pathway. In particular, the histories of a transactional interplay between genetic diathesis (e.g., family history of alcoholism and antisocial disorder) and early, chronic psychosocial stressors (e.g., deviant parental models, family discord) foster highly stable trajectories of aggression and deviance. By way of constitutional (e.g., biological proclivity toward alcohol), active (i.e., seeking out "like peers" as friends), and evocative (i.e., actively rejected by normal peers) processes, these children become increasingly involved in deviant activities, including drinking and heavy drug use, from early adolescence onward.

Adolescence

Periods of early and middle adolescence are characterized by substantial developmental changes across the major components of the biopsychosocial matrix of influences. In the social domain, adolescents face primary challenges of (1) coping with peer pressure; (2) undergoing transitions from the relatively intimate, personal confines of elementary school to ever larger and often more impersonal secondary schools; (3) successively renegotiating balances between autonomy and relatedness in the family; and (4) developing heterosexual friendships and relationships (Jacob & Leonard, 1994; Schulenberg, Maggs, & Hurrelmann, 1997). The process of resolving these tasks in the social domain is best conceptualized as transactional and bidirectional in nature. For example, the normative process of forging autonomy among adolescents precipitates new challenges for parenting, including integrating effective ways of monitoring and managing adolescent

activities and peer affiliations within the larger style of parenting characterized by consistent discipline and high levels of support.

Guided by the salience of this adolescent developmental task (forging
autonomy) and the associated parental demands, models have conceptualized parental alcoholism and the accompanying network of problems (e.g.,
parental psychopathology) as compromising parents' abilities to monitor
and manage adolescent activities. Poor parental monitoring, in turn, increases the risk of affiliation with deviant peers and, eventually, maladaptive outcomes (Dishion, Patterson, & Reid, 1988; Hawkins, Catalano,
& Miller, 1992; Jacob & Leonard, 1994). Consistent with this hypothesis,
both cross-sectional and longitudinal growth curve studies have documented a multichain pathway of risk posed by parental alcoholism whereby (1) parental alcoholism predicts decreases in parental monitoring; (2)
lax parental monitoring, in turn, predicts subsequent adolescent affiliation
with deviant peers; and (3) deviant peer affiliation is associated with concurrent adolescent substance use involvement and subsequent escalation of
substance use (Chassin, Pillow, Curran, Molina, & Barrera, 1993; Chassin,
Curran, Hussong, & Colder, 1996).

Illustrating the necessity of a multiple pathway conceptualization of
adolescent risk, the growing influence of peer, friendship, and intimate relations is likely to operate through complex transactional processes. Although *peer socialization* models posit the popular notion that peer
substance use is a proximal cause of adolescent substance use (Swaim,
Oetting, Edwards, & Beauvais, 1989), alternative explanations exist. *Peer
selection* models, for example, suggest that adolescents become increasingly
active in seeking out and selecting peer groups that are most consistent with
their attitudes and behaviors (Farrell, 1994). Contextual influences may
also serve as alternative, common variables (e.g., neighborhood or school
characteristics) that may account for the co-occurrence of both peer and
adolescent substance use by contributing to the development of both. A recent systematic test of possible peer-influenced pathways provided evidence
for both the peer selection and peer socialization models, thereby supporting a dynamic, bidirectional relationship between adolescent and peer substance use across 6-month intervals (Curran, Stice, & Chassin, 1997).
Specifically, parental alcoholism predicted greater adolescent and peer substance use which, in turn, predicted subsequent bidirectional changes
across time between adolescent and peer substance use.

Although adolescents are undergoing considerable physical and maturational changes as a result of puberty, these developmental processes and
their psychological and social correlates have yet to be systematically examined in the context of risk and protective models of adolescent substance
use. Findings from developmental research, however, indicate that maturational changes may play a critical role in shaping high-risk families. For
example, pubertal development has been associated with increases in parent–adolescent conflict (Steinberg, 1990) and a rise in depressive symptoms

and lower self-esteem in girls (Brooks-Gunn & Warren, 1989). Thus, one implication is that these biologically linked processes (i.e., pubertal development) may exacerbate preexisting vulnerabilities of adolescents with a family history of alcoholism and dysfunction, or function to increase family tension and parental stress (Steinberg, 1990). Such hypotheses remain speculative, particularly given the failure empirically to demonstrate that the combination of pubertal development and parental alcoholism synergistically increase parent–child relationship disturbances (Molina & Chassin, 1996).

In order to accommodate the multiple developmental changes across the organism–context coaction during adolescence, alcohol researchers have increasingly replaced conventional techniques of testing single, intervening variables with models of multiple, intervening variables. *Multiple mediator models* have been used to account for the complex matrix óf constitutional and psychosocial processes underlying the linkage between parental alcohol problems and adolescent vulnerability. For example, in predicting adolescent substance use, Chassin and colleagues (1996) reported a complex, but theoretically compelling, pattern of mediators of parental alcoholism involving lax parental monitoring, uncontrollable life stressors, negative affect, and affiliation with drug-using peers. *Multiple moderator models* may also be developed to incorporate principles of contextual and ecological relativism. In alcohol conceptualizations, protective factors such as a good parent–adolescent relationship have been tacitly treated as if they were static "traits" that retained their buffering power across contexts (Hawkins et al., 1992). More dynamic, contextual models, however, underscore that the nature of the moderating effect of any factor depends on the larger ecological context. For example, in a recent study, Andrews, Hops, and Duncan (1997) found that adolescents were more likely to model parental alcohol and substance use if they had a *good relationship* with their parent. Thus, in alcoholic or drug using families, strong bonds between parents and adolescents may increase, not decrease, their vulnerability, at least in certain domains of functioning, such as drug use.

Incorporating mediators and moderators into single research designs has also proven useful in capturing meaningful developmental phenomena in adolescence. The task of testing developmental psychopathology models of risk and protection is not simply complete after demonstrating that a particular factor such as parental support buffers (i.e., moderates) the risk posed by parental alcoholism to adolescents. Identifying the presence of a protective factor is only the first step toward ultimately understanding the protective processes (i.e., mediators) through which the factor ultimately impacts on the adolescent. For example, after finding that stress predicted significantly greater increases in psychological symptoms in adolescent COAs than adolescent non-COAs, Barrera, Li, and Chassin (1995) took the analyses one step further by identifying that family conflict played an important role in mediating the stress–symptomatology link for COAs only—a pathway supporting a *model of moderated mediation* (also see Baron & Kenny, 1986). This design not only showed that parental alcoholism status moderated the effects of stress but also explicated one of the mediating processes responsible for the interaction between alcoholism and stress in the form of family conflict.

Timing of Developmental Transitions

In addition to examining how normative developmental tasks may reshape mediator and moderator pathways in the dynamic diathesis–stress model, another critical theme in developmental psychopathology involves understanding the influence of the timing of developmental tasks in the expression of alcohol problems among children and adolescents. According to the pseudomaturity theory endorsed by Newcomb (1996), prematurely confronting developmental transitions hinders the ability to master adequately the psychosocial skills that are necessary to resolve subsequent developmental roles and tasks. Premature developmental transitions during adolescence consist not only of deviant events (e.g., age of initiation of drug involvement and deviant activities) but also of inherently positive or culturally valued events such as age of financial autonomy and independent living. Thus, in contrast to general deviance theory (e.g., Jessor & Jessor, 1977; McGee & Newcomb, 1992), pseudomaturity theory underscores the deleterious effects of the early timing of developmental transitions and not the maladaptive quality of the transition itself. Early empirical tests of this theory have been promising. For example, early establishment of financial autonomy, independent living, intimate relations, and deviant activities in adolescence were moderate to strong predictors of early transitions into alcohol involvement and drug use (Newcomb, 1996; also see the next section, "Young Adulthood," for evidence of long-term sequelae).

Although mapping the timing of the organization and clustering of multiple developmental transitions provides a promising foundation for understanding the context of alcohol and substance use development, an important, but neglected, task is to delineate the etiological substrates from which this constellation of early transitions develops. Particularly relevant to this chapter is the hypothesis that the stress accompanying exposure to parental alcoholism or heavy drinking may precipitate premature cycling into adult roles and, subsequently, vulnerability to alcohol and drug problems. For example, in keeping with the principle of multifinality, family systems models have proposed that family distress and dysfunction that accompany parental alcoholism may promote at least two different pathways that may increase risk for alcohol and drug problems. In the first pathway, the discord in alcoholic families may promote family "role reversal" whereby the adolescent prematurely assumes adult responsibilities such as taking care of the alcoholic parent. By adopting a parental role, the COA adolescent may simultaneously (and inadvertently) make transitions into other family distress and discord issues that may exhaust coping resources and precipitate the initiation or escalation of alcohol and drug use by the adolescent. In the second pathway, adolescents may cope with certain forms of discord in alcoholic families (e.g., parental rejection) by emotionally "detaching" themselves from the family. A consequence of this detachment from family may be that these adolescents are then forced into adult responsibilities prematurely and do not develop the competencies necessary to shield them from the deleterious effects of alcohol and substance use (Newcomb, 1996).

Developmental Pathways

The well-documented normative increase in alcohol involvement over the period between early and late adolescence is also accompanied by a less acknowledged process characterized by increases in the heterogeneity of change in alcohol involvement during this period (Johnstone, Leino, Ager, Ferrer, & Fillmore, 1996). This heterogeneity suggests that there is considerable interindividual variability in intraindividual change in alcohol patterns during adolescence. Stated differently, it underscores the multiplicity of different pathways of drinking patterns even during the early half of adolescence. Wills, McNamara, Vaccaro, and Hirky (1996) were able to reliably distinguish among five developmental trajectories on the basis of their pattern of level, stability, and escalation in drug use over a 3-year period from early to middle adolescence. Particularly pertinent to developmental psychopathology were their findings indicating that escalated substance use was predicted by a multivariate matrix of factors including parental substance use, life stress, low parental support, low levels of self-control, and greater affiliation with deviant peers. Given that these results held even after statistically controlling for differences in initial levels of substance use, it can be more confidently concluded that these factors predict change in developmental trajectories and not simply age of onset or level of substance use.

Attesting to the importance of a lifespan view of alcoholism, the roots of these developmental pathways during adolescence may date back to very early life. The principle of canalization posits that lengthier histories on a specific developmental course of adaptation or maladaptation increasingly limits the probability, degree, and nature of subsequent changes in adaptation (Cicchetti & Cohen, 1995; Waddington, 1957). In support of canalization, Zucker et al. (1995) reviewed a number of studies indicating that early development of maladaptation placed individuals in increasingly stable and crystallized patterns of deviance characterized by increasing differentiation and ranges of problems in the form of delinquency, criminal activity, alcohol problems, and substance use. Yet alcohol problems of individuals who were relatively free of prolonged bouts of psychological problems in earlier stages of the life span are more likely to be temporary and unstable (Zucker, 1994; Zucker et al., 1995).

Unraveling the Main Effects and Moderating Role of Gender

Recent historical trends have included an increase in the number of adolescent girls who use alcohol and engage in binge drinking episodes, thus fostering the notion that there is a convergence in drinking behavior between boys and girls during adolescence. However, more careful scrutiny of the data indicates that boys, relative to girls, drink more frequently and in larger quantities, and have more alcohol-related problems (e.g., White & Huselid, 1997). Although little is known about the origins of gender differences in many alcohol-related behaviors, there are several hypotheses that can be advanced from a developmental psychopathology framework. For example, it may be a by-product, in part, of the disproportionate risk among males to exhibit antisocial trajectories to alcoholism characterized by the persistent, early-development of conduct problems and early-onset alcohol involvement in early to middle adolescence. Developmental trajectories that are more commonly followed by girls are conceptualized as manifesting themselves in the form of alcohol problems much later in adolescence or adulthood (e.g., negative affect alcoholism; Zucker, 1994).

Guided by the gender intensification hypothesis, another possibility is that the physical differentiation between boys and girls is accompanied by increasing socialization pressures to conform to traditional gender roles (Petersen, Sarigiani, & Kennedy, 1991). Thus, boys may be socialized into valuing agency, exploration, independence, and risk taking, whereas girls may be socialized into valuing communal, interpersonal relationships with significant others. Since increased emotional autonomy has been associated with susceptibility to peer pressure and affiliation (Steinberg & Silverberg, 1986), one possible pathway is that middle-adolescent boys may be more apt to comply or accept normative peer behavior and values endorsing alcohol use and delinquency (Aseltine, 1995). By contrast, to the extent that girls increasingly assume traditional female roles, greater affiliation with the family and wariness of novelty may buffer or, at least delay, their involvement in alcohol and substance use experimentation and escalation in the peer group.

In addition to providing a useful foundation for explaining the origins of gender differences in alcohol involvement, the gender intensification theory may also provide evidence of gender differences in socialization pathways in alcoholic families (e.g., gender as a moderator). For example, although greater concern and caring in harmonious family relationships among girls may serve adaptive functions (e.g., Chase-Lansdale, Wakschlag, & Brooks-Gunn, 1995), greater concern and sensitivity in the face of discordant family conditions that commonly accompany parental alcoholism may lead to greater psychological burden and symptomatology, including depressed affect and alcohol problems (e.g., Davies & Windle, 1997; also see Russell, Cooper, & Frone, 1990). Although the research findings are inconsistent, gender socialization may also shape the form of problems exhibited by adolescent girls, as they may be especially susceptible to the development of internalizing symptoms (e.g., Chassin, Rogosch, & Barrera, 1991). Thus, although speculative, pathways between family histories of alcoholism, family discord, and adolescent outcomes may very well be stronger (or at least qualitatively different) for adolescent girls than boys.

Complex, but largely untested, models also posit that adolescent boys may be more prone to progressing along constitutionally driven trajectories of family alcoholism. For example, Pihl and Bruce (1995) have interpreted differences in P300 wave amplitude between sons of male alcoholics (SOMAs) and controls as reflecting mild impairments in the prefrontal cortex that may manifest themselves in terms of (1) poor planning abilities, and (2) generalized chronic arousal resulting from disturbances in the information processing of affective, threatening, and novel events. The resulting impulsivity and hyperactivity may restrict opportunities for achieving pleasant psychological states and may engender negative interpersonal reactions. Alcohol, which becomes increasingly accessible to adolescents, may be an ultimate means of coping with problems. However, the implicit assumption that boys may be more susceptible to temperamental risk associated with parental alcoholism may simply be an artifact of the overreliance on sons of alcoholics in the literature (Ohannessian & Hesselbrock, 1994). Thus, at the very least, recruiting female COAs and non-COAs is necessary to examine more adequately whether such pathways are gender-specific (for other temperament-based pathways, see Whipple & Noble, 1991).

Young Adulthood

In the aggregate, the transition between adolescence and young adulthood is characterized by normative declines in alcohol consumption (Bachman, Wadsworth, O'Malley, Johnston, & Schulenberg, 1997; Johnstone et al., 1996). In integrating role incompatibility theory within a developmental framework (Kandel, 1980; Yamaguchi, 1990), the role socialization hypothesis proffers that this decline is, in part, a by-product of assuming new developmental challenges and tasks centering around the establishment of (1) a stable, occupational trajectory; (2) an intimate, long-term, relationship; and (3) a family, by becoming a parent. Consistent with this theory, research has demonstrated that declines in alcohol involvement, especially drinking problems, accompany the successful transition from schooling into the full-time workforce (e.g., Gotham, Sher, & Wood, 1997; Temple et al., 1991); the establishment of close, romantic relationships (e.g., Bachman et al., 1997; Miller-Tutzauer, Leonard, & Windle, 1991; Sadava & Pak, 1994); and, to a lesser extent, the role of parenthood (Bachman et al., 1997).

A developmental process model of young-adult alcohol involvement draws attention to the importance of investigating not only the occurrence of stage-salient tasks (e.g., assuming occupational, marital, and family roles), but also the mediating and moderating processes that are linked to changes in drinking behaviors. Thus, the assumption is that it is not simply the changes in marital, parenting, or occupational status that are tied to changes in drinking. Such structural changes are conceptualized as only rough markers or proxies for more proximal mediating processes that guide, in part, modifications in drinking behaviors. For example, changes in residence (e.g., cohabitation) and increases in commitment to a partner may accompany transitions into serious relationships (e.g., engagement, marriage) that may reduce drinking by limiting the opportunities, leisure time, or motivation to become involved in contexts that are conducive to drinking (e.g., peer group from college, bar settings). A large part of this motivation may involve a purposeful attempt to develop a larger identity that is consistent with mature, adult roles (e.g., role of a supportive spouse and parent). Alternatively, a more global process (e.g., "maturing out," secure attachment representations) may actually be responsible for the adoption of these adult roles and the reduction in alcohol problems (Bachman et al., 1997).

Qualifying structural conceptualizations (e.g., change in marital status) as "rough" proxies also serves to underscore the importance of explicating the study of status variables by focusing on the process and quality of resolving important developmental tasks (for a further description of the influence of alcohol on the marital transition, see Leonard & Rothbard, in press). The simple adoption of the spousal or employee role is not sufficient to account for changes in drinking behaviors. Quite the contrary, relationship quality (e.g., conflict, support, intimacy, trust) with an intimate partner is likely to play an important role in drinking, irrespective of marital status. For example, increases in young adult drinking following divorce suggest that the distress of conflict and the dissolution of an intimate adult bond may be a key mediating process (Bachman et al., 1997).

Young-adult problem drinkers who do attempt to assume adult roles often experience greater problems in coping with the associated challenges (e.g., of parenting). For example, alcoholism is associated with a higher risk of impairments in fundamental parenting domains such as emotional unavailability, lax supervision and monitoring, and child maltreatment in the form of abuse and neglect (e.g., Chassin et al., 1993; Reich, Earls, & Powell, 1988; Sher, Gershuny, Peterson, & Raskin, 1997), and in marital domains such as marital distress, violence, and dissolution (e.g., Fitzgerald, Zucker, & Yang, 1995; Leonard, 1990). On the basis of existing research, the causal directionality of associations between alcohol use and role impairments is far from definitive and may vary by impairment and across time. Furthermore, these associations may be attributable to alternative, common variables (e.g., antisocial personality may cause impairments in adult roles and exacerbate drinking problems). Nevertheless, early empirical and theoretical work support a transactional conceptualization. Among the most definitive findings is the demonstration that heavy drinking among newlywed couples prospectively predicted marital violence even after statistically controlling for a host of relationship, personality, and demographic variables (Leonard & Senchak, 1993). Mediational analyses have further supported a pathway whereby the family stress created by living with an alcoholic husband disrupted marital adjustment and parent–child relationship quality (e.g., Dumka & Roosa, 1993). In the context of the greater tendency among women problem drinkers to marry problem-drinking spouses (Hall et al., 1983; Windle, 1997a), the dual impairments associated with drinking problems and living with a problem drinker may create a "double whammy" for women in particular as they meet the challenges of approaching marital and parenting tasks.

A developmental psychopathology perspective, however, does not view heavy drinking and alcoholism in young adulthood as a crystallized trait or disease, but rather as a dynamic, evolving, by-product manifested via interrelations between diathesis, stress, and *prior adaptational histories* (Sroufe, 1997). Thus, an increased risk for developing drinking problems in young adulthood has been linked to a proximal balance between risk and protective factors such as current diathesis (e.g., genetic vulnerability fully realized in developmental contexts in which there is easy access to alcohol) and stress (e.g., exposure to conflict and rejection in the family of origin) (e.g., Kendler, 1996). However, a narrow focus on only the proximal context in studying the etiology of alcohol (and other) disorders is often limiting and even misleading. Since experimentation and problems with alcohol begin as early as late childhood and become increasingly common in adolescence, significant adaptational histories have already been forged when individuals reach adulthood. The state of adaptational histories may be particularly relevant for young adult COAs, who continue to evidence greater vulnerability not only to drinking problems (e.g., Cavell, Jones, Runyan, Constantin-Page, & Velasquez, 1993), but also symptomatology that may serve to initiate or maintain adult drinking problems, including depressive symptoms (e.g., Jarmas & Kazak, 1992; Neff, 1994), aggression and antisocial disorder (e.g., Windle, 1990), and poor social competence (Ohannessian & Hesselbrock, 1994; Senchak, Greene, Carroll, & Leonard, 1996). More expansive assessments of adaptational histories have also revealed that young adult COAs report greater family discord, parental maltreatment, and direct exposure to parental drinking problems (Sher et al., 1997); experiential histories (e.g., stressful life events) also predict adult alcohol problems independent of family history of alcoholism (Beardslee, Son, & Vaillant, 1986; Jones & Houts, 1992).

Young adulthood provides a critical window for elucidating the etiology, course, and sequelae of alternative patterns of drinking. Because heavy and serious drinking problems are a defining part of the subculture for many individuals in early periods of young adulthood (Blane, 1979), it is difficult, without prospective research designs, to differentiate between developmental trajectories characterized by (1) serious drinking problems limited to late adolescence and early periods of adulthood (e.g., developmentally limited), and (2) chronic, serious drinking problems beginning in adolescence and continuing into adulthood (e.g., antisocial alcoholism) (Schulenberg, Wadsworth, O'Malley, Bachman, & Johnston, 1996; Zucker, 1994). Nor is it possible to detect the subsequent development of alcohol problems in later stages of young adulthood and beyond, that are proposed to be part of a larger constellation of symptomatology (e.g., depression, anxiety) and experiences (e.g., family conflict, neglect), particularly for women (Jacob & Leonard, 1994; Sher, 1991). Prospective measurements of heavy drinking and psychosocial adaptation across the transition from late adolescence into young adulthood are essential to capture the lawful heterogeneity of intraindividual change and stability of alcohol problems over time.

Middle and Late Adulthood

Our practice of subsuming middle and late adulthood into a single section in this chapter is due primarily to a paucity of research rather than any demonstrated lack of utility in differentiating the biopsychosocial contexts over these latter stages of adulthood. Alcohol involvement in the latter years of adulthood has been disproportionately neglected, due, at least in part, to the premature adherence among scientists to early theoretical claims that alcohol problems and heavy drinking evidenced marked declines after the age of 45 (Minnis, 1988). However, accumulating research and theory in several domains clearly indicate that alcohol use continues to play a key role in the quality of life during the latter half of the lifespan. Rates of alcohol problems in elderly samples are far from negligible, affecting between 2% and 10% of late middle-aged to elderly groups (Fillmore, 1987; Hilton, 1987). Moreover, these figures may very well be underestimates of alcohol problems in light of the difficulties associated with sampling and detecting alcohol problems among isolated, high-risk elderly people (Minnis, 1988). Furthermore, there are biological changes associated with aging (e.g., changes in percentage of body water) that may impact different definitions of alcohol use among the elderly.

Developmental trajectories (e.g., antisocial alcoholism) involve the progressive interplay and intermeshing between organismic (e.g., family history of alcoholism) and environmental (e.g., family dysfunction) risk factors across the lifespan. Across time, these processes impose some constraints on the potential plasticity in biological, psychological, and contextual systems and, as a result, have the effect of increasing the stability of alcohol use and psychosocial disturbances as individuals progress through later adulthood (see Zucker, Davies, Kincaid, Fitzgerald, & Reider, 1997). Consistent with this notion, earlier onset drinkers (i.e., before 50 years of age) reported more frequent intoxication and higher levels of emotional problems, life dissatisfaction, and physical withdrawal symptoms than later onset problem drinkers (Schonfeld & Dupree, 1991).

Even though some individuals follow a more malleable developmental trajectory and are able to overcome their alcohol problems and reduce their alcohol consumption during the later adult years, the accompanying course of biopsychosocial risk processes following earlier histories of alcohol problems may well persist into middle and older adulthood (e.g., Fillmore et al., 1991). Comparisons between elderly men with histories of heavy and nonheavy drinking histories have indicated that men with heavy drinking histories had more widespread developmental impairments in physical (e.g., substantial decreases in their ability to engage in self-care activities, more serious medical conditions, higher mortality rates), cognitive (e.g., sharper declines in recall memory), and social–emotional (e.g., lower life satisfaction) domains of functioning, even though the current drinking patterns between the two groups were statistically comparable (Colsher & Wallace, 1990). Indirect experiences of growing up in alcoholic families are similarly associated with differences in subsequent developmental trajectories in middle adulthood. For example, middle-aged female COAs, relative to non-COAs, have been found to report greater disturbances in current intrapersonal functioning (e.g., diminished self-esteem, depressive symptoms), marital relations (e.g., conflict, dissatisfaction), parenting roles (e.g., distress, helplessness), and family life as a whole (e.g., low cohesion) (Domenico & Windle, 1993).

Although developmental trajectories of alcohol use are hypothesized to become increasingly crystallized and stable throughout adulthood, vulnerability and resilience are dynamic, probabilistic processes rather than fixed, crystallized intrapersonal attributes. For example, modest differences between early- and late-onset elderly problem drinkers with regard to psychosocial, alcohol use, and demographic variables are, more than anything, a testimony to significant heterogeneity within developmental trajectories (Mulford & Fitzgerald, 1992). The dynamic balance between risk and protective factors is theorized to be a fundamental context for elucidating further the significant heterogeneity of drinking trajectories during late adulthood.

As an important first step in addressing these heterogeneity issues, Brennan and Moos (1990) delineated the concurrent associations between problem drinking, stressors in stage-salient life domains, and social resources in a sample of late-middle-aged adults. Problem drinkers reported more stressors in marital, financial, friendship, and neighborhood domains, and fewer social resources (e.g., support in key life domains). While the cross-sectional nature of the study precluded confident conclusions about directionality of relations, the authors interpreted the association within a transactional model, in which drinking problems were both (1) products of the scarce social resources and the accumulation of stressors, and (2) causes of subsequent stressors and diminished social support. Many of the interrelations between alcohol consumption, stress, and resources were found to differ across problem and nonproblem drinkers. For example, heightened conflict and low support predicted greater alcohol consumption for problem drinkers only, with one interpretation being that marital problems may trigger more alcohol consumption. By contrast, the authors interpreted the positive relationship between alcohol consumption and friendship stressors for nonproblem drinkers as support for the notion that the more conventional peer group of the nonproblem drinker may react to heightened alcohol consumption with disapproval in an effort to sanction it.

A limitation of Brennan and Moos (1990) study was that it did not exploit the range of methodological designs fostered by a developmental psychopathology perspective to address substantively important issues. Rather than exploring the dynamic balance between resources and stressors (i.e., considering them simultaneously), and the synergistic interplay (e.g., evaluating moderator effects) between stressors, symptomatology, social resources, and problem-drinking status on alcohol consumption, this study primarily tested a series of univariate, main effects models. As a result, main effect models may obscure more complex, contextual relationships among variables. Revisions of the tension-reduction hypothesis, for example, suggest that the moderating role of alcohol consumption in the link between stressful life events and psychological distress among older adults varies as a complex function of the perceived value of the social domain or role. Whereas alcohol consumption is hypothesized to be a stress-buffering mechanism only in the face of negative life events arising in less salient or valued roles, it is proposed to exacerbate the negative effects of stressful life events in salient social roles. The central premise underlying this prediction is that alcohol, as a means of escape, may be effective in coping with stressors that are less threatening to self-identity (i.e., less salient), but when the stressors are threatening to the self (i.e., in a salient role), alcohol consumption hinders the use of direct problem solving necessary to effectively alter the stressor and its negative effects. Consistent with this "double moderator" proposition, recent findings suggest that (1) the deleterious impact of salient role stressors on elderly emotional adjustment is exacerbated under conditions of high alcohol consumption, and, in contrast, (2) high alcohol consumption serves as a buffer or protective factor by lessening the impact of nonsalient stressors on elderly emotional adjustment (Krause, 1995). Therefore, alcohol use in an elderly sample cannot simply be conceptualized as a fixed, static protective or risk factor. Rather, it is best conceptualized as dynamic, with the risk or protective value of alcohol gaining meaning from the larger context in which it is embedded.

Lawful developmental changes during the latter half of adulthood may reconfigure the nature of alcohol involvement in the context of the diathesis–stress model. Although the marital and parenting domains remain salient as adults progress from the early to middle adult years, overlaid upon the functional role of raising children is also the challenge of readjusting family roles in the face of the growing autonomy and eventual departure of children from home. Stressful tasks in other domains involve coping with progressively limited career choices and opportunities for advancement, a loss of youthful attractiveness, and the onset of noticeable physical decline (Gomberg, 1994). Within lifespan conceptualizations, old age is accompanied by a different developmental context, characterized by increases in nonnormative negative events (e.g., physical illness, death of close companions), as well as age-graded influences (e.g., biological decline, retirement, loss of social status) (Meyers, Hingson, Mucatel, Heeren, & Goldman, 1985; Staudinger, Marsiske, & Baltes, 1993).

Against this developmental backdrop, it is not surprising to find very different relationships between organismic, contextual, and alcohol-related variables in old age. For example, since escaping stress does not appear to be a primary motive for alcohol consumption among elderly individuals (Meyers et al., 1985), sociodemographic (e.g., retirement, low socioeconomic status) and social-psychological (e.g., satisfaction and perceived efficacy in various social roles) variables are often unrelated to or associated with lower alcohol consumption (Krause, 1995; Meyers et al., 1985; Welte & Mirand, 1995). This pattern of findings is opposite to those found in samples of younger adults. The apparent developmental specificity of such findings underscores the importance of more systematic attempts to integrate the study of alcohol into lifespan models of aging. For example, within the aging model of "Selective Optimization with Compensation" (Baltes & Baltes, 1990; Staudinger et al., 1993), the efficiency with which elderly individuals may allocate their progressively limited resources to cope with increases in age-graded and negative, nonnormative events may be shaped by previous drinking histories and, via transactional processes, influence their subsequent drinking patterns.

Comparing and contrasting the precursors, correlates, and sequelae of alcohol consumption and heavy drinking for men and women may further serve to clarify inconsistencies and gaps in the literature. With the exception of findings that men continue to evidence greater alcohol consumption and problems than women as they grow older, little is definitively known about gender differences in alcohol involvement among the elderly. This gap becomes even more significant in the face of promising theoretical and empirical work that has recently emerged. For example, gender-specific stressors such as reproductive problems (e.g., miscarriage, hysterectomy) have been found to predate heavy drinking in retrospective analyses (Wilsnack, Klassen, & Wilsnack, 1986). A common, but untested, process hypothesis is that the accompanying distress mediates the influence of reproductive problems on drinking patterns (Gomberg & Nirenberg, 1993). "Sleeper effects" may emerge, with distress symptoms becoming especially pronounced as women approach middle age and the end of their reproductive span. As another related example, results from a research synthesis

provide support for the longstanding assumption that the pattern of reciprocal relations between alcohol consumption and depression is much stronger for women than men (see Wilsnack & Wilsnack, 1995). Nesting gender
within a lifespan developmental framework, Gomberg (1994) has also developed some interesting hypotheses concerning how the interrelations between successive life challenges (e.g., impact of "empty nest" syndrome,
loss of youthful attractiveness), interpersonal contexts (e.g., heightened
marital disruption, spousal alcoholism), and drinking patterns may be very
different for older women relative to older men (also see Gomberg &
Nirenberg, 1993).

Although additional research is needed to clarify the specific contexts
in which gender serves as a moderating variable, among adults (as well as
children and adolescents), these searches must be tempered by the recognition that (1) variability within each gender is commonly greater than the
variability between the genders; and (2) earlier documentation of gender
differences is being seriously challenged by more recent research (e.g., magnitude of genetic influences) (Heath, Sluske, & Madden, 1997). Furthermore, the historical erosion of gender-specific socialization pressures, social
roles, and norms may have the effect of increasing the resemblance of the
origins and consequences of alcohol use and alcohol problems among men
and women (Allan & Cooke, 1985; Wilsnack & Wilsnack, 1995).

RECENT METHODOLOGICAL ADVANCES

The developmental psychopathology model described previously has increased the demands on the level of methodological/statistical skills required to adequately conduct this research; that is, to conduct multiwave,
multivariable research necessitates greater knowledge and appreciation of
diverse methodologies and statistical models so as to optimally design research studies to address significant scientific questions. There has been a
fairly accelerated expansion of methodological approaches and statistical
models over the past 25 years or so, facilitated by changes in technology
(specifically in computers and electronics). We cite but two of these methodological advances that are relevant to the topic of this chapter (for a
more extensive, yet still selective presentation, see Bryant et al., 1997; Collins & Horn, 1991).

Sampling of Time Points

A vitally important methodological question in studies of developmental
psychopathology and substance use is the number and timing of occasions
of measurement in a prospective research design. If measurement occasions
occur too close in time, there may be insufficient time for any substantively
significant change in behavior to have occurred. If measurement occasions

occur too far apart, important processes underlying key dimensions of change (e.g., increases, decreases, termination of alcohol use) may be inadvertently excluded, thus yielding the findings suspect with regard to the underlying mechanisms or processes contributing to the changes in behavior. This problem is exacerbated when it is acknowledged that there are different rates of intraindividual growth (i.e., not everyone begins drinking at the same time; recovery patterns from treatment are variable across patients) and intraindividual decay (e.g., not all individuals are equally susceptible to medical conditions associated with the abusive use of alcohol, nor do they have the same rate of deterioration), thus precluding a simple answer to the number and spacing of occasions puzzle.

This methodological issue, which is central to a developmental psychopathology perspective, has only begun to be addressed substantively in the literature (though it has been recognized for some time as a significant issue in developmental psychology, see Wohlwill, 1973). Some investigators have utilized multiwave research designs and then analyzed their data by selecting different occasions of measurement to study a hypothesized set of relations. For example, Sher and Wood (1997) used data from all four occasions of measurement (with 1-year intervals between occasions of measurement) and analyzed a cross-lagged panel design model; then, they specified and evaluated a second model that used only the repeated-measures data available at the first and fourth occasions—the results of these two models were quite different substantively, even though both models included the same data at the first and fourth occasions.

At this time, there is no easy answer to the number and spacing of the measurement occasions issue, because, substantively, not enough is known about the underlying causal process to definitively state what the optimal measurement intervals should be. However, the consideration of the number and spacing of occasions of measurement should be a critical feature of prospective research designs, with some (albeit incomplete) rationale for the selection of intervals. Furthermore, this consideration should extend to the critical reading of the existing literature and to the substantive costs associated with an inadequate sampling of measurement occasions to make the kinds of causal (or plausible) explanations sought in many research designs.

Latent Growth Curves

An important feature of the developmental psychopathology perspective is the appreciation of variability in intraindividual growth (i.e., across-time, within-person changes). Two individuals may reach the same end point, such as a height of 6 feet, but one may have demonstrated a relatively linear, incremental pattern of growth across time, whereas the growth pattern of the other may have been characterized by nonsystematic, alternating periods of rapid growth and then near-zero growth (a further example of equifinality). Some researchers (e.g., Cloninger et al., 1981; Zucker, 1987) have suggested that lifetime alcohol disorders may be subtyped according to onset, with one subtype manifesting an early-onset, heavy drinking and antisocial behavior pattern, and another subtype manifesting a later-onset, heavy drinking, but no antisocial behavior pattern. Clearly, the intra-individual growth trajectories of alcohol use would be expected to differ across members from these two alcohol subtypes, as would predictors (e.g., family history of alcoholism) of changes in these trajectories; that is, child-hood conduct problems may be a significant predictor of early and rapid changes in alcohol use among the early-onset, antisocial group, but not among the late-onset, nonantisocial group.

Although the notion that individuals may vary in terms of their time-ordered patterns of manifesting alcohol (or other disordered) behaviors has not been ignored, there have been very few applications that have at-tempted to truly capture this source of variability in alcohol studies (e.g., McArdle, Hamagami, & Hulick, 1994; Windle, 1997b). Two relatively new statistical modeling approaches have emerged that are useful for modeling individual differences in intraindividual change. These two ap-proaches are latent variable (or covariance structure) growth curve model-ing (e.g., McArdle, 1988; Muthén, 1991) and hierarchical linear modeling (HLM) (e.g., Bryk & Raudenbush, 1992; Goldstein, 1995). More complete expositions on the details of specifying latent growth curve models (e.g., McArdle, 1988) and HLMs (e.g., Bryk & Raudenbush, 1992) are available elsewhere, and space constraints limit their explication in this chapter. However, it is worthwhile to note that such statistical models do exist and that they may be implemented on commercially available software. Such statistical modeling is essential to the adequate specification and evaluation of the complex relations often hypothesized to underlie features of develop-mental psychopathology and substance use and abuse.

SUMMARY

Using empirical studies selected from different portions of the lifespan, we have provided examples of how a developmental psychopathology perspec-tive may be of heuristic value in generating hypotheses about the origins and time course of alcohol-related behaviors. The developmental psycho-pathology perspective provides a broad conceptual lens for viewing individ-ual development and the time-ordered trajectories for various behaviors, including alcohol use, across the lifespan. A key element of the develop-mental psychopathology perspective is that individual development is char-acterized by an ongoing, evolving dialectic across levels of analyses (e.g., biological, psychological, social–cultural), across time, and across prior ad-aptational histories and emerging proclivities, challenges, and environmen-tal affordances.

A fundamental assumption among many prominent substance use theories, such as problem behavior theory, is that different problem symptoms such as delinquency, alcohol use, substance use, and precocious sexual behavior, are concrete manifestations of a larger syndrome of deviance or unconventionality (Jessor & Jessor, 1977; Donovan & Jessor, 1985). Although the strength of problem behavior theory lies in its parsimony, powerful simplicity, and heuristic utility, as a midlevel theory, it is not designed to explain fully the origins, development, and sequelae of alcohol involvement, substance use, or any other specific form of deviance. Additional theories are needed to fully elucidate the developmental psychopathology of diverse alcohol-related behaviors (e.g., alcohol problems, dependency symptoms) and their time course (e.g., onset, escalation). By underscoring the diversity and multidimensionality of alcohol-related behaviors and substance use with regard to origins, time course, and developmental trajectories, developmental process perspectives complement the emphasis on uniformity and homogeneity in broad-spectrum theories such as problem behavior theory. As our knowledge of alcohol and substance-related behaviors increases, our research questions become more sophisticated as we increasingly recognize the need to study the complexities involved. A developmental psychopathology perspective may prove fruitful in confronting the ensuing challenges to the alcohol research community.

REFERENCES

Allan, C. A., & Cooke, D. J. (1985). Stressful life events and alcohol misuse in women: A critical review. *Journal of Studies on Alcohol, 46,* 147–152.

Andrews, J. A., Hops, H., & Duncan, S. C. (1997). Adolescent modeling of parent substance use: The moderating effect of the relationship with the parent. *Journal of Family Psychology, 11,* 259–270.

Aseltine, R. H. (1995). A reconsideration of parental and peer influences on adolescent deviance. *Journal of Health and Social Behavior, 36,* 103–121.

Bachman, J. G., Wadsworth, K. N., O'Malley, P. M., Johnston, L. D., & Schulenberg, J. E. (1997). *Smoking, drinking, and drug use in young adulthood.* Mahwah, NJ: Erlbaum.

Baltes, P. B., & Baltes, M. M. (1990). Psychological perspectives on successful aging: The models of selective optimization with compensation. In P. B. Baltes & M. M. Baltes (Eds.), *Successful aging: Perspectives from the behavioral sciences* (pp. 1–34). New York: Cambridge University Press.

Baron, R. M., & Kenny, D. A. (1986). The moderator–mediator variable distinction in social psychological research: Conceptual, strategic, and statistical considerations. *Journal of Personality and Social Psychology, 51,* 1173–1182.

Barrera, M. J., Li, S. A., & Chassin, L. (1995). Effects of parental alcoholism and life stress on Hispanic and non-Hispanic Caucasian adolescents: A prospective study. *American Journal of Community Psychology, 23,* 479–507.

Beardslee, W. R., Son, L., & Vaillant, G. E. (1986). Exposure to parental alcoholism during childhood and outcome in adulthood: A prospective longitudinal study. *British Journal of Psychiatry, 149,* 584–591.

Begleiter, H., Porjesz, B., Bihari, B., & Kissin, B. (1984). Event-related brain potentials in boys at risk for alcoholism. *Science, 225,* 1493–1496.

Blackson, T., Tarter, R., Martin, C., & Moss, H. (1994). Temperament induced father–son family dysfunction: Etiological implications for child behavior problems and substance abuse. *American Journal of Orthopsychiatry, 64,* 280–292.

Blane, H. T. (1979). Middle-aged alcoholics and young drinkers. In H. T. Blane & M. E. Chafetz (Eds.), *Youth, alcohol, and social policy* (pp. 5–38). New York: Plenum.

Blane, H. T., & Leonard, K. E. (1987). *Psychological theories of drinking and alcoholism.* New York: Guilford Press.

Brennan, P. L., & Moos, R. H. (1990). Life stressors, social resources, and late-life problem drinking. *Psychology and Aging, 5,* 491–501.

Bronfenbrenner, U. (1977). Toward an experimental ecology of human development. *American Psychologist, 32,* 513–531.

Brook, J. S., Whiteman, M., Shapiro, J., & Cohen, P. (1996). Effects of parent drug use and personality on toddler adjustment. *Journal of Genetic Psychology, 157,* 19–35.

Brooks-Gunn, J., & Warren, M. P. (1989). Biological and social contributions to negative affect in young adolescent girls. *Child Development, 60,* 40–55.

Bryant, K., Windle, M., & West, S. G. (Eds.). (1997). *The science of prevention: Methodological advances from alcohol and substance abuse research.* Washington, DC: American Psychological Association Press.

Bryk, A. S., & Raudenbush, S. W. (1992). *Hierarchical linear models: Applications and data analysis methods.* Newbury Park, CA: Sage.

Cavell, T. A., Jones, D. C., Runyan, D., Constantin-Page, L. P., & Velasquez, J. M. (1993). Perceptions of attachment and the adjustment of adolescents with alcoholic fathers. *Journal of Family Psychology, 7,* 204–212.

Chase-Lansdale, P. L., Wakschlag, L. S., & Brooks-Gunn, J. (1995). A psychological perspective on the development of caring in children and youth: The role of the family. *Journal of Adolescence, 18,* 515–556.

Chassin, L., Curran, P. J., Hussong, A. M., & Colder, C. R. (1996). The relation of parent alcoholism to adolescent substance use: A longitudinal follow-up study. *Journal of Abnormal Psychology, 105,* 70–80.

Chassin, L., Pillow, D. R., Curran, P. J., Molina, B. S. G., & Barrera, M. (1993). Relation to parental alcoholism to early adolescent substance use: A test of three mediating mechanisms. *Journal of Abnormal Psychology, 102,* 3–19.

Chassin, L., Rogosch, F., & Barrera, M. (1991). Substance use and symptomatology among adolescent children of alcoholics. *Journal of Abnormal Psychology, 100,* 449–463.

Christiansen, B. A., Smith, G. T., Roehling, P. V., & Goldman, M. S. (1989). Using alcohol expectancies to predict adolescent drinking behavior after one year. *Journal of Consulting and Clinical Psychology, 57,* 93–99.

Cicchetti, D. (1984). The emergence of developmental psychopathology. *Child Development, 55,* 1–7.

Cicchetti, D. (1993). Developmental psychopathology: Reactions, reflections, projections. *Developmental Review, 13,* 471–502.

Cicchetti, D., & Cohen, D. (1995). Perspectives on developmental psychopathology. In D. Cicchetti & D. Cohen (Eds.), *Developmental psychopathology: Vol. 1. Theory and method* (pp. 3–20). New York: Wiley.

Cicchetti, D., Cummings, E. M., Greenberg, M. T., & Marvin, R. S. (1990). An organizational perspective on attachment beyond infancy: Implications for theory, measurement, and research. In M. T. Greenberg, D. Cicchetti, & E. M. Cummings (Eds.), *Attachment in the preschool years: Theory, research, and intervention* (pp. 3–49). Chicago: University of Chicago Press.

Cicchetti, D., & Rogosch, F. A. (1996). Equifinality and multifinality in developmental psychopathology. *Development and Psychopathology, 8,* 597–600.

Cloninger, C. R., Bohman, M., & Sigvardsson, S. (1981). Inheritance of alcohol abuse: Cross fostering analysis of adopted men. *Archives of General Psychiatry, 38,* 861–868.

Collins, L. M., & Horn, J. L. (Eds.). (1991). *Best methods for the analysis of change: Recent advances, unanswered questions, future directions.* Washington, DC: American Psychological Association Press.

Colsher, P. L., & Wallace, R. B. (1990). Elderly men with histories of heavy drinking: Correlates and consequences. *Journal of Studies on Alcohol, 51,* 528–535.

Cummings, E. M., & Davies, P. (1996). Emotional security as a regulatory process in normal development and the development of psychopathology. *Development and Psychopathology, 8,* 123–129.

Cummings, E. M., Davies, P. T., & Simpson, K. S. (1994). Marital conflict, gender, and children's appraisals and coping efficacy as mediators of child adjustment. *Journal of Family Psychology, 8,* 141–149.

Curran, P. J., Stice, E., & Chassin, L. (1997). The relation between adolescent alcohol use and peer alcohol use: A longitudinal random coefficients model. *Journal of Consulting and Clinical Psychology, 65,* 130–140.

Davies, P. T., & Windle, M. (1997). Gender-specific pathways between maternal depressive symptoms, family discord, and adolescent adjustment. *Developmental Psychology, 33,* 657–668.

Dishion, T. J., Patterson, G. R., & Reid, J. R. (1988). Parent and peer factors associated with drug sampling in early adolescence: Implications for treatment. *National Institute on Drug Abuse: Research Monograph Series, No. 77,* 69–93.

Domenico, D., & Windle, M. (1993). Intrapersonal and interpersonal functioning among middle-aged female adult children of alcoholics. *Journal of Consulting and Clinical Psychology, 61,* 659–666.

Donovan, D. M. (1988). Assessment of addictive behaviors: Implications of an emerging biopsychosocial model. In D. M. Donovan & G. A. Marlatt (Eds.), *Assessment of addictive behaviors* (pp. 3–48). New York: Guilford Press.

Donovan, J. E., & Jessor, R. (1985). Structure of problem behavior in adolescence and young adulthood. *Journal of Consulting and Clinical Psychology, 53,* 890–904.

Dumka, L. E., & Roosa, M. W. (1993). The role of stress and family relationships in mediating problem drinking and fathers' personal adjustment. *Journal of Studies on Alcohol, 56,* 528–537.

Eiden, R. D., & Leonard, K. E. (1996). Paternal alcohol use and the mother–infant relationship. *Development and Psychopathology, 8,* 307–323.

El-Sheikh, M., & Cummings, E. M. (1997). Marital conflict, emotional regulation, and the adjustment of children of alcoholics. In K. C. Barrett (Ed.), *New directions in child development: Emotion and communication* (pp. 25–44). San Francisco: Jossey-Bass.

Endler, N. S., & Magnusson, D. (1976). Toward an interactional psychology of personality. *Psychological Bulletin, 83,* 956–974.

Farrell, A. D. (1994). Risk factors for drug use in urban adolescents: A three-wave longitudinal study. *Journal of Drug Issues, 23,* 443–462.

Fillmore, K. M. (1987). Women's drinking across the adult life course as compared to men's. *British Journal of Addiction, 82*, 801–811.

Fillmore, K. M., Hartka, E., Johnstone, B. M., Leino, E. V., Motoyoshi, M., & Temple, M. T. (1991). Life course variation in drinking. *British Journal of Addictions, 86*, 1221–1268.

Fitzgerald, H. E., Zucker, R. A., & Yang, H.-Y. (1995). Developmental systems theory and alcoholism: Analyzing patterns of variation in high-risk families. *Psychology of Addictive Behaviors, 9*, 8–22.

Gaines, L., Brooks, P., Maisto, S., Dietrich, M., & Shagena, M. (1988). The development of children's knowledge of alcohol and the role of drinking. *Journal of Applied Developmental Psychology, 7*, 441–457.

Goldstein, H. (1995). *Multilevel statistical models* (2nd ed.). London: Edward Arnold.

Gomberg, E. L. (1994). Risk factors for drinking over a woman's life span. *Alcohol Health and Research World, 18*, 220–227.

Gomberg, E. L., & Nirenberg, T. D. (1993). Antecedents and consequences. In E. L. Gomberg & T. D. Nirenberg (Eds.), *Women and substance use* (pp. 118–141). Norwood, NJ: Ablex.

Gotham, H. J., Sher, K. J., & Wood, P. K. (1997). Predicting stability and change in frequency of intoxication from the college years to beyond: Individual difference and role transition variables. *Journal of Abnormal Psychology, 106*, 619–629.

Grych, J. H., Seid, M., & Fincham, F. D. (1992). Assessing marital conflict from the child's perspective: The children's perception of interparental conflict scale. *Child Development, 63*, 558–572.

Hall, R. L., Hesselbrock, V. M., & Stabenau, J. R. (1983). Familial distribution of alcohol use: I. Assortative mating in the parents of alcoholics. *Behavior Genetics, 13*, 361–372.

Hawkins, J. D., Catalano, R. F., & Miller, J. Y. (1992). Risk and protective factors for alcohol and other drug problems in adolescence and early adulthood: Implications for substance abuse prevention. *Psychological Bulletin, 112*, 64–105.

Heath, A. C., Sluske, W. S., & Madden, P. A. F. (1997). Gender differences in the genetic contribution to alcoholism risk and to alcohol consumption patterns. In R. W. Wilsnack & S. C. Wilsnack (Eds.), *Gender and alcohol: Individual and social perspectives* (pp. 114–149). New Brunswick, NJ: Rutgers Center for Alcohol Studies.

Heyman, R. E., O'Leary, K. D., & Jouriles, E. N. (1995). Alcohol and aggressive personality styles: Potentiators of serious physical aggression against wives? *Journal of Family Psychology, 9*, 44–57.

Hilton, M. E. (1987). Changes in American drinking patterns and problems, 1967–1984. *Journal of Studies on Alcohol, 48*, 515–522.

Huba, G. J., & Bentler, P. M. (1982). A developmental theory of drug use: Derivation and assessment of a causal modeling approach. In P. B. Baltes & O. G. Brim, Jr. (Eds.), *Life-span development and behavior* (Vol. 4, pp. 147–203). New York: Academic Press.

Jacob, T., & Leonard, K. (1994). Family and peer influences in the development of adolescent alcohol abuse. In R. Zucker, G. Boyd, & J. Howard (Eds.), *The development of alcohol problems: Exploring the biopsychosocial matrix of risk* (NIH Publ. No. 94-3495, pp. 123–155). Washington, DC: U.S. Government Printing Office.

Jarmas, A. L., & Kazak, A. E. (1992). Young adult children of alcoholic fathers: Depressive experiences coping styles and family systems. *Journal of Consulting and Clinical Psychology, 60,* 244–251.

Jessor, R., & Jessor, S. L. (1977). *Problem behavior and psychosocial development: A longitudinal study of youth.* New York: Academic Press.

Johnstone, B. M., Leino, E. V., Ager, C. R., Ferrer, H., & Fillmore, K. M. (1996). Determinants of life-course variation in the frequency of alcohol consumption: Meta-analysis of studies from the collaborative alcohol-related longitudinal project. *Journal of Studies on Alcohol, 57,* 494–506.

Jones, D. C., & Houts, R. (1992). Parental drinking, parent–child communication, and social skills in young adults. *Journal of Studies on Alcohol, 53,* 48–56.

Kandel, D. B. (1980). Drug and drinking behavior among youth. *Annual Review in Sociology, 6,* 235–285.

Kendler, K. S. (1996). Parenting: A genetic–epidemiologic perspective. *American Journal of Psychiatry, 153,* 11–20.

Krause, N. (1995). Stress, alcohol use, and depressive symptoms in later life. *Gerontologist, 35,* 296–307.

Leonard, K. E. (1990). Marital functioning among episodic and steady alcoholics. In R. L. Collins, K. E. Leonard, & J. S. Searles (Eds.), *Alcohol and the family: Research and clinical perspectives* (pp. 220–243). New York: Guilford Press.

Leonard, K. E., & Rothbard, J. C. (in press). Alcohol and the marriage effect. *Journal of Studies on Alcohol.*

Leonard, K. E., & Senchak, M. (1993). Alcohol and premarital aggression among newlywed couples. *Journal of Studies on Alcohol, 11*(Suppl.), 96–108.

Lerner, R. M. (1978). Nature, nurture and dynamic interactionism. *Human Development, 21,* 1–20.

Magnusson, D. (1988). *Individual development from an interactional perspective: A longitudinal study.* Hillsdale, NJ: Erlbaum.

McArdle, J. J. (1988). Dynamic but structural equation modeling of repeated measures data. In R. B. Cattell & J. Nesselroade (Eds.), *Handbook of multivariate experimental psychology* (2nd ed., pp. 561–614). New York: Plenum.

McArdle, J. J., Hamagami, F., & Hulick, P. (1994). Latent variable path models in alcohol use research. In *The development of alcohol problems: Exploring the biopsychosocial matrix of risk* (NIAAA Monograph No. 26, Department of Health and Human Services Publication No. NIH 94-3495, pp. 341–385). Washington, DC: U.S. Government Printing Office.

McGee, L., & Newcomb, M. D. (1992). General deviance syndrome: Expanded hierarchical evaluations at four ages from early adolescence to adulthood. *Journal of Consulting and Clinical Psychology, 60,* 766–776.

Meyers, A. R., Hingson, R., Mucatel, M., Heeren, T., & Goldman, E. (1985). The social epidemiology of alcohol use by urban older adults. *International Journal of Aging and Human Development, 21,* 49–59.

Miller-Tutzauer, C., Leonard, K. E., & Windle, M. (1991). Marriage and alcohol use: A longitudinal study of "maturing out. " *Journal of Studies on Alcohol, 52,* 434–440.

Minnis, J. R. (1988). Toward an understanding of alcohol abuse among the elderly: A sociological perspective. *Journal of Alcohol and Drug Education, 33,* 32–40.

Molina, B. S. G., & Chassin, L. (1996). The parent–adolescent relationship at puberty: Hispanic ethnicity and parent alcoholism as moderators. *Developmental Psychology, 32,* 675–686.

Mulford, H. A., & Fitzgerald, J. L. (1992). Elderly versus younger problem drinker profiles: Do they indicate a need for special programs for the elderly. *Journal of Studies on Alcohol, 53,* 601–610.

Muthén, B. O. (1991). Analysis of longitudinal data using latent variable models with varying parameters. In L. M. Collins & J. L. Horn (Eds.), *Best methods for the analysis of change* (pp. 1–17). Washington, DC: American Psychological Association Press.

Neff, J. A. (1994). Adult children of alcoholic or mentally ill parents: Alcohol consumption and psychological distress in a tri-ethnic community study. *Addictive Behaviors, 19,* 185–197.

Newcomb, M. D. (1996). Pseudomaturity among adolescents: Construct validation, sex differences, and associations in adulthood. *Journal of Drug Issues, 26,* 477–504.

Noll, R. B., Zucker, R. A., & Greenberg, G. E. (1990). Identification of alcohol by smell among preschoolers: Evidence for early socialization about drugs occurring in the home. *Child Development, 61,* 1520–1527.

O'Connor, M. J., Sigman, M., & Brill, N. (1987). Disorganization of attachment in relation to maternal alcohol consumption. *Journal of Consulting and Clinical Psychology, 55,* 831–836.

O'Connor, M. J., Sigman, M., & Kasari, C. (1992). Attachment behavior of infants exposed prenatally to alcohol: Mediating effects of infant affect and mother–infant interaction. *Development and Psychopathology, 4,* 243–256.

O'Connor, M. J., Sigman, M., & Kasari, C. (1993). Interactional model for the association among maternal alcohol use, mother–infant interaction, and infant cognitive development. *Infant Behavior and Development, 16,* 177–192.

Ohannessian, C. M., & Hesselbrock, V. M. (1994). An examination of the underlying influence of temperament and problem behaviors on drinking behaviors in a sample of adult offspring of alcoholics. *Addictive Behaviors, 19,* 257–268.

Petersen, A. C., Sarigiani, P. A., & Kennedy, R. E. (1991). Adolescent depression: Why more girls? *Journal of Youth and Adolescence, 20,* 247–271.

Pihl, R. L., & Bruce, K. N. (1995). Cognitive impairment in children of alcoholics. *Alcohol Health and Research World, 19,* 142–147.

Reich, W., Earls, F., & Powell, J. (1988). A comparison of the home and social environments of children of alcoholic and non-alcoholic parents. *British Journal of Addiction, 83,* 831–839.

Rodning, C., Beckwith, L., & Howard, J. (1989). Characteristics of attachment organization and play organization in prenatally drug-exposed toddlers. *Development and Psychopathology, 1,* 277–289.

Russell, M. (1990). Prevalence of alcoholism among children of alcoholics. In M. Windle & J. S. Searles (Eds.), *Children of alcoholics: Critical perspectives* (pp. 9–38). New York: Guilford Press.

Russell, M., Cooper, M. L., & Frone, M. W. (1990). The influence of sociodemographic characteristics on familial alcohol problems: Data from a community sample. *Alcoholism: Clinical and Experimental Research, 14,* 221–226.

Sadava, S. W. (1987). Interactional theory. In H. T. Blane & K. E. Leonard (Eds.), *Psychological theories of drinking and alcoholism* (pp. 90–130). New York: Guilford Press.

Sadava, S. W., & Pak, A. W. (1994). Problem drinking and close relationships during the third decade of life. *Psychology of Addictive Behaviors, 8,* 251–258.

Sameroff, A. L. (1983). Developmental systems: Contexts and evolution. In P. Mussed (Ed.), *Handbook of child psychology* (Vol. 1, pp. 237–294). New York: Wiley.

Schonfeld, L., & Dupree, L. D. (1991). Antecedents of drinking for early- and late-onset elderly alcohol abusers. *Journal of Studies on Alcohol, 52,* 587–592.

Schuckit, M. A. (1994). A clinical model of genetic influences in alcohol dependence. *Journal of Studies on Alcohol, 55,* 5–17.

Schulenberg, J., Maggs, J. L., & Hurrelmann, K. (Eds.). (1997). *Health risks and developmental transitions during adolescence.* New York: Cambridge University Press.

Schulenberg, J., Wadsworth, K. N., O'Malley, P. M., Bachman, J. G., & Johnston, L. D. (1996). Adolescent risk factors for binge drinking during the transition to young adulthood: Variable- and pattern-centered approaches to change. *Developmental Psychology, 32,* 659–674.

Senchak, M., Greene, M. W., Carroll, A., & Leonard, K. E. (1996). Global, behavioral, and self ratings of interpersonal skills among adult children of alcoholic, divorced, and control parents. *Journal of Studies on Alcohol, 57,* 638–645.

Shell, R. M., Groppenbacher, N., Roosa, M. W., & Gensheimer, L. D. (1992). Interpreting children's reports of concern about parental drinking: Indicators of risk status. *American Journal of Community Psychology, 20,* 463–489.

Sher, K. J. (1991). *Children of alcoholics: A critical appraisal of theory and research.* Chicago: University of Chicago Press.

Sher, K. J., Gershuny, B. S., Peterson, L., & Raskin, G. (1997). The role of childhood stressors in the intergenerational transmission of alcohol use disorders. *Journal of Studies on Alcohol, 58,* 414–427.

Sher, K. J., & Wood, P. K. (1997). Methodological issues in conducting prospective research on alcohol-related behavior: A report from the field. In K. J. Bryant, M. Windle, & S. G. West (Eds.), *The science of prevention: Methodological advances from alcohol and substance abuse research* (pp. 3–41). Washington, DC: American Psychological Association Press.

Sroufe, L. A. (1990). Considering normal and abnormal together: The essence of developmental psychopathology. *Development and Psychopathology, 2,* 335–347.

Sroufe, L. A. (1997). Psychopathology as an outcome of development. *Development and Psychopathology, 9,* 251–268.

Sroufe, L. A., & Rutter, M. (1984). The domain of developmental psychopathology. *Child Development, 55,* 17–29.

Staudinger, U. M., Marsiske, M., & Baltes, P. B. (1993). Resilience and levels of reserve capacity in later adulthood: Perspectives from life-span theory. *Development and Psychopathology, 5,* 541–566.

Steinberg, L. (1990). Autonomy, conflict, and harmony in the family relationship. In S. Feldman & G. Elliott (Eds.), *At the threshold: The developing adolescent* (pp. 255–276). Cambridge, MA: Harvard University Press.

Steinberg, L., & Silverberg, S. B. (1986). The vicissitudes of autonomy in early adolescence. *Child Development, 57,* 841–851.

Streissguth, A. P. (1986). The behavioral teratology of alcohol: Performance, behavioral, and intellectual deficits in prenatally exposed children. In J. R. West (Ed.), *Alcohol and brain development* (pp. 3–44). New York: Oxford University Press.

Streissguth, A. P., Barr, H. M., & Martin, D. C. (1983). Maternal alcohol use and neonatal habituation assessed with the Brazelton Scale. *Child Development, 54,* 1109–1118.

Streissguth, A. P., Barr, H. M., & Sampson, P. D. (1990). Moderate prenatal alcohol exposure: Effects on child IQ and learning problems at age 7½ years. *Alcoholism: Clinical and Experimental Research, 14,* 662–669.

Streissguth, A. P., Bookstein, F. L., Sampson, P. D., & Barr, H. M. (1995). Attention: Prenatal alcohol and continuities of vigilance and attentional problems from 4 through 14 years. *Development and Psychopathology, 7,* 419–446.

Swaim, R. C., Oetting, E. R., Edwards, R. W., & Beauvais, F. (1989). Links from emotional distress to adolescent drug use: A path model. *Journal of Consulting and Clinical Psychology, 57,* 227–231.

Tarter, R., Alterman, A., & Edwards, K. (1985). Vulnerability to alcoholism in men. A behavior–genetic perspective. *Journal of Studies on Alcohol, 46,* 329–356.

Temple, M. T., Fillmore, K. M., Hartka, E., Johnstone, B., Leino, E. V., & Motoyoshi, M. (1991). A meta-analysis of change in marital and employment status as predictors of alcohol consumption on a typical occasion. *British Journal of Addiction, 86,* 1269–1281.

von Bertalanffy, L. (1968). *General systems theory.* New York: Braziller.

Waddington, C. (1957). *The strategy of genes.* London: Allen & Unwin.

Welte, J. W., & Mirand, A. L. (1995). Drinking, problem drinking, and life stressors in the elderly general population. *Journal of Studies on Alcohol, 56,* 67–73.

Werner, E. E., & Smith, R. S. (1982). *Vulnerable but invincible: A longitudinal study of resilient children and youth.* New York: McGraw-Hill.

Whipple, E. E., Fitzgerald, H. E., & Zucker, R. A. (1995). Parent–child interactions in alcoholic and nonalcoholic families. *American Journal of Orthopsychiatry, 65,* 153–159.

Whipple, S. C., & Noble, E. P. (1991). Personality characteristics of alcoholic fathers and their sons. *Journal of Studies on Alcohol, 52,* 331–337.

White, H. R., & Huselid, R. F. (1997). Gender differences in alcohol use during adolescence. In R. W. Wilsnack & S. C. Wilsnack (Eds.), *Gender and alcohol: Individual and social perspectives* (pp. 176–198). New Brunswick, NJ: Rutgers Center of Alcohol Studies.

Wills, T. A., McNamara, G., Vaccaro, D., & Hirky, A. E. (1996). Escalated substance use: A longitudinal grouping analysis from early to middle adolescence. *Journal of Abnormal Psychology, 105,* 166–180.

Wilsnack, R. W., Klassen, A. D., & Wilsnack, S. C. (1986). Retrospective analysis of lifetime changes in women's drinking behavior. *Advances in Alcohol and Substance Abuse, 5,* 9–28.

Wilsnack, S. C., & Wilsnack, R. W. (1995). Drinking and problem drinking in US women: Patterns and recent trends. In M. Galanter (Ed.), *Recent developments in alcoholism: Vol. 12. Alcoholism and women* (pp. 29–60). New York: Plenum.

Windle, M. (1990). A longitudinal study of antisocial behaviors in early adolescence as predictors of late adolescent substance use: Gender and ethnic group differences. *Journal of Abnormal Psychology, 99,* 86–91.

Windle, M. (1997a). Mate similarity, heavy substance use, and family history of problem drinking among young adult women. *Journal of Studies on Alcohol, 58,* 573–580.

Windle, M. (1997b). Alternative latent variable approaches to modeling change in adolescent alcohol involvement. In K. Bryant, M. Windle, & S. G. West (Eds.), *The science of prevention: Methodological advances from alcohol and substance abuse research* (pp. 43–78). Washington, DC: American Psychological Association Press.

Windle, M., & Searles, J. S. (1990). Summary, integration, and future directions: Toward a life-span perspective. In M. Windle & J. S. Searles (Eds.), *Children of alcoholics: Critical perspectives* (pp. 217–238). New York: Guilford Press.

Windle, M., & Tubman, J. G. (in press). Children of alcoholics: A developmental psychopathology perspective. In W. K. Silverman & T. Ollendick (Eds.), *Developmental issues in the clinical treatment of children and adolescents*. Needham Heights, MA: Allyn & Bacon.

Wohlwill, J. F. (1973). *The study of behavioral development*. New York: Academic Press.

Yamaguchi, K. (1990). Drug use and its social covariates from the period of adolescence to young adulthood: Some implications from longitudinal studies. In M. Galanter (Ed.), *Recent development in alcoholism: Combined alcohol and other drug dependence* (Vol. 8, pp. 125–143). New York: Plenum.

Zucker, R. A. (1987). The four alcoholisms: A developmental account of the etiologic process. In P. C. Rivers (Ed.), *Alcohol and addictive behaviors: Nebraska Symposium on Motivation, 1986* (pp. 27–84). Lincoln: University of Nebraska Press.

Zucker, R. A. (1989). Is risk for alcoholism predictable? A probabilistic approach to a developmental problems. *Drugs and Society, 4,* 69–93.

Zucker, R. A. (1994). Pathways to alcohol problems and alcoholism: A developmental account of the evidence for multiple alcoholisms and for contextual contributions to risk. In R. Zucker, G. Boyd, & J. Howard (Eds.), *The development of alcohol problems: Exploring the biopsychosocial matrix of risk* (Research Monograph 26, pp. 255–289). Rockville, MD: National Institute on Alcohol Abuse and Alcoholism.

Zucker, R. A., Davies, W. H., Kincaid, S. B., Fitzgerald, H. E., & Reider, E. E. (1997). Conceptualizing and scaling the developmental structure of behavior disorder: The Lifetime Alcohol Problems Score as an example. *Development and Psychopathology, 9,* 453–471.

Zucker, R. A., Fitzgerald, H. E., & Moses, H. D. (1995). Emergence of alcohol problems and the several alcoholisms: A developmental perspective on etiologic theory and life course trajectory. In D. Cicchetti & D. J. Cohen (Eds.), *Developmental psychopathology: Vol. 2. Risk, disorder and adaptation* (pp. 677–711). New York: Wiley.

Zucker, R. A., Kincaid, S. B., Fitzgerald, H. E., & Bingham, C. R. (1995). Alcohol schema acquisition in preschoolers: Differences between children of alcoholics and children of nonalcoholics. *Alcohol: Clinical and Experimental Research, 19,* 1011–1017.

Zucker, R. A., & Noll, R. B. (1982). Precursors and developmental influences on drinking and alcoholism: Etiology from a longitudinal perspective. In *Alcohol consumption and related problems* (Alcohol and Health Monograph No. 1, Department of Health and Human Services Publication No. ADM 82-1190, pp. 289–330). Washington, DC: U.S. Government Printing Office.

6

Alcohol Expectancy Theory: The Application of Cognitive Neuroscience

MARK S. GOLDMAN
FRANCES K. DEL BOCA
JACK DARKES

INTRODUCTION

"The determinants of drinking behavior are diverse and complex."

(NIAAA, 1997, p. 33).

"Understanding the neurobiological mechanisms of addiction requires an integration of basic neuroscience with social psychology, experimental psychology, and psychiatry."

(Koob & Le Moal, 1997, p. 52).

"Addiction is a complex phenomenon with important psychological and social causes and consequences."

(Nestler & Aghajanian, 1997, p. 58).

The articles that contain these statements about the etiology of alcohol and drug use, abuse, and dependence, found in the most recent NIAAA report to Congress (1997), and in an issue of the journal *Science* (November 3, 1997), first acknowledge the operation of multiple determinants, but then quickly shift to an emphasis on a variety of genetic and neurobiological variables and processes that have been associated with substance use and addiction. These recent advances in the neurobiology of addiction have been nothing short of awe inspiring.

Nevertheless, much of this research falls short of full explanation, in part because of what we do not yet know, but also because, in many cases, it primarily has served only to identify and describe variables reliably associated with the target conditions. No matter how elaborate, description alone does not constitute explanation. Explanation requires specification of the theoretical processes by which variables influence one another. And even when the aforementioned research does emphasize neurobiological mechanisms and processes, these mechanisms are often variations of the normal substrate for learning, memory, motivation, and emotion, rather than some independent and specialized pathway(s) of drug abuse.

Put another way, these are the neurobiological mechanisms ("hardware") that support many of the information processing capacities ("software") of the brain. Hence, it may be possible to gain insight into these mechanisms from an information-processing perspective, in addition to the more reductionist perspective of neurobiology. The information-processing perspective also can provide pathways through which many biological, psychological, and environmental variables identified as antecedents of drinking and drug use exert their influence. This chapter proposes that full appreciation of the processes by which drinking and drug use is proximally determined is difficult, if not impossible, without consideration of information processing systems. In alcohol and drug research, these systems most often have been studied under the general rubric of expectancies. This chapter elaborates on these themes in the context of updating expectancy research since the 1987 edition of this book (Blane & Leonard, 1987; see also reviews by Brown, 1993; Connors, Maisto, & Derman, 1992; Goldman, 1989, 1994; Goldman, Brown, Christiansen, & Smith, 1991; Goldman, Darkes, & Del Boca, in press; Goldman & Rather, 1993; Leigh, 1989a; Stacy, Widaman, & Marlatt, 1990).

That earlier chapter (Goldman, Brown, & Christiansen, 1987) traced the evolution of the expectancy concept from Tolman (1932) up to the early 1980s. Tolman maintained the intellectual discipline of methodological behaviorism while arguing that a full appreciation of behavior requires concepts such as knowledge, thinking, and purpose. MacCorquodale and Meehl (1953) further systematized the theory by defining expectancy as a learned relationship among a stimulus, a response, and the outcome of the response. Within this framework, it was possible for an organism to learn an expectancy without ever performing the behavior or achieving the intended goal (i.e., vicarious learning). Rotter (1954) noted that performance of the response was dependent on the organism's subjective estimate of the likelihood of reinforcement, and that expectancies were not bound to a specific stimulus but could generalize along a gradient that could be predicted from "common sense" or cultural knowledge of situational similarities. In 1972, Bolles enlarged the scope of expectancy theory and finalized its inevitable merger with the "cognitive revolution" by calling for replacement of the entire concept of associative learning with the expectancy concept. Two kinds of expectancies were proposed: The first, S-S* (the asterisk denotes a stimulus functioning as a biologically important *consequence* rather than a cue), represented the organism's acquired knowledge of environment–outcome contingencies. The second, R-S*, represented the organism's knowledge of the relation between its own behavior and environmental outcomes. Bandura (1977) then theorized that humans also maintain higher order, "efficacy" ÿ2Dexpectancies of their ability (or inability) to execute particular behaviors in situations in which they would be reinforcing (e.g., a socially phobic individual's expectancy of his or her ability to give a speech).

Since the review in 1987, the expectancy concept has rapidly evolved as a consequence of its use within the emerging area of cognitive neuroscience and its capacity to link conceptually other cognitive and neural processes that have been recently articulated to explain complex behavior. At this point, expectancy does not seem best construed as a unitary construct, but instead as a unifying umbrella term for a variety of neurocognitive processes that serve a common function, namely, preparing the organism to respond to future circumstances. Hence, the term "expectancy" may be applied to the emerging conceptualizations of memory functions (Eichenbaum, 1997), to what sometimes are called more primitive habit-learning mechanisms, or even to the memory aspects of motivation and emotion, as long as what is emphasized is their capacity to use inborn or acquired information to prepare for behavioral adaptation to later circumstances.

An explosion of research applying the expectancy concept to alcohol use has also taken place since the 1987 review. This research has covered a wide variety of domains in alcohol studies and has highlighted a number of controversies. Some disagreements have resulted from different usages of the term "expectancy." Because of its heuristic utility, this term has found application in a variety of fields (e.g., animal and human learning, perception, personality, and social psychology), and its definition and usage have varied with the research traditions in these areas. Also, the use of this term in cognitive neuroscience again has expanded its meaning and provided somewhat of a shifting foundation upon which to base applications, such as those in alcohol research. In the remainder of this chapter, we survey the evolution of the expectancy concept in relation to emerging trends in cognitive neuroscience, and then review applications of the expectancy concept in alcohol research since 1987.

THE EXPECTANCY CONCEPT

To function adequately, organisms must reduce the degrees of freedom intrinsic to the information in the environment. Simple organisms receive limited inputs and are capable of limited outputs. Farther up the evolutionary ladder, however, sensory systems can receive information that would be overwhelming without some preexisting template for organizing such information and guiding ensuing behavior. Some aspects of this template are hardwired at birth. For example, the visual system is programmed to respond to complex stimulus configurations (i.e., lines in various orientations, patterns, movement; Maunsell, 1995). Because higher-order adaptive behavior requires plasticity, complex organisms also use templates that are acquired from experience (Grossberg, 1995) and adapt in response to relevant new information. Even aspects of the visual system, once thought to be hardwired, are apparently adaptable (Singer, 1995).

Tolman (1932) referred to this capacity to use information stored at one time point to organize and guide responses to information encountered later as expectancy. In Tolman's time, however, it was not clear to behavioral theorists how a nonsubstantive process (information processing) could produce movement. It is now abundantly evident that information-processing devices (computers) readily can control the actions of servomechanisms. In living organisms, some memory systems are so integrated with muscle (movement) systems that they are found to reside in the peripheral nervous system (Grillner, 1996).

This is just one example of how models taken from cognitive neuroscience, computer science, and artificial intelligence have become applicable to expectancy research (also see Goldman, in press). Furthermore, cognitive/expectancy models easily can be integrated with models of affect and emotion (Bower, 1981, 1992; Lang, 1979), because these domains are significantly, and perhaps seamlessly, related in the nervous system and routinely function together to influence behavior (Gray, 1990). As modern theories of personality structure have been articulated and related to theories of emotion, it also has become possible to tie together cognition, affect, and personality within a general model of expectancy operation.

This theoretical evolution over the last decade has made it even clearer than in 1987 that expectancy is not a narrow theoretical process but is best viewed as an umbrella term for processes that influence all behavior. The term "expectancy" may be generically applied to information templates stored in the nervous system and to the processing of this information to produce behavioral output. These templates and their associated processes are appropriately called expectancies in that they prepare the organism for future circumstances based on their degree of similarity to circumstances already encountered. Two interconnected classes of templates may be considered: those that are compared with incoming sensory input so as to organize and interpret this input, and ultimately to influence output, and those that structure this output.

The pervasiveness of expectancy processes is underscored by the recent movement toward expectancy-based neurocomputational models of brain functioning. Consider, for example, the comments of Grossberg (1995):

"Neural networks that match sensory input with learned expectations help explain how humans see, hear, learn and recognize information" (p. 438); and Schultz, Dayan, and Montague (1997): "Learning is driven by . . . expectations about future salient events . . . [and output of] . . . dopaminergic neurons . . . signals changes in the predictions of future salient or rewarding events" (p. 1593). Such models do not require complex deliberation and might be based on nothing more than the detection of information patterns that match previously stored patterns. When a sufficient match is achieved, information templates representing associated response patterns are activated in turn. These "response expectancies" then activate associated affective and motor pathways and may result in behavioral output. The term "may" reflects only a probability of output, because other information templates are almost certainly activated simultaneously; these multiplex activation patterns compete for influence over final behavioral output.

Expectancy systems are not solely passive, however. They actively influence the perception of incoming stimuli, sometimes quite selectively. Consider an example presented by Grossberg (1995, who credits Richard Warren): "Suppose that you hear a noise followed immediately by the words 'eel is on the . . . ' If that string of words is followed by the word 'orange,' you hear 'peel is on the orange.' If the word 'wagon' completes the sentence, you hear 'wheel is on the wagon.' If the final word is 'shoe,' you hear 'heel is on the shoe' " (p. 439). According to Grossberg, learned expectations that are activated by the final word in the sequence influence the perception of the first word in the sequence, which is held in a buffer (working memory).

The Computational Model

In 1950, Turing described the "universal machine" that would be programmable to perform an unlimited range of tasks. This work served as the model for the modern computer. The notion of a machine with flexible and adaptable functions, which, in some configurations, could be said to "learn" (alter its functioning in accord with external inputs), also provided a model for the nervous system. As suggested by Newell (1970), this model could be applied as an interesting metaphor, or could be the literal basis for cognition. Recent findings from neuroscience research have supported the latter view (see Maunsell, 1995; Singer, 1995).

The "biological computer" of the nervous system is, however, more complex than any electronic computer, due largely to having evolved in stages. Simpler systems developed earlier, some of which are still present in organisms lower on the phylogenetic scale. More sophisticated systems then evolved, often overlaying the simpler systems. For example, dopamine is released in the nucleus acumbens when stimuli are encountered that previously have been associated with reinforcement (Schultz et al., 1997). This is essentially a lower-order expectancy mechanism that does not require complex intervening cognitions. This system for the "attribution of incentive salience" (Robinson & Berridge, 1993, p. 249) may be directly activated by drugs that have abuse potential. Because these systems also receive input from the cortex, it is quite possible that they also can be activated by higher-order information templates of the sort described earlier.

To further explore the nervous system–computer connection, it is useful to consider the two basic architectures (structures) that have been developed as the substrate for computers (Newell, Rosenbloom, & Laird, 1989). The first architecture supports serial processing and appears in computers in everyday use. The second architecture supports parallel processing.

In a serial system, an addressable memory is separate from a central processing unit that runs the program. The program (designed by an external agent, a programmer) sequentially accesses designated information from memory and transforms it in a predetermined manner. Such computers are fast because their electronics are fast, but problems must be solved by brute force over many steps. Because neurons operate in milliseconds, human processes (the simplest of which take approximately 100 msecs) must only involve 100 or so steps (Feldman, 1985). Serial programs require many more steps to perform any function of consequence. Thus, parallel processing appears more consistent with nervous system operation; that is, in human neural functioning, the simultaneous activation of multiple information elements produces complex information patterns that guide output. The underlying architecture for such a parallel system may be construed as a network with highly interconnected elements or "nodes."

Evidence, in fact, is accumulating that complex memories (i.e., stored expectancy templates) are not maintained intact, but are assembled from parts when needed. Ungerleider (1995) writes, "Information about all the different visual attributes of an object is not stored in a unified fashion in any single area of the cortex. . . . [It] seems to be stored in a distributed cortical system in which information about specific features is stored close to regions of the cortex that mediate the perceptions of those features" (p. 771). The hippocampus first links cortical areas to form concepts, but, once formed, the prefrontal cortex jointly activates the multiple areas that constitute a concept. When assembled, complex associations correspond to the constructs of schemas (concepts at different levels of abstraction), and scripts (complex action patterns; "how to do something," such as preparing a meal, see Schank & Abelson, 1977). Although the terminology differs, these complex association networks conceptually and functionally overlap the expectancy concept. Both assist with organizing and interpreting incoming information, and guiding appropriate responses.

To simulate the operation of the nervous system, cognitive scientists have articulated two general computational network models. The first, the parallel distributed processing (PDP), or "connectionist" model, relates electronic elements in a manner thought similar to biological elements in the nervous system. In this "neurally inspired" (Rumelhart, 1989, p. 134) system, information resides in the rules (weights) that associate (connect) one electronic element to another. With a complex set of processing units (usually three hierarchically arranged levels of units), a connectionist network not only can perform complex functions, but also can appear to "learn"; that is, feedback loops can convey the discrepancy between actual and desired output so that, over many successive trials, a desired output will occur without external programming. This capacity to acquire a function without an outside agent has made connectionist models quite appealing. It is impossible, however, to understand how the network performs a task, since the solution resides in temporary activation patterns. In addition, these networks typically need an extraordinarily large number of trials to "learn" a predesignated output.

An alternative network architecture stores representations of the external world as codes or symbols. In symbolic network models, molecular concepts are represented as nodes that are closely or more distantly linked based on intrinsic meaning and learning history. Higher-order concepts are assembled when the network is triggered by appropriate stimuli. Because humans are capable of processing relations, and not just concrete stimuli, some experts (Pylyshyn, 1989) argue that human systems must include some form of symbol manipulation. For example, a child who learns to place a red ball in a blue box, will also know to place a blue ball in a red box. Pylyshyn (p. 62) points out that this characteristic is a natural consequence of symbol architectures but must be enforced in nonsymbol (e.g., connectionist) architectures. Human processing must occur at multiple levels that may include both connectionist and symbol networks, as well as higher-order semantic (knowledge) networks (Pylyshyn, 1989; Simon & Kaplan, 1989). Connectionist networks would correspond to the biological level of processing, which would serve as the substrate for symbol and semantic processing.

Mathematical Approaches from Cognitive Psychology

Cognitive psychologists have offered other approaches for modeling symbolic networks. Estes (1991) suggested that memory "traces can be viewed as vectors or lists, as nodes in a network, or as points in multidimensional space" (p. 12). These formal (mathematical) schemes are not mutually exclusive, however; each point in multidimensional space could serve as the representation of a node in a network. Each node modeled at one level of a network also may represent the activation of a subnetwork that reflects a collection or list of elementary characteristics of the concept. Due to this flexibility, Chang (1986; see McNamara, 1992) recommends network theory as a useful general theory of cognitive representation from which more specific theories can be developed.

Furthermore, formalizing symbolic or semantic memory models as networks implies a basis for memory process as well as structure. In the spreading activation model of Collins and Loftus (1975), distance between nodes reflects the level of association between concepts in memory. When triggered by an appropriate stimulus, activation is assumed to spread spatially and then to dissipate. The coactivated nodes represent a higher-order concept (e.g., schema, script). Although this network-based process has been considered part of declarative (episodic and semantic) memory, sequences of activated information that organize movement could also underlie procedural memory (simpler, repetitive, motor sequences), perhaps in a different brain location (e.g., cerebellum, motor strip: see Raymond, Lisberger, & Mauk, 1996; Squire, 1987, 1992).

The Expectancy Construct: Surplus Meaning

Because the expectancy construct has been so widely used, it has accumulated meanings that are, in the current context, superfluous. For example, within some psychological traditions, expectancy-guided behavior is seen as exclusively top-down in nature. The implication of this usage often goes unexamined, but it seems to suggest that an expectancy template is activated only at the "highest" levels of cognition. Top-down influences are contrasted with "bottom-up" processes, which are somehow "stimulus-driven." In the complex and hierarchical network environment that characterizes brain functioning, "top" and "bottom" are highly relative. In any particular function, the higher-up level may, in the absolute sense, be low in the processing architecture.

Often associated with the presumption of top-down influence is the view that expectancies are "conscious" and must use attentional resources. None of the models discussed earlier require conscious processes or focused attention. They assume only that previously stored information serves to organize incoming information. Given the amount of simultaneous information we must process, it may be argued that most perceptual and behavioral control systems are "automatic" in nature, operating without awareness. We constantly carry out behavioral sequences that we do not plan in advance, and to which we pay only marginal attention. (Consider the common experience of traveling home from work over an everyday route and not being able to recall just how we got there.) Berns, Cohen, and Mintun (1997) even have identified brain regions that are specifically responsive to environmental novelty in the absence of awareness. In this sense, Freud may have misled us; rather than treating behavior in the absence of awareness as requiring explanation (or even as pathological), such behavior is likely modal (see Banaji & Hardin, 1996; Bargh & Barndollar, 1996; Jacoby, Lindsay, & Toth, 1992). Some models of attention treat awareness as a limited resource (Shiffrin & Schneider, 1977). More consistent with expectancy models, however, are models that suggest that "performance is automatic when it can be supported by traces retrieved from memory instead of costly algorithmic computation" (Logan, 1995, p. 751). These traces essentially *are* expectancies.

Finally, in some areas of psychology (e.g., attitude theory in social psychology), the term "belief" has been linked with expectancies. This term often implies conscious, verbalizable (accessible) information, which certainly may derive from the larger set of information-processing mechanisms discussed earlier, but does not include all of them. In fact, the verbal expression of beliefs likely is influenced by a number of expectancy sets, working in both constructive and competitive fashion (e.g., constraints imposed by expectancies of appropriateness to particular settings, and by expectancies relating to interpersonal norms).

This argument for the pervasiveness of automatic information processing is not meant to imply that deliberative (conscious) processing is unimportant. From an evolutionary perspective, attention-demanding, "controlled" processing may be the most recent mechanism by which behavioral plasticity and adaptability are enhanced. Deliberative processing may increase survival potential by competing with automatic processes that may at times be maladaptive. Although the relative influence of controlled and automatic processing is not yet well articulated, the capacity of humans to make use of rule-based information-processing algorithms (e.g., logic, mathematics), and to plan over medium- to long-term intervals, has given us wide adaptability to environmental conditions. In fact, the capacity to consciously anticipate and plan for upcoming circumstances may be regarded as another level of expectancy processing. It is also these conscious, deliberative systems that are used in cognitive (and other) therapy to intrude into, and compete with, unwanted automatic behaviors; that is, psychotherapy may be regarded as an effort to influence expectancy processes.

Integrating Affect and Personality

In recent years, cognitive researchers have studied affect (e.g., Bower, 1981, 1992), and emotion researchers have begun to use cognitive models (e.g., Gray, 1990; Lang, 1979, 1995). Because expectancies anticipate reward and punishment, and these events are intimately tied to affective response, a neurocomputational model of expectancies should integrate cognition and affect. And, because recent theories of personality are built upon theories of affective responding, integration leads inevitably to an expectancy view of personality. The next two sections address these issues.

Affect

A pure information-processing model applied to organismic functioning fails in one major respect: There is no mechanism to provide goals in the absence of an outside agent. In living organisms, primary needs (e.g., hunger, thirst), allied with affect/emotion, play this role. Since life requires behavior, it is helpful to think of these systems as steering behavior (rather than inducing it), or making some behavioral options more salient in the face of a wide range of possibilities. This perspective on emotion can be readily coupled with an information-processing view of neural functioning; that is, affect may be seen as an internal governor of which computations are initiated, interrupted, or take precedence, among the competing possibilities available. Indeed, Gray (1982) has pointed out that neural systems underlying affect are so closely integrated with those that support cognition as to be virtually indistinguishable.

Two prevailing models of the basic mathematical dimensions of affect have been offered. One model includes two bipolar (and orthogonal) dimensions located in two-dimensional space: affective valence, ranging from pleasant to aversive; and arousal, ranging from extremely unaroused (or even asleep) to very aroused (e.g., Russell, 1979, 1980). The second model emphasizes two unipolar dimensions of positive and negative affectivity (Watson & Tellegen, 1985). Whereas Russell's model regards valence and arousal as independent (orthogonal), the Watson and Tellegen model combines valence and arousal on each of two unipolar dimensions. These dimensions can be distinguished by their different orientations in the same two-dimensional space (at a 45 degree rotation from the Russell dimensions). The latter two dimensions also have been called behavioral activation and inhibition (Fowles, 1980; Gray, 1982), or reward seeking and harm avoidance (Cloninger, 1987). The relative merits of these models and how they might be integrated have been debated (see Larsen & Diener, 1992), as has the time course of activation (tonic/phasic) of these systems. For example, some have argued that specific affects are distributed around the space defined by the two orthogonal dimensions with sufficient regularity, so as to be characterized more appropriately by a circumplex (circular dimension; Larsen & Diener, 1992). (See Figure 6.1.) A circumplex model has the additional advantage of subsuming different perspectives regarding the basic dimensions of affect. As shown in Figure 6.1, differing sets of opposing dimensions reflect axis rotations within the same two-dimensional space. There are also presumably individual differences in the tendency to experience and express these emotions. In fact, one way of understanding temperament would be to consider it an individualized predisposition to respond with one or another affective pattern.

Discussions over the "true" dimensions of affect and temperament take place because these dimensions are thought to reveal basic physiological processes (two or three at most) that are the substrate for affective response. For example, in the model espoused by Russell (1980; also advanced by Lang, 1995; see Figure 6.1), the valence dimension represents the operation of two opponent systems (approach/positive affect and withdrawal/ negative affect), located in related but separate brain areas. The nucleus accumbens, caudate nucleus, and putamen, are often cited as the substrate for approach behaviors, and the amygdala as the substrate for

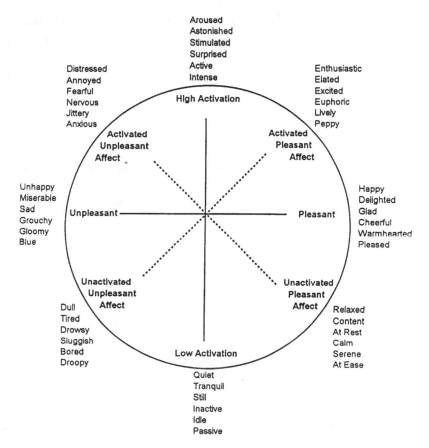

FIGURE 6.1. The domain of affective words (self-reported affect circumplex). From Larsen and Diener (1992). Copyright 1992 by Sage Publications, Inc. Reprinted by permission.

withdrawal reactions; alternatively, Davidson (1993) locates the substrate for approach-related affective responses in the left anterior cortex and withdrawal-related affective responses in the right anterior cortex. These systems are thought to operate at different levels of organismic arousal. The complex array of emotions we experience is thought to result from joint activation of these two or three basic systems. From this perspective, the wide array of emotions we experience has no unique existence; emotions are perceptual combinations (blends) in the same fashion that most colors are combinations of reception in three basic receptor types.

But since the nervous system seems to store traces of its own activation patterns, beginning at birth (and perhaps even earlier), a representation of each particular affective response, and the stimulus conditions within which it occurred, may be stored in memory, just as other expectancy information is stored (see Izard, 1993; Lang, 1979; LeDoux, 1995; Shaver, Schwartz, Kirson, & O'Connor, 1987). These affective memory networks remain linked to the subcortical systems that activate basic (primitive) affective responses (appetitive and defensive reactions; see Lang, 1995). Ongoing affective responding then results from both activation of the pathways that mediate primitive affective response, and activation of those same pathways via activation of the previously stored affective memory traces; that is, once the template of stimulus conditions relevant to an affective response is sufficiently matched by a newly encountered stimulus, then the stored representations of the previous affective response are activated, and in turn activate primary (physiological) affective systems. These conditions describe the operation of an expectancy system that influences affective responding.

Any given affective response may be either more or less a "raw" physiological event. Physiological activation triggered innately by a real external stimulus might be indistinguishable from physiological activation triggered by the stored representation of that affective response. This cognitive explanation for classical conditioning is not dissimilar to the Rescorla–Wagner model (1972; see Siegel & Allan, 1996), in which the organism is understood to learn correlations, rather than acquiring wired connections, between unconditional and conditional stimuli and responses. Models of this kind have become central in comprehensive accounts of affective functioning (see Bower, 1981, 1992; Lang, 1979, 1995; LeDoux, 1995).

Hence, we can use the previously described mathematical (graphic) models of affective space to model a working parallel processing network of affective activation. Nodes representing any stored affective experience can be located in this space with reference to the two dimensions thought to represent primary emotions. Those nodes located more closely together in this space are assumed to be more likely to coactivate. Figure 6.2 provides an example of such a model in the alcohol-expectancy realm. If a hypothetical threshold of activation of affective memories is achieved in this information storage system, activation then proceeds to the physiological systems that control affect expression, resulting in the experience of emotion. Once again, this essentially is an expectancy model of affective response.

Personality

To weave personality into the same expectancy (anticipatory information processing) scheme, we need only to view personality as a set of relatively consistent behavioral patterns that develop over time as manifestations of the aforementioned information/affective networks (see Meyer & Shack, 1989; Pervin, 1994; Revelle, 1995). Such a model reflects the consistency and changeability of behavior over time, as the networks accommodate changing life circumstances and physical maturation. The stability of per-

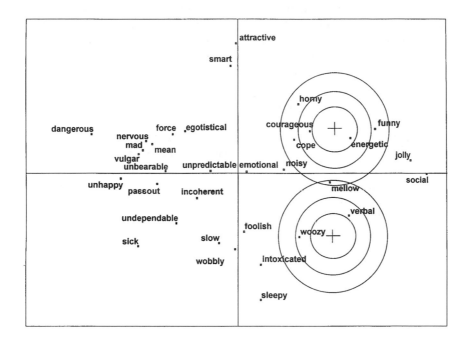

FIGURE 6.2. An example of alcohol-expectancy words in two-dimensional space as configured by multidimensional scaling (MDS). The horizontal dimension (axis) ranges from "bad" at the left of the figure to "good" at the right, and the vertical dimension (axis) from "sedated" at the bottom of the figure, to "aroused" at the top. Note that a rough circle could be drawn by connecting the words at the periphery of the configuration; this arrangement is one way of characterizing a circumplex organization. The axes drawn through the circumplex could be viewed as higher-order representations of the more basic elements (words).

Hypothetical starting points for activation of the expectancy network have been suggested based on auxilliary MDS methods (Rather & Goldman, 1994). The cross adjacent to "woozy" is the hypothetical starting point for light drinkers in this data set; the cross adjacent to "energetic" is the hypothetical starting point for heavy drinkers. Once activation begins, it may be presumed to spread as do ripples on a smooth lake (as characterized by the concentric circles).

sonality results from the centrality of the core information nets that begin developing at birth. Long-standing information patterns that are continually strengthened by inherited physiological predispositions are not easily changed.

Commonly identified traits and types, such as the "Big Five" (see Costa & McCrae, 1995), can be related with some consistency to locations in the affect space described earlier that reflect salient affective dimensions (see Goldman, in press; Larsen & Diener, 1992; Meyer & Shack, 1989).

Hence, by locating the behavioral concomitants of specific affective responses (which are described as traits and types) within the same kind of two-dimensional space, a graphic representation can be produced of a network model of personality in which spreading activation can serve as a heuristic for the process through which consistent behavioral response tendencies (i.e., personality) become manifest. Dimensions drawn through this same two-dimensional personality space can be construed as higher-order personality traits under which lower-order characteristics (or facets) are subsumed in a hierarchical arrangement (Costa & McCrae, 1995). For example, Larsen and Diener (1992) suggested that Extraversion can be located at the Activated-Pleasant Affect point along the circumplex (characterized in terms of feelings such as enthusiasm, liveliness, etc.; see Figure 6.1); similarly, Neuroticism corresponds to the Activated-Unpleasant Affect pole (typified by feelings of distress, anxiety, etc., as per Figure 6.1). In this conceptualization, part of the consistency in behavior we call personality derives from the repetitive processing of complex expectancy templates that have developed over years.

INTEGRATION AND APPLICATION
TO ALCOHOL RESEARCH

The pieces are now in place to explain how complex behaviors can be influenced either by actual experience, vicarious experience, or, in the absence of experience, guided by an acquired concept about appropriate behavior (e.g., "hypnotic" behavior based on the individual's knowledge of what hypnosis is *supposed* to do). The activation of an expectancy template can directly initiate a behavioral sequence (script) previously associated with that "recognized" stimulus. Such a template also can directly activate an affective experience. In a more indirect fashion, activation of an expectancy can produce a behavior that is associated with, or results from, the activation of an affective state. For example, persons may become more socially outgoing because they are affectively aroused. Expectancy operation can also produce the relatively stable behavior patterns we refer to as personality, with the same processes repeated over many occasions. This type of processing is the essence of modern conceptualizations of personality (see Revelle, 1995). Thus, expectancy processing can explain simple, time-limited behavioral and affective sequences, as well as more complex affective and stable behavior patterns.

Because these processes are theorized to influence all behavior, they obviously can be applied to alcohol consumption and alcohol-induced behavior. In this application, information that reflects the reinforcement value of alcohol acquired as a function of biological, psychological, and environmental risk variables is viewed as being stored as memory templates. The memory systems that retain this information are conceptualized as a kind of information-based "buffer." Once acquired, these templates have the capacity to influence alcohol use and its associated behavioral patterns over widely varying time periods. Because these memory templates anticipate the conditions under which particular behaviors are to be performed, they are appropriately called expectancies. Because we are describing what is essentially a mediational model, it becomes necessary to discuss an issue that has tended to blur understanding of the expectancy concept. Evidence in support of this model is then reviewed.

Mediators and Moderators

The concepts of mediation and moderation appear at two points in relation to the linkages between antecedent variables, alcohol expectancies, and drinking. First, genetic researchers have characterized expectancies as moderators of the relationship between drinking-related genetic influences and drinking itself. Second, some psychosocial researchers have referred to expectancies as moderators of the relationship between some other psychosocial variable and alcohol use (e.g., anxiety level only predicts drinking for those who expect alcohol to reduce anxiety). These characterizations of expectancies as moderators contrast with our view of expectancies as part of the causal process (i.e., as mediators).

The concept of moderation was originally invoked to increase the predictive relationship between one variable and another (e.g., Arnold, 1982; Saunders, 1956), that is, to show that prediction improved if a third variable was taken into account. In statistical terms, moderation referred to an interaction; nothing was implied about the mechanism or process responsible for the effect. And, consistent with an interaction, either variable could be understood as moderating the effect of the other. Baron and Kenny (1986), concerned about the interchangeable use of the terms "moderator" and "mediator," attempted to clarify the conceptual distinction and offered statistical designs that could be used to distinguish the two. Their definition of moderator retained an exclusively statistical denotation ("partitions a focal independent variable," p. 1173); however, mediators were given a process implication ("generative mechanism," p. 1173), that is, mediators carried the influence of (totally or partially) the antecedent variable upon the criterion.

While the Baron and Kenny (1986) article has justifiably become a classic, one consequence has been that concepts such as expectancy may become classified as mediators or moderators based solely on the choice of a particular statistical model. Often, there seems to be the associated inference that, once classified in this manner, variables are either mediators or moderators, but not both, and that moderators can carry no causal significance. Baron and Kenny addressed the possibility that variables could act as both; variables may serve as moderators by mediating a relationship at one level of the variable, but not at the other. For example, in the case of a neuron, a variety of excitatory and inhibitory inputs are processed at the presynaptic membrane and, if threshold is achieved, an action potential is carried down the neuron. Drugs show a similar pattern: Below an effective dose, no drug effect is apparent; once an appropriate dose is achieved, the drug shows an increasing influence. Without elaborating on the dynamic processes involved in both cases, note that both an on–off relationship and apparent causal influence might be observed depending on how the full mathematical relationship between the variables is broken down for analysis.

In addition to the thorough statistical analysis as suggested by Baron and Kenny (1986), we contend that inferences of causality are best based on a pattern of relationships (as in a construct validation network) obtained from multiple studies that include instances of true experiments. In the present context, we argue that the evidence supports the inference that expectancies serve as a (partial) mediator (a transmitter of causal influence), and that studies demonstrating moderation do not preclude their role as mediators; in fact, any observed moderation is inferred to be the result of a mediational process. For example, studies have found that expectancies of a certain type (e.g., tension reduction) moderate the relationship between other antecedent risk variables (e.g., anxious personality, family history of alcoholism) and drinking (e.g., Cooper, Russell, Skinner, Frone, & Mudar, 1992; Johnson & Gurin, 1994; Mann, Chassin, & Sher, 1987). Although the designs used in these studies cannot support a mediational interpretation, they also do not counter a mediational view.[1]

Furthermore, if expectancies are argued only to moderate (but not to mediate) a relationship between other antecedent variables (e.g., dysphoric states or heritable biological characteristics and alcohol use), a credible mediational pathway between the other variables and alcohol use must be theoretically articulated. Unless such a pathway can be theorized without the operational involvement of the learned reinforcing characteristics of alcohol, expectancies must be regarded as at least one mediator of the relationship. In fact, we argue that the expectancy process serves as one final-common-pathway to drinking and alcoholism.

Evidence Supporting a Mediational View of Expectancies

A construct validation network has become available over the past 20 years to support the inference that expectancies have a causal (mediational or process) influence on drinking. Central to this support is both the accumulating data base (our PsycINFO search of the literature from 1984 to 1996, using "alcohol" and "expectancies" as key words, identified 445 studies) and the use of research designs that offer effective logical support for a causal inference. Six increasingly stringent levels of evidence can be offered: (1) correlations between measured expectancies and reports of alcohol use; (2) measurement of expectancies in children before actual drinking begins;

(3) demonstrations that expectancies predict drinking prospectively; (4) the observation that drinking experience influences expectancy acquisition, in keeping with the notion that expectancies reflect learning; (5) findings consistent with the Baron and Kenny (1986) statistical method for demonstrating mediation; and finally (6) true experiments.

Correlations between Expectancies and Drinking

The body of studies that show a relationship between expectancies and drinking is now so large that some researchers have called for a moratorium on simple correlational research in favor of the investigation of moderators of the relationship (McCarthy & Smith, 1996). We add to this call an increased emphasis on process-oriented research. A number of reviews (Goldman, 1994; Goldman & Rather, 1993) show expectancies to be among the strongest predictors of drinking, even after other variables are controlled. Studies have used expectancy questionnaires of various types (e.g., the Anticipated Biphasic Alcohol Effects Scale [ABAES], Earleywine, 1994a; the Comprehensive Effects of Alcohol instrument [CEOA], Fromme, Stroot, & Kaplan, 1993; the Alcohol Outcome Expectancy Scale, Leigh & Stacy, 1993), related measured expectancies to a variety of drinking measures, including frequency (Fromme et al., 1993), amount consumed per occasion (Carey, 1995), and indices of alcoholism and drinking problems (Earleywine, 1994b; Werner, Walker, & Green, 1993), in age groups ranging from elementary-school-aged children (Miller, Smith, & Goldman, 1990), to older adults (Cooper, Russell, Skinner, & Windle, 1992), to alcoholics in treatment and in treatment follow-up (Connors, Tarbox, & Faillace, 1993; Gustafson & Engstrom, 1991). The relationship between expectancies and drinking has been estimated by simple correlations (Bogart, Yeatman, Sirridge, & Gear, 1995); multiple regression (Reese, Chassin, & Molina, 1993); covariance structure modeling (CSM), using latent variables (Henderson, Goldman, Coovert, & Carnevalla, 1994; Sher, Wood, Wood, & Raskin, 1996); and hierarchical linear modeling (Smith, Goldman, Greenbaum, & Christiansen, 1995).

A recent meta-analytic review indicated that the average amount of variance in drinking accounted for by expectancies is 12% cross-sectionally and 4% over time (McCarthy & Smith, 1996). Some studies have accounted for 50% or more of the drinking variance when well-developed instruments and analysis techniques were used (Goldman, Greenbaum, & Darkes, 1997; Leigh & Stacy, 1993). The McCarthy and Smith (1996) meta-analysis identified questionnaire length to be the major moderating influence on the size of the relationship between expectancies and drinking. Since expectancies presumably reflect accumulated information about drinking, it is no surprise that the availability of items reflecting a wide variety of alcohol effects might facilitate adequate assessment. Although percentages of variance accounted for are sometimes reported to be much lower (Leigh,

1989b), we found no instances in our review of failures to find a statistically significant relationship. Recently, methods for measuring expectancies arising from cognitive psychology have also been related reliably to drinking (Gustafson, 1989; Palfai, Monti, Colby, & Rohsenow, 1997; Stacy, 1997). Clearly, the relationship between measured expectancies and drinking is robust across participants, methods, and studies.

One potential problem suggested by the robust relationship between expectancies and drinking is that of criterion contamination; that is, to what extent is this relationship inflated by expectancy measurements that may reflect the indirect assessment of drinking experience (by assessing accumulated experience with alcohol use)? This issue echoes questions raised by early behaviorists about the measurement of any hypothetical construct, and particularly those measured by verbal report. As in other areas of science, the best support for a theory that uses unobservables is its effective organization and explanation of existing data, and suggestion of new approaches and experimental tests that would not be anticipated using other organizing principles. Expectancy formulations have begun to meet this goal, but much work remains to be done.

Expectancies Antedating Drinking

Cross-Sectional Designs. Expectancies or expectancy-like information has been detected in preschool children (Zucker, Kincaid, Fitzgerald, & Bingham, 1996; see Lang & Stritzke, 1993), elementary-school-aged children (Dunn & Goldman, 1996; Miller et al., 1990), and junior high school and high school students before they begin to drink (Christiansen & Goldman, 1983; Christiansen, Goldman, & Inn, 1982; Christiansen, Smith, Roehling, & Goldman, 1989). Hence, expectancies can be acquired vicariously, and prior to drinking, consistent with a causal process interpretation. As children mature toward drinking, expectancies change from being primarily negative (reflecting unpleasant and antisocial outcomes), to more elaborate and more reflective of positive social effects and arousal (Dunn & Goldman, 1996; Miller et al., 1990).

Longitudinal Designs. Longitudinal studies are more persuasive of a causal connection between expectancies and drinking. This work has predominantly involved adolescents (Christiansen et al., 1989; Newcomb, Chou, Bentler, & Huba, 1988) across the age range during which drinking is frequently initiated. Predrinking expectancies were found to predict the likelihood of drinking onset and consumption level, once drinking began. Similar findings have been reported over a longer time frame, ranging into young adulthood (Stacy, Newcomb, & Bentler, 1991). This study (Stacy et al., 1991) went further in supporting a causal role for expectancies by showing that expectancies measured at one time point predicted later drinking and drug use, beyond the level predicted by these same behaviors at the first time point (i.e., residual variance above the behavior-to-behavior relationship). In college students, expectancies predicted "high-risk drinking" 1 month later (Carey, 1995).

Expectancies of alcoholics in treatment have predicted posttreatment outcomes. Connors et al. (1993) found that expectancies decreased during an 18-month follow-up period in individuals whose drinking declined. Jones and McMahon (1994) reported that those individuals leaving treatment with the highest negative expectancies were the most successful in reducing their drinking.

Bidirectional Effects

Because theory suggests that expectancies are acquired through both vicarious and direct experience with alcohol's effects, expectancies should change as a function of drinking experience (see Goldman, 1994). Thus, expectancies measured in advance of drinking should predict later drinking, but changes in alcohol use should also anticipate changes in expectancies. Two recent studies confirmed this pattern. Smith et al. (1995) showed that, from early to midadolescence, higher scores on a social expectancy scale predicted more alcohol use 1 year later; greater drinking at that second time point, in turn, predicted higher expectancy scale scores after a subsequent year had passed. These results were noteworthy because the CSM procedures controlled for the spurious influence of autocorrelations, and results were cross-checked using hierarchical linear modeling (HLM; Bryk & Raudenbush, 1992).

Using CSM alone, Sher et al. (1996) evaluated the temporal sequencing of expectancies and drinking over 3 years, beginning with college admission. Reciprocal effects again were found, but in this case, declines in drinking predicted decreases in expectancies. The authors noted that their ability to discern such effects was highly dependent on the measurement interval used; short intervals tended to mask such effects, because drinking and expectancies were so highly correlated over brief time periods that little room was left for measuring effects beyond autoregressive effects.

These findings have implications for expectancy theory development. Drinking tends to increase into young adulthood and then to decrease for most individuals. Research tracking expectancies into young adulthood had shown them to elaborate and consolidate as drinking increased. Expectancies, however, had not been followed during the developmental period of general drinking decreases. A major question, therefore, was whether expectancies would remain high, or decrease, along with reductions in alcohol use. Expectancies might decrease because the enchantment with alcohol use diminishes with repeated exposure (hence, as a *consequence* of alcohol experience; see Sher et al., 1996). Or the emergence of other reward systems and their associated expectancies (e.g., school and career plans) might effectively compete with expectations of reward from alcohol use, thereby influencing drinking in a prospective fashion (expectancies again *anticipating* alcohol use). In any case, this study suggested that changes in expectancy parallel changes in drinking. At a process level, both effects likely occur reciprocally.

Mediational Models

Although consistent with mediation, longitudinal studies can only establish temporal sequencing; inferences about process require more demanding research designs. At the boundary between correlational designs and true experiments are tests of mediation using the Baron and Kenny (1986) design. Such studies have uniformly found expectancies to serve as a mediator of other antecedents; often, however, this mediation is partial, with the antecedent having a direct effect on drinking (e.g., Darkes, Greenbaum, & Goldman, 1996b; Henderson et al., 1994; Scheier & Botvin, 1997; Sher, Walitzer, Wood, & Brent, 1991; Smith & Goldman, 1990; Webb, Baer, Francis, & Caid, 1993). Antecedents partially mediated by expectancies have included personality variables such as sensation seeking/behavioral undercontrol and risk status based on peer and parental influences. Failure to find total mediation of the effects of these antecedents by alcohol expectancies is not surprising, given that these influences serve to place individuals in environments in which drinking is encouraged, independent of alcohol expectancies. Studies on reciprocal influences, however, have shown that such exposure may also result in delayed expectancy increases. Existing expectancy measures also may not assess all the expectancies that might be affected by drinking environments.

True Experiments

The most persuasive evidence for mediation comes from true experiments with random assignment of participants, manipulation of the hypothesized mediator, and inclusion of appropriate control groups to rule out the influence of alternative variables on the dependent variable. Several studies support the inference that expectancies influence drinking, but in these studies, the operational definition of expectancy must necessarily expand beyond psychometrically developed questionnaire responses. Manipulation of expectancies instead must be inferred from changes in observable variables, presumably, linked to expectancies. Procedures designed by cognitive psychologists to measure memory also have been recently applied to the study of expectancies. This expansion in the operational definition of alcohol expectancies does raise, of course, the question of whether the same processes are being measured.

In the first edition of this volume (Goldman et al., 1987), "balanced placebo" experiments were emphasized in this domain; these experiments demonstrated a dissociation between the pharmacological effects of consuming alcohol (at relatively low doses) and the instruction that alcohol was, or was not, to be consumed (see Hull & Bond, 1986). It is most parsimonious to assume that expectancies were activated by this set, but expectancies were not measured or manipulated directly. Since the earlier reviews, this design has both been criticized and defended with regard to its ability to effectively mask the true nature of the beverages (Collins & Searles, 1988; Knight, Barbaree, & Boland, 1986; Lyvers & Maltzman, 1991). Regardless of the ultimate judgment about this design, however, the relationship of expectancies to placebo effects remains well documented (see Vogel-Sprott & Fillmore, in press).

Part way toward true experiments, in which cognitions/expectancies were directly manipulated, were studies with subject groups defined by preexisting drinking characteristics. For example, Chenier and Goldman (1992) found that heavier-drinking college students completed more word fragments representing those expectancy words most associated with drinking when they were in a context that included alcohol advertising. In a series of studies, Stacy and colleagues showed that alcohol-related associations to ambiguous words (homophones such as pitcher or mug) and pictures were more frequently produced by heavier than by lighter drinkers (Stacy, Leigh, & Weingardt, 1994; Weingardt, Stacy, & Leigh, 1996). Stacy (1997) has suggested a mechanism in which memory associations influence drinking, and which is separate from expectancies. Because the ambiguity of these stimuli must be resolved using preexisting information stored in each individual, such associations also may reflect expectancies. (In fact, this issue may be one of definition rather than substance.) The utility of separating such cognitive processes versus combining them remains to be seen. Nevertheless these quasi-experimental investigations of expectancies (and memory associations) indicate that cognitively based methods produce a pattern of findings similar to correlational studies.

Six experiments conducted in our laboratory have directly manipulated expectancies and shown effects on self-reported and observed drinking (Darkes & Goldman, 1993, 1998; Henderson & Goldman, 1987; Massey & Goldman, 1988; Roehrich & Goldman, 1995; Stein, Goldman, & Del Boca, 1997). Equally important for supporting a causal inference, these manipulations have resulted in drinking decreases as well as increases. Reductions in drinking were shown by Darkes and Goldman (1993, 1998), Henderson and Goldman (1987), and Massey and Goldman (1988), using various placebo administration procedures to challenge expectancies. In the most recent studies (Darkes & Goldman, 1993, 1998), moderate- to heavy-drinking male college students were administered beverages that they were told might, or might not, contain alcohol and subsequently indicated who within their group had consumed alcohol. Their failure to identify actual drinkers at better than chance levels, coupled with information about alcohol expectancy effects, resulted in drinking decreases 6 weeks following the challenge procedure. These studies also suggested that expectancy challenge procedures might serve as prevention and intervention tools.

Relatively short-term (1–2 hour) increases in drinking following implicit priming of expectancy concepts (using a Stroop task) were first shown by Roehrich and Goldman (1995). Although this study did not measure cognitive changes associated with expectancy priming, a more recent study measured activation of expectancy concepts using a cognitive priming task and examined parallel changes in drinking behavior (Stein, Goldman, & Del Boca, 1997). This study also assessed the effects of a positive mood induction on alcohol consumption. Although both the measures of expectancy activation and mood showed changes appropriate to the experimental condition, alcohol consumption increased most in the cognitive priming condition, suggesting that a cognitive, and not a purely affective, process was the primary mediational pathway for the increases in drinking. Hence the available evidence indicates that priming of a cognitive system can induce increases in drinking. These findings are consistent with results reported by Stacy et al. (1994), who showed that experimental manipulation of cognitive processing could influence associative memory responses. Participants were more likely to provide alcohol as an associate to expectancy cues (e.g., "feeling more relaxed") when asked to generate an image pertaining to friends together on a Friday night than when the image was friends together on a Thursday morning. There was no attempt in this study to measure effects on drinking, however.

Summary of the Construct Validation Network

The consistency of findings provides strong support for the inference that an alcohol expectancy memory system is part of the causal pathway leading to alcohol use and alcoholism. In fact, although the inherent criterion contamination mentioned earlier increases the potential for overestimation of this influence, at this point, there is a relative absence of findings that would contradict the inference of causality. Instead, the major controversies in this area concern the structure of alcohol expectancies and issues associated with their measurement. These issues are now addressed after one brief diversion, followed by a discussion of the theoretical processes by which expectancies influence drinking.

Gender and Expectancies

Because of differences in subjects' customary drinking habits, and some intuitive differences in the behaviors shown while under the influence, a number of studies have been directed toward possible gender differences in expectancies. Although some differences have been found, these generally are minimal or nonexistent when differences in customary drinking are controlled. For example, Edgar and Knight (1994) found males to have higher expectancies for arousal and aggression, but Molina, Pelham, and Lang (1997) did not, nor have differences in expectancy factor structure been reported (George, Frone, Cooper, & Russell, 1995). In an effort to control for different levels of consumption, Lundahl, Davis, Adesso, and Lukas (1997) used a sample of heavy drinkers of both sexes to investigate factors associated with variations in alcohol expectancies and found interactions among gender, age, and family history of alcoholism. Females may be seen, by both males and females, as more sexually responsive while under the influence (George & McAfnee, 1987; Leigh, 1990). Method variations preclude definitive conclusions about this or other related variables, however.

Expectancy Structure

The "true" or best way to characterize the underlying structure of alcohol expectancies has been approached from two prevailing vantage points. The first, primarily psychometric, views issues of fit to statistical and predictive criteria as preeminent. The second, process-oriented approach focuses on how a theoretical structure might serve as the substrate for the process or mechanism of expectancy operation.

Psychometric Approach

Although the subject of many studies, the outlines of the fundamental structure of alcohol expectancies are only just beginning to come into focus, because measurement procedures have been intrinsically confounded with the search for structure. In fact, considering the variations in the operations used to measure expectancies and other closely associated concepts (e.g., motivations, reasons for drinking or not drinking, memory associations), it may be legitimate to ask whether the constructs being measured have any overlap at all. Careful scrutiny, we believe, reveals more similarities than differences, however, and the similar level of relationship to the criterion variable (alcohol consumption) suggests that whatever constructs are being measured should be considered together.

Some researchers have generated items from an implicit or explicit theory of the relevant domain (Bauman & Bryan, 1980; Earleywine & Martin, 1993; Farber, Khavari, & Douglas, 1980; Grube, Chen, Madden, & Morgan, 1995; Leigh & Stacy, 1993; McMahon & Jones, 1993; Mulford & Miller, 1960; Sher et al., 1991); others have obtained items by eliciting alcohol effects open-endedly from samples of the populations of interest (Brown, Goldman, Inn, & Anderson, 1980; Christiansen et al., 1982; Dunn & Goldman, 1996; Rather, Goldman, Roehrich, & Brannick, 1992; Young & Knight, 1989); still others have adapted items (and scales) from existing instruments, and perhaps added their own (Cooper, Russell, Skinner, & Windle, 1992; Fromme et al., 1993; Rohsenow, 1983; Wiers, Hoogeven,

Sergeant, & Gunning, 1997; Young & Knight, 1989); and a few investigators have used free associations directly (Gustafson, 1989; Stacy, 1997). The number of items included has varied widely from very few, for example, Effects of Drinking Alcohol (Leigh, 1987), to over 100 [e.g., Alcohol Expectancy Questionnaire—Adolescent Version (AEQ-A); Christiansen et al., 1982]. Response formats have ranged from binary agree–disagree judgments (e.g., Brown et al., 1980) to forced-choice adjective checklists (e.g., Southwick, Steele, Marlatt, & Lindell, 1981), to Likert scales (e.g., Leigh & Stacy, 1993), to similarity ratings (Rather & Goldman, 1994). Respondents have rated specific effects' subjective likelihood of occurrence (Stacy, 1997), frequency of occurrence (Rather et al., 1992), or strength (Collins, Lapp, Emmons, & Issac, 1990) or, in the case of motives or reasons for drinking, how frequently they drink to obtain an effect (Cooper, Russell, Skinner, & Windle, 1992).

In an effort to interpret underlying structure, these item sets have been subjected to exploratory factor analysis, and more recently, to confirmatory factor analysis (CFA). Given the diversity of methods, conceptual underpinnings, and sources of items, it is no surprise that a variety of factors have resulted. Before attempting an integration of these findings, several of the issues that researchers have chosen to highlight are reviewed.

Discriminant Validity of Expectancy Factors. Leigh (1989a) and Leigh and Stacy (1991) have criticized the Alcohol Expectancy Questionnaire (AEQ; Brown et al., 1980) for failing a confirmatory test of factor independence based on a criterion of perfect simple structure. This issue has since been addressed in a number of empirical and conceptual papers, beginning with Goldman et al. (1991) (see also Goldman, 1994; Goldman et al., 1997; Leigh & Stacy, 1993). Such a criterion emanates from classical test theory, in which the derivation of pure orthogonal variables is mandated to avoid ambiguity about what is being measured and redundancy in linear prediction. From a pure psychometric viewpoint, therefore, it might be advantageous to have expectancy scales that have simple structure. Some scales, in fact, have been shown to have simple structure (e.g., Earleywine, 1994a; Leigh & Stacy, 1993), but the number of confirmable factors tends to be very small and to reflect very global dimensions (e.g., positive–negative or arousal–sedation).

In contrast, the "fuzziness" inherent in the organization of information in the natural world (e.g., in human memory) suggests that simple structure often cannot be found (in psychometric terms, this means that some items may load on more than one factor; for example, is a minivan a truck or a car?). When participants generate expectancy items in response to open-ended inquiries about their subjective reactions to alcohol use and these items are directly subjected to factor analysis (without stringent efforts to eliminate natural item overlap), simple structure (especially perfect simple structure) will not be found. In fact, recent work using alternative grouping procedures such as multidimensional scaling (MDS) and cluster analysis (Rather & Goldman, 1994; Rather et al., 1992) demonstrated that natural expectancy structure is very similar to that found for dimensions of affect and personality (see Larsen & Diener, 1992), with a circumplex (circular) format arranged in two dimensional space (see Figure 6.2). This circumplex likely reflects an intrinsic hierarchical arrangement of natural categories. For example, concepts such as "funny" and "social" have unique meaning but also group together under the higher-order concept of positive outcomes. In fact, the application to the AEQ of recently developed CFA models, which recognize this more complex arrangement of the natural world, has supported the hierarchical nature of expectancies, as well as the discriminant validity of the AEQ scales (Goldman et al., 1997).

Hierarchical structure was also suggested by the earlier covariance structure models of Leigh and Stacy (1993). Such a structure is more consistent with the model of expectancies as information stored in memory than is simple structure. Ultimately, "the best assessment strategy may be that designed for a particular purpose, rather than a single 'all-purpose' strategy" (Goldman et al., 1997, p. 154; see Larsen & Diener, 1992). Confirmable simple-structure factors can be constructed for specific purposes but may not be a valid "window" into the full domain of alcohol expectancies.

Basic Expectancy Factors. A second issue concerns whether certain expectancy factors are more "basic," or in some way more closely match natural categories of expectancies. Three sets of constructs have emerged as candidates for the basic factors. First, positive versus negative outcomes refers to the valence of drinking consequences; for example, increased sociability versus increased belligerence. Second, positive–negative reinforcement (often called "reasons" or "motives" for drinking) refers to the positive outcomes that are most sought after (e.g., having fun), as well as to *relief from* aversive states that may exist prior to drinking (e.g., anxiety and depression). Third, arousing–sedating outcomes refer more directly to the observed pharmacological effects of alcohol (e.g., stimulation and sedation). As shall be seen, these constructs correspond to different locations of dimensions on an affect and personality circumplex.

The positive outcome dimension was always considered central to the understanding of alcohol effects and was included in early instruments such as the AEQ (Brown et al., 1980). Because the original AEQ did not include negative expectancies and became the assessment device of choice (Leigh, 1989a), the importance of negative expectancies began to be debated in the literature. A number of authors called for increased research on negative expectancies on theoretical grounds (e.g., Adams & McNeil, 1991; Leigh, 1989a; McMahon & Jones, 1993), and some additional work has been done (e.g., Grube et al., 1995; Jones & McMahon, 1994; Leigh & Stacy, 1993; Rather & Goldman, 1994; Rather et al., 1992). This research shows that if an effort is made to collect negative expectancies as items, positive and negative higher-order factors can be confirmed as independent, under which may be subsumed a number of other (lower-order) expectancies (Leigh & Stacy, 1993). Although negative expectancies predict drinking in adolescents and young adults, they typically account for far less variance than do positive expectancies (e.g., Leigh & Stacy, 1993; Rather & Goldman, 1994).

One exception to this pattern of findings is a study by McMahon, Jones, and O'Donnell (1994), and this study is difficult to interpret, because negative expectancies were found to correlate positively with drinking. This finding is inconsistent with the presumed rationale for the importance of negative expectancies in limiting drinking motivation. A likely basis for this finding is the inclusion in the Negative Alcohol Expectancy Questionnaire (NAEQ; McMahon & Jones, 1993) of severe negative consequences as might only appear in individuals with drinking problems and alcoholism (e.g., "If I went for a drink now, I would have memory lapses," or "If I went for a drink now, I would drink more than others in my company"); endorsement of such items is essentially a direct acknowledgment of very heavy drinking.

Grube et al. (1995) also reported a slight advantage (1% of variance) for negative expectancies in predicting adolescent drinking but did not report sample drinking levels. Adjustments made in their data analyses suggest these were quite low; hence, negative expectancies may have been associated primarily with their nondrinking adolescents. Higher expectancies of negative effects of drinking not surprisingly may predict short-term (3 months) treatment outcome in alcoholics (Jones & McMahon, 1994), but long-term (2 years) outcome has also been related to decreases in positive expectancies (Connors et al., 1993). Whether negative expectancies influence social drinking in adults over the age of 30 has not been investigated.

Several issues regarding negative expectancies remain unclear. Expectancies characterized as negative by researchers may not be so to all drinkers (Leigh, 1989a). Negative effects may be less predictive because they largely refer to delayed, or highly intermittent, consequences of drinking (e.g., trouble with the police), rather than proximal effects of alcohol use (e.g., have fun; Leigh, 1989a). Many negative effects may not be experienced by all drinkers (and certainly not the very severe effects measured by the McMahon and Jones, 1993, scale). What remains, however, is an underlying theoretical conundrum; from the early days of animal research on learning, it has been known that punishment (which is the consequence of negative effects) suppresses, but does not eliminate, behavior. Extinction instead requires removal of positive reinforcement. Reductions in drinking may also occur with a relative increase in the positively reinforcing effects of other behaviors (e.g., career and family).

Positive and negative *reinforcement* (to be distinguished from negative effects) were perhaps the earliest candidates for the basic factors (Farber et al., 1980). Positive reinforcement, of course, overlaps with the positive outcome factor described earlier. Tension relief as a negative reinforcer played a prominent role in early theories of drinking and alcoholism (Conger, 1956). While the tension-reduction view of alcohol effects has received mixed support (Cappell & Herman, 1972; Sher, 1985), this model has received renewed interest in the form of recent accounts of the effects of alcohol on affect (Stritzke, Patrick, & Lang, 1995). As noted later, hierarchical CFA of MDS solutions also suggests this factor (relief from negative affectivity) as a legitimate higher-order "basic" dimension of expectancy.

Positive and negative reinforcement also have reappeared recently as enhancement and coping "motives" or "reasons for drinking" (along with a third, social, motive) in work by Cooper, Russell, Skinner, and Windle (1992). Reasons for drinking and motives are included here because their operational definitions (items and instructions) reveal very little difference between them and expectancies. The primary distinction seems to be that reasons for drinking, and motive, items call upon respondents to indicate why they drink or how much they drink for various reasons; expectancy items merely ask what happens when they drink. Because the capacity of this information to influence future drinking would appear to be the critical issue, it remains to be seen whether this difference in wording taps into a different information set, or whether reliably different levels of prediction can be achieved based on the supposedly different constructs involved (i.e., independent of the differential capacity of any scale characteristics).

In an effort to measure the subjective aspects of the presumed biphasic effects of alcohol (stimulation at low doses followed by sedation at higher doses), Earleywine and colleagues developed and confirmed as independent two scales that measure arousing and sedating effects (Earleywine, 1994a; Earleywine & Erblich, 1996; Earleywine & Martin, 1993; Martin, Earleywine, Musty, & Perrine, 1993). Earleywine (1994b) has also suggested that these dimensions are related to alcoholism risk, in keeping with the differentiator model of Newlin and Thompson (1990). These dimensions also appear in MDS solutions of expectancy words (Rather et al., 1992), which, as will be seen, offer an organization that allows all the previously mentioned dimensions to be acceptable choices for basic structure.

Expectancy Value, Utility, and Strength. A third issue associated with the psychometric approach to expectancy measurement concerns the separate evaluation of value, utility, and strength. For example, some investigators have argued that solely measuring expectancies is insufficient because individuals may differ in the subjective value or utility they assign to outcomes (e.g., Fromme et al., 1993; Grube et al., 1995; Leigh, 1989a). Although sufficient research is not yet available to settle this issue, extant studies suggest that separate evaluations of value or utility add little beyond the predictive variance contributed by expectancy alone (Copeland, Brandon, &

Quinn, 1995, for smoking prediction; Fromme et al., 1993, and Grube et al., 1995, for alcohol), particularly if the expectancy scale used has sufficient predictive power alone. And because the drinking variance accounted for primarily by expectancies increases as the number of items increases (McCarthy & Smith, 1996), it remains to be seen whether adding value or utility judgments increases prediction beyond the addition of expectancy items.

A similar argument has been made for separate assessment of the subjective strength with which expectancies are held (Collins et al., 1990; Leigh, 1989a). Once again, research on this topic is sparse. Although Collins et al. (1990) reported empirical support for separate measurement, this support came from only a very limited subset of their analyses (most not showing an independent contribution). Also, separate comparisons were made for different alcohol-containing beverages (e.g., beer vs. wine); if, as one might anticipate, participants preferred one beverage over another, high scores on one index would tend to lower scores on another.

All these arguments (for separate assessment of value, utility, and strength) arise from theoretical developments in attitude theory and from psychometric considerations. If expectancy measurement taps an information-processing or memory system, separate assessment might not necessarily be helpful, however. Activation of particular outcomes in memory could be related inherently to their value and utility, because adaptive functioning should reflect real-world salience. And, because strength refers to likelihood of activation of a particular concept, accessibility should reflect strength. Hence, the expectancy response itself may implicitly reflect these other characteristics. Furthermore, because concepts that relate to real-world adaptive functioning intrinsically include these other aspects, separate assessment might call upon respondents to provide information on processes to which they have no access ("tell more than they can know"; Nisbett & Wilson, 1977).

A counterargument is, of course, that the preponderance of evidence supporting expectancies as an important construct is based on measurement using psychometrically based questionnaires. Whether responses to questionnaire items actually reflect memory processes has been a subject of debate. Many reasons to be skeptical of this possibility can be cited, all having to do with the fact that many psychological processes may influence responses to any scaled instrument, including those that produce error variance. Some of these processes may mask memory effects, and it is even possible to respond to such instruments without accessing long-term memory (see Hastie & Park, 1986; Rather & Goldman, 1994, p. 180). In connection with a construct based on stored information in memory, however, such influences would lower the relationship between the predictor and criterion, because they would introduce variation not related to the criterion. The robustness of the relationship observed between expectancies and drinking suggests otherwise; relevant person variation (presumably, information in memory) does seem to be tapped in some fashion.

Dose-Related Expectancies. A final issue regarding expectancy structure is the suggestion that people hold different expectancies for different doses of alcohol (Collins et al., 1990; Connors, O'Farrell, Cutter, & Thompson, 1987; Southwick et al., 1981; Wiers et al., 1997). As one might anticipate, expectancies for high-dose effects include behaviors more consistent with intoxication and drunkenness, and high-dose expectancies have been found to predict drinking in individuals who customarily drink a number of drinks at one sitting. The cross-sectional nature of these studies, however, makes it unclear whether these expectancies serve as an incentive for drinking at these levels, or reflect previous drinking experiences (see earlier discussion of criterion contamination). Furthermore, it is also unclear whether expectancies that are active when an individual initiates a drinking episode influence the total amount of alcohol that will be consumed on that occasion, or whether new or altered expectancies become activated after drinking has commenced, with these latter expectancies influencing the continuation of drinking to higher doses.

Structure from a Process Perspective

To begin development of a process model of alcohol expectancy operation, our laboratory (Rather et al., 1992; Rather & Goldman, 1994) applied MDS and hierarchical clustering methods to explicate expectancy structure. Unlike factor analysis, these methods do not assume that item responses are merely indicators of the operation of some unobserved and smaller set of variables that are opaque as to process (for a more detailed explication of these concepts, see Goldman, 1994; Goldman et al., 1997). For good psychometric reasons, factor-analytic methods assume that indicators that covary are manifestations of the same underlying construct (plus error). From the perspective of memory structure, however, it may be useful to recognize that items that humans can perceive as different *are* different (contain unique information), despite their tendency to covary in some circumstances. Hence, although MDS and clustering do not as effectively parse out error from the structural mapping process, they do permit a direct visual examination of relationships among items (information "nodes").

Items used in these analyses came from young adults and hospitalized alcoholics who were asked to generate as many adjectives as possible to complete the phrase, "Alcohol makes one _____." This process yielded 805 items (probably exhausting the category), which were reduced in successive steps to 33 groups of four words with overlapping meaning. We used a variety of MDS procedures to map these words in different participant samples, with consistent results: a two-dimensional solution, reflecting both a positive–negative dimension and arousal–sedation dimension. The pattern in which these items fell in two-dimensional space was striking. Items tended to fall in a circular (circumplex) arrangement, matching the circumplex arrangements found previously for both affect and personality (see Larsen & Diener, 1992). Since the orientation of axes (dimensions) in standard MDS is arbitrary, axes could be rotated to match all the basic dimensions noted earlier (although the mathematical algorithms "prefer" certain dimensional solutions due to considerations that are beyond the scope of this chapter).

The significance of these arrangements is that no group of dimensions may be more basic than any other. Axes could be drawn in expectancy multidimensional space to reflect any dimension a particular research group wished to emphasize. For example, in Figure 6.2, the item "funny" reflects both positive valence and arousal; an axis drawn through the origin and this word would correspond to positive reinforcement from alcohol and the dimension of positive affectivity described by Watson and Tellegen (1985) in their specification of the structure of mood. We have recently shown that with careful selection, word groups reflecting preferred higher-order constructs within the expectancy domain can be confirmed by factor analysis (Darkes, Greenbaum, & Goldman, 1996a) to allow for minimally redundant linear prediction of drinking. Hence, theories reflecting conceptions of basic alcohol effects can be operationalized and tested by choosing the appropriate words from the circumplex. In essence, researchers have already been doing so without realizing that their preferred conceptualization fits within a larger system in which many solutions are possible. Because these overall patterns so closely match those found in the general domains of affect and personality, it must be considered that alcohol expectancies are, at least in part, anticipated changes in affect and personality due to alcohol use. Note that the configuration of the expectancy words in Figure 6.2 constitutes an example of an expectancy circumplex.

Expectancy Process

To translate the aforementioned structure into a working model of expectancy process, one need only regard this structure as a still photograph of a dynamic, unfolding process. In such a model, unique expectancy concepts (nodes) reflecting outcomes of alcohol use (including images, memories of sensorimotor and affective experiences, specific behavior patterns, and the verbal representations of these concepts) are seen as comprising a network structure and as having some overall relationship to each other. In accord with this network structure, activation of particular nodes occurs in a predictable fashion when stimuli that match previously encoded material relevant to drinking are encountered. (Such material is also legitimately characterized as an expectancy, or on a larger scale, as part of the overall expectancy process that may lead to drinking.) Such previously encoded material may consist of external (situational) or internal (activation of other encoded information) stimuli.

Although a variety of activation algorithms could be hypothesized, one starting point is to assume simple "spreading activation" (Collins & Loftus, 1975), in which a wave of activation begins with a certain node, or group of nodes, and spreads outward in a symmetrical fashion to other nodes as a function of their proximity to the starting point (as do ripples in a pond when a pebble is dropped). Using the MDS plots as a visualization of the model (see Figure 6.2), empirically derived starting points may be estimated using procedures that find preferred locations in the network for particular drinking groups (the crosses and circles in Figure 6.2 provide a graphic example of how such a model might be visualized). So, as reported in Rather and Goldman (1994), heavy drinkers seem likely first to associate concepts related to positive arousal (upper right quadrant; e.g., happy talkative, horny, funny) to drinking stimuli, whereas light drinkers first activate concepts related to positive sedation (e.g., relaxed, sleepy). Because these concepts are assumed to influence the activation of affective and motor systems consistent with the activated information template, the result is more drinking accompanied by the associated behavioral patterns for heavy drinkers, and a dampening of drinking as a consequence of general slowing for the light drinkers.

Although these behavior patterns may reflect the actual pharmacological effects of alcohol for these individuals, prior research has shown that these pharmacological patterns are not inevitable in every instance of use, or at every dose. In any case, these information patterns may anticipate what might be the later onset of the pharmacological effects, thereby foreshadowing and influencing alcohol use and its associated behaviors. Furthermore, the full range of alcohol-related behaviors is unlikely to be a direct pharmacological effect, but instead a set of learned patterns associated with alcohol use. As we have seen, these patterns are likely learned in childhood, well before actual use. Hence, alcohol use may be reinforced by the activation of behaviors that are not necessarily pharmacologically based, but which are seen by the drinker to occur following use, in part, because acquired information templates make it so.

An MDS plot is not the only way of visualizing these hypothetical networks. We could also model activation using plots from cluster analyses. Hierarchical clustering algorithms use the same similarity data for input as does MDS but depict the relative distances among a set of objects in a treelike structure, or dendrogram. Objects that are judged "closest" are connected first, and the resultant groupings are joined successively with others using a criterion of increasing distance. Such plots may be even closer to the neurocomputational system being modeled, in that no assumptions need be made about dimensional organization. Activation may be presumed to begin at the individual nodes and to influence behavior most when activation from one node joins with another. Figure 6.3 presents separate cluster analyses of alcohol expectancy ratings obtained from light and heavy drinkers. This figure suggests that the most sought after effects of drinking are located more closely together in heavier drinkers, thereby facilitating activation for these individuals.

The availability of multiple ways to visualize these processes under-scores that these plots are not literal depictions of the hypothetical net-works, but are empirically-derived theoretical models (see Lehmann, 1992). Such models link expectancy research to recent developments in a host of related areas, including research on memory (Bower, 1992), and on the memory underpinnings of emotional and motor behavior (Bower, 1992; Goldman, 1999; Lang, 1985). Animal researchers have recently indicated that drug reinforcement is associated with activation of brain neuro-chemical systems that normally mediate appetitive (approach) behavior (Gray, 1990; Panksepp, 1990; Stewart, deWit, & Eikelboom, 1984; Wise, 1988). These same systems are thought to be the substrate for human affec-tive response. Alcohol expectancy structure has been found to overlap the dimensions found for human affective response (see Russell, 1980; Watson & Tellegen, 1985). It is these systems that presumably are activated by ex-pectancy information templates, perhaps stored in these same areas, or in cortical association areas. While network models have also been criticized for being too powerful (irrefutable; see Johnson-Laird, Hermann, & Chaffin, 1984), they have also been defended as useful working models from which more specific models can be developed (Chang, 1986).

Models of this type have the flexibility to carry out the tasks described earlier in this chapter of storing information about alcohol's effects on the affective and motor system, and activating this information to influence drinking at times, and in settings, that are also "programmed" into the sys-tem. The organization of such a system can reflect differing subjective expe-riences with alcohol that may be related to inherited biological differences in alcohol metabolism or processing. It can also reflect differences atten-dant to different personality patterns and affective styles. In the same way, it can store information about alcohol use acquired from observation of family members, or from the general behavior of individuals in one's cul-tural environment (including peer groups, ethnic and religious groups, or from media and advertising). In a sense, this information processing/mem-ory system acts as a storehouse for the potential to consume alcohol, which is then translated into manifest drinking in certain circumstances. As noted throughout this chapter, support for these models can come only from in-ferences based on patterns of findings from studies of various types.

Theorizing by Stacy and his colleagues (e.g., Stacy et al., 1994) over-laps considerably with the model discussed here. One difference is that Stacy (1997) distinguishes between expectancy processes and what he re-fers to as memory association, and between implicit and explicit memory processes as they are manifest in the different ways of measuring expectan-cies. We, on the other hand, include these processes within the general op-eration of an expectancy system. As these lines of research proceed, it appears that the operations overlap considerably, so that distinctions be-come less clear. For example, Stacy uses the term "expectancy" when refer-ring to outcomes of alcohol use, whereas we have used it with reference to

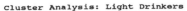

Cluster Analysis: Light Drinkers

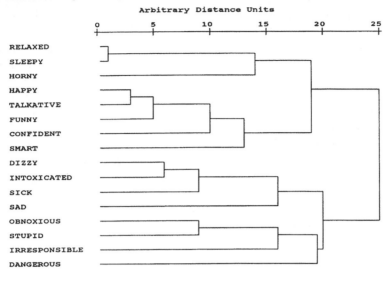

Cluster Analysis: Heavy Drinkers

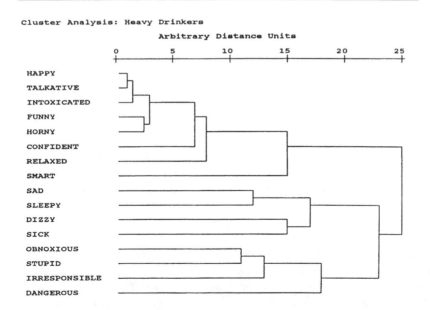

FIGURE 6.3. Cluster analyses of alcohol expectancy data were performed separately for light (top cluster) and heavy (bottom cluster) drinkers. Note that the words "happy," "talkative," "intoxicated," "funny," and "horny," are grouped much closer together for the heavy drinkers than the light drinkers. The light drinkers also most closely link "relaxed" and "sleepy" in relation to drinking, unlike the heavy drinkers, who most closely link "happy" and "talkative" in relation to drinking. From Rather and Goldman (1994). Copyright 1994 by American Psychological Association. Reprinted by permission.

all memory storage and activation processes connected with drinking. We have chosen this usage to reflect recent expectancy theories that address ongoing control of behavior in a real-life environment, and not just systems for storing and retrieving information in constrained settings, such as laboratory experiments. The expectancy concept also relates research with humans to behavioral pharmacological research with animals, which has shown changes in brain neurotransmitter systems (e.g., dopamine) to result from expectancies (Schultz et al., 1997). This usage is arbitrary, of course, and, as long as what is addressed is made clear, the distinctions may be more apparent than real.

Whether the arguments for distinct (qualitative) differences between memory processes that underpin implicit and explicit memory remain useful is yet to be resolved (see Eichenbaum, 1997; Neal & Hesketh, 1997, p. 34). Such arguments cannot be separated from the measurement operations associated with each supposed system; processing differences may be task-related, or truly a function of different systems. At present, we find ourselves in sympathy with a comment Reber (1997, p. 52) made as part of a recent symposium on implicit learning: "Psychologists just can't seem to resist dichotomies. . . . We like to be able to decide that one theory is right and another wrong. . . . We seem ineluctably drawn to setting up poles rather than recognizing continua. Alas, this tendency often functions as a hindrance to doing good science." We believe commonalities in the available findings serve as a basis for continuing advances that offer a new window on the problem of addiction.

CONCLUSION

Reber's comment might also apply to the apparent separation between genetic–neurobiological explanations of substance use and dependence, and the cognitive–psychological perspective presented in these pages. Nature is not divided into specialties or content areas. All levels of explanation may be (perhaps must be) woven together to provide comprehensive theories, particularly because the search for interventions into these extremely problematic behaviors may benefit from multiple potential points of entry into these systems. The inference that expectancies causally influence consumption is now based on a solid construct validation network, and working models of expectancy structure and process have been developed. Furthermore, such models offer considerable promise in terms of the development of theoretically grounded prevention and intervention strategies (see Brown, 1993; Connors, Maisto, & Derman, 1992; Goldman, 1994). Unlike previous atheoretical efforts that have typically emphasized the potential negative consequences of alcohol use, expectancy-based approaches logically target the incentive value of drinking (Goldman, 1994). The short-term reductions in alcohol consumption observed in the expectancy challenge studies described earlier provide preliminary empirical support for this approach. Expectancy formulations have additional, as yet untested, implications as well. For example, successful programs may require attention to automatic as well as deliberate cognitive processes that influence drinking. Promising prevention and intervention strategies based on expectancy models should be developed further.

ACKNOWLEDGMENT

Portions of this work were supported by National Institute on Alcohol Abuse and Alcoholism Grant No. R37 AA08333.

NOTE

1. A strong crossover interaction (graphed as a symmetrical X) might suggest that neither of two variables mediates the effect of the other, but this is not the pattern typically observed for expectancies.

REFERENCES

Adams, S. L., & McNeil, D. W. (1991). Negative alcohol expectancies reconsidered. *Psychology of Addictive Behaviors, 5*, 9–14.

Arnold, H. J. (1982). Moderator variables: A clarification of conceptual, analytic, and psychometric issues. *Organizational Behavior and Human Performance, 29*, 143–174.

Banaji, M. R., & Hardin, C. D. (1996). Automatic stereotyping. *Psychological Science, 7*, 136–141.

Bandura, A. (1977). *Social learning theory.* Englewood Cliffs, NJ: Prentice-Hall.

Bargh, J. A., & Barndollar, K. (1996). Automaticity in action: The unconscious as repository of chronic goals and motives. In P. M. Gollwitzer & J. A. Bargh (Eds.), *The psychology of action* (pp. 457–481). New York: Guilford Press.

Baron, R. M., & Kenny, D. A. (1986). The moderator–mediator variable distinction in social psychological research: Conceptual, strategic, and statistical considerations. *Journal of Personality and Social Psychology, 51*, 1173–1182.

Bauman, K. E., & Bryan, E. S. (1980). Subjective expected utility and children's drinking. *Journal of Studies on Alcohol, 41*, 952–958.

Berns, G. S., Cohen, J. D., & Mintun, M. A. (1997). Brain regions responsive to novelty in the absence of awareness. *Science, 276*, 1272–1275.

Blane, H. T., & Leonard, K. E. (Eds.). (1987). *Psychological theories of drinking and alcoholism.* New York: Guilford Press.

Bogart, C. J., Yeatman, F. R., Sirridge, S. T., & Gear, F. A. (1995). Alcohol expectancies and the personal and parental drinking patterns of women. *Women and Health, 22*, 51–66.

Bolles, R. C. (1972). Reinforcement, expectancy, and learning. *Psychological Review, 79*, 394–409.

Bower, G. H. (1981). Mood and memory. *American Psychologist, 39*, 129–148.

Bower, G. H. (1992). How might emotions affect learning? In S. Christianson (Ed.), *The handbook of emotion and memory: Research and theory* (pp. 3–31). Hillsdale, NJ: Erlbaum.

Brown, S. A. (1993). Drug effect expectancies and addictive behavior change. Special Section: Motivation and addictive behaviors. *Experimental and Clinical Psychopharmacology, 1*, 55–67.

Brown, S. A., Goldman, M. S., Inn, A., & Anderson, L. R. (1980). Expectations of reinforcement from alcohol: Their domain and relation to drinking problems. *Journal of Consulting and Clinical Psychology, 48*, 419–426.

Bryk, A. S., & Raudenbush, S. W. (1992). *Hierarchical linear models.* Newbury Park, CA: Sage.

Cappell, H., & Herman, C. P. (1972). Alcohol and tension reduction: A review. *Quarterly Journal of Studies on Alcohol, 33*, 33–64.

Carey, K. B. (1995). Alcohol-related expectancies predict quantity and frequency of heavy drinking among college students. *Psychology of Addictive Behaviors, 9*, 236–241.

Chang, T. M. (1986). Semantic memory: Facts and models. *Psychological Bulletin, 99*, 199–220.

Chenier, G., & Goldman, M. S. (1992, August). *Implicit priming of an alcohol expectancy network.* Paper presented at the meeting of the American Psychological Association, Washington, DC.

Christiansen, B. A., & Goldman, M. S. (1983). Alcohol-related expectancies versus demographic/background variables in the prediction of adolescent drinking. *Journal of Consulting and Clinical Psychology, 51*, 249–257.

Christiansen, B. A., Goldman, M. S., & Inn, A. (1982). Development of alcohol-related expectancies in adolescents: Separating pharmacological from social learning influences. *Journal of Consulting and Clinical Psychology, 50*, 336–344.

Christiansen, B. A., Smith, G. T., Roehling, P. V., & Goldman, M. S. (1989). Using alcohol expectancies to predict adolescent drinking behavior at one year. *Journal of Consulting and Clinical Psychology, 57*, 93–99.

Cloninger, C. R. (1987). Neurogenetic adaptive mechanisms in alcoholism. *Science, 236*, 410–416.

Collins, A. M., & Loftus, E. F. (1975). A spreading-activation theory of semantic processing. *Psychology Review, 82*, 407–428.

Collins, R. L., Lapp, W. M., Emmons, K. M., & Issac, L. M. (1990). Endorsement and strength of alcohol expectancies. *Journal of Studies on Alcohol, 51*, 336–342.

Collins, R. L., & Searles, J. S. (1988). Alcohol and the balanced-placebo design: Were experimenter demands in expectancy really tested? Comment on Knight, Barbaree, Boland (1986). *Journal of Abnormal Psychology, 97*, 503–507.

Conger, J. J. (1956). Reinforcement theory and the dynamics of alcoholism. *Quarterly Journal of Studies on Alcohol, 17*, 296–305.

Connors, G. J., Maisto, S. A., & Derman, K. H. (1992). Alcohol-related expectancies and their applications to treatment. In R. R. Watson (Ed.), *Drug and alcohol abuse reviews: Alcohol abuse treatment* (Vol. 3, pp. 203–231). Totowa, NJ: Humana Press.

Connors, G. J., O'Farrell, T. J., Cutter, H. S., & Thompson, D. L. (1987). Dose-related effects of alcohol among male alcoholics, problem drinkers and non-problem drinkers. *Journal of Studies on Alcohol, 48,* 461–466.

Connors, G. J., Tarbox, A. R., & Faillace, L. A. (1993). Changes in alcohol expectancies and drinking behavior among treated problem drinkers. *Journal of Studies on Alcohol, 53,* 676–683.

Cooper, M. L., Russell, M., Skinner, J. B., Frone, M. R., & Mudar, P. (1992). Stress and alcohol use: Moderating effects of gender, coping, and alcohol expectancies. *Journal of Abnormal Psychology, 101,* 139–152.

Cooper, M. L., Russell, M., Skinner, J. B., & Windle, M. (1992). Development and validation of a three-dimensional measure of drinking motives. *Psychological Assessment, 4,* 123–132.

Copeland, A. L., Brandon, T. H., & Quinn, E. P. (1995). The Smoking Consequences Questionnaire—Adult: Measurement of smoking outcome expectancies of experienced smokers. *Psychological Assessment, 7,* 484–494.

Costa, P. T., & McCrae, R. R. (1995). Domains and facets: Hierarchical personality assessment using the revised NEO personality inventory. *Journal of Personality Assessment, 64,* 21–50.

Darkes, J., & Goldman, M. S. (1993). Expectancy challenge and drinking reduction: Experimental evidence for a mediational process. *Journal of Consulting and Clinical Psychology, 61,* 344–353.

Darkes, J., & Goldman, M. S. (1998). Expectancy challenge and drinking reduction: Process and structure in the alcohol expectancy network. *Experimental and Clinical Psychopharmacology, 6,* 64–76.

Darkes, J., Greenbaum, P. E., & Goldman, M. S. (1996a, June). *Positive/arousal and social facilitation alcohol expectancies and concurrent alcohol use.* Paper presented at the meeting of the Research Society on Alcoholism, Washington, DC.

Darkes, J., Greenbaum, P. E., & Goldman, M. S. (1996b, August). *Disinhibition and alcohol use: The mediational role of alcohol expectancies.* Paper presented at the meeting of the American Psychological Association, Toronto.

Davidson, R. J. (1993). Parsing affective space: Perspectives from neuropsychology and psychophysiology. *Neuropsychology, 7,* 464–475.

Dunn, M. E., & Goldman, M. S. (1996). Empirical modeling of an alcohol expectancy network in elementary-school children as a function of grade. *Experimental and Clinical Psychopharmacology, 4,* 209–217.

Earleywine, M. (1994a). Confirming the factor structure of the Anticipated Biphasic Alcohol Effects Scale. *Alcoholism: Clinical and Experimental Research, 18,* 861–866.

Earleywine, M. (1994b). Anticipated biphasic effects of alcohol vary with risk for alcoholism: A preliminary report. *Alcoholism: Clinical and Experimental Research, 18,* 711–714.

Earleywine, M., & Erblich, J. (1996). A confirmed factor structure for the Biphasic Alcohol Effects Scale. *Experimental and Clinical Psychopharmacology, 4,* 107–113.

Earleywine, M., & Martin, C. S. (1993). Anticipated stimulant and sedative effects of alcohol vary with dosage and limb of the blood alcohol curve. *Alcoholism: Clinical and Experimental Research, 17,* 135–139.

Edgar, N. C., & Knight, R. G. (1994). Gender and alcohol-related expectancies for self and others. *Australian Journal of Psychology, 46,* 144–149.

Eichenbaum, H. (1997). How does the brain organize memories? *Science*, 277, 330–332.

Estes, W. K. (1991). Cognitive architectures from the standpoint of an experimental psychologist. *Annual Review of Psychology*, 42, 1–28.

Farber, P. D., Khavari, K. A., & Douglas, F. M. (1980). A factor-analytic study of reasons for drinking: Empirical validation of positive and negative reinforcement dimensions. *Journal of Consulting and Clinical Psychology*, 48, 780–781.

Feldman, J. A. (1985). Connectionist models and their applications: Introduction. *Cognitive Science*, 9, 1–2.

Fowles, D. C. (1980). The three arousal model: Implications of Gray's two-factor learning theory for heart rate, electrodermal activity, and psychopathy. *Psychophysiology*, 17, 87–104.

Fromme, K., Stroot, E., & Kaplan, D. (1993). Comprehensive effects of alcohol: Development and psychometric assessment of a new alcohol expectancy questionnaire. *Psychological Assessment*, 5, 19–26.

George, W. H., Frone, M. R., Cooper, M. L., & Russell, M. (1995). A revised Alcohol Expectancy Questionnaire: Factor structure confirmation and invariance in a general population sample. *Journal of Studies on Alcohol*, 56, 177–185.

George, W. H., & McAfnee, M. P. (1987). The effects of gender and drinking experience on alcohol expectancies about self and male versus female other. *Social Behavior and Personality*, 15, 133–144.

Goldman, M. S. (in press). Expectancy operation: Cognitive and neural models and architectures. In I. Kirsch (Ed.), *How expectancies shape behavior*. Washington, DC: APA Books.

Goldman, M. S. (1989). Alcohol expectancies as cognitive-behavioral psychology: Theory and practice. In T. Loberg, W. R. Miller, P. E. Nathan, & G. A. Marlatt (Eds.), *Addictive behaviors: Prevention and early intervention* (pp. 11–30). Amsterdam: Swets & Zeitlinger.

Goldman, M. S. (1994). The alcohol expectancy concept: Applications to assessment, prevention, and treatment of alcohol abuse. *Applied and Preventive Psychology*, 3, 131–144.

Goldman, M. S., Brown, S. A., & Christiansen, B. A. (1987). Expectancy theory: Thinking about drinking. In H. T. Blane & K. E. Leonard (Eds.), *Psychological theories of drinking and alcoholism* (pp. 181–226). New York: Guilford Press.

Goldman, M. S., Brown, S. A., Christiansen, B. A., & Smith G. T. (1991). Alcoholism and memory: Broadening the scope of alcohol expectancy research. *Psychological Bulletin*, 110, 137–146.

Goldman, M. S., Darkes, J., & Del Boca, F. K. (in press). Expectancy mediation of biopsychosocial risk for alcohol use and alcoholism. In I. Kirsch (Ed.), *How expectancies shape behavior*. Washington, DC: APA Books.

Goldman, M. S., Greenbaum, P. E., & Darkes, J. (1997). A confirmatory test of hierarchical expectancy structure and predictive power: Discriminant validation of the Alcohol Expectancy Questionnaire. *Psychological Assessment*, 9, 145–157.

Goldman, M. S., & Rather, B. C. (1993). Substance use disorders: Cognitive models and architectures. In P. Kendall & K. S. Dobson (Eds.), *Psychopathology and cognition* (pp. 245–291). Orlando, FL: Academic Press.

Gray, J. A. (1982). *The neuropsychology of anxiety: An inquiry into the function of the septo-hippocampal system*. Oxford, UK: Oxford University Press.

Gray, J. A. (1990). Brain systems that mediate both emotion and cognition. *Cognition and Emotion*, 4, 269–288.

Grillner, S. (1996). Neural networks for vertebrate locomotion. *Scientific American*, 274, 64–69.

Grossberg, S. (1995). The attentive brain. *American Scientist*, 83, 438–449.

Grube, J. W., Chen, M. J., Madden, P., & Morgan, M. (1995). Predicting adolescent drinking from alcohol expectancy values: A comparison of additive, interactive, and nonlinear models. *Journal of Applied Social Psychology*, 25, 839–857.

Gustafson, R. (1989). Self-reported effects of alcohol by nonalcoholic men and women. *Psychological Reports*, 64, 1103–1111.

Gustafson, R., & Engstrom, C. (1991). Alcohol-related expectancies for self and others reported by alcoholic men and women. *Psychological Reports*, 68, 555–562.

Hastie, R., & Park, B. (1986). The relationship between memory and judgment depends on whether the judgment task is memory-based or on-line. *Psychological Review*, 93, 258–268.

Henderson, M. A., & Goldman, M. S. (1987, November). *Effects of a social manipulation on expectancies and subsequent drinking*. Paper presented at the annual meeting of the Association for the Advancement of Behavior Therapy, Boston, MA.

Henderson, M. J., Goldman, M. S., Coovert, M. D., & Carnevalla, N. (1994). Covariance structure models of expectancy. *Journal of Studies on Alcohol*, 55, 315–326.

Hull, J. G., & Bond, C. F. (1986). Social and behavioral consequences of alcohol consumption and expectancy: A meta-analysis. *Psychological Bulletin*, 99, 347–360.

Izard, C. E. (1993). Four systems for emotion activation: Cognitive and noncognitive processes. *Psychological Review*, 100, 68–90.

Jacoby, L. L., Lindsay, D. S., & Toth, J. P. (1992). Unconscious influences revealed: Attention, awareness, and control. *American Psychologist*, 47, 802–809.

Johnson, P. B., & Gurin, G. (1994). Negative affect, alcohol expectancies and alcohol-related problems. *Addiction*, 89, 581–586.

Johnson-Laird, P. N., Hermann, D. J., & Chaffin, R. (1984). Only connections: A critique of semantic networks. *Psychological Bulletin*, 96, 292–315.

Jones, B. T., & McMahon, J. (1994). Negative and positive alcohol expectancies as predictors of abstinence after discharge from a residential treatment program: A one-month and three-month follow-up study in men. *Journal of Studies on Alcohol*, 55, 543–548.

Knight, L. J., Barbaree, H. E., & Boland, F. J. (1986). Alcohol and the balanced-placebo design: The role of experimenter demands in expectancy. *Journal of Abnormal Psychology*, 95, 335–340.

Koob, G. F., & LeMoal, M. (1997). Drug abuse: Hedonic homeostatic dysregulation. *Science*, 278, 52–58.

Lang, A. R., & Stritzke, W. G. K. (1993). Children and alcohol. In M. Galanter (Ed.), *Recent developments in alcoholism* (Vol. 11, pp. 73–85). New York: Plenum.

Lang, P. J. (1979). A bio-informational theory of emotional imagery. *Psychophysiology*, 16, 495–512.

Lang, P. J. (1985). The cognitive psychophysiology of emotion: Fear and anxiety. In A. H. Tuma & J. D. Maser (Eds.), *Anxiety and anxiety disorders*. Hillsdale, NJ: Erlbaum.

Lang, P. J. (1995). The emotion probe: Studies of motivation and attention. *American Psychologist*, 50, 372–385.

Larsen, R. J., & Diener, E. (1992). Promises and problems with the circumplex model of emotion. In M. S. Clark (Ed.), *Emotion* (pp. 25–59). Newbury Park, CA: Sage.

LeDoux, J. E. (1995). Emotion: Clues from the brain. *Annual Review of Psychology, 46*, 209–235.

Lehmann, F. (1992). Semantic networks. *Computers and Mathematical Applications, 23*, 1–50.

Leigh, B. C. (1987). Beliefs about the effects of alcohol on self and others. *Journal of Studies on Alcohol, 48*, 467–475.

Leigh, B. C. (1989a). In search of the seven dwarves: Issues of measurement and meaning in alcohol expectancy research. *Psychological Bulletin, 105*, 361–373.

Leigh, B. C. (1989b). Attitudes and expectancies as predictors of drinking habits: A comparison of three scales. *Journal of Studies on Alcohol, 50*, 432–440.

Leigh, B. C. (1990). The relationship of sex-related alcohol expectancies to alcohol consumption and sexual behavior. *British Journal of Addiction, 85*, 919–928.

Leigh, B. C., & Stacy, A. W. (1991). On the scope of alcohol expectancy research: Remaining issues of measurement and meaning. *Psychological Bulletin, 110*, 147–154.

Leigh, B. C., & Stacy, A. W. (1993). Alcohol outcome expectancies: Scale construction and predictive utility in higher order confirmatory models. *Psychological Assessment, 5*, 216–229.

Logan, G. D. (1995). The Weibull distribution, the power law, and the instance theory of automaticity. *Psychological Review, 102*, 751–756.

Lundahl, L. H., Davis, T. M., Adesso, V. J., & Lukas, S. E. (1997). Alcohol expectancies: Effects of gender, age, and family history of alcoholism. *Addictive Behaviors, 22*, 115–125.

Lyvers, M. F., & Maltzman, I. (1991). The balanced placebo design: Effects of alcohol and beverage instructions cannot be independently assessed. *International Journal of Addictions, 26*, 963–972.

MacCorquodale, K. M., & Meehl, P. E. (1953). Preliminary suggestions as to a formalization of expectancy theory. *Psychological Review, 60*, 55–63.

Mann, L. M., Chassin, L., & Sher, K. J. (1987). Alcohol expectancies and the risk for alcoholism. *Journal of Consulting and Clinical Psychology, 55*, 411–417.

Martin, C. S., Earleywine, M., Musty, R. E., & Perrine, M. W. (1993). Development and validation of the Biphasic Alcohol Effects Scale. *Alcoholism: Clinical and Experimental Research, 17*, 140–146.

Massey, R. F., & Goldman, M. S. (1988, August). *Manipulating expectancies as a means of altering alcohol consumption.* Paper presented at the meeting of the American Psychological Association, Atlanta, GA.

Maunsell, J. H. R. (1995). The brain's visual world: Representation of visual targets in cerebral cortex. *Science, 270*, 764–769.

McCarthy, D. M., & Smith, G. T. (1996, June). *Meta-analysis of alcohol expectancy.* Paper presented at the meeting of the Research Society on Alcoholism, Washington, DC.

McMahon, J., & Jones, B. T. (1993). Negative expectancy in motivation. *Addiction Research, 1*, 145–155.

McMahon, J., Jones, B. T., & O'Donnell P. (1994). Comparing positive and negative alcohol expectancies in male and female social drinkers. *Addiction Research, 1*, 349–365.

McNamara, T. P. (1992). Priming and the constraints it places on theories of memory and retrieval. *Psychological Review*, *99*, 650–662.

Meyer, G. J., & Shack, J. R. (1989). Structural convergence of mood and personality: Evidence for old and new directions. *Journal of Personality and Social Psychology*, *57*, 691–706.

Miller, P. M., Smith, G. T., & Goldman, M. S. (1990). Emergence of alcohol expectancies in childhood: A possible critical period. *Journal of Studies on Alcohol*, *51*, 343–349.

Molina, B. S. G., Pelham, W. E., & Lang, A. R. (1997). Alcohol expectancies and drinking characteristics in parents of children with attention deficit hyperactivity disorder. *Alcoholism: Clinical and Experimental Research*, *21*, 557–566.

Mulford, H. A., & Miller, D. E. (1960). Drinking in Iowa: III. A scale of definitions of alcohol related to drinking behavior. *Quarterly Journal of Studies on Alcohol*, *21*, 267–278.

Mulford, H. A., & Miller, D. E. (1960). Drinking in Iowa: IV. Preoccupation with alcohol and definitions of alcohol, heavy drinking and trouble due to drinking. *Quarterly Journal of Studies on Alcohol*, *21*, 279–291.

National Institute on Alcohol Abuse and Alcoholism. (1997). *Ninth special report to the U.S. Congress on alcohol and health*. Washington, DC: U.S. Government Printing Office.

Neal, A., & Hesketh, B. (1997). Episodic knowledge and implicit learning. *Psychonomic Bulletin and Review*, *4*, 24–37.

Nestler, E. J., & Aghajanian, G. K. (1997). Molecular and cellular basis of addiction. *Science*, *278*, 58–63.

Newcomb, M. D., Chou, C., Bentler, P. M., & Huba, G. J. (1988). Cognitive motivations for drug use among adolescents: Longitudinal tests of gender differences and predictors of change in drug use. *Journal of Counseling Psychology*, *35*, 426–438.

Newell, A. (1970). Remarks on the relationship between artificial intelligence and cognitive psychology. In R. Banerji & M. D. Mesarovio (Eds.), *Theoretical approaches to non-numerical problem solving* (pp. 363–400). New York: Springer-Verlag.

Newell, A., Rosenbloom, P. S., & Laird, J. E. (1989). Symbolic architectures for cognition. In M. I. Posner (Ed.), *Foundations of cognitive science* (pp. 93–131). Cambridge, MA: MIT Press.

Newlin, D., & Thompson, J. (1990). Alcohol challenge with sons of alcoholics: A critical review and analysis. *Psychological Bulletin*, *108*, 383–402.

Nisbett, R. E., & Wilson, T. D. (1977). Telling more than we know: Verbal reports on mental processes. *Psychological Review*, *84*, 231–259.

Palfai, T. P., Monti, P. M., Colby, S. M., & Rohsenow, D. J. (1997). Effects of suppressing the urge to drink on the accessibility of alcohol outcome expectancies. *Behaviour Research and Therapy*, *35*, 59–65.

Panksepp, J. (1990). Gray zones at the emotion/cognition interface: A commentary. *Cognition and Emotion*, *4*, 289–302.

Pervin, L. A. (1994). A critical analysis of current trait theory. *Psychological Inquiry*, *5*, 103–113.

Pylyshyn, Z. W. (1989). Computing in cognitive science. In M. I. Posner (Ed.), *Foundations of cognitive science* (pp. 49–91). Cambridge, MA: MIT Press.

Rather, B. C., & Goldman, M. S. (1994). Drinking-related differences in the memory organization of alcohol expectancies. *Experimental and Clinical Psychopharmacology, 2,* 167–183.

Rather, B. C., Goldman, M. S., Roehrich, L., & Brannick, M. (1992). Empirical modeling of an alcohol expectancy memory network using multidimensional scaling. *Journal of Abnormal Psychology, 101,* 174–183.

Raymond, J. L., Lisberger, S. G., & Mauk, M. D. (1996). The cerebellum: A neuronal learning machine? *Science, 272,* 1126–1131.

Reber, A. S. (1997). Implicit ruminations. *Psychonomic Bulletin and Review, 4,* 49–55.

Reese, F. L., Chassin, L., & Molina, B. S. G. (1993). Alcohol expectancies in early adolescents: Predicting drinking behavior from alcohol expectancies and parental alcoholism. *Journal of Studies on Alcohol, 55,* 276–284.

Rescorla, R. A., & Wagner, A. R. (1972). A theory of Pavlovian conditioning: Variations in the effectiveness of reinforcement and nonreinforcement. In A. H. Black & W. F. Prokasy (Eds.), *Classical conditioning II: Current research and theory* (pp. 64–99). New York: Appleton–Century–Crofts.

Revelle, W. (1995). Personality processes. *Annual Review of Psychology, 46,* 295–328.

Robinson, T. E., & Berridge, K. C. (1993). The neural basis of drug craving: An incentive sensitization theory of addiction. *Brain Research Reviews, 18,* 247–291.

Roehrich, L., & Goldman, M. S. (1995). Implicit priming of alcohol expectancy memory processes and subsequent drinking behavior. *Experimental and Clinical Psychopharmacology, 3,* 402–410.

Rohsenow, D. J. (1983). Drinking habits and expectancies about alcohol's effects for self versus others. *Journal of Consulting and Clinical Psychology, 51,* 536–541.

Rotter, J. B. (1954). *Social learning and clinical psychology.* Englewood Cliffs, NJ: Prentice-Hall.

Rumelhart, D. E. (1989). The architecture of mind: A connectionist approach. In M. I. Posner (Ed.), *Foundations of cognitive science* (pp. 133–159). Cambridge, MA: MIT Press.

Russell, J. A. (1979). Affective space is bipolar. *Journal of Personality and Social Psychology, 37,* 345–356.

Russell, J. A. (1980). A circumplex model of emotion. *Journal of Personality and Social Psychology, 39,* 1161–1178.

Saunders, D. R. (1956). Moderator variables in prediction. *Educational and Psychological Measurement, 16,* 209–222.

Schank, R. C., & Abelson, R. P. (1977). *Scripts, plans, goals, and understanding.* Hillsdale, NJ: Erlbaum.

Scheier, L. M., & Botvin, G. J. (1997). Expectancies as mediators of the effects of social influences and alcohol knowledge on adolescent alcohol use: A prospective analysis. *Psychology of Addictive Behaviors, 11,* 48–64.

Schultz, W., Dayan, P., & Montague, P. R. (1997). A neural substrate of prediction and reward. *Science, 275,* 1593–1599.

Seigel, S., & Allan, L. G. (1996). The widespread influence of the Rescorla–Wagner model. *Psychonomic Bulletin and Review, 3,* 314–321.

Shaver, P., Schwartz, J., Kirson, D., & O'Connor, C. (1987). Emotion knowledge: Further exploration of a prototype approach. *Journal of Personality and Social Psychology, 52,* 1061–1086.

Sher, K. J. (1985). Subjective effects of alcohol: The influence of setting and individual differences in alcohol expectancies. *Journal of Studies on Alcohol, 46,* 137–146.

Sher, K. J., Walitzer, K. S., Wood, P. A., & Brent, E. E. (1991). Characteristics of children of alcoholics: Putative risk factors, substance use and abuse, and psychopathology. *Journal of Abnormal Psychology, 100,* 427–448.

Sher, K. J., Wood, M. D., Wood, P. K., & Raskin, G. (1996). Alcohol outcome expectancies and alcohol use: A latent variable cross-lagged panel study. *Journal of Abnormal Psychology, 103,* 561–574.

Shiffrin, R. M., & Schneider, W. (1977). Controlled and automatic human information processing: II. Perceptual learning, automatic attending, and a general theory. *Psychological Review, 84,* 127–190.

Simon, H. A., & Kaplan, C. A. (1989). Foundations of cognitive science. In M. I. Posner (Ed.), *Foundations of cognitive science* (pp. 1–47). Cambridge, MA: MIT Press.

Singer, W. (1995). Development and plasticity of cortical processing architectures. *Science, 270,* 758–764.

Smith, G. T., & Goldman, M. S. (1990, August). *Toward a mediational model of alcohol expectancies.* Paper presented at the meeting of the American Psychological Association, Boston, MA.

Smith, G. T., Goldman, M. S., Greenbaum, P. E., & Christiansen, B. A. (1995). Expectancy for social facilitation from drinking: The divergent paths of high-expectancy and low-expectancy adolescents. *Journal of Abnormal Psychology, 104,* 32–40.

Southwick, L., Steele, C. M., Marlatt, G. A., & Lindell, M. (1981). Alcohol-related expectancies: Defined by phase of intoxication and drinking experience. *Journal of Consulting and Clinical Psychology, 49,* 713–721.

Squire, L. R. (1987). *Memory and brain.* Oxford, UK: Oxford University Press.

Squire, L. R. (1992). Memory and the hippocampus: A synthesis from findings with rats, monkeys, and humans. *Psychological Review, 99,* 195–231.

Stacy, A. W. (1997). Memory activation and expectancy as prospective predictors of alcohol and marijuana use. *Journal of Abnormal Psychology, 106,* 61–73.

Stacy, A. W., Leigh, B. C., & Weingardt, K. R. (1994). Memory accessibility and association of alcohol use and its positive outcomes. *Experimental and Clinical Psychopharmacology, 2,* 269–282.

Stacy, A. W., Newcomb, M. D., & Bentler, P. M. (1991). Cognitive motivation and problem drug use: A 9-year longitudinal study. *Journal of Abnormal Psychology, 100,* 502–515.

Stacy, A. W., Widaman, K. F., & Marlatt, G. A. (1990). Expectancy models of alcohol use. *Journal of Personality and Social Psychology, 58,* 918–928.

Stein, K. D., Goldman, M. S., & Del Boca, F. K. (1997, July). *Happy hour: The relative effects of alcohol expectancies and positive mood on drinking behavior.* Paper presented at the meeting of the Research Society on Alcoholism, San Francisco, CA.

Stewart, J., deWit, H., & Eikelboom, R. (1984). Role of unconditioned and conditioned drug effects in the self-administration of opiates and stimulants. *Psychological Review, 91,* 251–268.

Stritzke, W. G. K., Patrick, C. J., & Lang, A. R. (1995). Alcohol and human emotion: A multidimensional analysis incorporating startle–probe methodology. *Journal of Abnormal Psychology, 104,* 114–121.

Tolman, E. G. (1932). *Purposive behavior in animals and man.* New York: Appleton–Century–Crofts.

Turing, M. A. (1950). Computing machinery and intelligence. *Mind, 59,* 433–460.

Ungerleider, L. G. (1995). Functional brain imaging studies of cortical mechanisms for memory. *Science*, *270*, 769–775.

Vogel-Sprott, M., & Fillmore, M. T. (in press). Expectancy and behavioral effects of alcohol and caffeine. In I. Kirsch (Ed.), *How expectancies shape behavior*. Washington, DC: APA Books.

Watson, D., & Tellegen, A. (1985). Toward a consensual structure of mood. *Psychological Bulletin*, *98*, 219–235.

Webb, J. A., Baer, P. E., Francis, D. J., & Caid, C. D. (1993). Relationship among social and intrapersonal risk, alcohol expectancies, and alcohol usage among early adolescents. *Addictive Behaviors*, *18*, 127–134.

Weingardt, K., Stacy, A. W., & Leigh, B. C. (1996). Automatic activation of alcohol concepts in response to positive outcomes of alcohol use. *Alcoholism: Experimental and Clinical Research*, *20*, 25–30.

Werner, M. J., Walker, L. S., & Green, J. W. (1993). Alcohol expectancies, problem drinking, and adverse health consequences. *Journal of Adolescent Health*, *14*, 446–452.

Wiers, R. W., Hoogeven, K. J., Sergeant, J. A., & Gunning, W. B. (1997). High and low dose alcohol-related expectancies and the differential associations with drinking in male and female adolescents and young adults. *Addiction*, *92*, 871–888.

Wise, R. A. (1988). The neurobiology of craving: Implications for the understanding and treatment of alcoholism. *Journal of Abnormal Psychology*, *97*, 118–132.

Young, R. M., & Knight, R. G. (1989). The Drinking Expectancy Questionnaire: A revised measure of alcohol-related beliefs. *Journal of Psychopathology and Behavioral Assessment*, *11*, 99–112.

Zucker, R. A., Kincaid, S. B., Fitzgerald, H. E., & Bingham, R. C. (1996). Alcohol schema acquisition in preschoolers: Differences between children of alcoholics and children of nonalcoholics. *Alcoholism: Clinical and Experimental Research*, *19*, 1011–1017.

7

Cognitive Theory and Research

MICHAEL A. SAYETTE

INTRODUCTION

The past several decades have seen the emergence of cognitive theory in psychological research. During this period, much research has shifted away from a strict behaviorism toward a cognitive, or information-processing perspective. This "cognitive revolution in psychology" has affected the type of research conducted across many of the subfields within psychology (Baars, 1986; Dember, 1974). One area that has embraced a cognitive perspective is the field of psychopathology (Dobson & Kendall, 1993), including addictive behavior (Goldman & Rather, 1993; Marlatt & Gordon, 1985; Wilson, 1987). This chapter addresses cognitive theory and research in addiction, with an emphasis on the alcohol field. Although advances in neurobiology, psychophysiology, and neuropsychology have all contributed to our understanding of addictive behavior, they are beyond the scope of this chapter (see Fromme & D'Amico, Chapter 11, this volume). Memory-based alcohol expectancy research, while addressed in this chapter, is covered in detail by Goldman, Del Boca, and Darkes (Chapter 6).

Though many acknowledge the impact of this cognitive revolution, it has been difficult to describe precisely what is meant by "cognitive." At a metatheoretical level, the cognitive approach refers to a consideration of what constitutes acceptable scientific evidence. Both behaviorist and cognitive approaches rely on observable data. Unlike adherents to the former position, however, cognitive psychologists infer unobservable mental constructs on the basis of observed phenomena (Baars, 1986). Although the studies described herein cover a broad spectrum of phenomena associated with alcohol and drug use, they are linked by a shared use of objective and measurable data to draw inferences about internal mental processes.

A comprehensive account of drinking and the development of alcoholism requires an analysis of several general questions. Included among these is an examination of how one responds when alcohol is consumed, as well as when alcohol is desired. Applications of cognitive theory and methods to addiction research have led to substantial advances in our understanding of both questions. Inasmuch as the methodologies, and the inferences drawn from these methodologies, are unlike many other areas of psychology, this chapter begins by outlining some of the cognitive methods used in alcohol and drug research. Next, this chapter describes from a cognitive perspective the psychosocial effects of drinking. Three models are reviewed that, along with expectancy theory (see Goldman, Del Boca, & Darkes, Chapter 6, this volume), illustrate the importance of social-cognitive processes for understanding the effects of alcohol on psychosocial phenomena such as anxiety, aggression, risk taking, and prosocial behavior. The next section addresses research on craving and cue reactivity, and describes recent models that recognize the role of cognition in understanding these processes. This section is followed by a discussion of cognitive research that focuses on drugs other than alcohol. Finally, this chapter addresses a number of areas in which addiction research can continue to benefit from advances in cognitive science. Throughout the chapter, the focus is on acute effects rather than chronic effects associated with long-term use or dependence.

COGNITIVE METHODOLOGY IN ALCOHOL AND DRUG RESEARCH

Much cognitively oriented addiction research has relied on self-report introspections that require participants to articulate what they have experienced during a study. These are referred to as explicit cognitive tasks. Alternatively, researchers have assessed implicit cognition, in which information is revealed without awareness by the individual (Schacter, 1987). Measures of implicit cognition assess performance on tasks in order to form judgments about internal processes. Whereas self-report measures of introspection tend to focus on cognitive products, or the outcome of a series of different processes, performance measures permit examination of cognitive structures (i.e., the way information, or cognitive content, is represented in memory) and cognitive processes (i.e., the procedures executed by the organism) (Kendall & Dobson, 1993). Until recently, addictions research relied on self-report assessments of cognitive products (e.g., asking participants to rate how much attention they paid to an alcoholic beverage during cue exposure [Rohsenow et al., 1994[1]]). This type of assessment, while convenient, nevertheless suffers from a number of important limitations (Hammersley, 1994; Nisbett & Ross, 1980;

Nisbett & Wilson, 1977). The development of alternative measures of processes (e.g., attention, recall) and structures signals an important and emerging stage in the application of cognitive theory to addiction research and is the primary focus here.[2]

Before describing the various tasks that have been used by alcohol researchers to study cognition, two types of processing, automatic and nonautomatic, should be identified (Shiffrin & Schneider, 1977). A number of different criteria have been proposed to distinguish nonautomatic and automatic processing. Nonautomatic processing is said to draw upon limited-capacity resources. This type of processing requires effort, intentionality, or control, is modifiable, relatively slow, and subject to conscious awareness. In contrast, automatic processing does not require limited-capacity resources. Automatic processing is thought to be effortless, performed without intention or control, difficult to modify, and it operates without awareness (for a more extensive list of distinguishing criteria, see Shiffrin, 1988). To varying degrees, the following cognitive methodologies have been used to assess automatic and nonautomatic processes, as well as underlying structures associated with alcohol and drug use.

Judgments

Individuals are continually evaluating themselves and their environment. Such judgments often can be important in determining behavior (Segal & Cloitre, 1993). If an abstinent alcoholic, for example, judges the merits of having a few drinks to be especially compelling at a particular moment, then he or she may be in danger of relapse. Because the nature of these judgments may be influenced by a range of situational (e.g., one's current mood) and individual-difference factors (e.g., heavy vs. light drinkers), one approach to cognitive assessment is to measure these judgmental processes. According to Kahneman and Tversky (1972), judgments are affected by the relative accessibility of information in memory. To the degree that there are factors that influence judgments, inferences are made about the relative salience of different types of information. Examples of judgments include the expected probability or amount of reinforcement of future events, evaluations of self or others, and attributions about the causes of an event. Judgment studies have revealed that phobic or depressed persons are likely to increase the expected likelihood of negative outcomes, suggesting a selective processing of negative information (Segal & Cloitre, 1993). Although these judgments require self-report, they differ from self-report introspection measures. In the case of judgment methods, the self-reports themselves serve as the data to be interpreted.

Secondary Response Time Probes

Response time probes are one of a group of divided attention tasks that have been used to assess the extent to which performance on a primary task draws on nonautomatic resources (Kerr, 1973). The aim is to measure the amount of limited-capacity cognitive resources that is required during processing of a primary task by recording performance decrements (measured in milliseconds required to respond to a series of tones or probes) on a secondary task. When more capacity is required in a primary task, less capacity remains available for a secondary response time task. Thus, the longer the latency of response time to the probe, the more capacity is being consumed by the primary task (Britton & Tessor, 1982; Wickens, 1984). For example, performing tasks that demand limited-capacity processing resources, such as counting backwards from 100 in multiples of seven, or solving anagrams, should increase the time required to respond to auditory probes that are presented concurrently. Because researchers believe that alcohol or drug cues may draw upon limited-capacity processing resources in a similar manner, response time probes have provided a way to assess the processing demands of these cues on nonautomatic resources.

Cognitive Performance Measures

Cognitive performance tasks require the use of limited-capacity nonautomatic processing resources. Performance on these tasks is considered to be a function of the difficulty of the task and the processing resources available. For instance, a driver can operate a car effectively while chatting with a passenger, assuming the discussion is not especially engaging. Driving skills might deteriorate, however, if the conversation became especially compelling. This change in driving performance could be attributed to an increase in processing resources demanded by the now-interesting conversation (Wickens, 1984). Impaired performance on laboratory tasks, typically measured in errors or increased time to complete the task, presumably reflects a decrease in available resources. Examples of procedures that have been used to infer this shift in resource allocation are tracking tasks (see Moskowitz, 1973) and sentence reading tasks, in which the sentences vary in complexity (Daneman & Carpenter, 1980). In the latter paradigm, participants read a set of unrelated sentences and then recall the last word of each sentence. The investigator assesses the maximum number of sentences that can be read while still recalling the final word of each sentence. Presumably, reading sentences of varying complexity draws on limited-capacity processing resources, which affects the capacity available for holding a number of sentence–final words (Just & Carpenter, 1992).

Explicit Memory Tasks

Memory tasks often are considered to measure either explicit or implicit cognitive functioning. Research on explicit memory functioning includes the recall of a previously presented list of words, some of which are associated with a particular drug. Explicit memory requires conscious or deliberate recollection (Schacter, 1987). It is believed that good performance on these memory tasks reflects detailed and meaningful analysis of the stimulus. Studies of explicit memory have revealed individuals with various forms of psychopathology to recall words associated with their specific disorders more readily than others (Segal & Cloitre, 1993). More pertinent to the present chapter, Stacy (1997) has found explicit recall of alcohol expectancies to predict subsequent drinking levels.

Implicit Memory Tasks

Implicit memory tasks rely on information that is activated by a participant without conscious awareness and, in certain cases, can operate independently of explicit memory processes (Schacter, 1987). Instead of explicitly recalling information, participants perform a task, and memory is inferred through changes in task performance. Typically, these tasks present ambiguous information to participants, who, presumably, do not realize that they are relying on past experiences to respond. Examples of these tasks include word-stem completion tasks, in which one is provided with the beginning letters of a word and completes the word as quickly possible; perceptual identification tasks, in which one identifies rapidly presented (e.g., 35 msec) words, or words in which the letters are degraded; and categorization tasks, in which rapidly presented words are classified into one of a few categories. In each of these tasks, individuals are thought to have greater perceptual sensitivity to stimuli pertinent to their concerns and interests, and thus more accessible in memory, and will perform better when these ambiguous stimuli are associated with their disorder. Implicit memory tasks have examined situational and individual-difference factors that affect accessibility of different types of information stored in memory.

One implicit memory task that is popular among cognitive psychologists is the semantic priming paradigm. Semantic priming refers to a process in which concepts and their meanings in memory are activated by semantically associated information (Collins & Loftus, 1975). While different theories have been proposed to explain semantic priming, they generally agree that semantically related concepts are stored closer together in memory than unrelated concepts, and that activation of one word will activate semantically similar words more powerfully than unrelated words. For instance, when one makes a lexical decision on a letter string (e.g., deciding whether the letter string "boat" is an English word), the decision should be faster if the letter string is preceded, or primed, by a semantically related word (e.g., lake) than an unrelated prime (e.g., book). This has been found to be the case even when individuals are unaware that they have been presented with a prime (Fowler, Wolford, Slade, & Tassinary, 1981; Marcel, 1983). Semantic priming tasks have been used in alcohol research to provide insight into how information is stored in memory. Weingardt, Stacy, and Leigh (1996), for example, used a semantic priming task to show that, among heavy drinkers, alcohol-related targets (e.g., drink, booze) can be automatically activated in memory when preceded by positive drinking outcome primes (e.g., "They had fun after they had the . . . ").

Selective processing of relevant information in memory can also lead to impaired performance when the pertinent stimuli are designed to distract a participant from a task. An increasingly popular measure of interference is the Stroop color-naming task, sometimes called the emotional Stroop task (Williams, Mathews, & MacLeod, 1996). In this task, participants name the color of words while ignoring the word content. When words are personally or emotionally relevant, individuals are automatically drawn to them, and the latency to name the color of the word generally increases. For example, phobic patients take longer to color-name words describing phobic material, and this selective interference has been found using participants across a range of disorders (Williams et al., 1996). Color naming has predicted emotional distress better than explicit, self-report measures (MacLeod & Hagan, 1992), though the exact mechanism underlying the color-naming effect remains unclear (cf. de Ruiter & Brosschot, 1994; MacLeod & Rutherford, 1992; Mathews & Klug, 1993; Williams et al., 1996).

Before detailing how these different measures of the selective processing of information stored in memory have been applied to alcohol and drug research, some methodological limitations should be noted. One issue facing alcohol researchers using implicit priming tasks concerns the source of the prime. Investigators are often interested in detecting individual differences or underlying states (e.g., craving) that purportedly increase the salience of information related to drinking in memory, thereby facilitating the processing of this information. Yet priming also can result from alternative mechanisms that are independent of emotional states or preexisting individual-difference characteristics. Indeed, the bulk of priming research in cognitive psychology has ignored individual differences in mood state or familiarity with the topic. Basic cognitive research typically has experimentally introduced primes merely by presenting a prime and target in close temporal proximity. For example, response-time latency to pronounce the target "tiger" reliably decreases if it appears immediately after the prime "lion." This type of priming is powerful. In this case, one need not be a zookeeper or have just seen a safari film to show priming effects. Consequently, when participants are presented with a list of alcohol-related words, the first few words may prime subsequent identification of the remaining drinking-relevant words in the list (response chaining). Similarly, as soon as the first alcohol-related word on a word-stem completion task is generated, respondents may be primed to look for related words, regardless of their drinking patterns or current desire to drink.

A second problem for cognitively oriented alcohol researchers concerns response contamination, or the reciprocal influence that automatic and nonautomatic processes can have on each other. It is important to recognize that automaticity exists on a continuum and that automatic and nonautomatic processes operate in parallel together at different stages of information processing (Kahneman & Treisman, 1984). "The crucial point is that tasks are never wholly automatic or attentive [nonautomatic], and are always accomplished by mixtures of automatic and attentive [nonautomatic] processes" (Shiffrin, 1997, p. 50). Yet an assumption in most studies is that explicit tasks measure nonautomatic processes while implicit tasks assess automatic processes. This assumption has been criticized by those who argue that it is inappropriate to identify cognitive processes with particular tasks (e.g., Jacoby, Yonelinas, & Jennings, 1997). The trouble with linking task to process is that nonautomatic or conscious processing can affect implicit cognitive task performance and, in some cases, unconscious processes can even affect explicit cognitive tasks (Holender, 1986; Jacoby et al., 1997; Neely, 1991).

Though these artifactual concerns may not necessarily fatally confound studies using implicit memory tasks (see Williams et al., 1996), researchers still should attempt to minimize these potential problems. One approach to reducing the effects of these less interesting (from the perspective of alcohol research) sources of priming is to include a large number of words in the test list that are unrelated to drinking. The aim would be to prevent respondents from becoming aware that the stimuli are occasionally associated with alcohol (see Neely, 1991). Even with a large percentage of alcohol-irrelevant prime-target pairings, however, inadvertent priming may still occur. In the case of word-stem completions, it may be wise to focus on initial responses only (Stacy, Leigh, & Weingardt, 1994). In this case, there are no prior word stems to prime respondents and thus create a confound. For semantic priming tasks (e.g., lexical decision, word pronunciation, color naming), matching test words on length, frequency, and emotional valence or intensity may be indicated, as these dimensions can inadvertently affect response-time latencies (Lorch, 1982; Martin, Williams, & Clark, 1991).

ALCOHOL'S PSYCHOSOCIAL EFFECTS

In many instances, alcohol's effects on interpersonal behaviors (e.g., aggression) and intrapersonal processes (e.g., anxiety) are presumed to be due to a direct pharmacological impact of alcohol on the nervous system (Koob & Bloom, 1988; Room & Collins, 1983). This type of explanation has difficulty accommodating observations that alcohol's effects on anxiety, aggression, sexual behavior, and other psychosocial responses are extremely variable across persons and situations (Sayette, 1993; Taylor & Leonard, 1983; Wilson, 1977). To better explain these inconsistent findings, recent theories have proposed that alcohol's psychosocial effects are cognitively mediated. These different theories all share the position that alcohol pharmacologically alters cognitive processes, which in turn impact on a wide range of psychological states and social behaviors. These cognitive theories attempt to provide a framework for understanding the complex interplay of situational and individual-difference variables related to drinking.

Self-Awareness Model

One of the first cognitive theories that was proposed to understand the effects of alcohol on social behavior was the self-awareness model (Hull, 1981). This model applies a social-psychological theory of human behavior (Hull & Levy, 1979) to a range of phenomena related to drinking, including aggressive behavior, social anxiety, risk taking, sexual behavior, and risk for relapse (see Hull, 1987; Hull & Van Treuren, 1986). Two areas that have received particular emphasis are anxiety and aggression.

Anxiety

According to Hull's (1981) self-awareness model, alcohol's stress-reducing properties are cognitively mediated. By impairing the encoding of information in terms of its self-relevance, intoxication decreases self-awareness. The inhibition of encoding processes leads to a reduction in performance-based self-evaluation, which, in situations where such evaluation is unpleasant, dampens anxiety, thus increasing the probability of drinking. Hull's (1987) position that intoxication impedes the processing of information as self-relevant has been evaluated through attempts to show that alcohol reduces the use of self-focused statements during a speech, and that persons who are high in self-consciousness are more vulnerable to alcohol's anxiolytic effects.

Hull, Levenson, and Young (1981, unpublished manuscript cited in Hull, 1987) found that during a speech stressor, alcohol dampened the increased arousal experienced by highly self-conscious participants, compared to those low in self-consciousness. This finding suggested that alcohol was interfering with self-awareness. Subsequently, a series of experiments evaluated alcohol's impact more directly by including measures of self-awareness (Hull, Levenson, Young, & Sher, 1983). As predicted, alcohol consumption decreased the occurrence of self-focused statements. Further research tested whether magnitude of self-awareness reduction during intoxication was a function of change in self-evaluation (Hull et al., 1983). Participants were asked to rate a series of words according to either structural ("Is the word short or long?"), semantic ("Is the word meaningful?"), or self-relevant characteristics ("Does the word describe you?"). Based on research showing highly self-conscious individuals to be especially likely to recall words encoded according to self-relevance, Hull and colleagues predicted that alcohol would have the greatest impact on highly self-conscious participants. As expected, these individuals showed the greatest decrease in recall of the words encoded according to self-relevance, suggesting that alcohol reduces capacity to encode information according to self-relevance.

Antisocial or Aggressive Behavior

Hull's (1981) initial formulation of the self-awareness model of alcohol use linked alcohol consumption to decreased self-awareness. Noting that self-awareness increases the correspondence between behavior and both internal and external standards of comportment, Hull and Van Treuren (1986) broadened the scope of the model to assert that alcohol consumption should decrease self-regulation with respect to behavioral standards. In their review, they find indirect support for the view that alcohol inhibits the "propensity of an individual to use higher-order encoding and elaboration processes necessary for self-control" (p. 217). For example, Bailey, Leonard, Cranston, and Taylor (1983) reported that while a self-awareness manipulation reduced aggressive responding, alcohol consumption had the opposite effect. Moreover, instructions to increase self-awareness seemed to attenuate the effect of alcohol.

While support has been documented for the self-awareness model (Hull, 1981, 1987; Hull & Reilly, 1983; Hull, Young, & Jouriles, 1986), so too have data been reported inconsistent with this model (Chassin, Mann, & Sher, 1988; Sher, 1987). For example, some investigators have failed to find the predicted relationships between self-consciousness level and the anxiolytic effects of alcohol (Niaura, Wilson, & Westrick, 1988; Sher & Walitzer, 1986; Wilson, Brick, Adler, Cocco, & Breslin, 1989). Nor have all studies found alcohol consumption to reduce measures of self-awareness (Caudill, Wilson, & Abrams, 1987; Frankenstein & Wilson, 1984; Wilson et al., 1989). One difficulty in testing an individual's self-awareness level is that probes for self-awareness (e.g., Yankofsky, Wilson, Adler, Hay, & Vrana, 1986) may influence the cognitive processes being measured (Hull & Reilly, 1983). Despite these inconsistent findings, the self-awareness model has stimulated research on factors that may influence the effects of intoxication on cognition. In addition, this model provides a theoretical framework for examining the effects of intoxication during positive as well as negative events (Strizke, Lang, & Patrick, 1996).

Alcohol Myopia

Perhaps the most influential cognitive theory of alcohol's effects on social behavior to appear in recent years is that of alcohol myopia, "a state of shortsightedness in which superficially understood, immediate aspects of experience have a disproportionate influence on behavior and emotion, a state in which we can see the tree, albeit more dimly, but miss the forest altogether" (Steele & Josephs, 1990, p. 923). According to these authors, social behavior involves consideration of multiple cues. Though some of these cues are more salient than others, a sober individual can consider a range of information before responding. In many cases, less salient and more salient information may conflict. For example, upon noticing an unpleasant boss at a party, one initially may be inclined to behave rudely. Yet realizing that one's career is jeopardized by such behavior inhibits the impulse. Here, disrespectful or insulting behavior is provoked by salient cues, while simultaneously being inhibited by other cues that require additional processing. Steele and Josephs (1990) label this cognitive process *inhibition conflict* and propose that such conflict is reduced during intoxication. By impairing cognitive processing capacity, alcohol consumption is purported to interfere with the ability to consider more remote inhibiting cues, leading one to attend only to those cues that are most salient (see also Taylor & Leonard, 1983).

One implication of alcohol myopia theory is that under certain circumstances, intoxication, by reducing inhibition conflict, can cause responses to become more extreme. Because not all behavioral responses are conflictual, Steele and Southwick (1985) predicted an increase in excessive behavior only in situations in which inhibition conflict would otherwise be present. Thus, when a gambling study includes the possibility of large gains as well as large losses, conflict is high, whereas if the study provides an opportunity for a large gain, and only a small loss, inhibitory conflict is low, and the desire to gamble should not be affected by alcohol. Based on a meta-analysis of studies evaluating the effects of alcohol consumption on social behavior, these authors conclude that intoxicated behavior varied dramatically from sober behavior, but only during situations in which response conflict was high (Steele & Josephs, 1990; Steele & Southwick, 1985). According to alcohol myopia theory, intoxication can facilitate a wide range of emotional and interpersonal experiences. Data pertinent to several of these domains are addressed.

Anxiety

In their attention-allocation model, Steele and Josephs (1990) applied alcohol myopia theory to the study of alcohol's effects on anxiety. Like the self-awareness model, the attention-allocation model posits that alcohol affects anxiety indirectly through its impairment of cognitive processing (Josephs & Steele, 1990; Steele & Josephs, 1988). Alcohol's narrowing of perception to immediate cues, and its reduction of cognitive abstracting capacity, restricts attention to the most immediate, salient aspects of experience. Given this assumption, the concurrent activity in which an intoxicated person engages helps to determine alcohol's effects. Intoxication in the presence of concurrent distraction is predicted to attenuate stress responding, whereas, without a neutral or pleasantly distracting activity, intoxication is not predicted to relieve anxiety, and may even increase anxiety, by focusing attention on the then-salient stressor.

Tests of the attention-allocation model consistently have found that alcohol in conjunction with a pleasant distraction reduces self-reported anxiety associated with a stressor administration. Anxiolysis occurred when the stressor consisted of negative feedback from a test (Steele, Southwick, & Pagano, 1986) as well as anticipating the presentation of a self-disclosing speech (Josephs & Steele, 1990; Steele & Josephs, 1988). In the absence of distraction, however, alcohol no longer reduced anxiety (Josephs & Steele, 1990; Steele et al., 1986), and even increased anxiety (Steele & Josephs, 1988). To gain more direct evidence for this attention-allocation model, a study using a secondary response-time probe was conducted, which measured limited-capacity processing resources during varying levels of intoxication and distraction. Response-time data indicated that when participants had greater cognitive resources available (when they were sober or not distracted), they reported increased anxiety while anticipating the speech. In contrast, when participants were intoxicated and distracted, anxiety levels diminished and reaction time increased, suggesting less available cognitive capacity to focus on the stressor (Josephs & Steele, 1990).

The research by Steele and Josephs has produced multiple replications of the finding that in the presence of concurrent distraction, a moderate dose of alcohol will provide anxiolytic effects. Since most of the drinking that occurs outside the laboratory includes distractions, the attention-allocation model suggests that alcohol often will provide stress-attenuating effects (Josephs & Steele, 1990). Nevertheless, Steele and Josephs (1988) recognized the difficulty in reconciling their findings when distraction was absent with those from studies demonstrating stress-response dampening (e.g., Sayette, Smith, Breiner, & Wilson, 1992); that is, multiple studies conducted in different laboratories, using a variety of methods and measures, have sometimes found alcohol to reduce stress responding, even when no distraction was present (see Sayette, 1993), a finding inconsistent with Steele and Josephs's (1988) notion of "crying in one's beer." Still, the attention-allocation model is notable for identifying the critical role of cognitive processing in determining alcohol's effects on stress, and for providing a plausible explanation for both the anxiolytic and anxiogenic effects of alcohol. Moreover, because distractions are more common in the real world than in the laboratory, this model likely accounts for even more natural drinking behavior than experiments might suggest.

Antisocial Behavior

Several forms of antisocial behavior have been examined within the framework of alcohol myopia. They include drunk driving, risky sexual activity, and aggressive behavior. Steele and Josephs (1990) note that it is difficult to make predictions from alcohol myopia theory for activities, such as unprotected sex, in which it is hard to judge the relative strength and salience of response-relevant cues (e.g., sexual arousal, fear of disease) for a particular individual. Nevertheless, MacDonald, Zanna, and Fong (in press) have conducted both laboratory and field studies that provide support for alcohol myopia theory in the domains of condom use and drunk driving. In the former case, these authors found that alcohol consumption leads to a focus on the perceived benefits of sex rather than on the putatively less salient, negative consequences of forgoing condoms (MacDonald, Zanna, & Fong, 1996; see also Fromme, Katz, & D'Amico, 1997). In the latter domain, alcohol consumption was associated with improved attitudes and intentions to drive drunk only when compelling cues for driving were presented (MacDonald, Zanna, & Fong, 1995).

Leonard (1989) conducted a study testing the effects of alcohol on aggressive responding in which the salience of cues either to behave aggressively or to inhibit aggression was manipulated. Consistent with theory (Steele & Josephs, 1990; Taylor & Leonard, 1983), alcohol's effects on aggression depended on whether the cues to inhibit aggressive behavior were made salient. If participants were provided with explicit information inhibiting aggression, then intoxication did not lead to increased aggressive behavior. In contrast, if the cues for inhibiting aggression were subtler than initial, explicit cues to respond aggressively, then intoxicated participants responded significantly more aggressively than the sober participants.

Other Psychosocial Behaviors

Alcohol myopia theory can be invoked to understand the effects of alcohol on *self-evaluation*. Conflict arises when the wish to view oneself positively is contradicted by a distant awareness of less appealing characteristics. [The assumption here is that, at least among psychologically healthy individuals, positive information is more salient than negative information (Bannaji & Steele, 1989; Taylor & Brown, 1988)]. While sober, both the immediately available positive and less available negative aspects of self are accessible. Alcohol's myopic effects, however, can reduce this conflict. Accordingly, individuals who have consumed alcohol should readily access information associated with a positive self-image but not the negative information that is less salient. Several studies have found support for this model. Bannaji and Steele (1989) report that alcohol improved participants' self-ratings for high-conflict traits (i.e., a large discrepancy between their actual and ideal evaluations) but not for low-conflict traits. In a study requiring participants to make a self-disclosing speech about what they liked and disliked about their appearance, self-descriptions of intoxicated participants contained less negative information compared to those who were sober (Sayette, 1994).

Steele, Critchlow, and Liu (1985) created an experimental situation in which an initial impulse to engage in *helping behavior* would be inhibited by a desire to avoid participating in an unpleasant activity. In their study, participants were asked to perform a boring task for 17 minutes, after which they could relax for the remainder of the study. Following the task, they were asked to aid the experimenter by continuing to perform the task instead of relaxing. The study varied the degree of conflict between wanting to help and wanting to avoid further participation in the boring task. Consistent with the tenets of alcohol myopia, intoxication increased willingness of the participants to help out, but only in high-conflict conditions.

In summary, alcohol myopia theory provides a cognitive explanation for a variety of effects of alcohol on interpersonal behavior and intrapersonal processes. Importantly, this model has inspired a host of studies, across many different laboratories, designed to test its propositions. Further research is needed to examine relationships between different aspects of alcohol myopia theory. First, it is not clear whether the mechanism underlying attention allocation (a theory based on the proposition that alcohol consumption reduces attentional capacity) is the same mechanism underlying inhibition conflict. In theory it may be possible to experience high levels of inhibition conflict and also have reduced attentional capacity.[3] Second, it has been suggested that attention has both capacity and organizational components (Stadler, 1995). In addition to an attentional capacity framework, conceptualizations of attention that emphasize organizational processes may account for some of the findings supporting alcohol myopia. Indeed, recent evidence suggests that learning new information may depend more on organization and intention than on capacity (Stadler, 1995). Third, future research should distinguish between inhibition conflict and the concept of time-inconsistent preference. Investigators across different social sciences have observed that the ability to control impulses varies over time and across situations (Hoch & Loewenstein, 1991; Vuchinich & Tucker, 1988). According to this view, imminent rewards exert disproportionate effects on people. Intoxication may increase temporal discounting such that immediately available rewards become even more attractive relative to more delayed outcomes. Nevertheless, while specific aspects of alcohol myopia theory have been questioned (cf. Hull & Van Treuren, 1986; Ito, Miller, & Pollock, 1996; Sayette, 1993), a great deal of support has been established confirming alcohol's "myopic" effects.

Appraisal-Disruption Model

Although the appraisal-disruption model was initially formulated to address the relationship between alcohol and anxiety, it has also been applied to studies of alcohol and aggression.

Anxiety

Like the self-awareness and attention-allocation models, the appraisal-disruption model posits that alcohol affects stress indirectly through particular effects on cognitive processes (Sayette, 1993). Stress relief occurs to the degree that alcohol acts pharmacologically to interfere with one's appraisal of stressful information. Appraisal is defined as the act of classifying an event in terms of its impact for well-being and has been categorized as irrelevant, benign/positive, or stressful (Lazarus & Folkman, 1984). Stress appraisals involve encounters construed as aversive in that they concern either harm/loss or threat (Sher, 1987). According to models of associative recall, the appraisal of stressful information involves a spreading activation process resulting in the activation of information previously stored as nodes in a memory network, with related nodes sharing associated connections (Bower, 1981; Collins & Loftus, 1975).[4] The appraisal-disruption model proposes that alcohol acts pharmacologically to disrupt appraisal of stressful information by constraining the spread of activation of associated information previously established in memory; that is, alcohol impairs initial appraisal of stressful information by diminishing the power of a stressor to activate associated information stored in memory. The appraisal-disruption model predicts that alcohol will dampen stress responses in circumstances in which fewer associative connections related to a stressor are activated. Should a stressor be sufficiently appraised, however, alcohol is not expected to be anxiolytic.

The appraisal-disruption model is consistent with a body of research that indicates alcohol consumption impairs the storage of new information, and that this effect may be due in part to a diminished ability to elaborate or extract meaning from new material by integrating it with previously stored information (Birnbaum, Johnson, Hartley, & Taylor, 1980; Sayette, 1993). In contrast, when alcohol is consumed following the acquisition of new material, memory is not consistently impaired and may in some cases even show retrograde enhancement (Lister, Eckardt, & Weingartner, 1987; Mann, Cho-Young, & Vogel-Sprott, 1984; Parker et al., 1981). Accordingly, alcohol's stress-relieving effects should be most powerful when information is initially appraised during intoxication. A review of the human alcohol–stress literature revealed that descriptions of experimental methods provided in consent forms varied across studies. In some cases, detailed information was provided pertaining to the stressfulness of the upcoming manipulation, while, in other cases, this information was vague or absent. Consistent with predictions, alcohol reliably reduced stress in the latter but not in the former studies (Sayette, 1993). Moreover, three experiments that explicitly manipulated the temporal ordering of the drink and the administration of the stressor also found this same pattern of results (Noel, Lisman, Schare, & Meisto, 1992; Sayette, Wilson, & Carpenter, 1989; Sayette & Wilson, 1991).

The appraisal-disruption model is unique in its ability to explain the contradictory findings from past experiments, and it introduces an important methodological issue that often has been ignored: the temporal relationship between drinking and initial appraisal of a stressor. Nevertheless, at present, there remains a number of unresolved issues pertinent to the model. Most critical is the need to assess the cognitive mechanisms underlying these effects on stress. Data currently are being collected to test whether alcohol's effects on stress are mediated by disruption of cognitive processes. This research requires assessment of both stress responding and cognitive functioning in a group of intoxicated participants. With few exceptions (e.g., Peterson, Finn, & Pihl, 1992), rarely have both been measured in the same study. More research also is needed to determine if negative information is differentially sensitive to alcohol's effects on cognitive appraisal (Sayette, 1993; Strizke, Lang, & Patrick, 1996).

Antisocial or Aggressive Behavior

An enduring opinion among some researchers has been that alcohol's effects on aggression are mediated by anxiety (Dollard & Miller, 1950; Conger, 1956). Recently, Ito et al. (1996) argued that when the conditions for anxiolysis outlined by the appraisal-disruption model are met (i.e., that the stressful information is received during intoxication), the suppression of aggression is weakened. Their anxiolysis–disinhibition theory is reminiscent of the position adopted by early proponents of the tension-reduction model, who argued that anxiety reduction may provide a single mechanism that disinhibits a wide range of responses (see Wilson, 1988). In their meta-analysis, Ito et al. (1996) found that, as predicted, alcohol's facilitation of aggressive responding was greatest in studies that had the most anxiety-provoking cues. As these authors note, degree of anxiety elicited was strongly associated with level of inhibition conflict. Thus, it will require additional experimentation to disentangle these two theories. In any case, there appears to be strong support for the role of cognitive processing in determining the relationship between intoxication and aggression.

The appraisal-disruption model is similar to the self-awareness and alcohol myopia models in its emphasis on cognitive impairment. While the self-awareness and appraisal-disruption models share many assumptions and are not incompatible, the clearest distinctions between them rest in their specific predictions. The appraisal-disruption model does not necessarily predict that self-consciousness level would correspond to anxiolytic effects, nor would self-focused speech be considered a critical measure of appraisal deficits. The self-awareness model does not predict alcohol's differential effects on anxiety that occur as a function of the ordering of the stressor and the drink procedure. Nor is it clear from the self-awareness model (Hull, 1987) that the nature of the stressor (e.g., severity, complexity), so long as it is relevant to the self, should interact differently with alcohol (see Sayette, 1993).

Both the attention-allocation and appraisal-disruption models propose that alcohol's effects on stress depend on the salience of the stressor. When a stressor is sufficiently appraised, either because participants are not distracted (Josephs & Steele, 1990), or because the information is presented to participants initially while sober (Sayette & Wilson, 1991), alcohol is no longer expected to produce anxiolytic effects and may even cause an anxiogenic response (Steele & Josephs, 1988). Conversely, when information is made less salient, either because it was appraised during intoxication or because of concurrent distraction, alcohol is likely to help reduce anxiety. In this way, the two models can be seen as complementary.

The appraisal-disruption and alcohol myopia models differ, however, in the mechanisms posited to explain the cognitive impairment produced by alcohol. In contrast to alcohol myopia theory, the appraisal-disruption model considers the distinction between automatic and nonautomatic processing to be less important in understanding alcohol's effects on stress. While nonautomatic processes are especially affected by alcohol (e.g., Hashtroudi, Parker, DeLisi, Wyatt, & Mutter, 1984; Lapp, Collins, & Izzo, 1990; Moskowitz, 1973; Schneider, Dumais, & Shiffrin, 1984), it is also true that automatic processing can be impaired (Maylor & Rabbit, 1993, p. 315; Schneider et al., 1984). According to the appraisal-disruption model, alcohol's ability to impair the organization of information, perhaps by constraining the spread of activation of information associated with a stressor, provides the foundation for anxiolytic effects. The disruption is based on priming mechanisms that do not emphasize attentional capacity (Bower, 1987; MacLeod & Rutherford, 1992). The available data suggest that a decrease in attentional capacity may be sufficient, but not necessary, to disrupt the storage of information.

The self-awareness, alcohol myopia, and appraisal-disruption models all emphasize the critical role that cognition plays in mediating the effects of intoxication on inter- and intrapersonal experience. These theories suggest both situational (e.g., concurrent distraction, timing of drinking, and provocative cues) and individual-difference factors (e.g., self-consciousness) that help explain the variable effects of alcohol. Though these three models can be viewed as cognitive theories, it should be noted that each specifies that it is the pharmacological impact of alcohol consumption, rather than merely the belief that one has been drinking (dosage-set), that is principally responsible for cognitive effects.[5]

Application of cognitive constructs such as attentional capacity and organization have provided new directions for alcohol research. With a few exceptions (Hull et al., 1983; Josephs & Steele, 1990), it should be noted that most of the evidence relating to the various effects of alcohol on cognitive processing for these models has been indirect; that is, while we know that alcohol has important effects on cognitive processing, there is relatively little data to indicate whether these cognitive effects mediate the alcohol–behavior relationship. The ultimate validity of these models will depend in part on the outcome of future studies that directly relate these cognitive processes to the psychosocial phenomena of interest.

Future research also should include direct measures of more complex aspects of cognitive processing, such as the component social information processing skills known to affect social behaviors. For example, Sayette, Wilson, and Elias (1993) attempted to assess cognitive processes in a test of alcohol's effects on aggressive responding by measuring performance on a range of social information processing stages. Adapting a procedure outlined by Dodge (1986) to examine social information processing deficits in aggressive children, participants observed a series of videotaped scenes of potential interpersonal conflict. The videotapes were designed to examine the effects of alcohol on several distinct information-processing skills. Results indicated that alcohol consumption interfered with a range of social information processing skills, including generating interpersonally effective responses, anticipating the outcome of different solutions, selecting socially competent responses, and responding to an obstacle following an initial attempt to resolve the situation (Sayette et al., 1993). (Fromme et al., 1997, also have used videotaped stimuli and have found that alcohol affects risky decision making.) These data suggest that future research consider direct measurement of cognitive processes associated with input, throughput, and output stages of social information processing.

CRAVING

Researchers have long posited a relationship between craving and alcohol and drug dependence. While the nature of this relationship continues to be vigorously debated, interest in craving is rising (e.g., Baker, Morse, & Sherman, 1987; Kassel & Shiffman, 1992; National Institute on Alcohol Abuse and Alcoholism [NIAAA], 1997; National Institute on Drug Abuse [NIDA], 1998; Robinson & Berridge, 1993; Tiffany, 1990; Wise, 1988). Although craving typically is regarded as a strong desire, the literature is replete with multiple, alternative definitions (Kozlowski & Wilkinson, 1987). Adherents to a disease model of alcoholism have considered craving to reflect a biological need for alcohol and equate craving with physical withdrawal (Jellinek, 1960). Considerable evidence indicates, however, that the experience of craving does not require physical withdrawal (Kassel & Shiffman, 1992). This inconsistent relationship between craving and withdrawal has led in recent years to investigation of the role of cognitive factors in craving (Tiffany, 1995). Because most of this research has occurred in the laboratory, craving typically is induced experimentally (see Shiffman et al., 1997, for a field study of the relationship between craving and drug use).

One of the primary approaches to an experimental analysis of craving involves presenting drinkers or drug users with drug-related stimuli and then measuring their responses. Cue reactivity typically has been assessed while drinkers or drug users are exposed to their particular drug, while they observe others engaged in drug use, or during imaginal exposures in which they are asked to read scripts of drug use vignettes designed to elicit cravings. These procedures provide an opportunity to examine individuals while they are experiencing often strong desires to drink or to use other drugs.

Conditioning Models of Craving

Conditioned withdrawal models of cue reactivity view craving as the cognitive correlate of a conditioned subclinical withdrawal syndrome (Ludwig & Wikler, 1974). Through repeated pairing with drinking, alcohol cues are proposed to elicit a conditioned response to environmental stimuli associated with withdrawal. Exposure to drug cues would trigger the same (craving) responses elicited by withdrawal (such as increased salivation and increased heart rate). In contrast, Siegel (1983) posited craving to be a conditioned *compensatory* response to drug effects. According to Siegel, with repeated drug use, drug cues elicit a conditioned response, experienced as craving, that is opposite in direction to the unconditioned response to drug administration. This compensatory process presumably facilitates maintenance of homeostasis in an organism that would otherwise be disturbed by the effects of the drug. An opponent process model represents craving as an experience that is opposite in effect to the acute effects of drug use (Solomon & Corbit, 1973). According to this model, increased drug use strengthens the opponent process, and thus craving takes on an increasingly greater role in maintaining drug habits. Across these different models, craving is associated with a negative physical or emotional state of mind, and one's craving to drink is based on a desire to alleviate unpleasant symptoms. Although these models predict that unpleasant physical states elicited by drug cues would be linked most closely to craving, data on the determinants of relapse suggest other factors may be more predictive of craving (see Marlatt, 1985).

Conditioning models also have focused on positive reinforcing effects. These models propose that, over time, drug cues come to elicit a positive motivational state that approximates the actual effects of the drug (Stewart, de Wit, & Eikelboom, 1984). In this model, drug cues, through conditioning, provide an incentive, experienced as craving, to receive more of the drug. Once having been used, a drug may induce an appetitive motivational state featuring increases in thoughts associated with drug use and drug-seeking behavior (Niaura et al., 1988; Robinson & Berridge, 1993).

In summary, these models suggest that cues associated with drug use or withdrawal will trigger conditioned responses. Implicit in these models is the view that craving arises from the labeling of these conditioned physiological or affective states. This general approach to craving has been criticized on both conceptual and empirical grounds (Marlatt, 1985; Tiffany, 1995). (See Vogel-Sprott & Fillmore, Chapter 8, this volume, for further discussion of classical conditioning effects.)

Expectancy Models of Craving

A number of theories have been proposed that emphasize positive cognitive expectancies that arise while craving (Marlatt, 1985; Wise, 1988). These expectancies have both motivational (a desire to experience an anticipated positive outcome) and cognitive (recognizing which specific activity will prove satisfying) properties. According to Marlatt (1985), craving should (1) enhance positive expectancies about drinking or drug use, and (2) be associated with reduced self-efficacy to cope with high-risk situations (i.e., refrain from drug use).

Several lines of research are pertinent to an expectancy model of craving and drug use. Goldman and colleagues have proposed that the cognitive structure (i.e., the organization of expectancy representations in memory) differs between heavy and light drinkers, with the former tending more strongly to endorse positive alcohol expectancies (Rather, Goldman, Roehrich, & Brannick, 1992). Presumably, heavier drinkers would have a number of positive expectancies immediately accessible when information pertaining to alcohol is activated in memory. Stacy (1995; 1997) has found that alcohol-related information appears to be more accessible among heavier drinkers, suggesting a stronger relationship between alcohol cues and the alcohol concept than in lighter drinkers. College student volunteers were presented with a word list and asked to write down the first word they could think of for each word on the list. Some of these listed words (e.g., "pitcher") were ambiguously related to alcohol. Results indicated that memory associations to the ambiguous alcohol stimuli predicted self-reported level of drinking (Stacy, 1997). Similar findings emerged using ambiguous visual images (Stacy, 1997).

The color-naming task also has been used to infer selective processing of addiction-related material. Alcoholics have demonstrated increased color-naming latencies when presented with alcohol-related words (Johnson, Laberg, Cox, Vaksdal, & Hugdahl, 1994; Stetter, Ackerman, Bizer, Strauube, & Mann, 1995). Studies that provide participants with anxiety cues, which for some drinkers may be associated with alcohol consumption, find an increase in the salience of alcohol-related information (Stewart, 1996). Although these studies have not manipulated cue-elicited craving and thus may not permit analysis of craving on expectancies (Tiffany, 1995), they nevertheless provide a conceptual underpinning, emphasizing changes in cognitive structures, for understanding how craving may facilitate drinking or drug use (see Goldman, Del Boca, & Darkes, Chapter 6, for a more detailed account of expectancy theory).

There have been some attempts to examine the effects of cue exposure on expectancies. Cooney, Gillespie, Baker, and Kaplan (1987) compared the responses of alcoholics and nonalcoholics during alcohol cue exposure. These authors found that alcoholic participants reported an increased desire to drink following alcohol cue exposure. In addition, alcohol's effects were rated more positively during alcohol cue exposure, though the pattern of data was less clear for a more specific measure of anticipated effects (see Tiffany, 1995). Sayette and Hufford (1997) conducted a study in which smokers reported as many positive and negative aspects of smoking as they could during each of two experimental conditions. Results indicated that smokers were able to generate a greater number of positive, but not negative, aspects of smoking during the high-craving session (involving nicotine deprivation and exposure to smoking cues), compared to the low-craving session (involving a nondeprived state and exposure to a control cue). While the data do not permit analysis of whether the shift was due to cue exposure, nicotine deprivation, or both, they are consistent with the view that craving leads to increased salience of positive aspects of drug use. Others have found that craving affects how drug-related information is evaluated. Brandon, Wetter, and Baker (1996) reported that smokers who experienced stronger cravings evaluated smoking consequences in a more reinforcing manner than did those reporting weaker cravings. Taken together, these findings support Marlatt's (1985) position that craving should be associated with enhanced positive expectancies about drug use.

Kunda's (1990) social-cognitive theory of motivated reasoning suggests a mechanism by which motivations or impulses can alter cognitive representations that is consistent with expectancy theories. According to Kunda, motivations can fundamentally alter how relevant information is generated and evaluated. Even when trying to accurately process information, we may be subject to motivationally relevant biases. It may be that drug cue–elicited craving produces motivational changes that in turn affect cognitive processes (Sayette & Hufford, 1997).

Research has focused on the effects of craving on self-efficacy to refrain from drug use. In a study described earlier, Cooney et al. (1987) found that during alcohol cue exposure, alcoholics reported a decreased self-efficacy to resist future drinking. This decreased self-efficacy may be an accurate representation of the difficulty facing alcoholics during craving situations. Abrams et al. (1991) found that during alcohol-specific role plays, the urge to drink was associated with reduced effectiveness in performing the role plays. Not surprisingly, relapse episodes often have been associated with a failure to use coping skills (Brandon, Tiffany, Obremski, & Baker, 1990; Shiffman, 1982).

Although more data are needed before firm conclusions can be drawn, initial findings suggest that craving may influence the anticipated effects of drinking or drug use. Further specification of the mechanisms underlying this expectancy model is needed to understand better the relationship between craving, drug use expectancies, and self-efficacy (Tiffany, 1995).

Two-Affect Model of Craving

Baker et al. (1987) proposed a two-affect model of craving that emphasizes the cognitive structure of urges. Their model is based on a bioinformational processing theory in which both emotional and procedural information are accessed in parallel as part of an associated, propositional network (Lang, 1984). Baker et al. (1987) posit two distinct, mutually inhibitory, craving networks that become more articulated with increased drug use. Activation of each network reflects the instantiation of different motivational states, which can be observed via multiple response systems. In addition to affect-related elements, procedural information regarding drug use is considered to be coded into these urge networks. The positive-affect network is activated by stimuli that direct pursuit of appetitive consequences, while the negative-affect network is activated by aversive stimuli that increase the withdrawal–relief incentive for drug use.

Several factors are identified that influence the relative activation of these two craving networks. The positive-affect network is believed to be activated during positive emotional states, when the drug is available for use, and during nondeprived states. The negative-affect system is triggered during states of withdrawal, drug unavailability, and during negative emotional states (Baker et al., 1987). According to this model, both urge magnitude and response coherence are increased as a function of the match between the situation and the urge network (Zinser, Baker, Sherman, & Cannon, 1992). Furthermore, Baker et al. (1987) postulate greater coherence across response systems in heavier users.

Implications of this model include recognition of two distinct types of cravings and the prediction that stimuli will have differential effects on craving, depending on the context in which they occur. For example, a stressor should have a greater impact on negative-affect-based cravings than positive-affect-based cravings. Consistent with this hypothesis, Zinser et al. (1992) found that stress was more likely to increase cravings in drug-deprived rather than nondeprived individuals. Other findings have not supported the model (see Tiffany, 1995). For example, self-report data suggesting the simultaneous anticipation of positive and negative reinforcement is inconsistent with the notion of two mutually inhibitory networks. More research, especially studies that do not rely solely on self-reports of urge and affect to infer the cognitive structure of craving, is needed to test more comprehensively aspects of this model. At a minimum, the Baker et al. research is valuable by articulating a testable theory of craving that can account for both positive- and negative-affect-related urges and that provides a framework for understanding the relationships between the various response systems used to assess craving.

Tiffany's (1990) Cognitive Model of Urge Responding

In contrast to models that link cue-elicited craving to drug use, Tiffany (1990) has proposed that the mechanisms underlying the relationship between drug cues and drug use are different from the mechanisms underlying craving. With repeated use, the act of drinking or drug taking becomes increasingly well learned, and in the addict, drug use becomes automatized.

For example, the act of getting up from a living room chair, walking to the kitchen, opening the refrigerator, removing a beer, twisting off the cap, lifting the bottle, and taking an initial drink may require virtually no cognitive effort for someone who has performed this action sequence countless times. Moreover, the stimulus-bound nature of automatized behaviors suggests that once the sequence is initiated, it will move to completion without intention. According to Tiffany, among nonabstinent alcoholics, once the drinking action sequence is elicited, in most cases, the chain of behaviors required to complete the routine will be executed without relying on nonautomatic processing.

Unlike the automatized behavior associated with habitual drug use, cravings are defined as a collection of verbal, somatovisceral, and behavioral responses supported by nonautomatic cognitive processes (Tiffany, 1990). Craving only occurs when execution of a well-learned pattern of responses culminating in drug use is blocked. This may happen if one wants to drink but alcohol is unavailable (abstinence avoidance) (e.g., there is no more beer in the refrigerator), or if one wishes to abstain (abstinence seeking). Under conditions in which the drug use routine has been triggered (by internal or environmental cues) but is not completed, nonautomatic processing resources are mobilized either to support or prevent the completion of this action sequence. Returning to the previous example, activation of nonautomatic resources occurring during urge responding could be manifested through (1) overt behaviors associated with traveling to the store; (2) verbal reports associated with a desire and intention to drink, perhaps frustration at having run out of alcohol, and if asked, problem-solving descriptions possibly associated with figuring out the nearest place to buy beer; and (3) physiological responses associated with problem solving or the anticipation of action (Tiffany, 1992).

There are several propositions emanating from Tiffany's (1990) model that distinguish it from other approaches to craving. First, it is posited that most habitual drug use in the addict is under the control of automatic cognitive processes. One implication of this assertion is that craving is neither necessary nor sufficient for drug use. That craving does not provide a sufficient condition for drug use is unlikely to be disputed. Even theorists espousing a classical conditioning approach to craving have observed that cravings may not be sufficient for drug use (e.g., Ludwig & Wikler, 1974). An alcoholic who is craving a drink may still decide to abstain. Nevertheless, the claim that craving is not necessary for drug use does contrast with many (e.g., Ludwig, Wikler & Stark, 1974), though not all (e.g., Baker et al., 1987; Kassel & Shiffman, 1992), accounts of addiction. The notion of an absentminded relapse, occurring without any conscious desire, or craving, is easily accommodated by Tiffany's (1990) theory.

A second proposition of Tiffany's cognitive model is that cravings are associated with nonautomatic processes. Support for this hypothesis comes from a number of sources. Years ago, investigators found that food deprivation elicited a variety of cognitive changes, including preoccupation with food and impaired concentration (Keys, Brozek, Henschel, Mickelson, & Taylor, 1950; Sorokin, 1942). More recently, a number of studies have indicated that craving disrupts nonautomatic processes (Tiffany, 1995). Wetter, Brandon, and Baker (1992) report a relationship between urge to smoke and errors on a design-tracing task. Sayette et al. (1994) found that exposure to drinking cues led alcoholic inpatients to respond more slowly during a response-time probe, suggesting that limited-capacity nonautomatic processing resources were diverted during the craving manipulation. This effect also has been reported in populations of smokers using a variety of craving manipulations (Cepeda-Benito & Tiffany; 1996; Juliano & Brandon, 1998; Sayette & Hufford, 1994). These performance deficits found across tasks suggest a demand on processing resources during craving. Determining the content of these nonautomatic cognitions is a more difficult matter.

Most craving theories assume that when an organism is craving, information that is associated with a drug or a drug's effects is activated in memory (Goldman & Rather, 1993; Marlatt, 1985; Stacy, 1997; Wise, 1988). Moreover, it is often assumed that such information motivates drug use. In contrast, Tiffany's model posits that nonautomatic cognitive resources associated with craving are activated as a result of an interruption of a well-learned action sequence. These resources are mobilized to cope with this interrupted routine. Indeed, drug craving is not qualitatively different from responses to any other interrupted routines. So, for example, if a coworker parks in my customary spot in the parking lot, I nevertheless may absentmindedly walk toward my familiar spot at day's end. I would suddenly realize that my car is elsewhere (and thus the habitual "walk to car" routine is blocked), and would begin mobilizing nonautomatic processing resources toward the task of locating my car. According to Tiffany's model, the craving I experience in the parking lot is "probably not" qualitatively different from the craving that an addict experiences when a drug routine is blocked (Tiffany, personal communication, September 10, 1997). In this regard, Tiffany's (1990) conceptualization of craving is quite different from the other craving formulations that have been described.

The position expressed in this chapter is that Tiffany's (1990) cognitive model and theories of craving emphasizing motivation need not be mutually exclusive. While craving, nonautomatic resources are likely to be directed toward several functions including, but not necessarily limited to, procedures involved in coping with an interrupted action sequence. Craving may activate any of the following cognitions: monitoring the level of motivation or desire to use the drug (e.g., "I really want a beer"); the drug cues themselves (e.g., thoughts of a cold frosty mug); thoughts related to anticipated positive effects of drug use (e.g., "If I drink this beer, then I will feel better"); feelings associated with the event (e.g., frustration that the beer has run out); as well as problem-solving cognitions associated with completing the drinking action plan (e.g., "How can I hide this drink from my spouse?"). Because nonautomatic resources might be directed toward the processing of all of these different cognitions during craving, it is difficult to declare which are responsible for the multidimensional responses associated with a craving state.

In Tiffany's (1990) model, the physiological correlates of craving reflect the problem solving components of preparing to cope with the interrupted drug use sequence. Self-reported craving need not correlate with physiological arousal, because the demands of the situation are considered to be relatively independent of the motivation for drug use. In other words, how badly one wants to drink does not affect how difficult it will be to figure out the location of an open liquor store. This account stands in contrast to models that assume that physiological responses reflect a motivation to use a drug or to experience the effects of a drug. As noted earlier, however, physiological responses may be supported by nonautomatic resources associated with a variety of cognitions, only some of which pertain to executing the drug use routine. Presumably, physiological responses can reflect motivation to use as well as efforts to cope with the interrupted drug use routine.

A final implication of Tiffany's model to be addressed concerns the importance of desire in craving. Desire along with frustration and intention to use, appears to be just one of a number of features of craving. It is unclear from Tiffany's model whether desire is necessary for craving to be experienced. While desire does not appear to be a central feature of craving in Tiffany's model, it plays a critical role in most other definitions of craving, including those found in general dictionaries. Many theorists argue that desire is the essence of craving. Indeed, many have suggested that verbal reports of craving be restricted to measures of desire (e.g., Kozlowski, Pilliteri, Sweeney, Whitfield, & Graham, 1996).

Summary

Although there are important conceptual differences among the models of craving and cue reactivity described here (see also Tiffany, 1995), from a cognitive perspective, there are also important similarities. These models share the assumption that information pertaining to drinking and drug use resides in memory networks. When primed, these networks activate information related to drinking or drug use. The various models emphasize activation of different types of information. The information may relate to drug use procedures that coordinate particular behaviors necessary for drug use (Tiffany, 1990), as well as information associated with expected drinking outcomes and cues or emotions associated with drinking or drug use (Baker et al., 1987; Stacy, 1997). These hypothesized cognitive networks are heuristic for understanding how stimuli can elicit craving and cue reactivity. Moreover, these different frameworks all suggest that information processing is fundamentally altered during craving. The continued use of cognitive methods to assess the processes and structures associated with craving will likely lead to improved understanding of the role of craving in the etiology of addiction.

COGNITIVE THEORY AND RESEARCH ON SELECTED OTHER DRUGS

Acute Psychological Effects of Drug Administration

Most investigation of the cognitive effects of drugs has involved alcohol, with less attention directed at cognitive effects of drugs such as cocaine or opiates. Numerous studies, however, have examined the effects of nicotine on cognitive processes associated with performance (for recent reviews, see Heishman, Taylor, & Henningfield, 1994; Kassel, 1997). Investigators of nicotine's effects on cognitive processes face methodological challenges not encountered in alcohol research. First, identifying a neutral baseline state is difficult. On the one hand, it is important that participants have not recently smoked. On the other hand, it does not take long before smokers can begin to experience subtle effects of nicotine withdrawal. Consequently, much research on nicotine's effects cannot disentangle putative cognitive-enhancing effects of nicotine from cognitive-disrupting effects of nicotine withdrawal (Heishman et al., 1994; Hughes, 1991). Second, unlike alcohol, it is difficult to experimentally control nicotine levels (Pomerleau, Pomerleau, & Rose, 1989) without altering the typical route of administration (e.g., using a nasal spray [Perkins et al., 1995]). Moreover, in many cases, it may be inadvisable to prevent participants from tailoring their own nicotine levels to test cognitive effects. Nicotine doses that diverge from a smoker's normal level may produce cognitive effects unlike those usually experienced by these smokers. Despite these methodological challenges, findings suggest that nicotine enhances cognitive performance. For instance, a number of studies indicate that nicotine improves several different types of attentional processes (e.g., selective attention, divided attention, and sustained attention [Kassel, 1997]). Recently, Steele and Josephs's (1988) attention-allocation theory of alcohol use has been applied to cigarette smoking. As was found with alcohol consumption (Steele & Josephs, 1988), Kassel and Shiffman (1997) found that smoking reduced stress only when paired with distracting activity.

Cue-Elicited Craving

Research on cue-elicited craving has focused on a range of drugs (see Carter & Tiffany, in press; Rohsenow, Niaura, Childress, Abrams, & Monti, 1990–1991). In addition to alcohol, many theories of craving are based on studies involving tobacco, cocaine, opiates, and even food (e.g., Kassel & Shiffman, 1992). A number of cognitive studies have been conducted to examine the impact of nicotine deprivation on the selective processing of smoking-related information. Zeitlan, Potts, and Hodder (1994) report that abstinent smokers recalled more smoking-related words than did nonabstinent smokers or nonsmokers. Using a perceptual identification task, Jarvik, Gross, Rosenblatt, and Stein (1995) found that nicotine-deprived, but not nondeprived, smokers identified more smoking-related words than food-related or neutral words. These authors also used a categorization task, in which smoking- or food-related words were rapidly presented. Participants were required to categorize the word as being either food- or smoking-related. Results were comparable to those found for the perceptual identification task, with abstinent smokers more quickly categorizing the smoking-related words than the food-related words (Jarvik et al., 1995). A similar effect of nicotine deprivation has been reported using a word-stem completion task, in which only the initial letters of drug-related or control words are provided (Zeitlan et al., 1994). Finally, a version of the color-naming task has been used to infer selective processing of smoking-related material following nicotine deprivation (Gross, Jarvik, & Rosenblatt, 1993). The results of these different studies suggest that craving manipulations elicit similar cognitive effects for alcohol and smoking.

While there have been a number of cognitive studies examining cue-elicited craving, there has been relatively little focus on satiety. Recent evidence suggests that satiety to foods may be cognitively mediated. Habituation to food cues, as measured by salivary response, was inhibited by allocating processing resources to nonfood cues, in this case, a controlled cognitive search task requiring nonautomatic processing resources (Epstein, Paluch, Smith, & Sayette, 1997). Stated differently, these data account for why one may be more likely to polish off a large bucket of popcorn while engrossed in a movie in a theater than when home alone in a room devoid of distraction. Research is needed to determine whether similar psychological mechanisms also underlie craving and satiety for alcohol and drugs.

The Effects of Alcohol Consumption on Concurrent Drug Use

The widespread prevalence of polydrug use has prompted efforts to examine the effects of craving for one drug while under the influence of another substance. Research indicates that drug relapse frequently occurs in the presence of alcohol consumption. For example, relapse to smoking occurs more often after alcohol consumption than any other identified situational variable (Shiffman & Balabanis, 1995). In addition to neurobiological and conditioning explanations for the association between these two substances (Niaura & Shiffman, 1995; Pomerleau, 1995), there are several cognitive theories that may explain the relationship.

According to Tiffany (1990), alcohol consumption often is a stimulus that activates a smoking routine while simultaneously producing a cognitive load that may impede the nonautomatic processing required to cope with smoking urges (i.e., either by attempting or avoiding abstinence). To-gether, these dual cognitive effects of alcohol consumption should increase the likelihood of smoking. Alternatively, both alcohol intoxication and drug-cue exposure may restrict processing resources to the most salient cues. Consequently, alcohol consumption, through its myopic effects (Steele & Josephs, 1990), may enhance the cognitive effects typically asso-ciated with drug craving. Recent data from a study that repeatedly exposed smokers to smoking and neutral cues indicated that alcohol intoxication in-creases smoking urge during both types of cue exposure (Burton & Tiffany, 1997). Assuming that smoking information was more salient during the smoking cue than neutral cue exposures in this repeated measures design, the data do not support the hypothesis that alcohol restricts attentional fo-cus to the most salient cues; that is, one would not expect alcohol to in-crease smoking craving during the neutral cue exposures. These data may be consistent with Tiffany's (1990) cognitive-processing model, which pos-its that alcohol consumption engages part of the stimulus complex activat-ing automatized smoking behavior, although, presumably, the combination of alcohol and smoking cue exposure would be more likely to activate the smoking routine than intoxication alone.

Loss-of-Control Drinking

Discussion of the effects of alcohol consumption on other drug use may have relevance to the concept of loss-of-control drinking. Although this term has been loosely applied to a variety of drinking phenomena, it gener-ally is associated with Jellinek's (1952, 1960) disease concept formulation. According to this view, the ingestion of even a small amount of alcohol triggers in alcoholics a physical demand for alcohol that overwhelms their ability to control subsequent drinking. Loss-of-control drinking (e.g., drinking until severely intoxicated) follows naturally from the initial drink and is considered a hallmark of alcoholism. Empirical research has called this formulation into question (see Mello, 1978). A single drink does not seem to produce an invariant and involuntary loss of control (Marlatt, Demming, & Reid, 1973). Nevertheless, cognitive theories may suggest several explanations why, under certain conditions, a few drinks may facili-tate a drinking or drug use binge.

For the same reason that alcohol consumption may increase the chance of engaging in other drug use, it may also facilitate continued and excessive drinking. With each drink that is consumed, the routine of getting drunk becomes more activated and the action sequence is more likely to be com-pleted. As Tiffany (1990) notes, cognitive processing resources are needed to resist completing a well-learned behavior sequence that has been acti-vated in memory. At the very time that such resources are required, the al-cohol that has already been consumed impairs nonautomatic processing, thereby reducing the resources that are available. One would expect all behaviors associated with drinking (e.g., getting drunk, smoking, using other drugs) to be more likely.

Excessive drinking may also be accounted for by an alcohol myopia framework (Steele & Josephs, 1990). The conflict about whether to continue drinking through the point of intoxication can be appropriately described as a case of inhibition conflict. Here, the impulse to experience the immediate reinforcing effects of the next drink conflicts with more distant, negative consequences. As the initial effects of alcohol begin to restrict the range of information capable of being processed, the more salient cues associated with the imminent pleasures of continuing to drink become increasing more powerful. Accordingly, for some individuals, craving for alcohol could be enhanced after a few drinks. Another cognitive explanation for excessive drinking is offered by Marlatt (1985), who suggests that the unpleasant effects of alcohol experienced on the descending limb of the blood alcohol concentration curve may trigger a desire to persist in drinking in an attempt to cope with dysphoria. Finally, Baumeister, Heatherton, and Tice (1994) suggest a number of cognitive mechanisms to explain how alcohol's impairment of self-regulatory processes may impede a drinker's ability to control the amount that has been consumed.

Unlike the original formulations of loss of control, a perspective drawn from cognitive theories can accommodate data revealing that drinking to excess is not inevitable among alcoholics. Decisions to engage in excessive drinking simply become more likely following initial consumption. A full accounting of the cognitive effects produced by the initial drinks must be understood in the context of other features of the alcoholic's internal and external environment, such as the cognitive set of the drinker, the particular social setting, and the reinforcement contingencies present in that situation (Baumeister et al., 1994; Wilson, 1987). In this regard, excessive drinking can be viewed in a similar fashion to other relationships, such as those between alcohol and anxiety, or alcohol and aggression. In each case, it is alcohol's pharmacological effects on cognitive processing that, in conjunction with individual difference and situational factors, determine the outcome.

FUTURE DIRECTIONS

Cognitive theory and research in the addictions seem to lag behind basic psychological research (Tiffany, 1991). It therefore may be instructive to examine some basic cognitive issues currently being addressed, as they also may be important to those studying drinking and drug use and abuse.

Traditionally cognitive psychologists have not considered emotion to be especially relevant to their work (see Zajonc, 1980). Recently, however, there has been a growing consensus that a comprehensive analysis of information processing must account for both cognition and affect (Eich, 1995;

Izard, Kagan, & Zajonc, 1984). Models of information processing from perspectives as diverse as neurobiology, cognitive psychology, computer science, and social problem solving (cf. Bower, 1981; Damasio, 1994; D'Zurilla, 1986; Elias, Branden-Muller, & Sayette, 1991; Lang, 1984; Rumelhart, 1997; Shizgal & Conover, 1996) now incorporate affect into their theories. As alcohol research embraces cognitive theory, it should also attend to the relationship between cognition and affect. Alcohol research that accounts for affective, motivational, as well as cognitive changes will provide the most comprehensive analysis of information processing (Lister et al., 1987). Research indicates, for example, that the rising limb of the blood alcohol concentration curve is associated with positive affect (Lukas & Mendelson, 1988; Martin, Earleywine, Musty, Perrine, & Swift, 1993). Elevated mood in turn may impact cognitive tasks initially designed for processes as diverse as attention, memory and decision making (Isen, 1984; Salovey, 1992; Teasdale & Fogarty, 1979; see also Lang, Patrick, & Stritzke, Chapter 9, this volume).

Second, alcohol research that examines the complex relationship between automatic and nonautomatic processing will be especially valuable. Researchers interested in cognitive processes should recognize that automaticity exists on a continuum and that putative measures of automaticity often draw on nonautomatic resources as well (Jacoby et al., 1997). Jacoby, Toth, and Yonelinas's (1993) process-dissociation procedure, which permits examination of automaticity in the context of nonautomatic processing, has recently been used to study the effects of alcohol (von Hippel, Hawkins, & Fu, 1994) and holds promise for detecting the complex effects of alcohol on automatic and nonautomatic processing.

Third, research directed at nonautomatic processing should focus on organization as well as limited-capacity dimensions of processing. With some exceptions (Birnbaum et al., 1980; Jones & Jones, 1977), most alcohol research has focused on the effects of intoxication on cognitive capacity. Recent cognitive research suggests, however, that organization may be an especially important determinant of learning and memory (Stadler, 1995). Moreover, organization and capacity reciprocally influence each other (Stadler, 1995), and models of alcohol that integrate them may prove useful in developing a more comprehensive understanding of alcohol's cognitive effects.

Fourth, addiction research may benefit from studies emphasizing temporal factors (Zakay & Block, 1997). Studies evaluating changes in the perception of time (e.g., Lapp, Collins, Zywiak, & Izzo, 1994) will likely improve understanding of cognitive effects of alcohol consumption. As noted earlier, the relationship between time and the value of potential reinforcers may shift during intoxication, making immediate reinforcers not only more salient, but also more attractive than distal reinforcers. It also has been suggested that shifts in temporal perception may play a role in self-control and decision-making processes related to addiction (Hoch & Loewenstein, 1991; Loewenstein, in press).

Fifth, the exigencies of alcohol research require that investigators modify some of the tasks developed for basic cognitive research. In particular, the affective and motivational changes produced by alcohol consumption or alcohol cues may impact on concentration and thus confound the tasks. For example, in many cognitive studies, it is not uncommon for semantic priming studies to include as many as 400 word pairs, requiring close to 1 hour to administer (e.g., Myers & Lorch, 1980). If intoxication alters motivation to sustain attention for long periods of time, then it becomes difficult to interpret putative alcohol-induced cognitive deficits. Development of modified tasks that are relatively brief may be needed in order to study the effects of alcohol (e.g., Sayette, Hufford, & Thorson, 1996).

Sixth, relatively little research has focused on alcohol's effects on the processing of complex social information (Pandina, 1982). Rarely have measures been included that directly assess these higher-order cognitive processes. Application of such measures, which have been developed in other areas of psychology (e.g., Dodge, 1986), is necessary if alcohol researchers are to link persuasively cognitive impairment to changes in social behavior.

Seventh, more attention needs to be directed toward examining the role of ethnicity and gender in understanding cognitive research in addiction. Few studies using appropriate controls have contrasted male and female aggression, and those that have do not show a clear pattern (see Chermack & Giancola, 1997). Research on sexual behavior indicates that at relatively high doses, women may be more likely than men to perceive that they are aroused, perhaps due to different social learning histories (Wilson, 1977; see also Maisto, Carey, & Bradizza, Chapter 4, this volume). Initial studies with female samples reported gender differences for alcohol's anxiolytic effects (Abrams & Wilson, 1979; Thombs, Beck, & Maloney, 1993; Wilson & Abrams, 1977; Wilson et al., 1989). To date, however, these differences have not revealed a consistent pattern. In the largest studies conducted in this area (Josephs & Steele, 1990; Levenson, Oyama, & Meek, 1987; Sayette, Breslin, Wilson, & Rosenblum, 1994b; Steele & Josephs, 1988), gender did not influence alcohol's effects on anxiety across a range of physiological and self-report measures. It may be that other types of measures, such as the emotional Stroop task or analyses of facial expressive behavior, would be more sensitive to gender differences than traditional measures. These latter measures may capture elements of cognitive appraisal that are less subject to response biases, and, in the case of facial coding, provide an assessment of emotional responding that has previously detected gender differences (e.g., Walbott & Scherer, 1991).

Relatively little research has examined possible gender differences in cue-elicited craving. In most cases, alcohol cue reactivity studies rely on samples of exclusively male alcoholics. Potential gender differences in cue-elicited craving may result from multiple sources. In addition to differences in how craving is experienced, certain craving manipulations and measures may be differentially sensitive to gender. With regard to manipulations, men and women may respond differently, depending on type of craving stimuli (Monti, Rohsenow, Colby, & Abrams, 1995; Niaura et al., 1998; Rubonis et al., 1994). With respect to measurement, gender may impact on sensitivity to different response domains. Sayette and Hufford (1995) found that, during a cigarette cue exposure manipulation, women were more likely than men to respond with emotion-related facial reactions. It is difficult to determine whether women were experiencing a more emotional response than men, or if they were simply more expressive. Clearly, more research investigating ethnic and gender differences is needed.

Finally, further advances derived from the application of cognitive theory to understanding the etiology of alcoholism require a multidisciplinary effort (Lister et al., 1987). Progress in cognitive psychology, neurobiology, cognitive psychophysiology, and decision science can all contribute to this effort. Integrating the findings from these different disciplines provides the best opportunity to develop cognitive theories that will prove heuristic for the study of alcohol and drug use and abuse.

CONCLUSIONS

Cognitive research has begun to shape current conceptualizations of drinking and alcoholism. Using quantifiable and objective measures, tentative inferences can be drawn about cognitive processes and structures that are etiologically related to alcoholism and other addictions. Cognitive research has provided frameworks for understanding the variable effects of alcohol consumption on behaviors and emotional states such as anxiety, aggression, and other high-risk behaviors. It also has led to testable predictions regarding both individual-difference and situational factors that may relate to the power of environmental and internal stimuli to trigger craving or drinking.

In addition to providing conceptual advances, cognitive research on addiction has important clinical implications. Cognitive-behavioral therapies emphasize that one's cognitive biases and distortions can contribute fundamentally to a range of psychopathological behaviors. Often, treatment involves helping patients uncover and modify these biases. In the field of addiction, preventing relapse has been the greatest clinical challenge (Brownell, Marlatt, Lichenstein, & Wilson, 1986; Marlatt & Gordon, 1985). The application of cognitive science to the study of addiction provides possible approaches to this vexing problem. Consider the challenges awaiting alcoholics or smokers who have only recently quit. Data from cognitive studies suggest that when they walk down the street, there appears to be much that reminds them of a drink or a cigarette. Certainly, bars or other obvious triggers will be noticed, but even ambiguous cues may remind them of their habit. These ambiguous, yet ubiquitous, cues serve to activate well-practiced drinking or smoking routines. Once initiated, limited cognitive resources must be directed toward resisting the completion of this drinking–action sequence. In essence, under certain conditions, the world can become one big temptation, requiring a vigilant effort to resist its allure.

In the safety of a clinic, patients may be told that they will be confronted with these temptations, and will need to rationally dispute their distorted perceptions and judgments that follow. Perhaps writing down the advantages and disadvantages of returning to their habit may help them to regain perspective. If this list of pros and cons is generated while craving, however, it may not resemble one constructed in a more neutral state of mind. While tempted, the mix of pros and cons may shift and the reinforcing consequences of drug use might be strengthened (Brandon et al., 1996; Sayette & Hufford, 1997). Suddenly, the decision to resume drinking or smoking may not appear to be such a bad idea.

Pavlov's research suggested the potential of cue exposure/response prevention to extinguish previously conditioned appetites. Yet it is only recently that addiction researchers have begun to focus on the clinical implications of this research (Blakey & Baker, 1980; Heather & Bradley, 1990). Poulos, Hinson, and Siegel (1981) suggest that treatment programs would fare better if they altered their sterile environments to include the types of drug cues likely to elicit cravings. Recent controlled clinical studies suggest that alcohol cue exposure may be a valuable component of treatment (Drummond & Glautier, 1994; Monti et al., 1993). In addition to conditioning models, cognitive theories also may account for the utility of cue exposure treatment (e.g., Marlatt, 1985). Treatment should include helping patients prepare to refrain from drinking in the context of the often-powerful cognitive shifts that occur outside the clinic. Craving induction treatments in which drinking is prevented may help patients learn to cope with temptations while they are experiencing them. Coping skills taught in the context of a craving manipulation may be especially effective (e.g., Monti et al., 1993). In addition to developing skills to deal with high-risk situations, patients also may enhance their self-efficacy, so that they will be able to cope, which also may prove important for preventing relapse (Wilson, 1987).

Interest in the application of cognitive theory to the study of alcohol use and abuse continues to grow. Improved methodology has facilitated investigation of subtle cognitive changes that affect a wide range of social behaviors and emotional states pertinent to the study of drinking and alcoholism. A cognitive approach to the study of alcohol's effects can accommodate the seemingly inconsistent effects of alcohol consumption on anxiety, aggression, and other high-risk behaviors, as well as the individual and situational differences that impact on alcohol's affects. Likewise, understanding the relationship between drug or alcohol cue-elicited craving and addiction also is improved by considering the changes in cognitive processing that occur during craving states. Attempts to apply the methods of cognitive psychology to the study of addiction have already shown promise. Nevertheless, it is crucial that investigators appreciate possible methodological differences between basic psychological research and addiction studies that can otherwise lead to confounds and interpretive difficulties. The methods of cognitive psychology likely will prove as valuable to the field of addiction as they have to psychology in general, but only if they are used wisely.

ACKNOWLEDGMENT

Preparation of this chapter was supported in part by grants from the National Institute on Alcohol Abuse and Alcoholism (No. AA09918-04) and the National Institute on Drug Abuse (No. DA10605-03). I thank Chris Martin and Jonathan Schooler for their helpful comments.

NOTES

1. These investigators also have obtained nonverbal measures of cognitive processing (e.g., Sayette, Monti, et al., 1994).

2. Although the utility of drawing a conceptual distinction between cognitive structures and processes, or even of including mental structures in conceptualizations of cognition, is not universally held (Kolers & Roediger, 1984), this approach has proven heuristic in cognitive analyses across a range of psychopathology (Kendall & Dobson, 1993).

3. I thank Jonathan Schooler for this observation.

4. For heuristic purposes, a spreading activation model, which has proven useful for describing a range of memory tasks, is adopted here. Nevertheless, a number of alternative models of associative recall could be used, and, currently, data do not exist to distinguish among them.

5. In this regard, these theories differ from earlier accounts of alcohol's effects on social behavior that emphasized the belief that one has consumed alcohol (Marlatt & Rohsenow, 1980). Much of the data supporting the effects of dosage–set on emotional or social behavior stem from studies using the balanced placebo design, in which participants consume either an alcoholic or nonalcoholic beverage and are informed that they are drinking either an alcohol or a nonalcoholic beverage. Though this 2×2 factorial design is purported to isolate the separate and interactive effects of alcohol and dosage–set, investigation of this assumption reveals critical limitations (Hull & Bond, 1986; Lyvers & Maltzman, 1991; Martin & Sayette, 1993; Ross & Pihl, 1989; Sayette, Breslin, Wilson, & Rosenblum, 1994a). Differences in interpersonal and intrapersonal responding between alcohol and placebo conditions have provided the crucial data supporting the view held by the self-awareness, alcohol myopia, and appraisal-disruption models that alcohol's effects on cognition are pharmacologically mediated.

REFERENCES

Abrams, D. B., Binkoff, J. A., Zwick, W. R., Liepman, M. R., Nirenberg, T. D., Munroe, S. M., & Monti, P. M. (1991). Alcohol abusers' and social drinkers' responses to alcohol-relevant and general situations. *Journal of Studies on Alcohol, 52,* 409–414.

Abrams, D. B., & Wilson, G. T. (1979). Effects of alcohol on social anxiety in women: Cognitive versus physiological processes. *Journal of Abnormal Psychology, 88,* 161–173.

Baars, B. J. (1986). *The cognitive revolution in psychology.* New York: Guilford Press.

Bailey, D. S., Leonard, K. E., Cranston, J. W., & Taylor, S. P. (1983). Effects of alcohol and self-awareness on human physical aggression. *Personality and Social Psychology Bulletin, 9,* 289–295.

Baker, T. B., Morse, E., & Sherman, J. E. (1987). The motivation to use drugs: A psychobiological analysis of urges. In C. Rivers (Ed.), *The Nebraska Symposium on Motivation: Alcohol use and abuse* (pp. 257–323). Lincoln: University of Nebraska Press.

Bannaji, M. R., & Steele, C. M. (1989). Alcohol and self-evaluation: Is a social cognition approach beneficial? *Social Cognition, 7,* 137–151.

Baumeister, R. F., Heatherton, T. F., & Tice, D. M. (1994). *Losing control: How and why people fail at self-regulation.* San Diego: Academic Press.

Birnbaum, I. M., Johnson, M. K., Hartley, J. T., & Taylor, T. H. (1980). Alcohol and elaborative schemas for sentences. *Journal of Experimental Psychology: Human Learning and Memory, 6,* 293–300.

Blakey, R., & Baker, R. (1980). An exposure approach to alcohol abuse. *Behaviour Research and Therapy, 18,* 319–325.

Bower, G. H. (1981). Mood and memory. *American Psychologist, 36,* 129–148.

Bower, G. H. (1987). Commentary on mood and memory. *Behaviour Research and Therapy, 25,* 443–456.

Brandon, T. H., Tiffany, S. T., Obremski, K. M., & Baker, T. B. (1990). Postcessation cigarette use: The process of relapse. *Addictive Behaviors, 15,* 105–114.

Brandon, T. H., Wetter, D. W., & Baker, T. B. (1996). Affect, expectancies, urges, and smoking: Do they conform to models of drug motivation and relapse? *Experimental and Clinical Psychopharmacology, 4,* 29–36.

Britton, B. K., & Tessor, A. (1982). Effects of prior knowledge on use of cognitive capacity in three complex cognitive tasks. *Journal of Verbal Learning and Verbal Behavior, 21,* 421–436.

Brownell, K. D., Marlatt, G. A., Lichenstein, E., & Wilson, G. T. (1986). Understanding and preventing relapse. *American Psychologist, 41,* 765–782.

Burton, S. M., & Tiffany, S. T. (1997). The effect of alcohol consumption on craving to smoke. *Addiction, 92,* 15–26.

Carter, B. L., & Tiffany, S. T. (in press). Meta-analysis of cue reactivity in addiction research. *Addiction.*

Caudill, B. D., Wilson, G. T., & Abrams, D. B. (1987). Alcohol and self-disclosure: Analyses of interpersonal behavior in male and female social drinkers. *Journal of Studies on Alcohol, 48,* 401–409.

Cepeda-Benito, A., & Tiffany, S. T. (1996). The use of a dual-task procedure for the assessment of cognitive effort associated with cigarette craving. *Psychopharmacology, 127*, 155–163.

Chassin, L., Mann, L. M., & Sher, K. J. (1988). Self-awareness theory, family history of alcoholism, and adolescent involvement. *Journal of Abnormal Psychology, 97*, 206–217.

Chermack, S. T., & Giancola, P. R. (1997). The relation between alcohol and aggression: An integrated biopsychosocial conceptualization. *Clinical Psychology Review, 17*, 621–649.

Collins, A. M., & Loftus, E. F. (1975). A spreading–activation theory of semantic processing. *Psychological Review, 82*, 407–428.

Conger, J. (1956). Reinforcement theory and the dynamics of alcoholism. *Quarterly Journal of Studies on Alcohol, 17*, 296–305.

Cooney, N. L., Gillespie, R. A., Baker, L. H., & Kaplan, R. F. (1987). Cognitive changes after alcohol cue exposure. *Journal of Consulting and Clinical Psychology, 55*, 150–155.

Damasio, A. R. (1994). *Descartes' error: Emotion, reason, and the human brain.* New York: Putnam's Sons.

Daneman, M., & Carpenter, P. A. (1980). Individual differences in working memory and reading. *Journal of Verbal Learning and Verbal Behavior, 19*, 450–466.

Dember, W. N. (1974). Motivation and the cognitive revolution. *American Psychologist, 29*, 161–168.

de Ruiter, C., & Brosschot, J. F. (1994). The emotional Stroop interference effect in anxiety: Attentional bias or cognitive avoidance? *Behaviour Research and Therapy, 32*, 315–319.

Dobson, K. S., & Kendall, P. C. (Eds.). (1993). *Psychopathology and cognition.* San Diego: Academic Press.

Dodge, K. (1986). A social information processing model of social competence in children. In M. Perlmutter (Ed.), *Cognitive perspectives on children's social and behavioral development* (Minnesota Symposia on Child Psychology, Vol. 18, pp. 77–125). Hillsdale, NJ: Erlbaum.

Dollard, J., & Miller, N. E. (1950). *Personality and psychotherapy: An analysis in terms of learning, thinking, and culture.* New York: McGraw-Hill.

Drummond, C. D., & Glautier, S. P. (1994). A controlled trial of cue exposure treatment in alcohol dependence. *Journal of Consulting and Clinical Psychology, 62*, 809–817.

D'Zurilla, T. J. (1986). *Problem solving therapy: A social competence approach to clinical intervention.* New York: Springer.

Eich, E. (1995). Searching for mood dependent memory. *Psychological Science, 6*, 67–75.

Elias, M. J., Brandan-Muller, L. R., & Sayette, M. A. (1991). Teaching the foundations of social decision making and problem solving in the elementary school. In J. Baron & R. Brown (Eds.), *Teaching decision making to adolescents* (pp. 161–184). Hillsdale, NJ: Erlbaum.

Epstein, L. H., Paluch, R., Smith, J. D., & Sayette, M. (1997). Allocation of attentional resources during habituation to food cues. *Psychophysiology, 34*, 59–64.

Fowler, C. A., Wolford, G., Slade, R., & Tassinary, L. (1981). Lexical access with and without awareness. *Journal of Experimental Psychology: General, 110*, 341–362.

Frankenstein, W., & Wilson, G. T. (1984). Alcohol's effects on self-awareness. *Addictive Behaviors, 9*, 323–328.

Fromme, K., Katz, E., & D'Amico, E. (1997). Effects of alcohol intoxication on the perceived consequences of risk taking. *Experimental and Clinical Psychopharmacology, 5*, 14–23.

Goldman, M. S., & Rather, B. C. (1993) Substance use disorders: Cognitive models and architecture. In K. S. Dobson & P. C. Kendall (Eds.), *Psychopathology and cognition* (pp. 246–292). San Diego: Academic Press.

Gross, T., Jarvik, M., & Rosenblatt, M. (1993). Nicotine abstinence produces content-specific Stroop interference. *Psychopharmacology, 110*, 333–336.

Hammersley, R. (1994). A digest of memory phenomena for addiction research. *Addiction, 89*, 283–293.

Hashtroudi, S., Parker, E. S., DeLisi, L. E., Wyatt, R. J., & Mutter, S. A. (1984). Intact retention in acute alcohol amnesia. *Journal of Experimental Psychology: Learning, Memory, and Cognition, 10*, 156–163.

Heather, N., & Bradley, B. P. (1990). Cue exposure as a practical treatment for addictive disorders: Why are we waiting? *Addictive Behaviors, 15*, 335–337.

Heishman, S. J., Taylor, R. C., & Henningfield, J. E. (1994). Nicotine and smoking: A review of effects on human performance. *Experimental and Clinical Psychopharmacology, 2*, 345–395.

Hoch, S. J., & Loewenstein, G. F. (1991). Time-inconsistent preferences and consumer self-control. *Journal of Consumer Research, 17*, 492–507.

Holender, D. (1986). Semantic activation without conscious identification in dichotic listening, parafovial vision, and visual masking: A survey and appraisal. *Behavioral and Brain Sciences, 9*, 1–23.

Hughes, J. (1991). Distinguishing withdrawal relief and direct effects of smoking. *Psychopharmacology, 104*, 409–410.

Hull, J. G. (1981). A self-awareness model of the causes and effects of alcohol consumption. *Journal of Abnormal Psychology, 90*, 586–600.

Hull, J. G. (1987). Self-awareness model. In H. T. Blane & K. E. Leonard (Eds.), *Psychological theories of drinking and alcoholism* (pp. 272–304). New York: Guilford Press.

Hull, J. G., & Bond, C. F. (1986). Social and behavioral consequences of alcohol consumption and expectancy: A meta-analysis. *Psychological Bulletin, 99*, 347–360.

Hull, J. G., Levenson, R. W., Young, R. D., & Sher, K. J. (1983). Self-awareness reducing effects of alcohol consumption. *Journal of Personality and Social Psychology, 44*, 461–473.

Hull, J. G., & Levy, A. S. (1979). The organizational functions of the self: An alternative to the Duval and Wicklund model of self-awareness. *Journal of Personality and Social Psychology, 37*, 756–768.

Hull, J. G., & Reilly, N. P. (1983). Self-awareness, self-regulation, and alcohol consumption: A reply to Wilson. *Journal of Abnormal Psychology, 92*, 514–519.

Hull, J. G., & Van Treuren, R. R. (1986). Experimental social psychology and the causes and effects of alcohol consumption. In H. D. Cappell (Ed.), *Research advances in alcohol and drug problems* (Vol. 9, pp. 211–244). New York: Plenum.

Hull, J. G., Young, R. D., & Jouriles, E. (1986). Applications of the self-awareness model of alcohol consumption. *Journal of Personality and Social Psychology, 51*, 790–796.

Isen, A. M. (1984). Toward understanding the role of affect in cognition. In R. S. Wyer & T. K. Srull (Eds.), *Handbook of social cognition* (Vol. 3, pp. 179–236). Hillsdale, NJ: Erlbaum.

Ito, T. A., Miller, N., & Pollock, V. E. (1996). Alcohol and aggression: A meta-analysis on the moderating effects of inhibitory cues, triggering events, and self-focused attention. *Psychological Bulletin, 120*, 60–82.

Izard, C. E., Kagan, J., & Zajonc, R. B. (Eds.). (1984). *Emotions, cognitions, and behavior*. New York: Cambridge University Press.

Jacoby, L. L., Toth, J. P., & Yonelinas, A. P. (1993). Separating conscious and unconscious influences of memory: Attention, awareness, and control. *Journal of Experimental Psychology: General, 122*, 539–154.

Jacoby, L. L., Yonelinas, A. P., & Jennings, J. M. (1997). The relation between conscious and unconscious (automatic) influences: A declaration of independence. In J. D. Cohen & J. W. Schooler (Eds.), *Scientific approaches to consciousness* (pp. 13–48). Mahwah, NJ: Erlbaum.

Jarvik, M., Gross, T., Rosenblatt, M., & Stein, R. (1995). Enhanced lexical processing of smoking stimuli during smoking abstinence. *Psychopharmacology, 118*, 136–141.

Jellinek, E. M. (1952). The phases of alcohol addiction. *Quarterly Journal of Studies on Alcohol, 13*, 673–684.

Jellinek, E. M. (1960). *The disease concept of alcoholism*. New Brunswick, NJ: Hillhouse Press.

Johnson, B. H., Laberg, J., Cox, W. M., Vaksdal, A., & Hugdahl, K. (1994). Alcoholics' attentional bias in the processing of alcohol-related words. *Psychology of Addictive Behaviors, 8*, 111–115.

Jones, B. M., & Jones, M. K. (1977). Alcohol and memory impairment in male and female social drinking. In I. M. Birnbaum & E. S. Parker (Eds.), *Alcohol and human memory* (pp. 127–138). Hillsdale, NJ: Erlbaum.

Josephs, R. A., & Steele, C. M. (1990). The two faces of alcohol myopia: Attentional mediation of psychological stress. *Journal of Abnormal Psychology, 99*, 115–126.

Juliano, L. M., & Brandon, T. H. (1998). Reactivity to instructed smoking availability and environmental cues: Evidence with urge and reaction time. *Experimental and Clinical Psychopharmacology, 6*, 45–53.

Just, M. A., & Carpenter, P. A. (1992). A capacity theory of comprehension: Individual differences in working memory. *Psychological Review, 99*, 122–149.

Kahneman, D., & Treisman, A. (1984). Changing views of attention and automaticity. In R. Parasuraman & D. Davies (Eds.), *Varieties of attention* (pp. 29–62). New York: Academic Press.

Kahneman, D., & Tversky, A. (1972). Subjective probability: A judgment of representativeness. *Cognitive Psychology, 3*, 430–451.

Kassel, J. D. (1997). Smoking and attention: A review and reformulation of the stimulus filter hypothesis. *Clinical Psychology Review, 17*, 451–478.

Kassel J. D., & Shiffman, S. (1992). What can hunger teach us about drug craving? A comparative analysis of the two constructs. *Advances in Behaviour Research and Therapy, 14*, 141–167.

Kassel, J. D., & Shiffman, S. (1997). Attentional mediation of cigarette smoking's effect on anxiety. *Health Psychology, 16*, 359–368.

Kendall, P. C., & Dobson, K. S. (1993). On the nature of cognition and its role in psychopathology. In K. S. Dobson & P. C. Kendall (Eds.), *Psychopathology and cognition* (pp. 3–17). San Diego, CA: Academic Press.

Kerr, B. (1973). Processing demands during mental operations. *Memory and Cognition, 1,* 401–412.

Keys, A., Brozek, J., Henschel, A., Mickelsen, O., & Taylor, H. L. (1950). *The biology of human starvation: Volume 2.* Minneapolis: University of Minnesota Press.

Kolers, P. A., & Roediger, H. L. (1984). Procedures of mind. *Journal of Verbal Learning and Verbal Behavior, 23,* 425–449.

Koob, G. F., & Bloom, F. E. (1988). Cellular and molecular mechanisms of drug dependence. *Science, 242,* 715–723.

Kozlowski, L. T., Pillitteri, J. L., Sweeney, C. T., Whitfield, K. E., & Graham, J. W. (1996). Asking questions about urges or cravings for cigarettes. *Psychology of Addictive Behaviors, 10,* 248–260.

Kozlowski, L. T., & Wilkinson, D. A. (1987). Use and misuse of the concept of craving by alcohol, tobacco, and drug researchers. *British Journal of Addiction, 82,* 31–36.

Kunda, Z. (1990). The case for motivated reasoning. *Psychological Bulletin, 108,* 480–498.

Lang, P. (1984). Cognition in emotion: Concept and action. In C. E. Izard, J. Kagan, & R. B. Zajonc (Eds.), *Emotions, cognitions, and behavior* (pp. 192–226). New York: Cambridge University Press.

Lapp, W. M., Collins, R. L., & Izzo, C. V. (1990, November). *An interaction of the psychological and pharmacological effects of alcohol on the speed of retrieval from episodic memory.* Paper presented at the annual meeting of the Association for Advancement of Behavior Therapy, San Francisco, CA.

Lapp, W. M., Collins, R. L., Zywiak, W. H., & Izzo, C. V. (1994). Psychopharmacological effects of alcohol on time perception: The extended balanced placebo design. *Journal of Studies on Alcohol, 55,* 96–112.

Lazarus, R. S., & Folkman, S. (1984). *Stress, appraisal, and coping.* New York: Springer.

Leonard, K. E. (1989). The impact of explicit aggressive and implicit nonaggressive cues on aggression in intoxicated and sober males. *Personality and Social Psychology Bulletin, 15,* 390–400.

Levenson, R. W., Oyama, O. N., & Meek, P. S. (1987). Greater reinforcement from alcohol for those at risk: Parental risk, personality risk, and sex. *Journal of Abnormal Psychology, 96,* 242–253.

Lister, R. G., Eckardt, M. J., & Weingartner, H. (1987). Ethanol intoxication and memory: Recent developments and new directions. In M. Galanter (Ed.), *Recent developments in alcoholism* (pp. 111–126). New York: Plenum Press.

Loewenstein, G. F. (in press). A visceral account of addiction. In J. Elster & O. J. Skog (Eds.), *Getting hooked: rationality and addiction.* Cambridge, UK: Cambridge University Press.

Lorch, R. F. (1982). Priming and search processes in semantic memory. A test of three models of spreading activation. *Journal of Verbal Learning and Verbal Behavior, 21,* 468–492.

Ludwig, A. M., & Wikler, A. (1974). "Craving" and relapse to drink. *Quarterly Journal of Studies on Alcohol, 35,* 108–130.

Ludwig, A. M., Wikler, A., & Stark, L. H. (1974). The first drink: Psychobiological aspects of craving. *Archives of General Psychiatry, 30,* 539–547.

Lukas, S., & Mendelson, J. (1988). Electroencephalographic activity and plasma ACTH during ethanol-induced euphoria. *Biological Psychiatry, 23,* 141–148.

Lyvers, M. F., & Maltzman, I. (1991). The balanced placebo design: Effects of alcohol and beverage instructions cannot be independently assessed. *International Journal of the Addictions, 26,* 963–972.

MacDonald, T. K., Zanna, M. P., & Fong, G. T. (1995). Decision making in altered states: Effects of alcohol on attitudes toward drinking and driving. *Journal of Personality and Social Psychology, 68,* 973–985.

MacDonald, T. K., Zanna, M. P., & Fong, G. T. (1996). Why common sense goes out the window: Effects of alcohol on intentions to use condoms. *Personality and Social Psychology Bulletin, 22,* 763–775.

MacDonald, T. K., Zanna, M. P., & Fong, G. T. (1998). Alcohol and intentions to engage in risky health-related behaviours: Experimental evidence for a causal relationship. In J. Adair, D. Berlanger, & K. L. Dion (Eds.), *Advances in psychological science: Vol. 1. Social, personal, and cultural aspects* (pp. 407–428). Hore, UK: Psychology Press/Erlbaum.

MacLeod, C., & Hagan, R. (1992). Individual differences in the selective processing of threatening information, and emotional responses to a stressful life event. *Behaviour Research and Therapy, 30,* 151–161.

MacLeod, C. M., & Rutherford, E. M. (1992). Anxiety and the selective processing of emotional information: Mediating roles of awareness, trait and state variables, and personal relevance of stimulus materials. *Behaviour Research and Therapy, 30,* 479–491.

Mann, R. E., Cho-Young, J., & Vogel-Sprott, M. (1984). Retrograde enhancement by alcohol of delayed free recall performance. *Pharmacology, Biochemistry, and Behavior, 20,* 639–642.

Marcel, A. J. (1983). Conscious and unconscious perception: Experiments on visual masking and word recognition. *Cognitive Psychology, 15,* 197–237.

Marlatt, G. A. (1985). Cognitive factors in the relapse process. In G. A. Marlatt & J. R. Gordon (Eds.), *Relapse prevention: Maintenance strategies in the treatment of addictive behaviors* (pp. 128–200). New York: Guilford Press.

Marlatt, G. A., Demming, B., & Reid, J. B. (1973). Loss of control drinking in alcoholics: An experimental analogue. *Journal of Abnormal Psychology, 81,* 233–241.

Marlatt, G. A., & Gordon, J. R. (Eds.). (1985). *Relapse prevention: Maintenance strategies in the treatment of addictive behaviors.* New York: Guilford Press.

Marlatt, G. A., & Rohsenow, D. J. (1980). Cognitive processes in alcohol use: Expectancy and the balanced placebo design. In N. K. Mello, (Ed.), *Advances in substance abuse: Behavioral and biological research* (Vol. 1, pp. 159–199). Greenwich, CT: JAI Press.

Martin, C., Earleywine, M., Musty, R., Perrine, M., & Swift, R. (1993). Development and validation of the Biphasic Alcohol Effects Scale. *Alcoholism: Clinical and Experimental Research, 17,* 140–146.

Martin, C., & Sayette, M. (1993). Experimental design in alcohol administration research: Limitations and alternatives in the manipulation of dosage–set. *Journal of Studies on Alcohol, 54,* 750–761.

Martin, M., Williams, R. M., & Clark, D. M. (1991). Does anxiety lead to selective processing of threat-related information? *Behaviour Research and Therapy, 29,* 147–160.

Mathews, A., & Klug, F. (1993). Emotionality and interference with color-naming in anxiety. *Behaviour Research and Therapy, 31,* 57–62.

Maylor, E. A., & Rabbit, P. M. A. (1993). Alcohol, reaction time and memory: A meta-analysis. *British Journal of Psychology, 84,* 301–317.

Mello, N. K. (1978). A semantic aspect of alcoholism. In H. D. Cappell & A. E. LeBlanc (Eds.), *Biological and behavioral approaches to drug dependence* (pp. 73–87). Toronto: Addiction Research Foundation.

Monti, P. M., Rohsenow, D. J., Colby, S. M., & Abrams, D. B. (1995). Smoking among alcoholics during and after treatment: Implications for models, treatment strategies, and policy. In J. B. Fertig & J. P. Allen (Eds.), *Alcohol and tobacco: From basic science to clinical practice* (Research Monograph No. 30, pp. 187–206, National Institute on Alcohol Abuse and Alcoholism, NIH Publication No. 95-3931). Washington, DC: U.S. Government Printing Office.

Monti, P. M., Rohsenow, D. J., Rubonis, A. V., Niaura, R. S., Sirota, A. D., Colby, S. M., Goddard, P., & Abrams, D. B. (1993). Cue exposure with coping skills treatment for male alcoholics: A preliminary investigation. *Journal of Consulting and Clinical Psychology, 61,* 1011–1019.

Moskowitz, H. (1973). Laboratory studies of the effects of alcohol on some variables related to driving. *Journal of Safety Research, 5,* 185–199.

Myers, J. L., & Lorch, R. F. (1980) Interference and facilitation effects of primes upon verification processes. *Memory and Cognition, 8,* 405–414.

Neely, J. (1991). Semantic priming effects in visual word recognition: A selective review of current findings and theories. In D. Besner & G. W. Humphreys (Eds.), *Basic processes in reading: Visual word recognition* (pp. 264–336). Hillsdale, NJ: Erlbaum.

National Institute on Alcohol Abuse and Alcoholism. (1997, October). *National Institute on Alcohol Abuse and Alcoholism: Treatment and Alcohol Craving Workshop.* Washington, DC: Author.

National Institute on Drug Abuse. (1998, May). *National Institute on Drug Abuse: Craving Consensus Workshop.* Rockville, MD: Author.

Niaura, R. S., Rohsenow, D. J., Binkoff, J. A., Monti, P. M., Pedraza, M., & Abrams, D. B. (1988). Relevance of cue reactivity to understanding alcohol and smoking relapse. *Journal of Abnormal Psychology, 97,* 133–152.

Niaura, R., Shadel, W. G., Abrams, D. B., Monti, P. M., Rohsenow, D. J., & Sirota, A. (1998). Individual differences in cue reactivity among smokers trying to quit: Effects of gender and cue type. *Addictive Behaviors, 23,* 209–224 .

Niaura, R., & Shiffman, S. (1995). Overview of section 1: Psychological and biological mechanisms. In J. B. Fertig & J. P. Allen (Eds.), *Alcohol and tobacco: From basic science to clinical practice* (Research Monograph No. 30, pp. 159–168, National Institute on Alcohol Abuse and Alcoholism, NIH Publication No. 95-3931). Washington, DC: U.S. Government Printing Office.

Niaura, R., Wilson, G. T., & Westrick, E. (1988). Self-awareness, alcohol consumption, and reduced cardiovascular reactivity. *Psychosomatic Research, 50,* 360–380.

Nisbett, R. E., & Ross, L. (1980). *Human inference: Strategies and shortcomings of social judgment.* Englewood Cliffs, NJ: Prentice-Hall.

Nisbett, R., & Wilson, T. D. (1977). Telling more than we know: Verbal reports on mental processes. *Psychological Review, 84,* 231–259.

Noel, N. E., Lisman, S. A., Schare, M. L., & Maisto, S. A. (1992). Effects of alcohol consumption on the prevention and alleviation of stress-reactions. *Addictive Behaviors, 17,* 567–577.

Pandina, R. J. (1982). Effects of alcohol on psychological processes. In E. Gomberg, H. White, & J. A. Carpenter (Eds.), *Alcohol, science, and society revisited* (pp. 38–62). Ann Arbor: University of Michigan Press.

Parker, E. S., Morisa, J., Wyatt, R. J., Schwartz, B., Weingartner, H., & Stillman, R. C. (1981). The alcohol facilitation effect on memory: A dose response study. *Psychopharmacology, 74,* 88–92.

Perkins, K. A., Sexton, J. E., DiMarco, A., Grobe, J. E., Scierka, A., & Stiller, R. L. (1995). Subjective and cardiovascular responses to nicotine combined with alcohol in male and female smokers. *Psychopharmacology, 19,* 205–212.

Peterson, J. B., Finn, P. R., & Pihl, R. O. (1992). Cognitive dysfunction and the inherited predisposition to alcoholism. *Journal of Studies on Alcohol, 53,* 154–160.

Pomerleau, O. F. (1995). Neurobiological interactions of alcohol and nicotine. In J. B. Fertig & J. P. Allen (Eds.), *Alcohol and tobacco: From basic science to clinical practice* (Research Monograph No. 30, pp. 145–158, National Institute on Alcohol Abuse and Alcoholism, NIH Publication No. 95-3931). Washington, DC: U.S. Government Printing Office.

Pomerleau, O. F., Pomerleau, C. S., & Rose, J. E. (1989). Controlled dosing of nicotine: A review of problems and progress. *Annals of Behavioral Medicine, 11,* 158–163.

Poulos, C. X., Hinson, R. E., & Siegel, S. (1981). The role of Pavlovian processes in drug tolerance and dependence: Implications for treatment. *Addictive Behaviors, 6,* 205–211.

Rather, B. C., Goldman, M. S., Roehrich, L., & Brannick, M. (1992). Empirical modeling of an alcohol expectancy memory network using multidimensional scaling. *Journal of Abnormal Psychology, 101,* 174–183.

Robinson, T., & Berridge, K. (1993). The neural basis of craving: An incentive–sensitization theory of addiction. *Brain Research Reviews, 18,* 247–291.

Rohsenow, D. J., Monti, P. M., Rubonis, A. V., Sirota, A, Niaura, R. S., Colby, S., Wunschel, S., & Abrams, D. B. (1994). Cue reactivity as a predictor of drinking among male alcoholics. *Journal of Consulting and Clinical Psychology, 62,* 620–626.

Rohsenow, D. J., Niaura, R. S., Childress, A. R., Abrams, D. B., & Monti, P. M. (1990–1991). Cue reactivity in addictive behaviors: Theoretical and treatment implications. *International Journal of the Addictions, 25,* 957–993.

Room, R., & Collins, G. (Eds.). (1983). *Alcohol and disinhibition: Nature and meaning of the link* (Research Monograph No. 12, National Institute on Alcohol Abuse and Alcoholism, DHHS Pub. No. 83-1246). Washington, DC: U. S. Government Printing Office.

Ross, D. F., & Pihl, R. O. (1989). Modification of the balanced placebo design for use at high blood alcohol levels. *Addictive Behaviors, 14,* 91–97.

Rubonis, A. V., Colby, S. M., Monti, P. M., Rohsenow, D. J., Gulliver, S. B., & Sirota, A. D. (1994). Alcohol cue reactivity and mood induction in male and female alcoholics. *Journal of Studies on Alcohol, 55,* 487–494.

Rumelhart, D. E. (1997). Affect and neuromodulation: A connectionist approach. In J. D. Cohen & J. W. Schooler (Eds.), *Scientific approaches to consciousness* (pp. 469–477). Mahwah, NJ: Erlbaum.

Salovey, P. (1992). Mood-induced self-focused attention. *Journal of Personality and Social Psychology, 62,* 699–707.

Sayette, M. A. (1993). An appraisal-disruption model of alcohol's effects on stress responses in social drinkers. *Psychological Bulletin, 114,* 459–476.

Sayette, M. A. (1994). Effects of alcohol on self-appraisal. *International Journal of the Addictions, 29,* 127–133.

Sayette, M. A., Breslin, F. C., Wilson, G. T., & Rosenblum, G. (1994a). An investigation of the balanced placebo design in alcohol administration research. *Addictive Behaviors, 19,* 333–342.

Sayette, M. A., Breslin, F. C., Wilson, G. T., & Rosenblum, G. (1994b). Parental history of alcohol abuse and the effects of alcohol and expectations of intoxication on social stress. *Journal of Studies on Alcohol, 55,* 214–223.

Sayette, M. A., & Hufford, M. R. (1994). Effects of cue exposure and deprivation on cognitive resources in smokers. *Journal of Abnormal Psychology, 103,* 812–818.

Sayette, M. A., & Hufford, M. R. (1995). Urge and affect: A facial coding analysis of smokers. *Experimental and Clinical Psychopharmacology, 3,* 417–423.

Sayette, M. A., & Hufford, M. R. (1997). Effects of smoking urge on generation of smoking-related information. *Journal of Applied Social Psychology, 27,* 1395–1405.

Sayette, M. A., Hufford, M. R., & Thorson, G. (1996). Validating a brief measure of semantic priming. *Journal of Clinical and Experimental Neuropsychology, 18,* 678–684.

Sayette, M. A., Monti, P. M., Rohsenow, D. J., Bird-Gulliver, S., Colby, S., Sirota, A., Niaura, R. S., & Abrams, D. B. (1994). The effects of cue exposure on attention in male alcoholics. *Journal of Studies on Alcohol, 55,* 629–634.

Sayette, M. A., Smith, D. W., Breiner, M. J., & Wilson, G. T. (1992). The effect of alcohol on emotional response to a social stressor. *Journal of Studies on Alcohol, 53,* 541–545.

Sayette, M. A., & Wilson, G. T. (1991). Intoxication and exposure to stress: The effects of temporal patterning. *Journal of Abnormal Psychology, 100,* 56–62.

Sayette, M. A., Wilson, G. T., & Carpenter, J. A. (1989). Cognitive Moderators Of alcohol's effects on anxiety. *Behaviour Research and Therapy, 27,* 685–690.

Sayette, M. A., Wilson, G. T., & Elias, M. (1993). Alcohol and aggression: A social information processing analysis. *Journal of Studies on Alcohol, 54,* 399–407.

Schacter, D. (1987). Implicit memory: history and status. *Journal of Experimental Psychology: Learning, Memory and Cognition, 13,* 501–518.

Schneider, W., Dumais, S. T., & Shiffrin, R. M. (1984). Automatic and control processing and attention. In R. Parasuraman & D. R. Davies (Eds.), *Varieties of attention* (pp. 1–27). New York: Academic Press.

Segal, Z. V., & Cloitre, M. (1993). Methodologies for studying cognitive features of emotional disorder. In K. S. Dobson & P. C. Kendall (Eds.), *Psychopathology and cognition* (pp. 19–50). San Diego: Academic Press.

Sher, K. J. (1987). Stress response dampening. In H. T. Blane & K. E. Leonard (Eds.), *Psychological theories of drinking and alcoholism* (pp. 227–271). New York: Guilford Press.

Sher, K. J., & Walitzer, K. S. (1986). Individual differences in the stress-response-dampening effect of alcohol: A dose–response study. *Journal of Abnormal Psychology, 95,* 159–167.

Shiffman, S. (1982). Relapse following smoking cessation: A situational analysis. *Journal of Consulting and Clinical Psychology, 50,* 71–86.

Shiffman, S., & Balabanis, M. (1995). Associations between alcohol and tobacco. In J. B. Fertig & J. P. Allen (Eds.), *Alcohol and tobacco: From basic science to clinical practice* (Research Monograph No. 30, pp. 17–36, National Institute on Alcohol Abuse and Alcoholism, NIH Publication No. 95-3931). Washington, DC: U.S. Government Printing Office.

Shiffman, S., Engberg, J. B., Paty, J. A., Perz, W. G., Gnys, M., Kassel, J. D., & Hickox, M. (1997). A day at a time: Predicting smoking lapse from daily urge. *Journal of Abnormal Psychology, 106,* 104–116.

Shiffrin, R. M. (1988). Attention. In R. A. Atkinson, R. J. Herrnstein, G. Lindzey, & R. D. Luce (Eds.), *Steven's handbook of experimental psychology: Vol. 2. Learning and cognition* (pp. 739–811). New York: Wiley.

Shiffrin, R. M. (1997). Attention, automatism, and consciousness. In J. D. Cohen & J. W. Schooler (Eds.), *Scientific approaches to consciousness* (pp. 49–64). Mahwah, NJ: Erlbaum.

Shiffrin, R. M., & Schneider, W. (1977). Controlled and automatic human information processing: II. Perceptual learning, automatic attending and a general theory. *Psychological Review, 84,* 1127–1190.

Shizgal, P., & Conover, K. (1996). On the neural computation of utility. *Current Directions in Psychological Science, 5,* 37–43.

Siegel, S. (1983). Classical conditioning, drug tolerance, and drug dependence. In Y. Israel, F. Glaser, H. Kalant, R. Popham, W. Schmidt, & R. Smart (Eds.), *Research advances in alcohol and drug problems* (Vol. 7, pp. 207–246). New York: Plenum.

Solomon, R., & Corbit, J. (1973). An opponent process theory of motivation: II. Cigarette addiction. *Journal of Abnormal Psychology, 81,* 158–171.

Sorokin, P. A. (1942). *Man and society in calamity.* New York: Dutton.

Stacy, A. W. (1995). Memory association and ambiguous cues in models of alcohol and marijuana use. *Experimental and Clinical Psychopharmacology, 3,* 183–194.

Stacy, A. W. (1997). Memory activation and expectancy as prospective predictors of alcohol and marijuana use. *Journal of Abnormal Psychology, 106,* 61–73.

Stacy, A. W., Leigh, B. C., & Weingardt, K. R. (1994). Memory accessibility and association of alcohol use and its positive outcomes. *Experimental and Clinical Psychopharmacology, 2,* 269–282.

Stadler, M. A. (1995). Role of attention in implicit learning. *Journal of Experimental Psychology: Learning, Memory, and Cognition, 21,* 674–685.

Steele, C. M., Critchlow, B., & Liu, T. J. (1985). Alcohol and social behavior: II. The helpful drunkard. *Journal of Personality and Social Psychology, 48,* 35–46.

Steele, C. M., & Josephs, R. A. (1988). Drinking your troubles away: II. An attention-allocation model of alcohol's effect on psychological stress. *Journal of Abnormal Psychology, 97,* 196–205.

Steele, C. M., & Josephs, R. A. (1990). Alcohol myopia: Its prized and dangerous effects. *American Psychologist, 45,* 921–933.

Steele, C. M., & Southwick, L. (1985). Alcohol and social behavior: I. The psychology of drunken excess. *Journal of Personality and Social Psychology, 48,* 18–34.

Steele, C. M., Southwick, L., & Pagano, R. (1986). Drinking your troubles away: The role of activity in mediating alcohol's reduction of psychological stress. *Journal of Abnormal Psychology, 95,* 173–180.

Stetter, F., Ackerman, K., Bizer, A., Straube, E. R., & Mann, K. (1995). Effects of disease-related cues in alcoholic inpatients: Results of a controlled "alcohol Stroop" study. *Alcoholism: Clinical and Experimental Research, 19,* 593–599.

Stewart, J., de Wit, H., & Eikelboom, R. (1984). Role of unconditioned and conditioned drug effects in self-administration of opiates and stimulants. *Psychological Review, 91,* 251–268.

Stewart, S. H. (1996). Alcohol abuse in individuals exposed to trauma: A critical review. *Psychological Bulletin, 120,* 83–112.

Strizke, W. K., Lang, A. R., & Patrick, C. J. (1996). Beyond stress and arousal: A reconceptualization of alcohol–emotion relations with reference to psychophysiological methods. *Psychological Bulletin, 120,* 376–395.

Taylor, S. E., & Brown, J. D. (1988). Illusion and well-being: A social psychological perspective on mental health. *Psychological Bulletin, 103,* 193–210.

Taylor, S. P., & Leonard, K. E. (1983). Alcohol and human physical aggression. In R. G. Geen & E. I. Donnerstein (Eds.), *Aggression: Theoretical and empirical reviews* (Vol. 2, pp 77–101). San Diego: Academic Press.

Teasdale, J. D., & Fogarty, S. J. (1979). Differential effects of induced mood on retrieval of pleasant and unpleasant events form episodic memory. *Journal of Abnormal Psychology, 88,* 248–257.

Thombs, D. L., Beck, K. H., & Mahoney, C. A. (1993). Effects of social context and gender on drinking patterns of young adults. *Journal of Counseling Psychology, 40,* 115–119.

Tiffany, S. T. (1990). A cognitive model of drug urges and drug-use behavior: Role of automatic and nonautomatic processes. *Psychological Review, 97,* 147–168.

Tiffany, S. T. (1991). The application of 1980s psychology to 1990s smoking research. *British Journal of Addiction, 86,* 617–620.

Tiffany, S. T. (1992). A critique of contemporary urge and craving research: Methodological, psychometric, and theoretical issues. *Advances in Behaviour Research and Therapy, 14,* 123–139.

Tiffany, S. T. (1995). The role of cognitive factors in reactivity to drug urges. In D. C. Drummond, S. T. Tiffany, S. Glautier, & B. Remington (Eds.), *Addictive behaviour: Cue exposure theory and practice* (pp. 137–165). London: Wiley.

von Hippel, W., Hawkins, C., & Fu, V. (1994, August). Effects of alcohol intoxication on intentional and automatic processes. In G. T. Fong (Chair), *Effects of alcohol on social psychological processes.* Symposium conducted at the 102nd annual meeting of the American Psychological Association, Los Angeles, CA.

Vuchinich, R. E., & Tucker, J. A. (1988). Contributions from behavioral theories of choice to an analysis of alcohol abuse. *Journal of Abnormal Psychology, 97,* 181–195.

Walbott, H. G., & Scherer, K. R. (1991). Stress specificities: Differential effects of coping style, gender, type of stressor on autonomic arousal, facial expression, and subjective feeling. *Journal of Personality and Social Psychology, 61,* 147–156.

Weingardt, K. R., Stacy, A. W., & Leigh, B. C. (1996). Automatic activation of alcohol concepts in response to positive outcomes of alcohol use. *Alcoholism: Clinical and Experimental Research, 20,* 25–30.

Wetter, D. W., Brandon, T. H., & Baker, T. B. (1992). The relation of affective processing measures and smoking motivation indices among college-age smokers. *Advances in Behaviour Research and Therapy, 14,* 169–193.

Wickens, C. D. (1984). Processing resources in attention. In R. Parasuraman, R. Davis, & J. Beathy (Eds.), *Varieties of attention* (pp. 63–102). New York: Academic Press.

Williams, J. M. G., Mathews, A., & MacLeod, C. (1996). The emotional Stroop task and psychopathology. *Psychological Bulletin, 120,* 3–24.

Wilson, G. T. (1977). Alcohol and human sexual behavior. *Behaviour Research and Therapy, 15,* 239–252.

Wilson, G. T. (1987). Cognitive processes in addiction. *British Journal of Addiction, 82,* 343–353.

Wilson, G. T. (1988). Alcohol and anxiety. *Behaviour Research and Therapy, 26,* 369–381.

Wilson, G. T., & Abrams, D. (1977). Effects of alcohol on social anxiety and physiological arousal: Cognitive versus pharmacological processes. *Cognitive Therapy and Research, 1,* 195–210.

Wilson, G. T., Brick, J., Adler, J., Cocco, K., & Breslin, C. (1989). Alcohol and anxiety reduction in female social drinkers. *Journal of Studies on Alcohol, 50,* 226–235.

Wise, R. (1988). The neurobiology of craving: Implications for understanding and treatment of addiction. *Journal of Abnormal Psychology, 97,* 118–132.

Yankofsky, L., Wilson, G. T., Adler, J. L., Hay, W. M., & Vrana, S. (1986). The effect of alcohol on self-evaluation and perception of negative interpersonal feedback. *Journal of Studies on Alcohol, 47,* 26–33.

Zajonc, R. B. (1980). Feelings and thinking: Preferences need no inferences. *American Psychologist, 35,* 151–175.

Zakay, D., & Block, R. A. (1997). Temporal cognition. *Current Directions in Psychological Science, 6,* 12–16.

Zeitlan, S. B., Potts, A. J., & Hodder, S. L. (1994). *Implicit and explicit memory biases for smoking-related cues in nicotine abstinent and non-abstinent smokers* [Summary]. Convention Proceedings for the 28th Annual Meetings of the Association for the Advancement of Behavior Therapy, p. 160.

Zinser, M., Baker, T., Sherman, J., & Cannon, D. (1992). Relation between self-reported affect and drug urges and cravings in continuing and withdrawing smokers. *Journal of Abnormal Psychology, 101,* 617–629.

8

Learning Theory and Research

MURIEL VOGEL-SPROTT
MARK T. FILLMORE

INTRODUCTION

Alcohol has been used by humans throughout history and has been a common ingredient in social activities and religious ceremonies. Yet despite the integral role of alcohol in many cultural functions, it has proven to be a mixed blessing. It is now known that high consumption of alcohol over prolonged periods of time may pose serious health hazards. The risk of liver cirrhosis is high, and those who become physically dependent on alcohol may suffer life-threatening withdrawal symptoms when drug use is abruptly terminated. Although most drinkers do not harm themselves or others, alcohol consumption is often associated with hazardous or antisocial behavior that creates serious problems for an individual and society. Drinkers who encounter such alcohol-related behavioral problems may be referred to as "alcohol abusers." However, it is difficult to draw the line between abusers and social drinkers. Like social drinkers, abusers usually are not physically dependent upon alcohol and may not suffer withdrawal symptoms during periods of abstinence. As a result, alcohol abusers are usually identified only after the emergence of social or personal problems related to alcohol.

The detrimental consequences of alcohol abuse make it important to understand the physical and behavioral effects of the drug. Some important clues about how and where alcohol acts in the brain have been provided by studies showing that alcohol alters membrane functions that can affect such processes as ion movements and neurotransmitter interactions with their receptors (e.g., Didly-Mayfield & Harris, 1995). However, no direct causal relationship has been demonstrated between any specific biological change induced by alcohol and any particular behavioral response to the drug (e.g., Hunt, 1993). It is becoming increasingly apparent that behavioral responses to alcohol cannot be explained solely by the pharmacological effects of the drug. Thus, it is important to identify other factors that can affect behavior under the drug.

This chapter discusses some contributions that learning research and theory have made to understanding behavioral responses to drugs. In the chapter, a drug-taking situation is analyzed in terms of learned associations between important environmental and response events. This analysis provides the framework for understanding and predicting a behavioral response to a drug. The chapter gives a background to associative learning by describing traditional Pavlovian conditioning and instrumental training paradigms. We consider learning to be an associative cognitive process that produces an "expectancy," consisting of acquired information about the relationship between events. An analysis of expectancies in drug-taking situations using Pavlovian conditioning and instrumental training procedures is presented, and the research strategy for testing behavioral effects of the expectancies is described. Particular attention is given to the role of learning in the display of behavioral tolerance to alcohol and individual differences in the response to the drug. Practical implications for reducing harmful behavior associated with alcohol consumption are also considered.

BACKGROUND TO ASSOCIATIVE LEARNING

There is good agreement on the effective experimental methods that produce learning. One training procedure, termed "Pavlovian" or "classical" conditioning, derives from Pavlov's (1927) research on reflexive responses to stimuli and the acquisition of anticipatory responses to such stimuli. According to this paradigm, learning occurs whenever a neutral stimulus is paired with an important stimulus, such as food. The other training procedure is used primarily to investigate how behavior changes as a function of its environmental outcome and is known as "instrumental" learning or "operant" conditioning. According to this paradigm, learning occurs whenever an important event is contingent upon a particular response.

Although the two training methods involve different procedures and seemingly different types of behavior, considerable research now indicates that a reliable, predictive relationship between events is crucial for learning in both training paradigms (e.g., Rescorla, 1987; Rescorla & Colwill, 1989). The process of learning about reliable relationships is referred to as "associative learning," and many theorists consider the process to consist of the acquisition of information about the relationship between events (e.g., Bolles, 1972; Rescorla, 1990). A brief description of Pavlovian conditioning and instrumental training procedures indicates how they both involve associative learning.

Pavlovian Conditioning and Instrumental Training

A Pavlovian conditioning procedure arranges a relationship between two stimuli, so that the first stimulus reliably predicts the second one. The second stimulus, of the pair is commonly termed an "unconditional" stimulus because its presentation will elicit the response of interest. Food is one example of an unconditional stimulus that elicits salivation. The first stimulus might be the sound of a bell, or some other "neutral" stimulus that elicits no relevant response (e.g., no salivation) prior to training. After a number of paired presentations of the stimuli, learning is typically tested by measuring the response to the first stimulus when it is presented alone. Learning is inferred when the previously neutral stimulus comes to elicit the relevant response.

An instrumental training procedure arranges a reliable relationship between some behavioral response (e.g., bar press) and an important environmental outcome (e.g., food). At the outset of training, the response typically has a low probability of occurring in the situation. After a number of response–outcome pairings, learning is tested by the degree to which the response has increased. An outcome that increases responding is commonly called a "reinforcer." Reinforcers can be classified into one of two broad categories: positive or negative. Positive reinforcers are those whose *presentation* increase responding, as food does for a hungry animal. Those whose *removal* increase responding, as does electric shock, are called negative reinforcers.

Pavlovian conditioning and instrumental training both allow some event to predict another, so that associative learning occurs. But the events that are related in each training procedure are different; therefore, different information is acquired. Pavlovian conditioning is designed to provide an opportunity to learn what stimulus event predicts another stimulus: The bell signals food. Instrumental training is designed to provide an opportunity to learn what response event predicts a stimulus event: The bar press results in food.

The environment in which events become associated can also contribute to learning. A number of investigators have pointed out that the background stimuli in Pavlovian and instrumental training situations may provide an additional source of learned associations (e.g., Bolles, 1979). Although a Pavlovian conditioning procedure only manipulates the relationship between two stimulus events, information about this relationship may also be associated with the contextual setting. For example, a dog trained in the laboratory to salivate at the sound of a bell is less likely to salivate to that sound heard in the street. The stimulus context is also important in instrumental training. Although instrumental training only manipulates the relationship between a response and an outcome, this association occurs in a particular situation. For example, rats learn to bar press for food in the presence of many contextual stimuli, such as the sights, smells, and sounds of the training chamber. Research indicates that the stimulus context associated with a response–outcome relationship may come to convey important information, such as when the response is most likely to produce the outcome (e.g., Rescorla, 1990; Rescorla & Colwill, 1989). In short, regardless of whether relationships between events are acquired through Pavlovian conditioning or through instrumental training, the situation-specific nature of such learning is well recognized.

Expectancy

Because the learning process cannot be directly observed, it has the status of an intervening variable that must be inferred. Over half a century ago, Tolman (1932) argued that learning was a cognitive process that depended on learning signs, signals, and expectancies. As contemporary research on associative learning identified information about predictable relationships between events as a crucial factor in the learning process, its cognitive nature has become more widely accepted.

The use of "expectancy" as a cognitive intervening variable to conceptualize learning was advocated by Bolles (1972). He proposed a learning theory in which an expectancy was operationally defined by the relationship between events in a situation. An expectancy was considered to represent learned information about an association between events. The information was understood to be of an "if–then" nature; if a certain event is presented, then a certain event is expected to follow. Once acquired, an expectancy was considered to mediate behavior based on learned information (Bolles, 1972). The ability of expectancies to affect behavior has received considerable attention in social and clinical psychology. In this literature, the terms "attitude," "belief," "attribute," and "expectancy" have often been used interchangeably (e.g., Bandura, 1977; Rotter, 1981; Shapiro & Morris, 1978). Irrespective of the particular term, the conceptualizations of this intervening cognitive variable are fairly similar. It is customarily understood to be if–then information about the relationship between events in the real world. Researchers usually intend a close link between a cognitive expectancy and the related events that give rise to it. However, a review of clinical and social studies indicates that expectancies are sometimes inferred in situations where the relevant events are not always specified, or the relationship between these events is unknown (Goldman, Brown, & Christiansen, 1987). Without such information inferences about an expectancy and its influence on behavior cannot be tested. The next section explains how associative learning in a drug-taking situation provides a framework for identifying relationships between observable events, so that drug-related expectancies can be verified.

EXPECTANCIES IN A DRUG-TAKING SITUATION

Principles of associative learning that identify expectancies have developed primarily through studies of behavior under drug-free conditions using Pavlovian and instrumental training. However, the same principles may be applied to a drug-taking situation. This can be illustrated by identifying the events in a drug-taking situation, how they may be associated, and the predictive information that these associations convey.

Pavlovian Conditioning

This paradigm investigates the effect of stimulus events that reliably precede the administration of a drug. The training situation usually pairs some neutral stimulus event with the administration of a drug and measures a response that is unconditionally elicited by the drug, such as a change in body temperature. These events and their sequential relationship are illustrated in Figure 8.1. The S represents a stimulus event that is reliably associated with the administration of a drug. The presentation of S signals the drug (S_d), and the acquisition of this predictive information provides the expectation of receiving the drug. The effect of this expectancy can be investigated by presenting the S when the drug is absent and measuring the response. The stimulus context in which drug taking occurs provides a rich source of stimulus events (S) that may act as cues for the drug. Drug paraphernalia or contextual cues, such as the location where the drug is usually

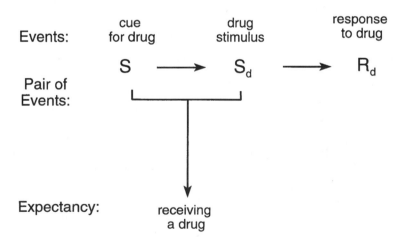

FIGURE 8.1. The sequential occurrence of events in a drug-taking situation in a Pavlovian conditioning paradigm: S represents the cue for the drug; S_d is the drug stimulus; and R_d is the response to drug. The association between S and S_d provides the information relevant to the expectancy of receiving a drug.

administered, are some examples of stimulus events that can be associated with the drug and thus come to predict its administration.

Instrumental Training

The drug-taking situation investigated in an instrumental training paradigm involves the three events in the Pavlovian conditioning procedure and adds an environmental outcome (S*) that is contingent upon the response to the drug (R_d). The events in this situation are illustrated in Figure 8.2. Instrumental training procedures can be used to investigate a variety of responses, depending on the type of activity that is performed. The reliable relation between a particular response and an outcome in a given situation conveys information that provides an opportunity to acquire a response–outcome expectancy (i.e., the expected consequence of the response). The instrumental training paradigm tests the effect of this expectancy on the response (R_d) by manipulating the outcome (S*) associated with R_d.

Three Expectancy Model

Figure 8.1 shows the association between events (S–S_d) that are investigated in Pavlovian conditioning. This association is identified as the expectation of receiving the drug. Figure 8.2 shows the associated events (R_d–S*) that are the

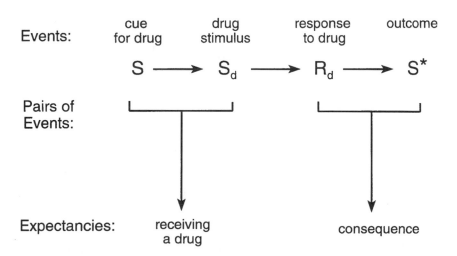

FIGURE 8.2. The sequential occurrence of events in a drug-taking situation in an instrumental training paradigm: S represents the cue for the drug; S_d is the drug stimulus; R_d is the response to drug; and S* represents the outcome of R_d. In addition to the pair of events that determine the expectation of the drug, the association between R_d and S* provides the information relevant to the expected consequence of R_d.

focus of instrumental training. This relation defines the expected consequence of the response to a drug. Figure 8.2 also reveals an association between the middle pair of events, the drug stimulus (S_d) and a response to the drug (R_d). Drug-taking situations in which the same activity is repeatedly performed provide an opportunity to associate the drug stimulus with a particular type of response. The reliable relationship between the drug stimulus and a particular response conveys information about the type of effect that the drug will have on a given activity. The acquisition of this information may be defined as an expected type of effect. This additional expectancy is illustrated in Figure 8.3, along with the other two expectancies, to show that three expectancies may be acquired in a drug-taking situation.

In summary, the events in a drug-taking situation illustrated in Figure 8.3 show that the sequential combination of pairs of events provide an opportunity to acquire three expectancies:

1. The expectation of receiving a drug, defined as $S-S_d$, is determined by the association between a predrug stimulus event and the drug.
2. The expected type of effect, defined as S_d-R_d, is determined by the relation between the drug and a particular response on a given activity.
3. The expected consequence of the response, defined as R_d-S^*, is determined by the relationship between the response to a drug and its outcome.

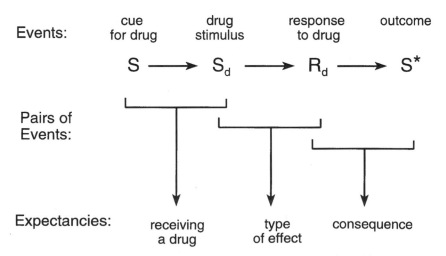

FIGURE 8.3. A learning analysis of three expectancies in a drug-taking situation based on four events: cue for drug (S); drug stimulus (S_d); response to drug (R_d); and outcome (S^*). The model shows how successive pairs of these events provide three expectancies that concern receiving a drug, the type of response, and its consequence.

The acquisition of each expectancy is assumed to depend upon a reliable association between a pair of events in a drug-taking situation. The events necessarily occur in a temporal sequence, beginning with the S–S_d pair. Therefore expecting a drug is a logical prerequisite for expecting some type of drug effect and some consequence of the response to a drug. These expectancies are also specific to the situational context. The expectation of the drug depends on predrug cues in the drug-use setting. The expected type of effect depends on the activity being performed in the situation, and the expected consequence depends on the particular environmental outcome that is likely to occur in the environment.

RESEARCH STRATEGIES

The relationships between pairs of events in a drug-taking situation (Figure 8.3) indicate that associative learning provides an opportunity to acquire three expectancies, each of which may affect the response to a drug (R_d). As a result, different research strategies are required to investigate the effect of each expectancy on the R_d.

Testing Effects of an Expectancy

The effect of expecting a drug has usually been investigated in a Pavlovian conditioning paradigm (e.g., Figure 8.1). Here, some distinctive stimulus (S) is reliably paired with the administration of the drug when no outcome is associated with the response. Under these conditions, the effect of expecting to receive a drug is tested by comparing the R_d displayed in the presence of the distinctive stimulus versus a novel stimulus.

Instrumental learning paradigms typically test the effect of a particular outcome on some response (e.g., Figure 8.2). These training situations manipulate the association between an environmental outcome (S^*) and a response to a drug. Because a drug needs to be expected before any outcome of a drugged response could be expected, tests of the effect of the expected outcome require that the expectation of receiving a drug is present and held constant. Thus only the environmental outcome (S^*) associated with a response (R_d) is manipulated.

The expected type of effect is defined by the S_d–R_d association, and thus includes events involved in both Pavlovian (Figure 8.1) and instrumental training (Figure 8.2). Because the expectation of receiving a drug is a logical precursor for expecting some type of drug effect, experiments testing the expected type of effect require that the expectation of the drug is present and held constant. The experimental situation also must exclude any environmental outcome for R_d, so no expected consequence would be present to affect behavior. In this respect, the situation resembles a Pavlovian conditioning paradigm.

Tolerance

In order to examine how drug-related expectancies can affect behavior under a drug, some measure of the response to a drug must be obtained. The types of responses that are studied can vary considerably and may range from complex, skilled activities, such as the performance of a hand–eye coordination task, to basic physiological regulatory behaviors, such as core body temperature. The response to a drug is commonly identified by a change in some ongoing behavior. The degree of change is of particular interest because it provides information on the intensity or potency of the drug effect.

The intensity of a response to a drug often diminishes with continued drug use. This reduction in the drug effect is referred to as tolerance. As tolerance develops, higher doses of the drug may be needed to reinstate the initial effect. Thus, tolerance has become recognized as a factor that may threaten the efficacy of long-term medication and contribute to drug abuse and dependence by encouraging the use of escalating doses (American Psychiatric Association, 1994). As a result, the phenomenon of tolerance has been the subject of a massive amount of research.

Some drug-induced adaptive reaction that compensates for, or counteracts the drug effect, is assumed to underlie tolerance. Traditionally, a compensatory response has been assumed to increase each time the drug is administered and to wane gradually during periods of abstinence. Centrally acting drugs, such as opiates or alcohol, are presumed to exert their effects in the brain, and information is rapidly accumulating on the effects of these drugs and the occurrence of tolerance at cellular and neuronal levels. For example, opiates act at central endorphin receptors, and neurochemical alterations induced by repeated drug administrations may account for tolerance. However, there has been no in vivo demonstration of a direct causal relationship between any drug-induced biological change and any particular behavioral response (e.g., Hunt, 1993). Indeed, it is becoming apparent that a recipient's behavioral response to a drug cannot be explained solely by pharmacological principles. Thus, it is important to know what factors in a drug-taking situation, in addition to the chemical stimulation of the drug, can affect behavioral tolerance.

A number of investigators have conducted repeated-dose experiments to test the possibility that associative learning interacts with drug effects to determine the tolerance displayed by animals or humans. Initial evidence suggesting that learning could affect the response to drugs was obtained in Pavlovian conditioning experiments during the 1930s. These findings focused attention on the learned expectation of receiving a drug as a factor that could affect tolerance. Three decades later, studies of drug tolerance using an instrumental training paradigm implicated the role of learned expectations about the consequence of behavior under the drug. The next two sections trace the historical development of research on each of these expectancies.

EXPECTATION OF RECEIVING A DRUG

The use of drugs as unconditional stimuli in a Pavlovian conditioning paradigm was initiated by Pavlov (1927), who demonstrated that the characteristic effects of a dose of apomorphine in dogs could be produced in lesser degree by a tone that predicted the administration of the drug. Such an anticipatory, "drug-like" reaction to the cue for the drug was consistent with Pavlov's theory of conditioning. However, subsequent research on dogs with a long history of epinephrine exposure showed that the cue for the drug would elicit a response that was antagonistic to the drug effect (e.g., Subkov & Zilov, 1937). The explanation for such a "drug-opposite" response was not apparent at the time. However, the potential adaptive value of such reactions was noted by a number of authors, who proposed that drug-induced disturbances of the homeostatic level of functioning may elicit "counterreactions" or "opponent-processes" to restore homeostasis (Solomon & Corbitt, 1974).

The potential adaptive advantage of counterreactions that occur just before the pharmacological effects of the drug had also been considered (e.g., Wikler, 1973). Pavlovian conditioning provides the experimental paradigm for investigating such preparatory responding based on associative learning. Siegel (1975) noted that a drug-administration situation resembles a Pavlovian conditioning paradigm: The drug stimulus unconditionally elicits some response, and distinctive environmental events precede and signal the administration of the drug. These predrug cues convey information that provides an opportunity to acquire an expectation of receiving the drug. During initial pairings of the predrug cues with the drug administration, the expectancy should elicit an anticipatory unconditional (i.e., drug-like) response, similar to Pavlov's (1927) findings with apomorphine. However, continuing administrations of the drug may result in a swifter, and stronger, drug-opposite compensatory response that could increasingly attenuate the drug-induced response, so that tolerance becomes evident. When tolerance is established, the drug stimulus would elicit a compensatory (i.e., drug-opposite) response, and the predrug cues would then be associated with this compensatory response. At this stage, the presentation of these cues alone should elicit an anticipatory drug-compensatory reaction that opposes the drug effect. On the basis of Siegel's analysis, the amount of tolerance displayed cannot be predicted solely from repeated drug exposures. Greater tolerance should be evident when the drug is administered in the context of the usual predrug cues (i.e., when the drug is expected). This is because the cues for the drug result in anticipatory drug-compensatory reactions that attenuate the drug effect. When these cues are not present, the drug is not expected and the anticipatory compensatory reaction is absent, so less tolerance (i.e., a stronger drug effect) is displayed.

Findings

A Pavlovian conditioning procedure investigating the effect of expecting a drug typically ensures that some distinctive cues reliably signal each administration of a drug. In the case of animals, these predrug cues could be the injection procedure in a distinctive cage. Drug administrations are repeated until tolerance is observed in some unconditional response to the drug, such as an analgesic, sedative, or thermic response. After tolerance is established, the expectation of receiving the drug is manipulated by administering the drug in the presence or the absence of the distinctive predrug cues.

Early research showed that tolerant rats with identical morphine treatment histories displayed greater tolerance to the analgesic effect of the drug when it was administered in the context of the usual predrug cues than when it was administered in the context of alternative cues (Siegel, 1976). These findings concerning the effect of expecting a drug on tolerance have been confirmed and extended to other unconditional effects of morphine and to a variety of centrally acting nonopiate substances, ranging from alcohol (Le, Poulos, & Cappell, 1979) to haloperidol (Poulos & Hinson, 1982). A review of the many drugs, dosages, and species that have been used in research showing that the expectation of receiving a drug affects tolerance is available elsewhere (Siegel, 1983). Although the majority of the evidence is based on animals, a few studies measuring heart rate and cognitive performance in humans have reported greater tolerance in the presence of predrug cues for alcohol (Dafters & Anderson, 1982; Shapiro & Nathan, 1986).

Much research has shown that Pavlovian conditioning procedures that determine the acquisition and extinction of signal properties of stimuli will also affect drug tolerance (for a review, see Siegel, 1989). Studies have also tested the assumption that the tolerance-enhancing effect of environmental cues for a drug is attributable to a learned, anticipatory drug-compensatory response. This has been done by administering an inert placebo substance to drug-tolerant subjects in the context of the usual predrug cues. For example, animals tolerant to the analgesic effects of morphine may display hyperalgesia when the predrug cues are presented without the drug (Krank, Hinson, & Siegel, 1981; Siegel, 1975). Thus, when a drug is administered, predrug cues that lead to the expectation of the drug result in anticipatory drug-compensatory responses that function adaptively to attenuate the pharmacologically induced disturbance. However, when the environmental cues for a drug occur without the drug, its effects are absent and the ensuing anticipatory drug-compensatory responses are unabated. Moreover, these drug-anticipatory responses do not simply abate with the passage of time. Pavlovian conditioning studies of drug-tolerant animals have shown that the extinction of signal properties of predrug cues and their impact on tolerance requires repeated presentations of these cues without the drug (Siegel, 1989). In other words, the situation must be changed so that the organism can learn that these cues no longer predict the administration of a drug.

Drug-compensatory responses oppose the drug effects. In this respect, they resemble withdrawal-like symptoms that also appear opposite to the effects of the drug. This has led to the suggestion that anticipatory drug-compensatory responses not only contribute to tolerance, but also may contribute to withdrawal distress and play a role in fostering relapse after a period of abstinence (e.g., Siegel, 1983; Wikler, 1948). Relapse may occur because withdrawal symptoms can be alleviated by taking the drug again, so that drug-use becomes negatively reinforced by the removal of withdrawal distress. Hinson and Siegel (1980) have proposed that the occurrence of drug-compensatory responses to cues for a drug in abstinent drug users may explain why they are more likely to relapse if they return to the same environment in which they were originally addicted. While such an explanation is difficult to test with humans, it is consistent with the situation-specific nature of associative learning.

Other researchers agree that the expectation of a drug based on predrug cues plays an the important role in relapse to drug taking, but they have offered a different interpretation that emphasizes the positive reinforcing influence of these cues (Stewart, de Wit, & Eikelboom, 1984; Wise, 1988). These investigators report that opiate drugs activate anatomically different brain areas that may represent neural mechanisms of reward and distress, and that drug tolerance develops readily to the distressing effects, but not to the rewarding effects. Thus, repeated drug administrations could result in tolerance to the distressing, undesirable drug effects, and no change in the rewarding, desirable effects. As a consequence, the net positive effects of the drug would increase, and environmental events signaling the drug would become more consistently associated with the drug-induced activation of brain mechanisms of reward. This association could result in the development of anticipatory drug-like rewarding effects that may summate with the positive effects of a drug and increase its incentive value.

This positive-incentive interpretation of predrug cues suggests that relapse to drug taking is encouraged by drug-like, positive reinforcing effects of the drug. Evidence that relapse to drug taking may be produced by the positive-incentive effects of opiates and cocaine has been provided, using addicted animals that had been withdrawn from the drug, and whose drug-taking response had extinguished (de Wit & Stewart, 1981, 1983). When a "priming" injection of a drug was administered, the animals' drug-taking response was reinstated. Considerable research with opiate and stimulant drugs has led investigators to suggest that relapse to drug taking after a period of abstinence may be prompted by anticipatory activation of brain reward mechanisms to predrug cues, rather than by relief from withdrawal distress in animals (Stewart et al., 1984). Although the conclusion has been extended to alcohol, similar evidence on its action has been difficult to obtain, possibly because alcohol has no specific receptor site (Didly-Mayfield

& Harris, 1995). The effects of alcohol are widespread and involve alterations in neural membranes, ion channels, and numerous neurotransmitters, including dopamine, which is considered to be important in the activation of neural brain mechanisms of reward (Gessa, Muntoni, Vargui, & Mereu, 1985; Hunt, 1990; Imperato & Di Chiara, 1986)

Implications and Limitations

Evidence from Pavlovian conditioning showing that associative learning can affect drug tolerance provided the first definitive challenge to the notion that the response to a drug was determined solely by its pharmacological action. The findings also stimulated interest in the potential of predrug cues to promote relapse in abstinent drug users. This has led to studies investigating the types of responses (drug-opposite withdrawal distress or drug-like positive incentive) that are displayed by former drug users when they are presented with environmental cues associated with drug taking.

Studies that examine the ability of drug-related cues to elicit reactions in abstinent drug users are broadly referred to as "cue reactivity" studies. This research is based on the assumption that prior drug use has resulted in learning what cues predict the drug. The studies rely on a drug user's prior learning to produce a reaction when predrug cues are presented in a laboratory. The experimental procedure usually involves the presentation of some predrug cue to an abstinent drug user. A syringe is an example of a cue that might be presented to opiate users, whereas the smell and sight of alcohol may be presented as cues to alcoholics. These studies have usually assessed some physiological reaction (e.g., heart rate, skin conductance, blood pressure, skin temperature, salivation), as well as self-reports of sensations. Studies concerned with alcohol may measure the responses to predrug and neutral cues within the same individual, or they may compare the responses of alcoholics with social drinkers (e.g., Cooney, Gillespie, Baker, & Kaplan, 1987; Greeley, Swift, Prescott, & Heather, 1993). The cues presented for alcohol vary across studies and range from generic stimuli (e.g., visual slide presentations of liquor bottles) to specific stimuli, such as the sight and smell of an individual's preferred alcoholic beverage (cf. Eriksen & Gotestam, 1984; Monti et al., 1987).

Early cue reactivity experiments with abstinent animals and humans who had been physically dependent on opiates indicated that predrug cues signaling the drug led to drug-opposite responses resembling withdrawal symptoms (O'Brien, 1976; Wikler, 1948). However, results of cue reactivity studies of abstinent alcoholics and smokers have been mixed. A review of this research indicates that heightened reactivity to predrug cues may be displayed, but the direction of responses (e.g., drug-like vs. drug-opposite) is not consistently observed in studies (Niaura et al., 1988). Even within the same individual, both drug-like and drug-opposite responses to predrug cues for alcohol have been observed (Staiger & White, 1988).

It is unclear why studies of cue reactivity to alcohol yield inconsistent results in abstinent drug users. It may be that drug-opposite responses to predrug cues are only displayed by individuals who have been physically dependent upon the drug (Glautier & Drummond, 1994), and many cue reactivity studies include drug users who may not have been physically drug dependent. Another difficulty in obtaining reliable results with humans may stem from a lack of control over their drug use histories. The types of predrug cues and the degree to which they have been previously associated with drug administration may vary greatly among individuals. Other investigators also have suggested that individual differences in prior experience with alcohol may produce different reactions to cues for the drug (Staiger & White, 1991). The more reliable findings in abstinent animals may be due to the experimental control of their prior drug exposures and the types of predrug cues associated with drug administrations.

While there appears to be good agreement that the expectation of receiving a drug will affect behavior, it has proven difficult to predict whether drug-like or drug-opposite responses will be displayed in the presence of cues for a drug. Some researchers have attempted to attribute this inconsistency to the particular physiological locus of the drug action (e.g., Eikelboom & Stewart, 1982). However, research indicates that the same physiological response to the expectation of a drug by a given individual can be drug-like or drug-opposite, depending on the particular predrug cue that is present (Staiger & White, 1988). Thus, it seems that an adequate explanation requires a consideration of more than the physiological locus of drug action.

Of particular interest is the finding that repeated doses of a drug in a Pavlovian conditioning situation occasionally fail to produce tolerance in animals. Tolerance to the hypothermic effect of alcohol is one example. When repeated drug administrations are conducted under normal room temperature, tolerance to the hypothermic effect develops and predrug cues elicit a drug-opposite (hyperthermic) response in animals (Le et al., 1979). However, under warmer ambient temperature, the same doses of alcohol result in no tolerance to the hypothermic effect, and no drug-opposite hyperthermic response to predrug cues when they are presented alone (Alkana, Finn, & Malcolm, 1983; Hjeresen, Reed, & Woods, 1986). One possible explanation for this inconsistent occurrence of tolerance can be offered by considering the outcome of a hypothermic response to alcohol when room temperature is manipulated. Under normal room temperature, a hypothermic response may result in an aversive drop in body temperature, and tolerance to this effect could be positively reinforced by a restoration of normal body temperature. Conversely, in a warmer environment, a hypothermic response could result in a beneficial cooling that restores normal body temperature, and thus tolerance to this effect would not be reinforcing. Generally speaking, this type of explanation implies that tolerance might be affected by events that occur after the drug is administered, such as the outcome of the response to a drug. The next section provides some historical background concerning this idea and reviews research on tolerance that examines the effects of the outcome of the response to a drug.

EXPECTED CONSEQUENCES

The idea that the events after drinking alcohol can affect behavioral tolerance has a long history. For example, more than 100 years ago, a physician reported:

> The mind exercises a considerable effect upon drunkenness, and may control it powerfully. When in the company of a superior whom we respect, or of a woman in whose presence it would be indelicate to get intoxicated, a much greater portion of liquor may be withstood than in societies where no such restraints operate. (MacNish, 1832, p. 45)

More that just providing a commentary on 19th-century etiquette, MacNish asserted that tolerance to alcohol may be affected by the anticipated standards of acceptable behavior. This notion has been advanced during the 20th century as well. MacAndrew and Edgerton (1969) noted that drinking orgies in aboriginal cultures resulted in gross intoxication in some societies and tolerance in others. They attributed these variations in behavior to learned conformity to different, culturally specific standards of acceptable conduct under alcohol. Goldberg (1943) speculated that the tolerance displayed by alcoholics was due to "psychic compensation" for the impairing effect of the drug. A few decades later, Dews (1962) proposed that drinkers' tolerance might result from new learned behavior that compensates for alcohol's impairing effects.

The possibility that events after drinking alcohol can affect tolerance also is suggested by anecdotes about grossly inebriated drinkers who displayed nonimpaired behavior when they believed it important to do so. The ability of drinkers to "sober up" apparently provided the impetus for introducing the Breathalyser to measure blood alcohol levels for forensic purposes. Before the Breathalyser was available, a medical examination of suspected intoxicated drivers was required to support the charge. Goldberg and Havard (1968) reported that these clinical assessments were completely unreliable, because suspects faced with a doctor called in by the police often were quite capable of "pulling themselves together" to pass all the clinical tests. However, after a suspect satisfied the police physician and was free to leave, signs of intoxication often reappeared. As a result, the police frequently had to assist suspects from the station and escort them home. Tolerance on the part of intoxicated suspects appeared to depend on the expectation of a reward for displaying sober behavior. The suspects exhibited sober behavior (i.e., tolerance) when they anticipated a payoff for its display, but lost it in the absence of a rewarding outcome for compensating for alcohol's effect. In this respect, their tolerance resembled a goal-directed (i.e., instrumental) response that became dominant when associated with an immediate reward and extinguished when the reward was withdrawn.

Research on drug tolerance using an instrumental training paradigm began to appear during the 1960s. Animal research showed that the development of tolerance to the stimulating effect of amphetamine on bar pressing for reinforcement varied abruptly within an animal depending upon the reinforcement schedule (Schuster, Dockens, & Woods, 1966). In this particular experiment, animals received repeated injections of amphetamine and bar pressed for food reinforcement under a fixed-interval schedule that alternated with a low-rate schedule. Under the fixed-interval schedule, reinforcement was maintained by responding any time during the interval. Under the low-rate schedule, reinforcement was maintained by infrequent, periodic responding. Amphetamine initially stimulated (increased) responding. This produced no change in reinforcement under the fixed interval schedule but decreased reinforcement under the low-rate schedule. With repeated doses, tolerance to the stimulant effect was displayed when the low-rate schedule was in effect, and no tolerance was evident when the reinforcement switched to a fixed-interval schedule. Thus, the display of tolerance by the animal appeared to be goal-directed and dependent on the outcome of its behavior. More recent research with animals has examined the effects of many different drugs under a variety of schedules of reinforcement. While the results show that the development of tolerance can be affected by different schedules of reinforcement, the findings have not led to any integrating theoretical explanation (Branch, 1984; Wolgin, 1989).

However, an associative learning account of events in a drug-taking situation offers a framework for predicting behavior (Vogel-Sprott, 1992). This theory has led to research testing predictions about the tolerance-inducing effect of the outcome of behavior after a drug is received. The model, illustrated in Figure 8.2, shows that the outcome of a response is the final event in a drug-taking situation. The important methodological implication of the model is that the effect of different learned associations between a response and its outcome can be tested only in experimental situations where the outcome of the response is the sole factor that is manipulated. The stimulus context for the response, such as the cues signaling the drug, the number of repetitions of the dose, and the ongoing activity being measured, must be held constant.

Experiments adopting this experimental procedure have primarily aimed to determine the degree to which associative learning principles that predict an instrumental (i.e., goal-directed) response can predict a drug-tolerant response. Thus, most studies have compared the tolerance displayed by groups of subjects whose treatment differs only with respect to the outcome of their performance under a drug. Research to date has focused on the behavioral tolerance to alcohol of social drinkers. A detailed review of the evidence has been presented (Vogel-Sprott, 1992), and some of the results have also been summarized elsewhere (e.g., Vogel-Sprott, 1997; Vogel-Sprott & Fillmore, in press; Wolgin, 1989). This section provides a general overview of the methodology and results, and discusses some of the more recent findings of this research.

The studies have used simple and complex psychomotor tasks to investigate the development of behavioral tolerance to a moderate dose of alcohol (peak blood alcohol levels of 80 mg/100 ml). Alcohol-induced impairment on such tasks is characterized by reduced accuracy or speed of performance. Groups of male social drinkers are typically trained on a task and then attend a series of four or five 2.5 hour sessions in which they receive a moderate dose of alcohol (0.62 g/kg) and perform the task at intervals while their blood alcohol concentrations (BACs) rise and decline. The intensity of the impairing effect of the dose is measured on each session by the difference between a subjects' drug-free (i.e., sober) proficiency on the task and their average performance under the dose of alcohol. The development of tolerance is inferred from a reduction in impairment as the drinking sessions are repeated. Different outcomes of performance are administered to different groups, and comparisons among the groups provide information on the tolerance-inducing effect of the various outcomes.

Findings

A number of experiments have demonstrated that tolerance is readily acquired in drinking situations that train drinkers to expect immediate positive reinforcement for sober (i.e., nonimpaired) behavior (e.g., Beirness & Vogel-Sprott, 1984; Sdao-Jarvie & Vogel-Sprott, 1991, 1992). These studies trained the expectancy using a positive reinforcement procedure that administered an immediate reward, in the form of money or approving verbal feedback (e.g., "Yes, good"), whenever drinkers' performance under alcohol equaled their sober level of proficiency. Groups of subjects receiving this reward treatment displayed a progressive increase in tolerance as drinking sessions were repeated. No such trend was evident in control groups whose treatment was identical except that they had no opportunity to associate tolerant behavior with positive reinforcement (i.e., they received either no reward or equivalent rewards that were unrelated to sober performance).

Learning research has shown that a response trained with positive reinforcement will extinguish when the reinforcer is withdrawn (Domjan & Burkhard, 1986). When a response is immediately rewarded, subsequently withholding the reward creates an obvious change in the situation that fails to confirm the expected rewarding consequence, and this may account for the fairly swift extinction of a response. Similarly, research using an immediate reward treatment to develop tolerance has shown that it readily extinguishes if the reward is subsequently withheld, even though drinkers continue to expect, and to consume alcohol (e.g., Mann & Vogel-Sprott, 1981; Zack & Vogel-Sprott, 1993).

More recent experiments show that behavioral tolerance to repeated doses of alcohol also is readily developed by negative reinforcement (i.e., where the removal of an aversive outcome serves as a reward; Zack & Vogel-Sprott, 1995, 1997). Drinkers in this research received unfavorable verbal feedback (e.g., "No, bad") whenever they displayed impaired performance under alcohol. Whenever they displayed drug-tolerant performance, no unfavorable or other verbal feedback was received. Learning studies of avoidance responding in animals indicates that when a response is trained under negative reinforcement, it tends to be very resistant to extinction when the reinforcement is withheld (e.g., Domjan & Burkhard, 1986). This may be attributed to the fact that negative reinforcement during training and during extinction are both characterized by the absence of the aversive outcome when the appropriate response is displayed. There is no obvious change in the situation, so the expectation of reinforcement for the response remains unchallenged. In accord with the results of learning studies, Zack and Vogel-Sprott (1995, 1997) showed that when negative reinforcement is used to train tolerance in social drinkers, their tolerance is well retained when the reinforcement is withheld during subsequent drinking sessions.

Research on the transfer of tolerance has also indicated that the expectation of a reward for drug-tolerant behavior plays a mediating role (Rawana & Vogel-Sprott, 1985). When drinkers were trained to expect an immediate reward for sober performance on one task, their tolerance transferred to a similar task performed for the first time under alcohol in a situation where drug-tolerant performance was rewarded. However, if the reward was absent, no transfer of tolerance was observed.

Taken together, the results are consistent with associative learning theory, in which acquired expectancies about the consequence of a response are assumed to mediate behavior. In the studies described here, drinkers were shown to display greater tolerance in situations where they expected sober behavior to yield a more favorable outcome than impairment. In theory, other types of responses under alcohol also should increase when a drinker expects them to yield the most favorable consequence in the situation. For example, associating gross impairment under alcohol with a reward should increase behavioral impairment. Such an intensification of a drug effect is termed "sensitization." Although it is seldom observed to occur with a depressant drug, such as alcohol, recent experiments have shown that the expectation of a reward for flagrant impairment under alcohol intensifies this response (Zack & Vogel-Sprott, 1995, 1997). In this research, drinkers displayed intense psychomotor impairment when it was rewarded under repeated doses of alcohol. In contrast, other drinkers displayed tolerance when the same reward was associated with sober performance.

Speaking casually, it seems that whether a drinker will display tolerance or gross impairment under alcohol depends upon which response is expected to yield the more favorable consequence.

Tolerance is commonly attributed to a drug-compensatory response. In the case of behavioral tolerance, a compensatory response should act to change behavior in a direction opposite to the drug effect. Thus, if a drinker performs a task more slowly under alcohol, a compensatory response should speed performance. Tests for such a compensatory response have been conducted by surreptitiously substituting a placebo for alcohol after a series of drinking sessions in which groups of drinkers who were rewarded for sober performance displayed tolerance, and no tolerance was evident in groups receiving control treatments (Beirness & Vogel-Sprott, 1984; Sdao-Jarvie & Vogel-Sprott, 1991, 1992). After drinking the placebo, the groups that had a history of reward for drug-tolerant behavior showed the greatest compensatory improvement in performance. These group differences could not be attributed to differences in the expectation of receiving the drug, because the same predrug cues were associated with the alcohol and placebo administered to all subjects.

Additional insight on the mechanism underlying tolerance to alcohol-induced psychomotor impairment has been obtained by considering the similarity between the acquisition of tolerance and the learning of a new motor skill. Studies using psychomotor tasks to assess the effect of rewarding tolerant behavior indicate that this training results in a progressive development of alcohol tolerance as doses are repeated. This gradual recovery from impairment resembles the improvement that characterizes the learning of a motor skill. Research on motor learning indicates that rewarding efficient performance provides feedback that helps the learner identify the alterations in behavior required to perform more skillfully (e.g., Schmidt, 1988). As training continues, the changes in behavior that yield a reward are maintained, and those that do not are discarded. The possibility that the development of drinkers' behavioral tolerance may similarly reflect the acquisition of some behavioral strategy to compensate for drug-impaired behavior is a long-standing notion (e.g., Dews, 1962). However, this possibility has resisted investigation because of the recognition that task practice under repeated doses of a drug confounds the contribution of learning and drug effects to behavioral tolerance (Wolgin, 1989).

Some recent research has been designed to separate the learning and drug effects. This was done by administering drug-free training of a motor skill task under environmental conditions that induced impairment resembling the impairing effect of alcohol, and subsequently testing task performance under alcohol (Easdon & Vogel-Sprott, 1996; Zinatelli & Vogel-Sprott, 1993). These studies showed that individuals with prior drug-free training to overcome environmental impairment displayed robust resistance to the impairing effects of an initial dose of alcohol. Task practice under environmental impairment apparently resulted in the acquisition of a compensatory behavioral strategy that could subsequently be applied to enhance behavioral tolerance to alcohol. These findings are in line with the idea that drinkers' behavioral tolerance may reflect learned behavioral strategies to compensate for the effects of alcohol (e.g., Dews, 1962).

In the case of motor skills, it appears that an expectation of reward for drug-tolerant behavior mediates the acquisition of a behavioral strategy to compensate for alcohol impairment, and the gradual acquisition of tolerance may reflect the gradual learning of the requisite strategy. One implication of this conclusion is that the expectation of a reward for sober performance may develop tolerance more swiftly (i.e., with fewer drug doses) in activities that are less likely to require the learning of some new motor skill to compensate for alcohol impairment. Examples of such activities are ones that depend more on cognitive processes than on motor skills. Accordingly, some recent research using an information-processing task has shown that rewarding sober (i.e., nonimpaired) performance under alcohol dramatically enhances drinkers' resistance to the impairing effect of an initial dose of alcohol (Fillmore & Vogel-Sprott, 1997).

The ability of expected consequences of behavior to affect the degree of alcohol impairment in cognitive performance requires further investigation. However, the findings suggest that the expected consequences of behavior under a drug may affect many types of activities. The ability to inhibit an undesirable response under alcohol is another type of behavior that also appears to be affected by the expected consequence. A moderate dose of alcohol has been shown to impair the ability of male and female social drinkers to inhibit a response (Mulvihill, Skilling, & Vogel-Sprott, 1997), and some preliminary studies indicate that associating response inhibition with a favorable outcome increases tolerance to the disinhibiting effect of the drug (Mulvihill, 1997).

Implications and Limitations

Results of studies reviewed in this section identify the environmental outcome of behavior under a drug as an important determinant of drug-tolerant behavior. Experiments with social drinkers showed that behavioral tolerance to alcohol readily developed whenever this behavior was reliably associated with a favorable outcome. The acquisition of this information (i.e., the expectation of a favorable consequence for tolerance) appeared to be the important mediating factor, because withholding the reward, so that the expectancy was no longer confirmed, extinguished tolerance even though alcohol continued to be consumed. In contrast, tolerance was well retained in drinking situations where no clues were provided to indicate that the reward was withheld. This evidence and interpretation is in accord with associative learning theory accounts of the acquisition and extinction of instrumental (i.e., goal-directed) behavior. The findings imply that explanations of drug-tolerant behavior will require a consideration of the expected consequence of behavior under a drug, as well as the expectation of receiving a drug.

In accord with the notion that a drug-opposite compensatory response underlies tolerance, studies showed that drinkers who were trained to expect a reward for tolerant behavior subsequently displayed a more intense compensatory response (i.e., improved performance) to a placebo when alcohol was expected. However, the results also indicated that this compensatory response could not be attributed to some physiological change induced by prolonged or high drug exposures. Three or four repetitions of a moderate dose were sufficient to develop tolerance to the impairing effect of alcohol on psychomotor performance. Moreover, the necessity to repeat these doses seemed to be due to the gradual learning of some compensatory behavioral strategy to counteract psychomotor impairment under alcohol. Two major findings point to this conclusion. Prior drug-free training to overcome environmentally induced impairment of psychomotor performance appears to allow individuals to learn a compensatory behavioral strategy that can be subsequently applied to enhance their resistance to the impairing effect of an initial dose of alcohol. In addition, rewarding outcomes for nonimpaired performance of cognitive tasks that require little motor skill results in robust tolerance to the impairing effect of an initial dose of alcohol.

Evidence that drug-tolerant behavior depends on the expectation of a favorable consequence has been based on moderate doses of alcohol (peak BACs of 80 mg/100 ml). It is obvious that the tolerance-enhancing effect of this expectancy must be limited to BACs lower than those that induce coma or stupor. Although nothing is yet known about how high BACs must be to override the effect of the expectancy, some studies of alcoholics suggest that the expected consequence of behavior still influences tolerance when BACs are in excess of 250 mg/100 ml (Mello & Mendelson, 1965). Subjects in these studies performed a task to obtain alcoholic drinks. Because the task was performed while drinking occurred, drug-tolerant performance was rewarded by the continuing attainment of alcohol. Under these conditions, the alcoholics continued to perform the task with good accuracy and rarely displayed any symptoms of intoxication in spite of their high BACs.

To date, tests of the effects of environmental outcomes of human behavior under a drug have provided evidence on the effects of alcohol on psychomotor and cognitive behavior of male social drinkers. Although this information is of practical and theoretical importance in its own right, the findings carry implications that should apply generally to the behavioral effects of centrally acting drugs in animals and humans. Continued research on expected consequences of behavior under a drug may contribute more knowledge on how environmental events associated with behavior in drug-taking situations influence the performance of a variety of activities. The generality of the findings may be tested in future research that examines female social drinkers. The results may also be extended to animals, using a variety of drugs that could not ethically be administered to humans.

EXPECTED TYPE OF EFFECT

Single-dose experiments occasionally have been used to compare the tolerance of habitual and naive drug users. A classic example is Goldberg's (1943) experiment that compared social drinkers and alcoholics in terms of the behavioral impairment each group displayed under a dose of alcohol. The results of that study showed that the BAC associated with onset and the offset of impairment was higher for alcoholics than for social drinkers. The greater resistance to the effect of a dose on the part of alcoholics is commonly considered to support the notion that they have developed more tolerance as a result of greater drug exposures.[1]

Although some studies have aimed to investigate tolerance in relation to prior drug use, the goal of most single-dose studies has been to identify the typical behavioral effects of a moderate dose of alcohol displayed by social drinkers. These studies commonly measure the drug effect by the degree to which task performance under alcohol differs from predrinking performance. Reviews of such research usually conclude that alcohol can impair cognitive and motor performance to some extent, and that the degree of impairment bears some relation to the dose or BAC (e.g., Carpenter, 1962; Koelega, 1995; Linnoila, Stapleton, Lister, Guthrie, & Eckardt, 1986; Mitchell, 1985; Wallgren & Barry, 1971). Although the main focus of single-dose studies has been on the average impairing effect of alcohol displayed by a group of drinkers, individual differences in the degree of behavioral impairment have been noted for some time (e.g., Jellinek & McFarland, 1940; Vogel, 1958; Wallgren & Barry, 1971). These differences are of particular interest, because they do not appear to be explained by factors that might normally be thought to affect impairment. For example, drinkers may differ in the degree to which alcohol impairs their task performance despite having common attributes such as BACs at the time of testing, prior drinking history, and sober performance skill.

One explanation for such individual differences in alcohol impairment is offered by the associative learning analysis of a drug-taking situation presented in this chapter. The experimental procedure of single-dose studies resembles a Pavlovian conditioning situation (Figure 8.1). The receipt of the drug is preceded by stimuli (S) that are reliably associated with the administration of the drug (S_d), and no environmental outcome (S*) is contingent upon the response (R_d). The S–S_d association determines the expectation of a drug, and the absence of any outcome (S*) for R_d provides no opportunity to acquire a response–outcome expectancy that could affect behavior. Although the experimental procedure controls the expectation of receiving the drug, and the expected consequence of the response, the situation includes another pair of associated events (S_d–R_d) that are ignored. This relationship determines the expected type of effect, and is labeled in Figure 8.3. Just like the other two expectancies, the expected effect derived from associating S_d–R_d should also affect behavior. The next section explains how drinkers may acquire different expectations about the type of effect that alcohol exerts on an activity and reviews research showing that these expectations can contribute to individual differences in response to the drug.

Responses to Alcohol

Social drinkers engage in a variety of activities after drinking, and the repeated performance of a given activity under alcohol provides opportunities to associate alcohol with a particular type of effect. A reliable relationship between the drug (S_d) and a particular response (R_d) provides information that determines the type of effect that will be expected when the activity is performed under a drug. The expectation may be based on drinkers' own performance of an activity under alcohol. In addition, the expectancy may be acquired from information based on various reports about the effect of alcohol on an activity (e.g., Goldman et al., 1987). It is generally known that alcohol impairs behavior; thus, most individuals may expect impairment from alcohol. However, because their expectations may be based on different sources of information, the degree of impairment that each drinker expects may differ.

A number of experiments have examined the relationship between the degree of impairment drinkers expect from alcohol and their behavioral impairment under the drug (Fillmore, Carscadden, & Vogel-Sprott, 1998; Fillmore & Vogel-Sprott, 1994, 1995b). This research has used psychomotor and cognitive tasks to test the relationship between male social drinkers' expected and actual impairment under alcohol. Subjects in these studies performed a task alone in a laboratory room, where no outcome was associated with any response on the task. After they were familiarized with the task, they rated the expected effect of alcohol (two beers drunk in 1 hour) on their task performance using a scale that ranged from extreme impairment to extreme improvement. They subsequently performed the task under a moderate dose of alcohol, and the impairment was measured by the pre- to postalcohol change in a subject's performance. This research has shown that individuals differ in their expectations about the degree to which alcohol will impair their performance of psychomotor and cognitive tasks. Moreover, these differences predict the degree of impairment they display under alcohol. Those who expect less impairment display less impairment and thus appear more tolerant to the behavioral effects of the drug. In contrast, those who expect more impairment display greater impairment (i.e., less behavioral tolerance).

The relationship between expected and actual drug effects has also been extended to caffeine, a socially used stimulant in the form of coffee (Fillmore, 1994; Fillmore & Vogel-Sprott, 1994). In this research, subjects rated the effect they expected caffeinated coffee would have on their performance of a psychomotor task and subsequently performed the task under caffeine. The results showed that individual differences in the type and degree of effects expected from caffeine predicted the type of response displayed under the drug. Although caffeine tended to improve performance, individuals who expected less improvement performed more poorly.

According to associative learning principles, the repeated association of the drug with a particular behavioral effect strengthens the relationship between these events, so that the resulting expected type of effect should more reliably predict the actual effect displayed under the drug. In the case of alcohol, more repetitions occur as drinkers regularly use alcohol over time, allowing them to acquire expectancies that should better predict their response to the drug. This possibility was tested in a study that classified social drinkers in terms of the length of time they had been using alcohol regularly (Fillmore & Vogel-Sprott, 1995a). "Novices" had been drinking socially for 20 months or less, and "experienced" individuals had been drinkers for 24 months or more. The subjects rated the degree to which alcohol was expected to impair their performance of a motor skill before they performed the task under alcohol. The results were consistent with an associative learning account of the expectancy. The expectancies of the experienced drinkers predicted their actual impairment, and expectancies of novice drinkers were not related to their impairment.

Correlations between drinkers' expected and actual impairment under alcohol are consistent with the notion that the expected type of effect plays a role in mediating the degree of behavioral impairment displayed by drinkers. However, such correlations do not necessarily indicate a causal influence of the expected type of effect. Therefore, other research has adopted a different strategy that provides clearer evidence on the causal role of this expectancy. This approach eliminates the pharmacological effect of the drug by measuring the response to a placebo when subjects expect a drug. The next section reviews the results of this research.

Responses to Placebos

Reviews of placebo studies of social drinkers who perform many different social, cognitive, and psychomotor activities indicate that the receipt of a placebo when alcohol is expected does not reliably affect a behavioral response (e.g., Hull & Bond, 1986). Factors that may account for the failure to observe reliable or consistent placebo response in these studies remain unclear. Some researchers have speculated that certain types of activities may be more susceptible to placebo effects (e.g., Hull & Bond, 1986). Others have pointed to procedural differences among studies in the administration of the placebo (e.g., Rohsenow & Marlatt, 1981). The possibility that individual differences in a variety of expectancies about alcohol might contribute to inconsistent placebo responses has also been suggested (e.g., Marlatt & Rohsenow, 1980).

Research on placebo responses typically employs the methodology used in single-dose studies that investigate the response to a drug. Thus predrug cues (S) signaling the administration of the drug are presented to ensure that the subject expects the drug, and no environmental outcome is associated with the response. This experimental procedure controls the expectation of receiving a drug and the expected consequence, but the expected type of effect is uncontrolled. Thus individual differences in this expectation could affect responses to a placebo in the same way that they affect responses to the drug. Because the drug is expected, but its effects are absent in placebo studies, the behavioral response can be attributed to the influence of the expected type of effect.

Placebo research testing the influence of individual differences in the expected type of drug effect is a relatively new undertaking (Fillmore et al., 1998; Fillmore & Vogel-Sprott, 1994, 1995b). Drinkers in these studies rated the expected effect of alcohol on their performance. Then, they received a placebo and performed a psychomotor or cognitive task. The results showed that drinkers who expected greater impairment from alcohol performed more poorly under a placebo. Thus, just as expectancies about alcohol impairment related to changes in psychomotor and cognitive behavior under the drug, these expectancies also predicted changes in response to a placebo when drinkers expected alcohol. The relationship between expected types of drug effects and placebo responses also has been extended to a socially used stimulant drug (Fillmore, 1994; Fillmore & Vogel-Sprott, 1994). In those studies, individual differences in psychomotor performance under placebo caffeine (decaffeinated coffee) were predicted by the type of effect the subjects expected caffeine to have on their performance.

Implications and Limitations

The methodology of studies described in this section is similar to traditional, single-dose studies of alcohol and placebo effects on behavior: Alcohol is expected and some response is tested after the drug or a placebo has been received. However, traditional studies have focused on the average response of groups of subjects. The novel feature of the research reviewed in this section is the investigation of individual differences in response, and its link to expectations concerning the effect of the drug on behavior. This research was guided by the associative learning analysis of a drug-taking situation that identified the particular events defining the expected type of effect and the particular circumstances under which this expectation should predict the response to the drug or to a placebo. The associative learning model is generic, because it is based on principles that should apply to many behavioral activities and to other drugs and placebos. The potential of the model to contribute to understanding individual differences in response to drugs and to placebos is suggested by findings showing that the expected type of drug effect predicts responses to alcohol and to caffeine. These two drugs are generally considered to have opposing effects on the central nervous system; thus, it seems that the effects of expectancies may not be limited to one particular class of psychoactive drug. Moreover, evidence that the expected type of effect can influence both cognitive and psychomotor activities suggests that this expectancy may affect individual differences in a broad range of activities in drug-taking situations.

The findings have important implications for interpreting the results of placebo studies. When no consistent change in response to a placebo is observed in a group of individuals, such observations usually lead to the conclusion that the placebo does not alter behavior. However, the evidence presented in this section indicates that the lack of a consistent change in response to a placebo among individuals does not necessarily mean that the placebo is ineffective. Individual differences in response to a placebo can be systematically related to differences in the type of drug effect that is expected, and this relationship can occur regardless of whether some consistent placebo response is displayed by a group of individuals. In short, evidence that the response to a placebo can be unique to a person challenges traditional methods of testing placebo effects that ignore differences among individuals.

The expected type of effect has only recently been formally identified in associative learning analyses of drug-taking situations (Vogel-Sprott & Fillmore, in press). While the evidence to date provides support for an associative learning model, many gaps in the evidence remain unfilled. One important question concerns the feasibility of changing people's expectations about drug effects to alter their behavior under a drug. Little is known about methods that might be applied to change individuals' expectancies about drug effects. One possibility is to provide them with new information about a particular drug effect, with the intention of revising their expectations in accordance with the new information. Some studies have adopted this procedure to provide groups of subjects with the expectation that alcohol will either improve or impair their performance on a motor skills task (Fillmore, Mulvihill, & Vogel-Sprott, 1994; Fillmore & Vogel-Sprott, 1996). This research has shown that changing individuals' expectancies can alter their responses to the drug and to the placebo, but the responses are not always consistent with the intended expected effect (e.g., Fillmore et al., 1994). There may be several reasons for this finding. Expectancies acquired through extensive prior drug use are likely to be well learned and therefore more resistant to change by the provision of new information. In addition, if new information does change the type of drug effect that an individual expects, it may "prime" other expectancies relevant to the drug-taking situation, such as those concerning the outcome of the response, that also may affect behavior. As yet, it is unclear whether new information can override prior learning of expectancies, or selectively alter a particular expectancy without changing others.

The research reviewed in this section was based on moderate doses of alcohol and caffeine. Another interesting, and yet untested, question concerns the influence of the expected type of effect under different doses of a drug. The pharmacological action of very high doses of a drug may have overwhelming behavioral effects. As doses are increased, expectancies may exert less influence and thus contribute less to individual differences in response to the drug.

Finally, studies to date have used only men as subjects. The applicability of the findings to women is not known. Future research including both men and women would allow a comparison of the types of effects they expect from a drug and the degree to which these expectancies influence their responses to drugs and placebo.

RELEVANCE

The general purpose of learning theory and research is to understand the factors that promote new behavior or change it. The learning studies reviewed in this chapter have a similar aim and are directed at understanding drug-related behavior and how it may be changed. The hazardous and harmful behavior associated with alcohol consumption and drug abuse has created problems in urgent need of solutions. Society has responded with a number of initiatives, but much remains to be accomplished. This section discusses some ways of conceptualizing and dealing with these problems by drawing on an understanding of the role of learning in the development of behavioral tolerance to alcohol and individual differences in drug-related responses.

Behavioral Tolerance and Physical Dependence

Behavioral tolerance to alcohol has often been regarded as a drug-induced symptom associated with a risk of alcohol abuse or physical dependence (e.g., American Psychiatric Association, 1994). Tolerance and dependence are customarily attributed to a single, adaptive mechanism. Under a drug, this reaction restores homeostasis so that tolerance is observed. When the drug is withheld, the reaction is observed as withdrawal distress. However, the learning research in this chapter has shown that social drinkers can display remarkable degree of behavioral tolerance, with no vestige of withdrawal distress that could be considered to indicate physical dependence. Moreover, events in the situation can affect the degree of tolerance drinkers display. In short, their behavioral tolerance resembles adaptive learning and appears to be a normal phenomenon.

The involvement of learning has ramifications for understanding the role that behavioral tolerance may play in promoting physical dependence. Although it is only possible to speculate about the nature of the adaptive processes underlying tolerance, the evidence on social drinkers implies that learning mechanisms must be involved. This conclusion appears to be at odds with the traditional view of tolerance as an involuntary, adaptive reaction that restores biological homeostasis in the presence of alcohol, and with the opinion that alcohol tolerance and physical dependence are closely related phenomena that essentially develop in parallel (Kalant, 1975). The traditional assumption of a common compensatory process underlying tolerance and physical dependence implies that the same process initiates tolerance and sustains it during all stages of alcohol use. However, learning research indicates that tolerance developed by social drinkers during early stages of alcohol use may depend, importantly, and possibly chiefly, upon learning processes. This interpretation does not necessarily replace traditional assumptions about tolerance. Rather, it raises the possibility that the tolerance might depend on a number of different processes. Those accounting for tolerance during early stages of alcohol use may differ from those that sustain tolerance after dependence is established.

The findings reviewed in this chapter also have implications for interpreting the degree of behavioral tolerance to a dose of alcohol as a possible marker for the risk of the alcohol-related problems (e.g., Schuckit, 1994). Most learned responses are situation-specific. This also appears to apply to the display of alcohol tolerance, because social drinkers can display either tolerance or impairment, depending on the events in the situation. The adaptive, changeable nature of a drinker's behavioral tolerance to alcohol makes it unlikely to be a reliable diagnostic symptom of risk for alcohol-related problems.

Individual Differences and Alcohol Abuse

Although the majority of adults in Western society use alcohol, only a small percentage engage in heavy, addictive drinking. Understanding individual differences in susceptibility to the abusive use of alcohol and physical dependence has been a long-standing puzzle. Some explanations for addictive use have been based on the biological actions of drugs in activating brain mechanisms of reward (e.g., Robinson & Berridge, 1993; Stewart et al., 1984; Wise & Bozarth, 1987). However, addictive drugs would presumably activate the same brain mechanisms in all individuals. Therefore, an explanation based solely on biological actions of a drug may not explain individual differences in susceptibility to addictive, high alcohol consumption.

Other explanations that may account for differences among individuals in the abusive use of alcohol have linked consumption to expectancies about the drug (e.g., Goldman et al., 1987). Studies have shown that heavier drinkers tend to report more favorable expectancies about alcohol than do lighter drinkers (e.g., Goldman et al., 1987). In addition, some research with heavy drinkers shows that efforts to challenge their favorable expectations about alcohol may reduce their consumption of alcohol (Darkes & Goldman, 1993). The association between individual differences in expectancies about alcohol and the extent of alcohol consumption suggests that expectancies may play a role in the susceptibility to abusive use of alcohol. This possibility warrants further investigation in light of evidence that drug-related expectancies are learned and can be changed by altering the association between events in drug-taking situations. Studies to date have only investigated the relation of alcohol consumption to expectancies in general and have not examined the separate contribution of expectancies about effects of the drug and expectancies concerning consequences. The degree to which alcohol use is mediated by one or the other of these expectancies is not known, but such information may contribute to more effective treatments that aim to reduce alcohol consumption by manipulating drug-related expectancies.

Individual Differences and Alcohol Impairment

Society has implemented many strategies to protect drinkers from the hazards of alcohol-induced impairment. Some prevention strategies aim to restrict the accessibility of alcohol (e.g., increasing the cost or raising the legal drinking age). Concern over the prevalence of alcohol-related accidents and injuries also has led to efforts to reduce the risk of impairment by legislating maximum BAC limits for performing activities, such as driving. Such a policy may misleadingly imply that BACs within the legal limit are "safe," and that the onset of impairment depends solely on reaching a particular BAC. However, individual differences in threshold BACs for impairment are noted in many types of mental and psychomotor tasks (National Institute on Alcohol Abuse and Alcoholism, 1994). Research reviewed in the chapter indicates that learned expectancies about the behavioral effects of alcohol and its consequences may account for some of these individual differences. Alcohol impairment may be reduced in situations where drinkers expect a favorable consequence for compensating for impairment. In contrast, impairment may be intensified in situations that provide reasons to expect that compensation yields no favorable consequence. Thus, a consideration of drinkers' expectations about the consequence of an activity in different drinking contexts may increase our understanding of the types of situations that are associated with high and low risk of impairment.

Expectancies about the effect of alcohol also may contribute to the risk of alcohol-related accidents and injuries in other ways. Such expectancies may influence a drinker's decisions about how much to drink and what activities to undertake while drinking. For example, a drinker who expects alcohol to induce little impairment of an activity, such as driving, may decide to drink more alcohol and may be more inclined to engage in this activity after drinking. Investigations of the potentially pervasive effects of expectancies on decision making in drug-taking situations may identify an important source of risk that has received little attention.

Alcohol, Antisocial Behavior, and Harm Reduction

Drinkers perform many types of activities under alcohol, some of which may be harmful or antisocial. The link between the expression of such behavior and alcohol use poses serious problems for society in general, and the individual in particular. To the extent that such behavior is attributed to the intoxicating chemical action of alcohol, individuals are not held personally accountable for their actions. However, pardoning antisocial activities that occur under the influence of alcohol on the grounds that the drug is responsible may foster the expectation of minimal or nonexistent adverse consequences for antisocial behavior. The removal of a penalizing outcome for such behavior makes the expected consequence more favorable than it would otherwise be. As a result, the undesirable behavior may be more likely to occur.

Harm-reduction strategies aim to diminish the deleterious effects of drug abuse. With respect to alcohol, harm reduction recognizes the difficulties in achieving abstinence and emphasizes the importance of any intervention that can reduce the harm associated with alcohol use (Marlatt, Larimer, Baer, & Quigley, 1993). Examples of such strategies are treatments that promote moderate alcohol use, and educational programs that promote awareness of hazards associated with alcohol intoxication. The common goal of harm-reduction strategies is to change and control alcohol-related behavior. Evidence that learned expectancies play an important role in determining alcohol-related behavior offers a perspective to complement harm-reduction initiatives. In general, an individual is more likely to display a response if the consequence is expected to be favorable. By clearly targeting socially acceptable drinking behavior for approval and consistently penalizing antisocial or hazardous behavior, the net outcome of socially acceptable behavior would be more favorable. These conditions could provide drinkers with an opportunity to learn that responsible drinking behavior consistently yields a more rewarding consequence than antisocial drinking behavior. Such expectancies may help to reduce the occurrence of undesirable, harmful, alcohol-related behavior.

SUMMARY AND CONCLUSIONS

An associative learning model of events in a drug-taking situation identifies relationships between three pairs of events. The acquisition of information conveyed by each association identifies three different expectancies: receiving a drug, the type of drug effect, and its environmental consequence. Evidence that these expectancies mediate behavior was provided by showing that the response to a drug could be changed by manipulating the association between the events determining each expectancy. Taken together, the results of the research indicate how the general principle of associative learning offers a basis for understanding how each of the drug-related expectancies can be acquired and what specific events must be changed in order to alter behavior mediated by these expectancies.

Behavioral responses to drugs remain a complex phenomenon, and research from different theoretical perspectives and different levels of analysis are needed to provide a more complete understanding. Environmental events are appropriately excluded in research examining the action of a drug on organ tissues and cells. However, in behaving organisms, environmental events are not extraneous factors that obscure the "true" pharmacological effect of a drug. Events, through their history of association with drug exposure and with behavior, participate in the selective expression of drug-related behavior.

ACKNOWLEDGMENT

Preparation of this chapter was supported, in part, by grants from the Natural Sciences and Engineering Research Council and the Alcoholic Beverage Medical Research Foundation.

NOTE

1. Although such differences may be loosely interpreted as differences in tolerance, evidence on the acquisition of tolerance can actually only be provided in repeated-dose studies that measure the initial drug effect and its attenuation after a series of drug exposures. Nonetheless, determining the degree of behavioral impairment to a single dose is important and has been the aim of many studies in the area of behavioral pharmacology.

REFERENCES

Alkana, R. L., Finn, D. A., & Malcolm, R. D. (1983). The importance of experience in the development of tolerance to ethanol hypothermia. *Life Sciences, 32,* 2685–2692.

American Psychiatric Association. (1994). *Diagnostic and statistical manual of mental disorders* (4th ed.). Washington, DC: Author.

Bandura, A. (1977). *Social learning theory*. Englewood Cliffs, NJ: Prentice-Hall.

Beirness, D. J., & Vogel-Sprott, M. (1984). Alcohol tolerance in social drinkers: Operant and classical conditioning effects. *Psychopharmacology, 84,* 393–397.

Bolles, R. C. (1972). Reinforcement, expectancy and learning. *Psychological Review, 79*, 394–409.

Bolles, R. C. (1979). *Learning theory* (2nd ed.). New York: Holt, Reinhart & Winston.

Branch, M. N. (1984). Rate dependency, behavioral mechanisms, and behavioral pharmacology. *Journal of the Experimental Analysis of Behavior, 42*, 511–522.

Carpenter, J. A. (1962). Effects of alcohol on some psychological processes. *Quarterly Journal of Studies on Alcohol, 23*, 274–314.

Cooney, N. L., Gillespie, R. A., Baker, L. H., & Kaplan, R. F. (1987). Cognitive changes after alcohol cue exposure. *Journal of Consulting and Clinical Psychology, 55*, 150–155.

Dafters, R., & Anderson, G. (1982). Conditioned tolerance to the tachycardia effect of ethanol in humans. *Psychopharmacology, 78*, 365–367.

Darkes, J., & Goldman, M. S. (1993). Expectancy challenge and drinking reduction: Evidence for a mediational process. *Journal of Consulting and Clinical Psychology, 61*, 344–353.

de Wit, H., & Stewart, J. (1981). Reinstatement of cocaine: Experimental reinforced responding in the rat. *Psychopharmacology, 75*, 134–143.

de Wit, H., & Stewart, J. (1983). Drug reinstatement of heroin- reinforced responding in the rat. *Psychopharmacology, 79*, 29–31.

Dews, P. B. (1962). Psychopharmacology. In A. J. Bachrach (Ed.), *Experimental foundations of clinical psychology* (pp. 423–441). New York: Basic Books.

Didly-Mayfield, J. E., & Harris, R. A. (1995). Neurobiology of alcohol's actions and the addiction process. In B. Tabakoff & P. Hoffman (Eds.), *Biological aspects of alcoholism* (pp. 189–223). Seattle: Hogrefe & Huber.

Domjan, M., & Burkhard, B. (1986). *The principles of learning and behavior* (2nd ed.). Monterey, CA: Brooks/Cole.

Easdon, C. M., & Vogel-Sprott, M. (1996). Drug-free behavioral history affects social drinkers' tolerance to a challenge dose of alcohol. *Journal of Studies on Alcohol, 57*, 591–597.

Eikelboom, R., & Stewart, J. (1982). Conditioning of drug-induced physiological responses. *Psychological Review, 89*, 507–528.

Eriksen, L. M., & Gotestam, K. G. (1984). Conditioned abstinence in alcoholics: A controlled experiment. *International Journal of the Addictions, 19*, 287–294.

Fillmore, M. T. (1994). Investigating the behavioral effects of caffeine: The contribution of drug-related expectancies. *Pharmacopsychoecologia, 7*, 63–73.

Fillmore, M. T., Carscadden, J. L., & Vogel-Sprott, M. (1998). Alcohol, cognitive impairment, and expectancies. *Journal of Studies on Alcohol, 59*, 174–179.

Fillmore, M. T., Mulvihill, L. E., & Vogel-Sprott, M. (1994). The expected drug and its expected effect interact to determine placebo responses to alcohol and caffeine. *Psychopharmacology, 115*, 383–388.

Fillmore, M. T., & Vogel-Sprott, M. (1994). Psychomotor performance under alcohol and under caffeine: Expectancy and pharmacological effects. *Experimental and Clinical Psychopharmacology, 2*, 319–328.

Fillmore, M. T., & Vogel-Sprott, M. (1995a). Behavioral effects of alcohol in novice and experienced drinkers: Alcohol expectancies and impairment. *Psychopharmacology, 122*, 175–181.

Fillmore, M. T., & Vogel-Sprott, M. (1995b). Expectancies about alcohol-induced motor impairment predict individual differences in responses to alcohol and placebo. *Journal of Studies on Alcohol, 56,* 90–98.

Fillmore, M. T., & Vogel-Sprott, M. (1996). Evidence that expectancies mediate behavioral impairment under alcohol. *Journal of Studies on Alcohol, 57,* 598–603.

Fillmore, M. T., & Vogel-Sprott, M. (1997). Resistance to impaired information processing under alcohol: The role of environmental consequences of cognitive performance. *Experimental and Clinical Psychopharmacology, 5,* 251–255.

Gessa, G. L., Muntoni, F., Vargui, L., & Mereu, G. (1985). Low doses of ethanol activate dopaminergic neurons in the ventral tegmental area. *Brain Research, 348,* 201–203.

Glautier, S., & Drummond, D. C. (1994). Alcohol dependence and cue reactivity. *Journal of Studies on Alcohol, 55,* 224–229.

Goldberg, L. (1943). Quantitative studies of alcohol tolerance in man: The influence of ethyl alcohol on sensory, motor, and psychological functions referred to blood alcohol in normal and habituated individuals. *Acta Physiologica Scandinavica, 5*(Suppl. 16), 1–128.

Goldberg, L., & Havard, J. (1968). *Research on the effects of alcohol and drugs on driver behavior and their importance as a cause of road accidents.* Paris: Organization for Economic Cooperation and Development.

Goldman, M. S., Brown S. A., & Christiansen, B. A. (1987). Expectancy theory: Thinking about drinking. In H. Blane & K. Leonard (Eds.), *Psychological theories of drinking and alcoholism* (pp. 181–226). New York: Guilford Press.

Greeley, J. D., Swift, W., Prescott, J., & Heather, N. (1993). Reactivity of alcohol-related cues in heavy and light drinkers. *Journal of Studies on Alcohol, 54,* 359–368.

Hinson, R. E., & Siegel, S. (1980). The contribution of Pavlovian conditioning to ethanol tolerance and dependence. In H. Rigter & J. C. Crabbe (Eds.), *Alcohol tolerance and dependence* (pp. 181–199). Amsterdam: Elsevier/North-Holland Biomedical Press.

Hjeresen, D. L., Reed, D. R., & Woods, S. C. (1986). Tolerance to hypothermia induced by ethanol depends on specific drug effects. *Psychopharmacology, 89,* 45–51.

Hull, J., & Bond, C. (1986). Social and behavioral consequences of alcohol consumption and expectancy: A meta-analysis. *Psychological Bulletin, 99,* 347–360.

Hunt, W. A. (1990). Brain mechanisms that underlie the reinforcing effects of ethanol. In W. M. Cox (Ed.), *Why people drink: Parameters of alcohol as a reinforcer* (pp. 71–91). New York: Gardner.

Hunt, W. A. (1993). Neuroscience research: How has it contributed to our understanding of alcohol abuse and alcoholism? A review. *Alcoholism: Clinical and Experimental Research, 17,* 1055–1065.

Imperato, A., & Di Chiara, (1986). Preferential stimulation of dopamine release in the nucleus accumbens of freely moving rats by ethanol. *Journal of Pharmacology and Experimental Therapeutics, 239,* 219–228.

Jellinek, E. M., & McFarland, R. A. (1940). Analysis of psychological experiments on the effects of alcohol. *Quarterly Journal of Studies on Alcohol, 1,* 272–371.

Kalant, H. (1975). Biological model of alcohol tolerance and physical dependence. In M. M. Gross (Ed.), *Psychopharmacology of alcohol* (pp. 107–120). New York: Raven Press.

Koelega, H. S. (1995). Alcohol and vigilance performance: A review. *Psychopharmacology, 118,* 233–249.

Krank, M., Hinson, R. E., & Siegel, S., (1981). Conditional hyperalgesia is elicited by environmental signals of morphine. *Behavioral and Neural Biology, 32,* 148–157.

Le, A. D., Poulos, C. X., & Cappell, H. (1979). Conditioned tolerance to the hypothermic effect of ethyl alcohol. *Science, 206,* 1109–1110.

Linnoila, M., Stapleton, J., Lister, R., Guthrie, S., & Eckardt, M. (1986). Effects of alcohol on accident risk. *Pathologist, 40,* 36–41.

MacAndrew, C., & Edgerton, R. B. (1969). *Drunken comportment: A social explanation.* Chicago: Aldine.

MacNish, R. (1832). *The anatomy of drunkenness* (4th ed.). Glasgow: W. R. McPhun Press.

Mann, R. E., & Vogel-Sprott, M. (1981). Control of alcohol tolerance by reinforcement in nonalcoholics. *Psychopharmacology, 75,* 315-320.

Marlatt, G. A., Larimer, M. E., Baer, J. S., & Quigley, L. A. (1993). Harm reduction for alcohol problems: Moving beyond the controlled drinking controversy. *Behavior Therapy, 24,* 461–504.

Marlatt, G. A., & Rohsenow, D. (1980). Cognitive processes in alcohol use: Expectancy and the balanced placebo design. In N. K. Mello (Ed.), *Advances in substance abuse* (pp. 159–199). Greenwich, CT: J.A.I. Press.

Mello, N. K., & Mendelson, J. H. (1965). Operant analysis of drinking patterns of chronic alcoholics. *Nature, 206,* 43–46.

Mitchell, M. C. (1985). Alcohol-induced impairment of central nervous system function: Behavioral skills involved in driving. *Journal of Studies on Alcohol, Suppl. 10,* 109–116.

Monti, P. M., Binkoff, J. A., Abrams, D. B., Zwick, W. R., Nirenberg, T. D., & Liepman, M. R. (1987). Reactivity of alcoholics and nonalcoholics to drinking cues. *Journal of Abnormal Psychology, 96,* 1–5.

Mulvihill, L. (1997). *Reducing alcohol-impairment of inhibitory control: The effects of feedback and incentive.* Unpublished manuscript, University of Waterloo, Waterloo, Ontario.

Mulvihill, L. E., Skilling, T. A., & Vogel-Sprott, M. (1997). Alcohol and the ability to inhibit behavior in men and women. *Journal of Studies on Alcohol, 58,* 600–605.

National Institute on Alcohol Abuse and Alcoholism. (1994). *Alcohol alert: Alcohol-related impairment* (Public Health 351 No. 25). Rockville, MD: Author.

Niaura, R., Rohsenow, D. J., Binkoff, J. A., Monti, P. M., Pedraza, M., & Abrams, D. B. (1988). Relevance of cue reactivity to understanding alcohol and smoking relapse. *Journal of Abnormal Psychology, 97,* 133–152.

O'Brien, C. P. (1976). Experimental analysis of conditioning factors in human narcotic addiction. *Pharmacological Reviews, 27,* 533–543.

Pavlov, I. P. (1927). *Conditioned reflexes* (G. V. Anrep, Trans.). London: Oxford University Press.

Poulos, C. X., & Hinson, R. E. (1982). Pavlovian conditional tolerance to haloperidol catalepsy: Evidence of dynamic adaptations in the dopaminergic system. *Science, 218,* 491–492.

Rawana, E., & Vogel-Sprott, M. (1985). The transfer of alcohol tolerance, and its relation to reinforcement. *Drug and Alcohol Dependence, 16*(1), 75–83.

Rescorla, R. A. (1987). A Pavlovian analysis of goal-directed behavior. *American Psychologist, 42,* 119–129.

Rescorla, R. A. (1990). The role information about the response–outcome relation in instrumental discrimination learning. *Journal of Experimental Psychology: Animal Behavior Processes, 16,* 262–270.

Rescorla, R. A., & Colwill, R. M. (1989). Associations with anticipated and obtained outcomes in instrumental learning. *Animal Learning and Behavior, 17,* 291–303.

Robinson, T. E., & Berridge, K. C. (1993). The neural basis of drug craving: An incentive-sensitization theory of addiction. *Brain Research Reviews, 18,* 247–291.

Rohsenow, D., & Marlatt, G. A. (1981). The balanced placebo design: Methodological considerations. *Addictive Behaviors, 6,* 107–122.

Rotter, J. B. (1981). The psychological situation in learning theory. In D. Magnusson (Ed.), *Toward a psychology of situations: An interactional perspective.* Hillsdale, NJ: Erlbaum.

Schmidt, R. A. (1988). *Motor control and learning: A behavioral emphasis* (2nd ed.). Champaign, IL: Human Kinetics.

Schuckit, M. (1994). Low level of response to alcohol as a predictor of future alcoholism. *American Journal of Psychiatry, 151,* 184–189.

Schuster, C. R., Dockens, W. S., & Woods, J. H. (1966). Behavioral variables affecting the development of amphetamine tolerance. *Psychopharmacologia, 9,* 170–182.

Sdao-Jarvie, K., & Vogel-Sprott, M. (1991). Response expectancies affect the acquisition and display of behavioral tolerance to alcohol. *Alcohol, 8,* 491–498.

Sdao-Jarvie, K., & Vogel-Sprott, M. (1992). Learning alcohol tolerance by mental or physical practice. *Journal of Studies on Alcohol, 53,* 533–540.

Shapiro, A. K., & Morris, L. A. (1978). Placebo effects in medical and psychological therapies. In S. L. Garfield & A. K. Bergin (Eds.), *Handbook of psychotherapy and behavior change* (2nd ed., pp. 369–410). New York: Wiley.

Shapiro, A. P., & Nathan, P. E. (1986). Human tolerance to alcohol: The role of Pavlovian conditioning processes. *Psychopharmacology, 88,* 90–95.

Siegel, S. (1975). Evidence from rats that morphine tolerance is a learned response. *Journal of Comparative and Physiological Psychology, 89,* 498–506.

Siegel, S. (1976). Morphine analgesic tolerance: Its situation specificity supports a Pavlovian conditioning model. *Science, 193,* 323–325.

Siegel, S. (1983). Classical conditioning, drug tolerance and drug dependence. In Y. Israel, B. F. Glaser, H. Kalant, R. E. Popham, W. Schmidt, & R. G. Smart (Eds.), *Research Advances in Alcohol and Drug problems* (Vol 7, pp. 207–246). New York: Plenum.

Siegel, S. (1989). Pharmacological conditioning and drug effects. In A. J. Goudie & M. W. Emmett-Oglesby (Eds.), *Psychoactive drugs: Tolerance and sensitization* (pp. 115–180). Clifton, NJ: Humana Press.

Solomon, R. L., & Corbitt, J. D. (1974). An opponent–process theory of motivation. *Psychological Review, 81,* 119–145.

Staiger, P. K., & White, J. M. (1988). Conditioned alcohol-like and alcohol-opposite responses in humans. *Psychopharmacology, 95,* 87–91.

Staiger, P. K., & White, J. M. (1991). Cue reactivity in alcohol abusers: Stimulus specificity and extinction of the responses. *Addictive Behaviors, 16,* 211–221.

Stewart, J, de Wit, H., & Eikelboom, R. (1984). Role of unconditioned and conditioned drug effects in the self-administration of opiates and stimulants. *Psychological Review, 91,* 251–268.

Subkov, A. A., & Zilov, G. N. (1937). The role of conditioned reflex adaptation in the origin of hyperergic reactions. *Bulletin de Biologie et de Medécine Expérimentale, 4,* 294–296.

Tolman, E. C. (1932). *Purposive behavior in animals and men.* New York: Century.

Vogel, M. (1958). Low blood alcohol concentrations and psychological adjustment as factors in psychomotor performance: An exploratory study. *Quarterly Journal of Studies on Alcohol, 19,* 573–589.

Vogel-Sprott, M. (1992). *Alcohol tolerance and social drinking: Learning the consequences.* New York: Guilford Press.

Vogel-Sprott, M. (1997). Is behavioral tolerance learned? *Alcohol Health and Research World, 21,* 161–168.

Vogel-Sprott, M., & Fillmore, M. T. (in press). Expectancy and behavioral effects of socially-used drugs. In I. Kirsch (Ed.), *Expectancy, experience and behavior.* Washington, DC: American Psychological Association Press.

Wallgren, H., & Barry, H., III. (1971). *Actions of alcohol.* Amsterdam: Elsevier.

Wikler, A. (1948). Recent progress in research on the neurophysiological basis of morphine addiction. *American Journal of Psychiatry, 105,* 329–338.

Wikler, A. (1973). Conditioning of successive adaptive responses to the initial effects of drugs. *Conditioned Reflex, 8,* 193–210.

Wise, R. A. (1988). The neurobiology of craving: Implications for the understanding and treatment of addiction. *Journal of Abnormal Psychology, 97,* 118–132.

Wise, R. A., & Bozarth, M. A. (1987). A psychomotor stimulant theory of addiction. *Psychological Review, 94,* 469–492.

Wolgin, D. L. (1989). The role of instrumental learning in behavioral tolerance to drugs. In A. J. Goudie & M. W. Emmett-Oglesby (Eds.), *Psychoactive drugs: Tolerance and sensitization* (pp. 17–114). Clifton, NJ: Humana Press.

Zack, M., & Vogel-Sprott, M. (1993). Response outcomes affect the retention of behavioral tolerance to alcohol: Information and incentive. *Psychopharmacology, 113*(2), 269–273.

Zack, M., & Vogel-Sprott, M. (1995). Behavioral tolerance and sensitization to alcohol in humans: The contribution of learning. *Experimental and Clinical Psychopharmacology, 3*(4), 396–401.

Zack, M., & Vogel-Sprott, M. (1997). Drunk or sober? Learned conformity to behavioral standards. *Journal of Studies on Alcohol, 58,* 495–501.

Zinatelli, M., & Vogel-Sprott, M. (1993). Behavioral tolerance to alcohol in humans is enhanced by prior drug-free treatment. *Experimental and Clinical Psychopharmacology, 1,* 194–199.

9

Alcohol and Emotional Response: A Multidimensional– Multilevel Analysis

ALAN R. LANG
CHRISTOPHER J. PATRICK
WERNER G. K. STRITZKE

> We all know, from what we experience with and within ourselves, that our conscious acts spring from our desires and our fears. . . . We all try to escape pain and death, while we seek what is pleasant . . . these primary impulses . . . are the springs of man's actions. . . . All such action would cease if those powerful elemental forces were to cease stirring within us.
> —ALBERT EINSTEIN (1956/1990, p. 15)

INTRODUCTION

Einstein's observation suggests that, whatever the arena of human behavior, emotion is at the center of it. Is there any reason to believe that it is otherwise as far as alcohol consumption is concerned? The very definition of a psychoactive substance, of which alcohol is one, revolves around its connection with altered states of emotion and/or consciousness. The DSM-IV description of simple alcohol intoxication includes "mood lability" as a core feature and, although subjective distress is not a diagnostic criterion specific to alcohol abuse or dependence, it is one of the principal attributes of any mental disorder. Moreover, virtually all major theories of drinking behavior and alcohol problems include an important role for emotional factors. Goldman, Brown, and Christiansen (1987) went so far as to say, "If any characteristic has been seen as a central, defining aspect of alcohol use, it is the presumed capacity of alcohol to alter anxiety, depression, and other moods" (p. 200). This does not mean, of course, that all alcohol consumption is governed by exclusively emotional motives or that it invariably exerts a direct influence on emotional reactions. Heath (1995a, 1995b), for example, asserted that most drinking throughout the cultures of the world is first and foremost a social act, shaped by norms, rituals, and ceremonies pertinent to sociability, social cohesion, and social structure. Yet it is evident that affect permeates many social interactions, particularly those in which alcohol is present. Thus, an assumption underlying the psychophysiological approach advanced in this chapter is that understanding the alcohol–emotion nexus is fundamental to understanding drinking and its problems.

We begin with a summary of the key role that emotion seems to play in a wide range of theories of drinking and alcoholism. We then proceed to develop a multidimensional–multilevel model of emotion and describe alcohol's effects on the psychophysiological indices that underlie it, reviewing recent, pertinent literature within this framework. Our primary focus is on laboratory analogue investigations of one particular aspect of the alcohol–emotion relationship: the impact of acute alcohol intoxication on human psychophysiological response to emotional stimuli. In the concluding sections, we provide an illustration of how our approach can be applied, using the example of fear responding, and offer recommendations for future research.

THE ROLE OF EMOTION IN THEORIES OF DRINKING

The idea that emotion, in one way or another, occupies a pivotal position in nearly all major theories of drinking and alcohol problems seems almost axiomatic, but it may be instructive to reflect for a moment on just how prominent that position is. Selected examples, spanning biological, sociocultural, and psychological realms, are offered to support this assertion. Further evidence of the pervasiveness of this theme will be apparent to any reader willing to peruse the other chapters in this volume, with the construct of emotion in mind.

Emotion and Biological Theories

Besides extensive research on the health consequences of chronic heavy drinking, a major theme in theories with a strong biological orientation has been elucidation of the genetics and associated markers of risk for alcoholism (see McGue, Chapter 10, and Sher, Trull, Bartholow, & Vieth,

Chapter 3, this volume). But, considerable attention has also been directed toward analysis of the nature of acute intoxication. Much of this work has revolved around the biochemical bases and brain mechanisms of reinforcement from alcohol (e.g., Hunt, 1990a, 1990b, for a review; Chapter 11 by Fromme & D'Amico, this volume). Brain systems, of course, are dynamic and interactive, and the complexities of dose variables and pharmacokinetics add difficulty to the understanding and prediction of alcohol effects. Yet whatever the exact substrates and processes may be, it seems clear that changes in emotional state and/or emotional response are closely tied to alcohol effects. One prominent theme in this literature is that alcohol's physiological action may be "biphasic."

It is widely acknowledged that the primary action of alcohol, like that of sedative–hypnotics, is as a central nervous system (CNS) depressant, but it has been recognized for some time that this effect is not necessarily linear across dose or time (e.g., Mello, 1968; Pohorecky, 1977). Rather, despite some null findings (e.g., McCollam, Burish, Maisto, & Sobell, 1980; Turkkan, Stitzer, & McCaul, 1988; for a review, also see Tucker, Vuchinich, & Sobell, 1982), it appears that particularly while blood alcohol concentration (BAC) is rising shortly after administration, alcohol can have a stimulant effect, weaker than, but similar to, that caused by amphetamines. This stimulation is apparent in the initially increased spontaneous motor activity of lower animals exposed to alcohol (e.g., Lewis & June, 1990) as well as in the increased cortical activity of humans early in an episode of intoxication (e.g., Lukas, Mendelson, Benedikt, & Jones, 1986). Perhaps more important for our purposes is that the stimulation is correlated with self-reported experiences of positive emotions such as elation and euphoria, as well as increased arousal described as energy and vigor (e.g., Lukas et al., 1986; Martin, Earleywine, Musty, Perrine, & Swift, 1993). Based on the additional observation that the slope of rising BAC seems to influence the magnitude of stimulation and positive affect, Newlin and Thomson (1990) have speculated further that the rate of *transition* from sobriety to intoxication may influence reinforcement more than the absolute level of BAC. Other evidence suggests that alcohol-induced psychomotor activation is associated with facilitation of brain reward systems, and a number of theorists (e.g., Wise & Bozarth, 1987) have suggested that a wide range of addictive drugs (including alcohol) exert their power through actions on dopaminergic fibers projecting into areas of the brain that mediate reinforcement, emotional state, and approach behavior.

At the other end of the emotional spectrum, alcohol is also known to produce sedation and dysphoria at high BACs and on the declining limb of the BAC curve. It is perhaps more in connection with these actions that substantial effort has been devoted to investigation of the possible anxiolytic effect of alcohol (for reviews, see, e.g., Cappell & Greeley, 1987; Pohorecky, 1991; Sher, 1987; West & Sutker, 1990; Wilson, 1988). This extensive and complex literature has been somewhat disappointing in its equivocation and in its relative inattention to neurobehavioral mechanisms that might underlie those effects (e.g., a tendency for alcohol-intoxicated organisms to resolve approach–avoidance conflicts in the approach direction) that have been observed with some consistency. The contemporary analysis of alcohol and tension reduction available in this volume (Chapter 2 by Greeley & Oei) should help bring better order to this area.

Related work on what some (Sher, 1987) have called a "minitheory" of tension reduction, limited to the hypothesis that response to stress is dampened in alcohol-intoxicated persons, has also attracted attention. But, here, too, results from pertinent research have not been altogether clear, particularly where measures of autonomic reactivity are concerned (e.g., Sayette, 1993a). We address this area in some detail in later sections, introducing a broader perspective and new research on how alcohol might influence response to emotional stimuli. For the moment, suffice it to say that almost regardless of the empirical evidence from laboratory studies, the possible alleviation or dampening of negative emotion by alcohol remains a time-honored theory of why people drink.

A third category of biobehavioral theory in which emotional state is central is opponent process theory (Solomon, 1977). Indeed, Donegan, Rodin, O'Brien, and Solomon (1983) described the opponent processes in terms of "affective contrast," and argued that they represent a common feature of many addictive and habitual behaviors. The essence of the theory is that the nervous system is organized to oppose or suppress the unconditioned, hedonic effects of alcohol [and other addictive drugs] that provide intrinsic reinforcement. Perhaps in an effort to maintain homeostasis, these unconditioned stimuli (UCS) or operant reinforcers automatically elicit opposing physiological processes and accompanying affective states. The result is a biphasic process of another sort: one in which a pleasant, phasic "a-process," occasioned by acute intoxication, builds up and subsides rapidly, with little sensitization or habituation. However, it is inevitably followed by an affectively negative "b-process" of equal magnitude, but having much longer latency and slower decay. With repeated presentations of the UCS—particularly if the intertrial interval is not long enough to allow the organism to return to baseline—the unpleasant b-process increases in intensity (cf. withdrawal) and is more readily elicited by the UCS, thereby diminishing the drug's intrinsically pleasant effects (cf. tolerance). As a result, drinking or other drug taking becomes motivated more by a desire to relieve dysphoria than by a desire to attain euphoria. In either case, it is clear that modulation of emotional state is the force driving the indulgence.

Naturally, the processes of affective contrast are subject to a variety of conditioning phenomena that can also influence drinking and its effects (Chapter 8 by Vogel-Sprott & Fillmore, this volume). These are especially evident in the reactions of addicts to cues associated with their problem substance or other habit. Once again, these "cue reactivity" effects have a decidedly emotional flavor to them (for a review, see Drummond, Tiffany, Glautier, & Remington, 1995).

Emotion and Sociocultural Theories

At the other extreme from the micro-level of biological analysis, sociocultural theories of drinking attempt to describe the integration and function of alcohol use within the social fabric of a society or culture as a whole. Bales's (1946) classic cross-cultural model of drinking and its associated problems exemplifies this tradition. He posited that the rate of drinking and alcoholism in a society can be estimated from the level of stress in that society and the available means to cope with stress, along with the prevailing norms for drinking. Clearly, Bales regarded the emotional state of a people and their access to alternate means for modifying it as crucial determinants of alcohol use, assuming such use is an available option. Other influential sociocultural theorists (e.g., MacAndrew & Edgerton, 1969) have described intoxication as a "time out" from constraints that ordinarily govern social behaviors, especially affect-laden behaviors such as aggression and sexual expression. Because such disinhibition is usually accompanied by a marked change in mood, the potential mediating role of emotion in key behavioral consequences of drinking is implicit in this theory.

Among sociologists, two other theorists (Gusfield, 1987; Orcutt, 1993) have pursued a somewhat different version of the "time out" model by emphasizing more positive concomitants of drinking. They argue that the mood-setting properties of alcohol derive, in part, from its ritualized association with transitions between work and play, or, more generally, between serious and playful periods. Thus, alteration of emotion again appears to figure prominently in drinking behavior, even if it is not altogether clear whether it is a cause, consequence, or simple covariate of alcohol use.

Emotion and Psychological Theories

Because contemporary psychological theories of drinking and alcoholism typically acknowledge, if not incorporate, biological and sociocultural variables, it is difficult to discuss such theories without reference to the two broad perspectives introduced previously. Indeed, several approaches that can be inferred to be "psychological" by virtue of their inclusion in this book have already been mentioned in connection with biological and sociocultural theories. Others, including developmental (Chapter 5 by Windle & Davies, this volume) and social learning (Chapter 4 by Maisto, Carey, & Bradizza, this volume) approaches, also involve biological concepts such as dispositional temperament and sociocultural concepts such as modeling/imitation in their analyses. Although emotion probably plays a major role in the processes outlined by such theorists, its focal position is even more evident in psychological theories emphasizing expectations about alcohol effects and motives for drinking.

As already noted, Goldman et al. (1987) concluded from their early work on expectations about alcohol effects that alteration of mood and affective reaction are probably the most prevalent and pivotal of the beliefs. Subsequent research by this team (Rather & Goldman, 1994; Rather, Goldman, Roehrich, & Brannick, 1992; Chapter 6 by Goldman, Del Boca, & Darkes, this volume) has applied multidimensional scaling, hierarchical clustering, and other sophisticated analytic techniques to fortify this position. Results consistently pointed to arousal (activation vs. sedation) and affective/social valence (positive vs. negative) as the primary dimensions along which alcohol expectancies are distributed, and further showed these dimensions can be used to distinguish between heavy and light drinkers. These findings indicate that emotions are at the center of expectations about alcohol effects.

From a psychological perspective, the next logical question is whether such expectancies and the memory networks presumed to underlie them map onto important motives for drinking. Recent work by Cooper and her colleagues (e.g., Cooper, Frone, Russell, & Mudar, 1995) suggests that they do. Their model, which is in many ways consistent with the more elaborate "incentive motivation" approach of Cox and Klinger (1990), proposes that desire to regulate both positive and negative emotions is the major motivation for alcohol consumption. Furthermore, Cooper et al. (1995) maintain that relatively distinct antecedents and consequences (not only emotions, but also alcohol expectancies and other individual differences) are associated with drinking to enhance positive emotions versus to cope with negative ones. Analyses of large, longitudinal data sets collected on both adolescent and adult samples provide convincing support for each of the major premises of this model. They show, for example, that enhancement drinkers are apt to be sensation seekers who hold strong expectations that alcohol will facilitate positive emotional experience, whereas coping drinkers are liable to be depressed, rely on avoidance and other maladaptive coping strategies, and hold strong beliefs in the tension-reducing properties of alcohol. The authors assert, we think justifiably, that "the emotion management perspective offers a potentially heuristic framework for understanding drinking behavior" (p. 1004).

There are, of course, other domains to which this brief survey of the role of emotion in major theories of drinking and alcohol problems could be extended. For example, certainly, alcoholism is frequently comorbid with other mental disorders (e.g., anxiety, mood, and antisocial personality disorders) in which affective response, or lack thereof, is critical (e.g., Regier et al., 1990). Or, we could review work on negative emotional traits and states often associated with alcoholic relapse (e.g., Hodgins, el-Guebaly, & Armstrong, 1995; Vuchinich & Tucker, 1996). However, the preceding summary should be sufficient to make it evident that understanding the many connections between alcohol and emotion is probably critical to understanding drinking and its attendant problems more broadly. Research to date has only scratched the surface, but it now appears that we are poised to advance our knowledge significantly. The need to integrate a complex array of diverse variables and mechanisms makes this task challenging, but we believe that psychology is the discipline best equipped to make such a contribution because of its potential and inclination to bridge the artificial boundaries between biological, social, and psychological approaches. Let us set out on that path by outlining a multidimensional–multilevel approach to analysis of the construct of emotion.

THEORIES OF EMOTION IN ALCOHOL RESEARCH

Alcohol and Emotion: A Dimensional and Hierarchical Framework

Definition and description of a complex hypothetical construct such as emotion is always difficult and sometimes controversial (Ekman & Davidson, 1994). Nonetheless, we believe that the theoretical and empirical foundation for the multidimensional–multilevel conceptualization of emotion, upon which our work is predicated, is both broad and deep. But before proceeding further, a brief clarification of what distinguishes "emotion" or "affect" (which are used synonymously throughout this chapter) from mood is in order. For our purposes, an emotion is defined as a relatively brief complex of responses to evocative stimuli, typically biasing the organism toward action. In contrast, a mood is sustained over a longer time span and serves to modulate cognition (cf. Ekman, 1984). In a sense, some kind of mood, however weak, is always present and provides a background for emotion. The responses elicited by controlled, time-limited laboratory manipulations of affect that form the data base for this review can generally be characterized as emotions. The implications of a temporal (specifically, phasic vs. tonic) dimension of emotion for adequate resolution in psychophysiological measurement are addressed later.

Our basic approach holds that emotion or affective state involves central activation of "action dispositions" or response tendencies that prepare an organism to act (Izard, 1993; P. Lang, 1995; Plutchik, 1984). Consistent with P. Lang (1995), Larsen and Diener (1992), Russell (1980), and others, we organize these action dispositions along dimensions of *arousal* (degree of activation) and *valence* (pleasant or unpleasant) to represent two primary brain motivational systems: an aversive system governing defensive reactions, and an appetitive system governing consummatory and other approach behaviors (cf. Konorski, 1967; P. Lang, 1995). This view can be reconciled with Gray's (1987) model, which includes a nonspecific arousal system that is driven by both appetitive and aversive motive systems (also see Fowles, 1980). In any event, we presume that these motivational systems are subcortically based, but that through reciprocal connections to higher cortical regions, they can influence and be influenced by more complex cognitive processes such as attention, perception, declarative memory, and imagery (P. Lang, 1994a; LeDoux, 1995). Thus, we maintain that emotional action dispositions should be represented within a two-factor framework, defined by the primary, or what some (P. Lang, Bradley, & Cuthbert, 1990) have called the "strategic," affective dimensions of valence and arousal.

An alternative perspective is that positive affect (PA) and negative affect (NA) dimensions represent the primary axes of emotional space (Tellegen, 1985; Watson, Clark, & Tellegen, 1988). This viewpoint derives from a somewhat different data base (viz., mood reports) and has been applied to psychophysiological measurement only recently (Witvliet & Vrana, 1995). Although some analyses of the putative independence of PA and NA suggest that it may be an artifact of measurement error (Green, Goldman, & Salovey, 1993), many contemporary theorists (Larsen & Diener, 1992; P. Lang, 1995; Russell, Weiss, & Mendelsohn, 1989) embrace the notion but are inclined to view it as complementary to rather than incompatible with the arousal/valence model. In any case, we assert that the processes involved in emotion are best understood with reference to potentially interactive cognitive processes.

In contrast to the dimensional and hierarchical view we are proposing, most work on alcohol and emotion, at least prior to about 1990, seems to have been guided by more narrowly defined theories of action and process. For example, "tension reduction" and "stress response dampening" models have historically focused almost exclusively on alcohol's possible effects as a moderator of *negative* affective states and reactions. Moreover, the relevant responses have generally been operationalized mainly in terms of nonspecific arousal indices, with intermittent self-reports as the only index of valence. Overall, theorists and investigators in this tradition seem to have assumed that any alcohol effects were direct, selective, and at the level of primary brain motive systems (for reviews, see Cappell & Greeley, 1987; Pohorecky, 1991; Sher, 1987). From this perspective, an alcohol-induced reduction of anxiety or dampening of response to stress is inferred primarily from any significant attenuation of physiological arousal (e.g., decreased heart rate), with self-reports sometimes applied to assist in interpretation. Although this approach has generated important contributions, the application of concepts and measures emanating from contemporary theories of emotion appears to have the potential to expand and refine them.

One area in need of attention is the smaller but parallel body of literature on alcohol and emotion that relates elevated levels of arousal at particular positions on the blood alcohol curve to stimulation or enhancement of *positive* affect (e.g., Marlatt, 1987; Mello, 1968; Pohorecky, 1977). Unfortunately, experimental manipulations of positively valenced emotions are rare in alcohol research (for an exception, see early work by Vuchinich, Tucker, & Sobell, 1979), perhaps because they are relatively difficult to execute and control (West & Sutker, 1990). Still, considering the hypothesized major role of both negative *and* positive affect in drinking behavior and its consequences, it is puzzling that so few investigators have sought to study the full range of affect and to measure emotional valence specifically. Incorporation of both arousal and valence dimensions in future research should facilitate development of a better integrated, or at least, more precise understanding of the alcohol–affect relationship.

We are, of course, cognizant of the fact that the contextual or "tactical" (P. Lang et al., 1990) demands of a situation can shape specific expressions of basic aversive or appetitive motivational dispositions and account for much of the variation in the expression of distinct emotions (e.g., fear vs. anger). However, even if the psychophysiological measures we advocate here cannot capture subtle distinctions between emotions very well, there is abundant evidence that they can reliably index the underlying strategic dimensions of affect. In any case, it is not our intention to try to reduce all emotional phenomena to arousal and valence coordinates alone, nor to assume that all the important distinctions among discrete emotions (cf. Buck, 1988; Izard, 1972; Tomkins, 1984) can be understood in terms of just two dimensions. Rather, our position is that a full understanding of emotional experience and expression will require examination of other variables and processes that may interact with primary brain motivational systems.

Accordingly, we wish to highlight another major theme evident in contemporary theories of emotion: Affective reactivity involves the interplay of primitive action mobilization systems and higher brain processes. There is mounting evidence to suggest that emotional phenomena involve a hierarchy of neural, sensorimotor, motivational, and cognitive processes (Izard, 1993; LeDoux, 1989; 1995). Information-processing theories of emotion (e.g., Bower, 1981; P. Lang, 1979) maintain that emotional episodes are represented in associative networks, which differ from other memory structures in that they include links between cortical processing regions and the subcortical systems that govern primitive appetitive and defensive reactions (P. Lang, 1994a). In general, more complex emotion-eliciting stimuli or situations are more likely to entail higher-order processing. Provocative data accumulated recently by alcohol researchers interested in emotional behavior also seem to challenge the assumption that alcohol acts directly on primary motivational (i.e., approach or defensive) systems. Instead, there are indications that its impact is characterized by nonspecific changes in arousability and concomitant alterations in higher-level cognitive functions—including attention, appraisal, and declarative memory—that normally participate in affective processing and expression (e.g., Chapter 1 by Leonard & Blane, this volume; Marlatt, 1987; Sayette, 1993b; Steele & Josephs, 1990; Stritzke, A. Lang, & Patrick, 1996). An additional alternative line of research that dovetails with the primarily psychophysiological approaches reviewed here, has used verbal methods. Applying them in an associative-cognitive network theory to investigate of the role of alcohol expectancies in predicting alcohol use, a multidimensional framework involving arousal and valence has emerged (see Chapter 6 by Goldman, Del Boca, & Darkes, this volume; Rather et al., 1994; Rather, Goldman, Roehrich, & Brannick, 1992; Stacy, 1995; Stacy, Leigh, & Weingardt, 1994)

Having outlined this multidimensional–multilevel perspective, and bearing in mind that the complexities of dose and pharmacokinetics have not been systematically explored in the relevant research to date, we now identify several key methodological considerations and then proceed to examine the current state of knowledge regarding the impact of acute alcohol intoxication on the arousal and valence dimensions of emotional response.

Methodological Issues in the Multidimensional Analysis of Emotion in Alcohol Research

It has been recognized for some time that thorough assessment of emotional response ordinarily involves attention to three loosely coupled response systems: physiological, self-report, and behavioral expression (P. Lang, 1968). There is also abundant evidence to indicate that these systems are often dyssynchronous, changing at different rates and sometimes even moving in different directions (Hodgson & Rachman, 1978; P. Lang, 1968). This, of course, poses a dilemma for all research on emotion but can be especially troublesome for alcohol research in this area, because alcohol might affect two or more of the three response systems in different ways (e.g., elevating heart rate, but diminishing overt behavioral activity), thus adding an additional level of complexity. Indeed, a review by Stritzke et al. (1996) indicates that inconsistency across the domains of psychophysiological and subjective response is the rule rather than the exception in experiments examining how alcohol intoxication affects emotional reactions. However, valid inferences about critical psychological processes need not depend on simple convergence as long as explicit and meaningful a priori hypotheses about patterns of responding can be formulated. As we shall see, this is also the case within the limited domain of psychophysiological indices of arousal and valence that are the focus here.

Another critical point raised by Stritzke et al. (1996) is a temporal one. Emotions in general, and their psychophysiological manifestations in particular, are dynamic events; thus, the time frame in which they are considered is important. Moreover, part of what may make drugs such as alcohol especially reinforcing is their ability to induce sudden alterations in brain physiology and in concomitant affective states (Lukas et al., 1991). Levenson (1987) noted that the grain of physiological measurement has often been too coarse (20–30 second averages) to allow precise tracking of the effects of alcohol on emotional processes as they unfold over time. Alcohol, for example, may not only modify the initial impact of affect-laden stimuli, but may also influence higher-order cognitive processing of those stimuli which, in turn, may prompt secondary affective reactions (Wilson, 1988). This means that the typical alcohol–emotion study, which uses a protracted period (often several minutes) of threat of an impending aversive stimulus, introduces opportunities for many variables and processes to influence psychophysiological activity. Thus, temporal parameters become significant determinants of what inferences can be drawn from the data.

From a temporal perspective, the patterning of bodily responses is often divided into *tonic* and *phasic* activity (P. Lang, 1971; Stern & Sison, 1990), the former referring to persistent, ongoing physiological activity, and the latter to discrete responses evoked by specific stimulus events. In alcohol challenge studies, particularly those focusing on arousal, level of tonic activity is itself of interest, because standard autonomic indices such as heart rate and skin conductance tend to be directly affected by alcohol ingestion (Naitoh, 1972; Sher, 1987). This can introduce "initial values" problems that make it difficult to separate actual alcohol–affect interactions from those that are artifacts of baseline differences (for a detailed discussion of this issue and suggestions for managing related problems, see Sayette, 1993a).

Consideration of the effects of alcohol on phasic responding to very brief, circumscribed affect manipulations has been more limited than that given to tonic response, but it has virtue in that it permits repeated measures of alcohol effects on emotional response, thereby increasing the reliability of the assessment. Focus on phasic reactions also minimizes confounding by uncontrollable or unknown variables and affords the opportunity to sample responses to affective stimuli that vary on the valence dimension. For example, in contrast to the equivocation and uncertainty of research addressing alcohol effects on reactions to tonic affective manipulations, there is reasonable consistency in the finding that intoxication tends to dampen phasic autonomic and electromyographic reactivity to a diverse array of discrete emotional stimuli, including pleasant and unpleasant words known to elicit an electrodermal response (Coopersmith, 1964; Lienert & Traxel, 1959; Smith, 1922), aversive auditory stimuli (e.g., Greenberg & Carpenter, 1957; McGonnell & Beach, 1968; Stewart & Pihl, 1994); electric shock (e.g., Finn & Pihl, 1987; Levenson, Oyama, & Meek, 1987; Levenson, Sher, Grossman, Newman, & Newlin, 1980; Stewart, Finn, & Pihl, 1992), and affective slides (Stritzke, Patrick, & A. Lang, 1995). This is encouraging, but to advance our knowledge, we must take steps to integrate the study of tonic and phasic reactions as well as arousal and valence dimensions of emotion. After reviewing research that examines these dimensions separately, we show how psychophysiological indices of them can be integrated and also used to analyze cognitive processes that might mediate alcohol's effects on emotional responding.

Alcohol and Arousal

The study of the effects of alcohol on arousal reactions to emotional stimuli has a long and venerable history dating back to Smith (1922), who regarded the "psychogalvanic reflex" as a true measure of the intensity of emotion aroused. He found that alcohol diminished electrodermal response to affect-laden words in an association test but was careful to note that this observation revealed little about the specific type of emotion involved (e.g., fear vs. joy). In other words, the changes were understood to reflect primarily the *nonspecific* arousal that might be associated with any kind of emotional excitement, positive or negative.

In the ensuing decades, Smith's finding of alcohol-attenuated electrodermal response to affective stimuli was replicated several times, using both verbal (e.g., Lienert & Traxel, 1959) and sensory (e.g., Carpenter, 1957) stimuli, but his cautions about interpretation went largely unheeded. Then, Doctor and Perkins (1960) conducted a study of alcohol effects using multiple measures of autonomic reactivity (heart rate and pulse volume, as well as skin conductance) to assess reactivity to venipuncture and cold-pressor stressors. Rather than diminished arousal, they found evidence of increased response variability—including *heightened* activation or stimulation—among intoxicated participants. There was also some dyssynchrony among the various measures of arousal. Although it never attracted much attention, this early work not only pointed out the need for dose–response studies, but also offered a reminder that exclusive reliance on one, or even multiple, measures of arousal alone may be of limited utility in the assessment of affective state.

The liabilities of exclusive dependence on the construct of arousal to relate complex physiological response patterns to psychological phenomena was detailed in Lacey's (1967) classic critique and dismissal of activation theory. He derived his conclusion from evidence that (1) somatic and behavioral arousal do not necessarily covary, particularly after pharmacological manipulations; (2) different physiological indices of activation are dissociable; and (3) specific situations prompt unique patterns of physiological response, depending on the nature of the stimulus and task requirements. The complexities involved in the last of these points are evident, for example, in the observation that during a task involving the viewing of affectively distressing pictures, heart rate tends to decelerate; but remembering and thinking about the same unpleasant material results in heart rate acceleration (P. Lang et al., 1990). Thus, interpretation of psychophysiological data from autonomic responses must take into account patterning across and within response systems, and their transactional context as well (Lacey, 1959; P. Lang, 1971).

The implications of these theoretical advances for the study of alcohol–emotion relationships were recognized by Naitoh (1972), whose review of psychophysiological approaches to alcoholism urged researchers to move beyond simplistic, activation-based studies of tension reduction to development of a perspective permitting exploration of possible connections between alcohol-induced physiological arousal and the experience of "pleasant drunkenness." His recommendations resonated with Valins's (1966) revised and elaborated version of Schachter and Singer's (1962) classic work on arousal and emotion, which emphasized the malleability of affect in persons exposed to nonspecific arousal manipulations. Naitoh proposed that interpretation of alcohol-mediated changes in the relatively ambiguous, altered state of arousal occasioned by intoxication may be either pleasant or unpleasant, depending upon the context.

Unfortunately, few alcohol researchers have pursued this insightful hypothesis in experimental analogue studies. Apparently, Dengerink and Fagan (1978) were the first to seriously consider the role of environmental cues and cognitive factors in the effects of drinking on emotional response, and they did so only in a post hoc attempt to explain an unexpected finding. Contrary to prediction, they observed that alcohol intoxication caused increased levels of heart rate and electrodermal activity, and higher self-reported anxiety, during anticipation and receipt of electric shock. This prompted them to consider the possibility that interpretation of the situation was critical, arguing that maybe the context was so threatening that it deprived participants of the sense of optimism or power that they might ordinarily get from alcohol and left them feeling even more helpless than they would have felt had they been sober. It is difficult to evaluate the validity of this interpretation, but given the provocative results of the study that spawned it, it is perhaps more difficult to understand why we could find no experiment designed specifically to evaluate how the cognitive processes underlying interpretation of external (or internal) cues might influence psychophysiological indices of the full range of emotional response during alcohol intoxication.

Although there is fairly clear evidence that the environment in which drinking occurs (e.g., social vs. solitary) can have a significant impact on self-reports and observed behaviors correlated with affective state (e.g., Pliner & Cappell, 1974), context alone cannot reliably predict whether drinking will increase or decrease physiological activity associated with a particular affect manipulation. In conjunction with the obvious influences of dose and manner of consumption, other variables such as ongoing mood and individual differences (e.g., sensation seeking vs. harm-avoiding temperament, or personal and family drinking history) may interact with pharmacological effects of alcohol to determine both physiological arousal and interpretation of the valence of the associated affect. Perhaps with these complexities in mind, Russell and Mehrabian (1975) renewed the call for better description of affective response as a domain of fundamental interest to alcohol research and theory. Based on factor-analytic studies, they suggested adoption of a two-dimensional (arousal/valence) space as an important step for analyses aimed at unraveling the alcohol–emotion nexus.

Despite periodic calls for incorporation of more sophisticated concepts of emotion and relevant research advances into the study of alcohol and affective responding, progress has been gradual. The best alcohol–emotion experiments of the 1980s (e.g., Levenson et al., 1980) brought a new level of methodological sophistication to the research. The use of balanced-placebo designs (Marlatt & Rohsenow, 1980) meant drinking variables were better controlled. Multiple psychophysiological measures (e.g., heart rate, blood pressure, and skin conductance) were typically taken continuously, thereby allowing for control of baseline differences and fine-grained analyses of response patterns and changes over time. Even if initial enthusiasm was later tempered by failures to replicate (e.g., Sayette, Breslin, Wilson, & Rosenblum, 1994; Sher & Walitzer, 1986), some of these experiments generated excitement by suggesting the possibility of systematic individual variation in alcohol-induced stress-response dampening (SRD) that might represent a risk factor for problem drinking (e.g., Levenson, et al., 1987; Peterson & Pihl, 1990; Sher & Levenson, 1982). Recent work along similar lines, (e.g., Kushner et al., 1996) is also intriguing in its demonstration that alcohol intoxication can reduce the frequency and intensity of reactions to panic challenges (breathing 35% carbon dioxide) in individuals with diagnosed panic disorders.

Nonetheless, continued concentration of alcohol–emotion research on SRD risks perpetuation of a relatively narrow focus that seeks mainly to identify the conditions under which alcohol intoxication influences the impact of anxiety-provoking stimuli or stressful situations on nonspecific psychophysiological measures of autonomic arousal and self-reports (cf. Sayette, 1993b; Sher, 1987; Wilson, 1988). There is merit to this approach, but its potential seems greater if it can be incorporated into an expanded perspective that capitalizes on recent advances in the conceptualization of emotion, measurement of its valence dimension, and attention to how alcohol might interact with manipulations of positive affect. These possibilities and their implications for a reinterpretation of the existing alcohol–emotion literature are explored in the remaining sections.

Alcohol and Valence

Psychophysiological Measurement of Emotional Valence

Although self-report measures of emotional valence have been available and widely used in emotion research for many years, there is good reason to be skeptical about their validity, because they are easily influenced by experimental demand and highly susceptible to intentional manipulation. These simple facts provided a major impetus for the development of psychophysiological indices of emotion thought to be tied more closely to underlying dispositions and less amenable to spontaneous efforts at volitional control. Still, there is some uncertainty about the extent to which psychophysiological activity can identify and distinguish among specific emotions. Although differences among response patterns for some emotions have been demonstrated using autonomic measures (Ekman, Levenson, & Friesen, 1983; Levenson, 1992; Schwartz, Weinberger, & Singer, 1981), as well as facial electromyography (P. Lang, Greenwald, Bradley, & Hamm, 1993; Schwartz, Fair, Salt, Mandel, & Klerman, 1976; Vrana, 1993), the total variance associated with fine distinctions among the emotions tends to be small and unreliable (P. Lang, 1994a; Levenson, 1992; Tassinary & Cacioppo, 1992). However, there is ample evidence that global differentiations along the pleasant/approach versus unpleasant/withdrawal dimension of affective valence can be made. Several psychophysiological methods, including facial electromyographic (EMG) activity, hemispheric brain physiology, and startle-reflex patterns, have shown considerable promise in this regard, and some behavioral measures (e.g., coded facial expression) have also proved useful under certain circumstances.

Facial EMG recordings provide a sensitive tool for discriminating pleasant from unpleasant emotional reactions to a variety of internal and external stimuli (for recent reviews, see Dimberg, 1990a; Tassinary & Cacioppo, 1992). In particular, increases in EMG activity over the corrugator supercilium muscle (which produces frowning) and increases over the zygomaticus major muscle (involved in smiling) have consistently covaried with unpleasant and pleasant emotions, respectively, regardless of whether emotion is evoked by imagery (Schwartz et al., 1976; Vrana, 1993), aversive conditioning (Dimberg, 1987), viewing of affect-laden pictures (Cacioppo, Petty, Losch, & Kim, 1986; Dimberg, 1982; Greenwald, Cook, & P. Lang, 1989; P. Lang, Greenwald, et al., 1993) and films (Hubert, & de Jong-Meyer, 1990), or listening to tones or environmental sounds that varied in pleasantness (Bradley, Zack, & P. Lang, 1994; Dimberg, 1990b, 1990c). Furthermore, EMG analysis can be useful in detecting differential facial muscle patterns for normal and clinical mood states (Schwartz et al., 1976) as well as for specific fears (Dimberg, 1990d).

Levenson (1987) has also shown that alcohol reduces the overall intensity of visually distinctive, observable facial behaviors, including signs of fear and attempts at emotional control. This approach is appealing because the videotape recordings on which these measures are based can be made unobtrusively. Using coded facial expression, Sayette, Smith, Breiner, and Wilson (1992) further showed that alcohol intoxication reduced negative emotional reactivity to manipulated stress. However, because drugs generally seem to blunt facial expressiveness, even fine-grained observational coding schemes (e.g., Ekman & Friesen, 1978) may sometimes lack the resolution necessary to reveal drug-induced emotional processes that are subtle or transient. Surface EMG recording may thus be preferable because it can extend the range of investigation to emotional events and affective states that are not accompanied by visible actions or significant visceral changes (Cacioppo, Tassinary, & Fridlund,

1990). For example, a recent study found that, even when drinking resulted in a dramatic suppression of arousal across several physiological response modalities (e.g., startle reactivity, electrodermal response, and heart rate), EMG indices of activity in the corrugator region were unaffected by alcohol and showed reliable differentiation in reactions to pleasant, neutral, and unpleasant pictorial stimuli in both intoxicated and sober participants (Stritzke et al., 1995).

Recording of cortical activity over various scalp regions is another psychophysiological method that has been related to the dimensional structure of emotion. Neuropsychological evidence has accumulated to suggest that the two dimensions of valence and arousal involve different patterns of hemispheric activation (Davidson, 1984, 1992, 1993; Heller, 1990, 1993). According to this model, changes in cortical and autonomic arousal are associated with corresponding shifts in activation of the right parietal region relative to the left, irrespective of the valence of the perceived emotion. In contrast, asymmetries in frontal lobe activity are proposed to reflect the valence of the emotional experience, with the left anterior region more activated during pleasant, approach-oriented emotion, and the right anterior region more activated during unpleasant, withdrawal-related emotion. We are not aware of any published studies that have examined the effects of alcohol on patterns of hemispheric asymmetry. However, diazepam has been found to shift frontal asymmetry toward a pattern of greater left hemispheric activation in stressed rhesus monkeys (Davidson, Kalin, & Shelton, 1992) and in humans (Mathew, Wilson, & Daniel, 1985). If, as hypothesized, alcohol–emotion effects involve a cortical component, exploring changes in frontal brain asymmetry may prove to be especially useful in determining whether alcohol simply reduces overall affective intensity, or under what circumstances it may act selectively to attenuate negative affect, enhance positive affect, or both.

One especially promising index of emotional valence is variation in startle-reflex strength and speed. Human research by Peter Lang and his associates (P. Lang et al., 1990) has demonstrated that when processing of emotional information is interrupted by a brief startle "probe" (i.e., a sudden, intense sensory stimulus such as a loud noise), the magnitude and latency of the eyeblink component of the human startle reflex varies monotonically with the pleasantness of the ongoing affective state. Larger, faster blinks are elicited by probes that occur when the foreground stimulus is aversive, whereas smaller, slower blinks occur during exposure to a pleasant stimulus, both relative to a neutral foreground. This valence-related startle modulation effect was initially observed in individuals viewing affective pictures but has been replicated with evocative film clips (Jansen & Frijda, 1994), as well as during olfactory stimuli of different valences (Miltner, Matjak, Braun, Diekmann, & Brody, 1994). Similarly, startle-reflex potentiation is observed if probes are introduced when unpleasant images (Vrana & P. Lang, 1990) or cues signaling electric shock are being processed (Grillion, Ameli, Woods, Merikangas, & Davis, 1991; Hamm, Stark, & Vaitl, 1990).

A key point is that this startle modulation can covary with emotional valence, independent of arousal. As unpleasant pictorial stimuli are rated higher in arousal and are accompanied by greater sympathetic activation, startle *potentiation* is intensified; but as arousal increases for pleasant pictorial materials, greater startle-reflex *inhibition* is prompted (Cuthbert, Bradley, & P. Lang, 1996). P. Lang et al. (1990) theorized that this effect occurs due to synergistic response matching or antagonistic response mismatching: The defensive startle reaction to an unexpected probe is augmented if the ongoing affective state is defensive, and attenuated if the ongoing state is appetitive. Because valence-modulated startle is a robust phenomenon across a wide array of stimulus-processing tasks, it has the potential to be a particularly useful tool in the examination of alcohol-induced changes in emotional response.

The use of startle to index valence is, of course, not without some limitations. In particular, although a credible theory exists to explain the phenomenon of startle potentiation during aversive cueing, the mechanisms underlying inhibition of probe reactions during the processing of pleasant stimuli are less well understood. Consequently, most of the discussion here revolves around fear-potentiated startle. Moreover, further exploration is needed to clarify the influences of modality, context, and attention on affect-related startle modulation and the results of such studies may have implications for optimal utilization of the phenomenon in alcohol–emotion research. For example, there is evidence that startle inhibition during pleasant affective activation may occur more reliably in the context of perceptual processing (e.g., of a picture foreground) than during imaginal processing (P. Lang, 1995). With these limitations in mind, let us summarize the insights gained from the application of startle methods to examination of the effects of alcohol and other drugs on emotional response.

Experimental Manipulation of the Valence Dimension

Laboratory tests of alcohol's purported anxiolytic effects have typically involved the exposure of participants to some physical or social stressor. Because most designs have not included appropriate affective control conditions, negative affect and general arousal are often confounded. Thus, when alcohol is found to attenuate autonomic stress responses, it is impossible to determine whether this effect is specific to aversive stimuli or secondary to a general dampening of *all* emotional processing. It is therefore desirable to compare at least two emotional states and an emotionally neutral reference condition, and to match the elicited emotions for level of intensity (Davidson, Ekman, Saron, Senulis, & Friesen, 1990). Other than a recent study in our own laboratory (Stritzke et al., 1995), we could uncover only one published alcohol study (Gabel, Noel, Keane, & Lisman, 1980) that appeared to conform to these criteria, and in it, alcohol consumption was the dependent rather than an independent variable.

In the first and, thus far, only experiment to manipulate positive as well as negative affect in a design based explicitly on a multidimensional (arousal/valence) model of emotion, participants received either a moderate dose of alcohol or no alcohol prior to viewing pleasant, neutral, and unpleasant slide stimuli, with the affect-laden slides matched for arousal (Stritzke et al., 1995). Eyeblink reactions to acoustic startle probes were used to index the valence of the response disposition evoked by the slides (cf. Vrana, Spence, & P. Lang, 1988). Changes in emotional valence were also assessed using EMG recording of corrugator ("frown") activity, while skin conductance responses were included as an index of physiological arousal. Heart rate responses during slide viewing were also recorded.

Results indicated that alcohol diminished the *overall* magnitude of both startle and phasic skin conductance response, regardless of the valence of the foreground slides. However, the normal affective *modulation* of startle remained intact in the alcohol condition. In other words, although mean startle magnitude during slide viewing was lower in the alcohol group, intoxicated subjects (like controls) showed comparatively greater reactions for aversive slides and smaller reactions for pleasant slides, both relative to neutral. A similar valence effect (i.e., unpleasant → neutral → pleasant) for corrugator EMG reactions was also found in both groups. These valence results were contrary to the prediction, derived from the tension reduction or stress-response dampening perspectives, that alcohol would selectively block reactions to aversive slides. On the other hand, the nonspecific suppressant effects of alcohol on electrodermal and overall startle reactivity suggested that "response dampening" by alcohol may be a general phenomenon that can occur in the context of pleasant as well as unpleasant stimuli.

The heart rate data from this study were also interesting. Following slide onset, there was an initial deceleration (i.e., an orienting response; see Graham & Clifton, 1966) that, although somewhat greater in intoxicated individuals, was marked in all participants. This indicated that everyone attended to the slide stimuli. However, analysis of complete waveforms revealed a dramatic failure of intoxicated participants to show normal secondary acceleration of heart rate later in the slide presentation. This could reflect alcohol's well-documented interference with higher cognitive processing, particularly elaborative encoding of visual and verbal information (Lister, Eckhardt, & Weingartner, 1987) and thereby suggest a mechanism for its impact on emotional responding.

The only other study to analyze pleasant, neutral, and unpleasant stimuli focused on how arousal elicited by these stimuli might affect alcohol consumption (Gabel et al., 1980). Participants viewed erotic, mutilation, or neutral slides *prior to* an ad lib drinking opportunity. Skin conductance levels confirmed that, relative to neutral slides, both erotic and aversive slides produced elevated physiological arousal, a pattern that was corroborated by self-report. However, contrary to the prediction that participants would drink relatively more alcohol after viewing aversive slides, presumably to derive its putative tension-reducing effects, alcohol consumption was highest after exposure to sexually arousing stimuli. The amount of drinking that occurred following unpleasant arousal did not differ from that in the neutral slide condition, thus calling into question the popular notion that people drink to reduce distress. These results should also alert researchers to the problems of inferring valence from arousal.

Further evidence that bears on the question of whether alcohol selectively alters negatively valenced emotions or modifies stimulus processing more broadly has emerged from research investigating the effect of alcohol on the acquisition and exhibition of conditioned aversive emotional states. To test the hypothesis that alcohol reduces conditioned anxiety development and reactivity in humans, McGonnell and Beach (1968) paired electric shock with a tone, controlling for generalized sensitization due to the UCS and for reactivity to novelty by incorporating a pseudoconditioning group and a neutral light stimulus. Alcohol was found to inhibit the acquisition and maintenance of the conditioned galvanic skin response in *both* the experimental and the control conditions. Similarly, in a study of psychophysiological reactivity in men at risk for alcoholism, alcohol both dampened cardiovascular reactivity to aversive shock and diminished skin-conductance-orienting responses to nonaversive tones (Finn, Zeitouni, & Pihl, 1990). These findings suggest that alcohol produces a general dampening of reactivity (cf. Stritzke, et al., 1995), which may be described as anxiolytic if it occurs in a stressful context.

The startle reflex was included as the primary dependent variable among several psychophysiological measures in another, more recent examination of the mechanisms involved in the apparent anxiolytic effects of alcohol in people exposed to stressful situations (Curtin, A. Lang, Patrick, & Stritzke, 1998). Using a procedure adapted from Grillon et al. (1991), sober or moderately intoxicated students were presented with a series of 2-minute light cues denoting either (1) the possibility that an electric shock could be delivered at any instant (red light = "threat"), or (2) that no shock would be administered (green light = "safe"). During half of the cue intervals of each type, participants were exposed to periodic presentations of pleasant photographic slides designed to serve as distracters. Acoustical startle probes were introduced at varied and unpredictable points during the threat and safe intervals, with some during the distracting slide presentations and some in the absence of any distraction. Autonomic activity (skin conductance and heart rate), corrugator EMG, and magnitude of eyeblink startle reactions to the multiple probes were monitored throughout the experiment.

Results of this study showed that threat of shock provoked predictable increases in arousal, self-reported distress, EMG indices of facial frowning, and startle-response magnitude. Yet, despite evidence of a general suppressant effect of alcohol on startle (i.e., overall startle reactivity was lower in intoxicated participants compared to sober ones), there was no overall Threat X Beverage Condition interaction to suggest a selective effect of alcohol on stress. However, fear-potentiated startle was not observed among alcohol-intoxicated participants when a pleasant distracter was interposed with the threat cue. This, of course, was the condition that placed the greatest cognitive demands on participants, particularly in terms of simultaneous allocation of attention to, or processing of, competing stimuli. Such results, obtained using a direct and potent manipulation of threat, are consistent with those of Stritzke et al. (1995) in suggesting that alcohol's anxiolytic effects may be easily confused with reduced arousal and limited to complex stimulus-processing contexts.

Startle-reflex potentiation is an especially compelling index of fear activation because of the robustness of the effect, and because it is known that inputs from the subcortical amygdaloid complex to the brain-stem acoustic startle circuit mediate this effect (Davis, 1986; 1988). Given that intoxicated participants show fear-potentiated startle under simple cueing conditions, it can be inferred that activity in the amygdala, which is perhaps the core of the defensive motivational system (LeDoux, 1995), is not directly influenced by alcohol. This is in marked contrast to effects observed for the well-known anxiolytic, diazepam, which has specific binding sites in the amygdala (Amaral, Price, Pitkanën, & Carmichael, 1992). Davis (1979) found that fear-potentiated startle in animals was blocked by doses of diazepam that produced no significant reduction of overall startle reactivity. We recently obtained the same result for humans (Patrick, Berthot, & Moore, 1996).

The Patrick et al. (1996) study was important in another way: It served to allay concern that typical human startle paradigms might not be sensitive to the fear-reducing effects of common psychoactive substances. It also offered an opportunity for comparison of the effects and possible mechanisms of a drug specifically prescribed as an anxiolytic with those of alcohol, a substance that has acquired its reputation by other means. The methodology of this experiment paralleled that used by Stritzke et al. (1995), with two main exceptions: (1) Participants received either a placebo or one of two doses (10 or 15 mg) of diazepam instead of alcoholic or nonalcoholic beverages, and (2) psychophysiological responses, including startle, were recorded in connection with neutral or aversive slides, but not pleasant ones. This latter fact limits comparisons to the fear-potentiation, neglecting possible appetite-attenuation, effects assessed in Stritzke et al. The results were quite striking nonetheless.

The main effect of drug condition on startle was not significant, indicating that diazepam did not dampen *general* startle reactivity. However, the predicted dose-related reduction in *fear-potentiated* startle was observed. In other words, diazepam selectively reduced the startle potentiation normally present in the context of aversive slides—without dampening overall startle reactivity. This pattern was the converse of that observed for alcohol in Stritzke et al. (1995), wherein overall startle was diminished but affective modulation (fear potentiation) was not. This suggests that a distinctively different mechanism probably underlies whatever anxiety-reducing or stress-response dampening effects alcohol may have. In particular, it provides reason to believe that, unlike diazepam, alcohol probably does not act directly and selectively at the level of the aversive or fear system but must traverse other pathways, perhaps at higher levels of the brain.

It is worth noting in this context that the general suppressant effect of alcohol on physiological reactivity to startle probes has been known for some time (e.g., Greenberg & Carpenter, 1957). In addition to the recent human eyeblink studies cited earlier (Curtin et al., 1998; Stritzke et al., 1995), ethanol challenge has also been shown to reduce substantially general startle reactivity, as indexed by whole-body motor reactions, in lower animals (Pohorecky, Brick, & Carpenter, 1986; Pohorecky, Cagan, Brick, & Jaffe, 1976; Pohorecky & Roberts, 1991; Rassnick, Koob, & Geyer, 1992). In direct contrast to these effects, the anxiolytic drug, diazepam, effectively blocks fear-potentiated startle without diminishing overall startle reactivity in subhuman species as well as humans (Davis, 1979; Patrick et al., 1996). In summary, available data indicate that, unlike diazepam, alcohol does not appear to operate selectively on the fear system. However, at least at moderate doses, it can exert a nonspecific dampening effect on physiological reactivity (including electrodermal and startle-probe responding). Interpretation of this effect may well be subject to higher-level cognitive processing.

Two important themes emerge from the literature reviewed thus far. The first is the need to advance beyond an exclusive focus on alcohol–distress relations and nonspecific measures of general arousal. Very few alcohol studies have provided for adequate manipulation and measurement of affective valence, and even fewer have simultaneously explored both ends of this dimension. To be maximally fruitful, future research designs must be more conceptually informed, reflect the multidimensional nature of affective experience, and incorporate tests of the specificity of hypothetical alcohol–emotion interactions. A second point is that despite the wide range of affect manipulations and the varied experimental paradigms, subject populations, alcohol dosages, and measures used in these studies, none has demonstrated an alcohol effect that was specific to aversive emotional reactions. The implication is that alcohol's effects on emotion may not be due to a direct pharmacological influence on primary motivational systems in the brain, and that alternative mechanisms need to be explored. In this regard, recent work, although still within the somewhat restrictive bounds of a unidimensional stress/arousal framework, offers some promising leads by placing greater emphasis on alcohol's known ability to impair cognitive functioning (Holloway, 1994).

Alcohol Intoxication and the Processing of Emotional Information

If alterations in consciousness or cognitive functioning mediate the effect of drinking on response to emotional stimuli, how exactly does this work? Hull (1981, 1987) proposed a relatively narrow focus in his "self-awareness" model, which holds that alcohol specifically impairs the cognitive processing of self-relevant information, thereby providing relief from unpleasant feedback about oneself. Although this approach raises some intriguing possibilities, its data base is somewhat limited and equivocal, particularly where psychophysiological measures are concerned, so it is not addressed further here (see Stritzke et al., 1996, for a more extended discussion and critique).

The main alternatives in the existing literature seem to resonate with the suggestion of Levenson et al. (1980) that alcohol may act as an anxiolytic by disrupting attention to stressors or altering evaluation of the aversiveness of threatening events. At least two important theoretical models consistent with this broad cognitive-disruption perspective have emerged: the attention-allocation model (Steele & Josephs, 1988, 1990) and the appraisal-disruption model (Sayette, 1993b). To date, the predictive scope of these models has been limited to the effects of alcohol on stress response. However, Sayette (1993b) did acknowledge that alcohol may differentially affect processing of aversive versus benign/positive information, and that future models might profitably consider both phenomena. The remainder of this section provides a brief overview of the status of attention-allocation and appraisal-disruption approaches. Special consideration is given to how psychophysiological measures have contributed to empirical tests of these models, and to how incorporation of the valence dimension of emotion might increase the variance explained. More comprehensive reviews of the pertinent evidence can be found elsewhere (Sayette, 1993b; Chapter 7, this volume).

Attention Allocation

The attention-allocation model (Steele & Josephs, 1988, 1990) posits that alcohol intoxication modulates affective experience through its effects on information processing. Alcohol's pharmacological action on the brain is thought to impair cognitive activity that requires controlled, effortful processing and restrict attention to the most immediate internal and external cues. The theory proposes that psychological stress can be reduced as a result of a complex interaction between this modified information processing and several features of the situation. Although near-ataxic doses of alcohol can obviously prevent worry about an upcoming stressor by disrupting thought of any sort (Steele & Josephs, 1990), the extent to which lower doses reduce anxious response may depend on the combined effects of how much intoxication reduces attentional capacity and the presence and nature of distracting stimuli and task demands that may capture some of the available attentional resources. The more that attentional resources are occupied by nonaversive distractions, the greater the potential for anxiety reduction. In fact, if a distracting activity is highly demanding, worry over an impending or concurrent negative event can be diminished even without alcohol (Josephs & Steele, 1990). But, importantly, alcohol-induced reduction in attentional capacity is regarded as essential to its effects on emotion. In the absence of concurrent distraction, moderate intoxication is not predicted to attenuate stress responding, and indeed, it may even increase the impact of the stressor by intensifying attention to it.

Several studies by Steele and his colleagues have provided some support for the model, although generally the data have been limited to self-reports of state anxiety. Only in their first experiment (Steele, Southwick, & Pagano, 1986) was an attempt made to monitor physiological arousal in response to negative feedback from a test. Heart rate and skin conductance measures, however, "gave rise to inconsistent results" (p. 174) and were omitted from the report. Just one other published study relevant to the attention-allocation model has included a physiological measure of stress response to test its predictions. Sayette and Wilson (1991) found a significant alcohol-induced increase in heart rate reactivity during a countdown leading up to the delivery of a self-disclosing speech when instructions about the upcoming stressor *preceded* intoxication (i.e., before alcohol could impair the encoding of the stressful information). In contrast, when information about the stressor *followed* alcohol consumption, a stress-dampening effect was observed. The anxiogenic effect seen in the stress-followed-by-alcohol condition was consistent with an attention-allocation interpretation because the unimpaired encoding of information regarding the stressor and absence of a concurrent distracting activity should make the stressor more salient. However, alcohol should not have attenuated cardiac response in the alcohol-followed-by-stress condition, unless there was a distracter. Thus, the attention-allocation model cannot fully account for the heart rate patterns observed in this study.

Psychophysiological data from a recent experiment in our own laboratory provide some support for the attention-allocation perspective and address one weakness of prior efforts (Curtin et al., 1998). As described earlier, this study involved recording of skin conductance and facial EMG activity, as well as eyeblink responses to intermittent startle probes, while social drinkers alternated between periods of exposure to "threat" of shock and "safe" periods in which no shock was possible. During half of the intervals of each type, participants were distracted by exposure to pleasant photographic slides known to engage viewers' attention, as indexed by heart rate deceleration, ad lib viewing times, and interest ratings (e.g., Bradley, Cuthbert, & P. Lang, 1990). Because measures of phasic response were taken simultaneous with the distraction, this design offered a better test of the model than previous studies using delayed assessments of attentional effects. Results for all relevant measures supported the efficacy of the threat manipulation, and the finding that alcohol selectively suppressed fear-potentiated startle *only* when it was combined with distraction is consistent with predictions derived from the attention-allocation perspective. Although this initial psychophysiological exploration of interactions between the effects of alcohol, distraction, and the processing of stressful information was encouraging, available data are limited at this time, and a number of the theory's key assumptions remain untested.

One concern revolves around the assumption that in order for the combined effects of alcohol and distraction to alleviate negative affect, the distracting activity must be pleasant or at least affectively neutral (Steele et al., 1986). The theory predicts that if the distraction has a negative valence, alcohol may actually *increase* negative affect. In this connection, to act as a suitable distracter from psychological stress, an activity cannot be so complex and demanding that it becomes a source of frustration and anxiety (Josephs & Steele, 1990). Although, no studies have systematically varied both the valence and attentional demands of distracting activity in a single design to test these assumptions, there is evidence that both dimensions may *interact* with alcohol to produce differential affective outcomes. For example, Weaver, Masland, Kharazmi, and Zillmann (1985) suggested that the effect of intoxication on humor appreciation changes as a function of the cognitive skills needed to decipher humorous information. They found that the perceived "funniness" of blunt humor appears to increase after drinking, whereas subtle humor tends to be perceived as less funny after intoxication. Similarly, under conditions of high attentional demand, alcohol reduced physiological and self-reported arousal in men listening to erotic stories, but under conditions with low attentional demand, alcohol increased sexual arousal (Wilson, Niaura, & Adler, 1985). In summary, assumptions implicit in the attention-allocation model regarding the required valence and attentional properties of a suitable distracter still await empirical validation.

Appraisal Disruption

The appraisal-disruption model shares many of the tenets of the attention-allocation model, but concurrent distraction during processing of emotion information is viewed merely as one way in which appraisal of that information can be disrupted (Sayette, 1993b). The appraisal-disruption model proposes more generally that alcohol acts pharmacologically to interfere with the initial appraisal of stressful information by constraining the spread of activation of associated information previously established in long-term memory. A central prediction of the model is that participants who are naive as to the details of an imminent stressor when consuming alcohol are more likely to show stress-response dampening than those who learn about the nature of the stressor before drinking. In the latter situation, alcohol may even enhance stress responses. In support of his hypothesis, Sayette (1993b) noted that none of the psychophysiological studies providing details of a stressor to participants before intoxication found stress-response dampening effects (e.g., Ewing & McCarty, 1983; Keane & Lisman, Study 1, 1980; Sutker, Allain, Brantley, & Randall, 1982; Thyer & Curtis, 1984), and several studies reported an increase in physiological stress responses (e.g., Keane & Lisman, Study 2, 1980; Sayette, Wilson, & Carpenter, 1989). Psychophysiological results were less consistent when participants drank without prior, detailed knowledge of the stressor. Some studies yielded stress-response dampening effects (e.g., McGonnell & Beach, 1968; Sayette & Wilson, 1991; Wilson, Abrams, & Lipscomb, 1980), whereas others failed to do so (e.g., Abrams & Wilson, 1979; Bradlyn, Strickler, & Maxwell, 1981; Sayette et al., 1992). Thus, conclusions about the mediation of alcohol–emotion effects by disruption of appraisal must remain tentative.

Sayette (1993b) further speculated that intoxication may selectively constrain the spread of negative versus positive information, although this assertion is not altogether consistent with his own review of the literature, which indicated that alcohol reliably impairs encoding and storage, and thus appraisal, of a variety of stimuli—including pleasantly valenced information (e.g., Lansky & Wilson, 1981). Consequently, we concur with Sayette's call for studies that assess reactions of intoxicated individuals to both pleasant and unpleasant stimuli, and anticipate that the results of such research will lead to further refinements of the appraisal-disruption model.

Although currently limited in their data bases, these two recently developed cognitive models of alcohol–emotion relations converge on the view that alcohol's influence on affective reactivity does not occur directly at the level of primary brain motivational systems, but rather through its effect on higher information-processing centers that participate in emotional regulation in a "top-down" manner (LeDoux, 1995). Innovative conceptual approaches and research paradigms are needed to explore the impact of alcohol on higher associative processes and to specify relevant psychophysiological concomitants. The sections that follow offer some perspective on what these might entail.

THEORETICAL INTEGRATION AND DIRECTIONS FOR FUTURE RESEARCH

Emotional Processing: Dimensions, Levels, and Systems

Our thesis throughout this chapter has been that research on alcohol and affective response can profit a more sophisticated conceptualization of emotion that recognizes the multidimensional–multilevel nature of the phenomena and considers the functional significance of physiological responses within this framework. We have noted that the valence dimension of affect has been largely ignored in alcohol research, with very few studies addressing enhancement of pleasant emotion and almost none addressing the entire range of valence within the same study. We do not wish to minimize the importance of this neglect, but we acknowledge that it is not likely to be dramatically reversed until better paradigms for manipulating and assessing positive emotion are developed. Indeed, we have made only one preliminary foray into this area ourselves (Stritzke et al., 1995). Nonetheless, we are optimistic that the conceptual framework we outline, although illustrated here only in terms of what is known about fear processing, can inform future research on the positive as well as negative affective concomitants of drinking.

Based on the foregoing analysis, it appears that a viable theory of alcohol and emotional response must accommodate and incorporate the following observations: (1) Alcohol does not seem to directly diminish defensive or appetitive responses to simple, explicit emotional cues; (2) alcohol produces conspicuous disruptions in higher "cognitive" operations, such as selective attention, appraisal, and spatial and declarative memory; and (3) alcohol affects some physiological indices of affective reactivity (e.g., electrodermal response), whereas others (e.g., fear-potentiated startle; corrugator EMG response) are not affected. Our position is that alcohol's effects on emotion and emotional behavior are closely tied to its impact on information processing, and that constraints on its effects can be understood in these terms.

A prominent theme in contemporary theories of emotion is that affective processing can take place at different brain levels through varying mediational pathways. The core motivational systems that govern defensive and appetitive behavior are based in subcortical brain centers (P. Lang, Bradley, et al., 1993), but these centers are interconnected with both lower and higher brain regions. At the most elementary level, neural projections between sensory input systems and subcortical motivation centers permit automatic, "quick and dirty" processing of emotional stimuli (LeDoux, 1995)—possibly without conscious awareness (Öhman & Soares, 1993). However, pathways from higher cortical regions to core motive centers provide opportunities for emotional reactions to be influenced by higher cognitive activities, such as detailed selective attention, perceptual processing, and episodic memory (P. Lang, 1994b).

This multilevel perspective on affective processing has been most clearly developed for the emotion of fear. Considerable neuroscientific evidence indicates that the subcortical amygdaloid complex is the core of the defensive motivational system (Davis, 1992; Fanselow, 1994; LeDoux, 1995). The central nucleus of the amygdala is regarded as the motor output system because it projects to brain structures such as the central gray and the lateral hypothalamus, which participate directly in fear expression. The lateral nucleus of the amygdala is considered to be its input substation. It receives multimodal projections from the sensory thalamus and from perceptual processing regions of the neocortex. Importantly, it also receives projections from higher associational systems—including the hippocampus, well-known for its role in complex functions including declarative memory (Squire, 1992) and affiliated spatial, contextual, and associative processes (e.g., Nadel & Willner, 1980; Rudy & Sutherland, 1992).

Connections between the amygdala and higher brain regions such as the hippocampus provide a means whereby higher-order cognitive activities can activate or modify emotional reactions in a "top-down" fashion (LeDoux, 1995). Where the hippocampus is concerned, recent research has demonstrated interesting dissociations among distinct fear-learning capacities in animals following surgical ablations of this structure. In particular, animals with lesions of the hippocampus show impairments in contextual fear conditioning but not in explicit-cue conditioning (Kim, Rison, & Fanselow, 1993; Phillips & LeDoux, 1992). Unlesioned control rats that are placed in an unfamiliar cage and shocked in the presence of a tone CS learn to fear, not only the tone, but also the learning context itself, as evidenced by behavioral freezing. In contrast, hippocampal-lesioned rats under the same circumstances acquire a freezing response to the tone CS, but not to the novel context per se. These findings have been interpreted to mean that connections between sensory processing regions (thalamus, auditory cortex) and the amygdala are sufficient to mediate fear conditioning to a simple tone cue, but that pathways from the hippocampus to the amygdala are required for fear to be elicited through more complex information processing (LeDoux, 1995).

Also relevant, and of particular interest to the present discussion, is the fact the amygdala plays a key role in the phenomenon of fear-potentiated startle. As noted earlier, the eyeblink startle reflex is enhanced in humans during exposure to a range of aversive situations and stimuli. Similarly, in animals, the whole-body startle reflex is potentiated during exposure to a conditioned fear cue (Brown, Kalish, & Farber, 1951; Davis, 1989). Davis (1989, 1992) and his colleagues have further demonstrated that fear-potentiated startle in animals is mediated by a neural pathway from the central nucleus of the amygdala to the pontine reticular node of the primary, brain-stem startle circuit (Davis, 1989). Through this pathway, fear-relevant stimuli that activate the amygdala also prime the startle response. The finding that the anxiolytic drug, diazepam, blocks this effect in humans (Patrick et al., 1996) as well as animals (Davis, 1979) suggests that fear-potentiated startle is mediated similarly in both species.

The observation that startle reflex potentiation in humans normally occurs for complex aversive cues (including fearful text scenarios and environmental contexts; Grillon, 1996; Vrana & P. Lang, 1990) as well as explicitly fearful stimuli (e.g., unpleasant pictures, warning signals, and conditioned fear stimuli; P. Lang, Bradley, Cuthbert, & Patrick, 1993) is consistent with evidence from animal studies indicating that fear can be instigated in various ways. On the one hand, there can be instigation by simple sensory cues that activate the amygdala via direct thalamo–amygdaloid pathways. On the other hand, it can be based on more complex cues that operate through "top-down" connections. Parallel cortical–subcortical circuits are presumed to underlie positive emotional reactions (P. Lang, 1994a), but substantial work remains to be done in this area (LeDoux, 1995).

Emotion, Cognition, and Alcohol

This multilevel model of emotion provides a useful framework for thinking about the existing literature on alcohol and affective response, and for generating further hypotheses. Our review of the available evidence suggests that the emotional impact of alcohol is diffuse and nonselective, and stems from its effects on higher brain functions that ordinarily modulate affective processing at more basic, subcortical levels. This was particularly evident in our recent human studies using the startle reflex potentiation as an index of fear activation (Curtin et al., 1998; Stritzke et al., 1995). Recall that we found no evidence that moderate alcohol administration blocked defensive reactions to simple aversive cues (i.e., unpleasant pictures and warning signals), although it markedly attenuated overall startle reactivity. This finding is especially striking in view of the divergent effects observed for the anxiolytic drug, diazepam, which selectively blocked fear-potentiated startle without dampening overall reflex reactivity (Patrick et al., 1996). The implication is that diazepam directly suppressed fear, but alcohol did not.

The reader is also reminded that alcohol and diazepam produced differing effects on electrodermal response. At a dose that effectively blocked fear-potentiated startle, diazepam produced no significant reduction in skin conductance response to unpleasant slides (Patrick et al., 1996), whereas a moderate dose of alcohol significantly suppressed electrodermal reactions to aversive and pleasant slides, both relative to neutral ones (Stritzke et al., 1995). Moreover, similar effects have been demonstrated in previous alcohol studies cited earlier. In conjunction with the results for startle measures (contrasting fear potentiation with overall reactivity), the findings for phasic electrodermal response suggest that alcohol exerts a nonspecific effect on arousability, whereas the effect of diazepam is specific to the defensive (negative valence) component of emotion.

Also of interest in this context are findings from a recent human conditioning study that compared aversive and nonaversive classical conditioning in terms of their impact on physiological measures, including startle-reflex modulation and skin conductance response (Hamm & Vaitl, 1996). Conditioned startle potentiation developed consistently in the context of aversive learning, regardless of participants' knowledge of the contingency between the CS and UCS stimulus. In contrast, significant electrodermal conditioning was observed for nonaversive as well as aversive conditioning procedures, but only among participants who were able to accurately identify the CS–UCS contingency on a poststudy questionnaire. These data indicate that potentiated startle reflexes and skin conductance responses are mediated in different ways.

Hamm and Vaitl (1996) hypothesized that the conditioning of fear-potentiated startle develops automatically through direct sensory–subcortical pathways, whereas electrodermal conditioning depends more heavily on higher-order, elaborative processing. Consistent with this formulation, other research has indicated that awareness is necessary for skin conductance conditioning (Dawson & Schell, 1985) and that cortical systems play a direct, mediational role in electrodermal activity (Tranel & Damasio, 1994). In addition, it has been shown that skin conductance responses to emotional pictures habituate with repeated exposures, whereas startle modulation effects persist (Bradley, P. Lang, & Cuthbert, 1993), thus providing further evidence that different mechanisms underlie these two response systems.

Considered from this perspective, the finding of normal affective modulation of startle, but diminished electrodermal response, in moderately intoxicated subjects exposed to affective stimuli suggests that alcohol influences emotional response indirectly, by compromising higher elaborative functions required for complex cue processing. When the emotional stimuli are simple and unambiguous, appetitive and defensive response priming is unaffected by alcohol (Curtin et al., 1998; Stritzke et al., 1995). However, when affective cues are remote or complex and higher-level processing is required for stimulus detection or ongoing elaboration, emotional priming is vulnerable to impairment by alcohol. The research of Curtin et al. (1998) is pertinent here. They found that alcohol blocked fear-potentiated startle only under conditions of compound cueing (i.e., threat cue accompanied by distracter). Parallel effects were evident in experiments reviewed previously in connection with the cognitive perspectives of attention allocation and appraisal disruption.

Also relevant is the demonstration by Melia, Corodimas, Ryabinin, Wilson, and LeDoux (1994) of "dissociations" in fear learning in animals as a function of alcohol administration. These investigators examined explicit cue and contextual fear conditioning in rats administered low and moderate doses of ethanol, using behavioral freezing as an index of fear. The drug did not affect conditioning to a tone cue explicitly paired with the shock, but it blocked learning of the association between the situational context (novel cage) and aversive stimulation (shock). Although this study focused on alcohol's effects on the acquisition of contextual fear, other evidence indicates that alcohol impairs both the acquisition and the expression of spatial learning (Matthews, Simson, & Best, 1995; Vandergriff, Matthews, Best, & Simson, 1995), an activity that is also mediated by the hippocampus (Mayford et al., 1996). If spatial memory and processing of contextual fear cues are related phenomena (cf. Matthews et al., 1995), one would expect that ethanol should also interfere with the expression of contextual aversive learning.

The findings of Melia et al. (1994) are also consistent with the hypothesis that alcohol reduces sensitivity to fear cues by interfering with higher-order processing, rather than by directly suppressing subcortical defensive systems. As described earlier, disruption of hippocampal functioning is one potential mechanism by which alcohol produces such effects. Although apparently not essential to explicit fear learning, input from the hippocampus to the amygdala is clearly critical for contextual fear learning (LeDoux, 1995). Because alcohol has well-documented effects on a variety of cognitive functions, including vigilance and attention (Holloway, 1994; Lamb & Robertson, 1987; Zeichner, Allen, Petrie, Rasmussen, & Giancola, 1993), that reflect its impact on neural systems probably not intimately involved with the hippocampus, it seems likely that other systems are involved as well. For instance, Davis and colleagues (Davis, 1992; Davis, Walker, & Lee, in press;) have recently suggested that the bed nucleus of the stria terminalis comprises the basic substrate of an anxiety system analogous to, but functionally distinct from, the amygdaloid fear system. This could represent another avenue by which alcohol exerts its effects on emotional response.

Promising Avenues for Further Study

A multidimensional–multilevel perspective on emotion encourages consideration of variables not traditionally attended to in alcohol research: the valence and intensity of emotion-eliciting cues, the context of affective stimulation, the brain systems required to register and process cues of different sorts, and the functional significance of different physiological measures vis-à-vis these other parameters. In a previous paper (Stritzke et al., 1996), we outlined a broad research agenda based on these considerations. Here, we highlight a few particularly salient research questions and briefly outline strategies that might be used to address them.

As noted earlier, at least two studies conducted in our laboratory (Curtin et al., 1998; Stritzke et al., 1995) indicate that alcohol does not directly suppress defensive or appetitive reactivity. However, these studies involved only moderate doses of alcohol and unselected participants. It is possible that more direct suppression of fear reactivity, as indexed by startle potentiation, might be observed at higher BAC levels, if they produced more pervasive effects on brain systems. Thus, systematic dose–response evaluations are needed. Another possibility is that individuals with particular dispositional tendencies might show atypical fear suppression under the influence of alcohol. For instance, such a prediction might derive from prior research indicating that individuals at risk for alcohol abuse by virtue of a multigenerational family history of alcoholism showed enhanced cardiovascular "stress-response dampening" under the influence of alcohol (Finn & Pihl, 1987). It should be noted, however, that interpretation of these original findings was complicated somewhat by group differences in baseline cardiac response. In any case, further research examining the impact of alcohol on fear-potentiated startle as a function of trait dispositions is clearly warranted.

Additional research is also needed to determine the mechanisms by which alcohol impairs processing of fear cues under conditions of distraction. In the study by Curtin et al. (1998), pleasant, arousing pictures were used as distracters, raising the possibility that the fear-reducing impact of alcohol in this case was tied to enhanced appetitive responsivity. This study also included no direct index of attentional allocation. An interesting follow-up experiment would involve comparison of the defensive reactions to fear cues (indexed by startle potentiation) elicited when those cues were presented either explicitly or incidentally in the context of an affectively neutral task performance or other distraction. For example, the task might require discrimination between rare target stimuli and frequently-occurring nontargets (along with rare nontarget threat cues). This is a paradigm often used to study information processing (Donchin, 1979) and would provide an opportunity to use event-related potentials record an on-line index of differential attention to threat versus nonthreat stimuli. Our proposal of this kind of experiment illustrates how physiological measures with differing functional significance (e.g., startle reflex and Event-Related Potentials) might be used in tandem to assess alcohol's effects on complex links in cognitive and emotional processing.

Comparisons of explicit versus contextual fear conditioning in humans as a function of alcohol intoxication would be of interest as well. Recently, Grillon (1996) demonstrated an increase in baseline startle reactivity among student participants during a follow-up session in which they reentered a fear-conditioning chamber. Grillon interpreted this effect as evidence of contextual fear. Besides the increase in baseline startle, participants also showed enhanced reflex potentiation in the presence of a visual cue (CS+) that had been explicitly paired with shock. A strong prediction from the animal literature (Melia et al., 1994) would be that alcohol administration should eliminate the context-related enhancement of startle but have no effect on startle potentiation to the explicit CS+. A potentially complicating factor in this type of experiment is the main effect of alcohol in reducing overall startle reactivity. However, if it could be demonstrated that individuals administered alcohol in both sessions showed no baseline startle enhancement in Session 2, despite significant startle potentiation during exposure to the explicit CS+, this would provide impressive evidence of a differential impact of alcohol as a function of the complex cognitive processes involved in context cueing.

To pursue another option, it has been noted that alcohol dampens general startle reactivity in both humans (Curtin et al., 1998; Stritzke et al., 1995) and lower animals (Pohorecky et al., 1986; Rassnick et al., 1992). The implication of this observation is that alcohol exerts a reliable influence on the primary, brain-stem startle circuit (i.e., cochlear nucleus

→ nucleus reticularis pontis caudalis → orbicularis [blink] effectors). An important, unanswered question concerns the locus of alcohol's impact on the basic startle circuit. The fact that auditory brain-stem evoked potentials are unaffected by moderate doses of alcohol (McRandle & Goldstein, 1973) indicates that this effect is not attributable to a simple decrease in sensory sensitivity. In view of alcohol's demonstrable effects on motor functioning (Holloway, 1994), the startle-suppression effect might be due to an alteration in the responsivity of peripheral (including facial) musculature. This hypothesis could be tested by assessing the impact of alcohol on muscular reflexes elicited directly, via electrical stimulation.

Another intriguing possibility is that the decrement in startle reactivity associated with alcohol administration reflects a general decrease in brain-stem activation. The reticular system, with which the primary startle circuit intersects, plays an important role in mediating overall alertness and cortical processing efficiency (Morruzzi & Magoun, 1949; Routtenberg, 1968). In this respect, the observed effect of alcohol in diminishing overall startle reactivity could be linked to its effects on higher (cortical) processing activities and on electrodermal responsivity. The hypothesis that alcohol's effects on the primary startle circuit occur via the pontine reticular node could be tested in humans by assessing the impact of ethanol administration on an acoustical reflex involving similar input–output pathways, but which bypasses the nucleus reticularis pontis caudalis (e.g., postauricular reflex; cf. Hackley, 1993).

A final suggestion for future research derives from the obvious contrast between the present conceptualization of alcohol–emotion relations as indirect and the traditional view that alcohol directly reduces fear. In his highly influential treatise on fear, Gray (1987) stated that the effects of alcohol on emotional behavior "can be attributed to a single mechanism of action—that of reducing fear" (p. 191). This conclusion was based in part on the observation that alcohol appears to disrupt passive avoidance learning (i.e., inhibition of previously rewarded behavior in the presence of cues for punishment). Recently, however, LeDoux (1995) has argued that passive avoidance learning can be regarded as a form of contextual learning that is dependent upon the hippocampus. In light of this assertion, it would be interesting to see whether humans or animals sufficiently intoxicated to exhibit deficient passive avoidance learning would show normal fear (as evidenced by startle potentiation) in the presence of explicit aversive cues. A demonstration of this sort would lend indirect support to LeDoux's position and call for a reinterpretation of long-held notions concerning alcohol and emotion.

CONCLUSION

Returning now to the theme introduced at the beginning of this chapter, let us briefly consider the implications that the concepts and data reviewed here might have for the key position that emotion occupies in most major theories of drinking and alcohol-related problems. Our review indicates that the relationship between alcohol and affective response is by no means a simple one. Evidence of intrinsic reward or selective stress reduction seems neither powerful enough nor reliable enough to account for the widespread appeal of alcohol and the prevalence of alcoholism. Rather than exerting emotion-specific effects, the critical pharmacological action of alcohol where emotion is concerned appears to revolve around its ability to constrain perception and processing of context. When intoxicated, people respond differently to cues within and around them. The immediate and tangible assume greater importance relative to the nuances and implications of events.

This analysis is consistent with the observations of sociocultural theorists, concerned primarily with interpersonal effects of drinking. They have argued that a major impact of alcohol is that it leaves one in a malleable state, more responsive to the immediate social environment (cf. MacAndrew & Edgerton, 1969). If that environment supports a "time out" from the constraints that ordinarily govern behavior, the probability of aggressive, sexual, and other normally inhibited expression is increased. If that environment conveys a clear message that disinhibition of such behaviors will not be tolerated, they tend not to occur. Our thesis is that similar mechanisms can be applied more broadly to explain alcohol's effects on emotion as well as social behavior.

Basically, we hold that the emotional effects of alcohol are interwoven with its effects on cognitive functioning, including attention and memory. Intoxication compromises complex processing, leaving the individual less able to attend to and integrate subtle and distal cues. The result is a somewhat temporally constrained focus on a reduced number of proximal and explicit cues. This can facilitate appetitive tendencies, for example, opportunistic pursuit of sexual gratification without regard for possible adverse consequences in the long term. It can also produce an attenuation of negative affect by enabling one to set aside worries about the past or future if the immediate drinking context contains explicit cues that are more favorable. This model can accommodate individual differences in the depth and pervasiveness of indulgent or escapist motivations, or both, that people bring to each drinking episode. It also provides avenues to incorporate the many variables that can affect the likelihood that people will come to use drinking as a maladaptive coping response as opposed to an occasional diversion. However, it emphasizes the impact of alcohol in diminishing complex cognitive processing and suggests its pivotal role in understanding any of these motivations and their related actions.

Consequently, there is every reason to continue to develop a multidimensional–multilevel framework for conceptualizing the alcohol–emotion nexus and its implications for drinking and alcohol-related problems. We have offered such model, applied it to the existing literature, and outlined future research initiatives that derive from it. Only time will tell if this approach advances understanding and prediction of the connections between alcohol and emotion, but they seem too important to neglect.

ACKNOWLEDGMENT

Preparation of this manuscript was supported, in part, by National Institute on Alcohol Abuse and Alcoholism Grant AA09381 and National Institute of Mental Health Grants MH48657 and MH52384.

REFERENCES

Abrams, D. B., & Wilson, G. T. (1979). Effects of alcohol on social anxiety in women: Cognitive versus physiological processes. *Journal of Abnormal Psychology, 88,* 161–173.

Amaral, D.G., Price, J.L., Pitkanèn, A., & Carmichael, S.T. (1992). Anatomical organization of the primate amygdaloid complex. In J. P. Aggleton (Ed.), *The amygdala: Neurobiological aspects of emotion, memory, and mental dysfunction* (pp. 1–66). New York: Wiley.

Bales, R. F. (1946). Cultural differences in rates of alcoholism. *Quarterly Journal of Studies on Alcohol, 6,* 480–499.

Bower, G. H. (1981). Mood and memory. *American Psychologist, 36,* 129–148.

Bradley, M. M., Cuthbert, B. N., & Lang, P. J. (1990). Startle reflex modification: Emotion or attention? *Psychophysiology, 27,* 513–522.

Bradley, M. M., Lang, P. J., & Cuthbert, B. N. (1993). Startle reflex habituation in human beings: Emotion, novelty, and context. *Behavioral Neuroscience, 107,* 970–980.

Bradley, M. M., Zack, J., & Lang, P. J. (1994). Cries, screams, and shouts of joy: Affective responses to environmental sounds. *Psychophysiology, 31*(Suppl. 1), S29.

Bradlyn, A. S., Strickler, D. P., & Maxwell, W. A. (1981). Alcohol, expectancy and stress: Methodological concerns with the expectancy design. *Addictive Behaviors, 6,* 1–8.

Brown, J. S., Kalish, H. I., & Farber, I. E. (1951). Conditioned fear as revealed by magnitude of startle responses to an auditory stimulus. *Journal of Experimental Psychology, 32,* 317–328.

Buck, R. (1988). *Human motivation and emotion.* New York: Wiley.

Cacioppo, J. T., Petty, R. E., Losch, M. E., & Kim, H. S. (1986). Electromyographic activity over facial muscle regions can differentiate the valence and intensity of affective reactions. *Journal of Personality and Social Psychology, 50,* 260–268.

Cacioppo, J. T., Tassinary, L. G., & Fridlund, A. J. (1990). The skeletomotor system. In J. T. Cacioppo & L. G. Tassinary (Eds.), *Principles of psychophysiology: Physical, social, and inferential elements* (pp. 325–384). New York: Cambridge University Press.

Cappell, H., & Greeley, J. (1987). Alcohol and tension reduction: An update on research and theory. In H. T. Blane & K. E. Leonard (Eds.), *Psychological theories of drinking and alcoholism* (pp. 15–54). New York: Guilford Press.

Carpenter, J. A. (1957). Effects of alcoholic beverages on skin conductance. *Quarterly Journal of Studies on Alcohol, 18,* 1–18.

Cooper, M. L., Frone, M. R., Russell, M., & Mudar, P. (1995). Drinking to regulate positive and negative moods: A motivational model of alcohol use. *Journal of Personality and Social Psychology, 69,* 990–1005.

Coopersmith, S. (1964). The effects of alcohol on reactions to affective stimuli. *Quarterly Journal of Studies on Alcohol, 25,* 459–475.

Cox, W. M., & Klinger, E. (1990). Incentive motivation, affective change, and alcohol use: A model. In W. M. Cox (Ed.), *Why people drink: Parameters of alcohol as a reinforcer* (pp. 291–314). New York: Gardner.

Curtin, J. J., Lang, A. R., Patrick, C. J., & Stritzke, W. G. K. (1998). Alcohol and fear potentiated startle: A test of stress response dampening and attention allocation theories. *Journal of Abnormal Psychology, 107,* 547–557.

Cuthbert, B. N., Bradley, M. M., & Lang, P. J. (1996). Probing picture perception: Activation and emotion. *Psychophysiology, 33,* 103–111.

Davidson, R. J. (1984). Hemispheric asymmetry and emotion. In K. R. Scherer & P. Ekman (Eds.), *Approaches to emotion* (pp. 39–57). Hillsdale, NJ: Erlbaum.

Davidson, R. J. (1992). Emotion and affective style: Hemispheric substrates. *Psychological Science, 3,* 39–43.

Davidson, R. J. (1993). Cerebral asymmetry and emotion: Conceptual and methodological conundrums. *Cognition and Emotion, 7,* 115–138.

Davidson, R. J., Ekman, P., Saron, C. D., Senulis, J. A., & Friesen, W. V. (1990). Approach–withdrawal and cerebral asymmetry: Emotional expression and brain physiology I. *Journal of Personality and Social Psychology, 58,* 330–341.

Davidson, R. J., Kalin, N. H., & Shelton, S. E. (1992). Lateralized effects of diazepam on frontal brain electrical asymmetries in rhesus monkeys. *Biological Psychiatry, 32,* 438–451.

Davis, M. (1979). Diazepam and flurazepam: Effects on conditioned fear as measured with the potentiated startle paradigm. *Psychopharmacology, 62,* 1–7.

Davis, M. (1986). Pharmacological and anatomical analysis of fear conditioning using the fear-potentiated startle paradigm. *Behavioral Neuroscience, 100,* 814–824.

Davis, M. (1988). The potentiated startle as a measure of conditioned fear and its relevance to the neurobiology of anxiety. In P. Simon (Ed.), *Selected models of anxiety, depression, and psychosis* (pp. 61–89). Basel, Switzerland: Karger.

Davis, M. (1989). Neural systems involved in fear-potentiated startle. In M. Davis, B. L. Jacobs, & R. I. Schoenfeld (Eds.), *Annals of the New York Academy of Sciences, Vol. 563: Modulation of defined neural vertebrate circuits* (pp. 165–183). New York: Author.

Davis, M. (1992). The role of the amygdala in conditioned fear. In J. Aggleton (Ed.), *The amygdala: Neurobiological aspects of emotion, memory and mental dysfunction* (pp. 255–305). New York: Wiley.

Davis, M., Walker, D. L., & Lee, Y. (in press). Amygdala and bed nucleus of the stria terminalis: Differential roles in fear and anxiety measured with the acoustic startle reflex. In L. Squire & D. Schacter (Eds.), *Biological and psychological perspectives on memory and memory disorders.* Washington, DC: American Psychiatric Press.

Dawson, M. E., & Schell, A. M. (1985). Information processing and human autonomic classical conditioning. In P. K. Ackles, J. R. Jennings, & M. G. H. Coles (Eds.), *Advances in psychophysiology* (Vol. 1, pp. 89–165). Greenwich, CT: JAI Press.

Dengerink, H. A., & Fagan, N. J. (1978). Effect of alcohol on emotional responses to stress. *Journal of Studies on Alcohol, 39,* 525–539.

Dimberg, U. (1982). Facial reactions to facial expressions. *Psychophysiology, 19,* 643–647.

Dimberg, U. (1987). Facial reactions, autonomic activity and experienced emotion: A three component model of emotional conditioning. *Biological Psychology, 24,* 105–122.

Dimberg, U. (1990a). Facial electromyography and emotional reactions. *Psychophysiology, 27,* 481–494.

Dimberg, U. (1990b). Facial electromyographic reactions and autonomic activity to auditory stimuli. *Biological Psychology, 31,* 137–147.

Dimberg, U. (1990c). Perceived unpleasantness and facial reactions to auditory stimuli. *Scandinavian Journal of Psychology, 31,* 70–75.

Dimberg, U. (1990d). Facial reactions to fear-relevant stimuli for subjects high and low in specific fear. *Scandinavian Journal of Psychology, 31,* 65–69.

Doctor, R. F., & Perkins, R. B. (1960). The effects of ethyl alcohol on autonomic and muscular responses in humans. *Quarterly Journal of Studies on Alcohol, 22,* 374–386.

Donchin, E. (1979). Event-related potentials: A tool in the study of information processing. In H. Begleiter (Ed.), *Evoked brain potentials and behavior* (pp. 13–88). New York: Plenum.

Donegan, N. H., Rodin, J., O'Brien, C. P., & Solomon, R. L. (1983). A learning theory approach to commonalities. In P. Levison, D. Gerstein, & D. Maloff (Eds.), *Commonalities in substance abuse and habitual behavior* (pp. 111–156). Lexington, MA: Lexington Books.

Drummond. D. C., Tiffany, S. T., Glautier, S., & Remington, B. (1995). *Addictive behaviour: Cue exposure theory and practice.* New York: Wiley.

Einstein, A. (1990). *Out of my later years.* New York: Bonanza Books. (Original work published 1956)

Ekman, P. (1984). Expression and the nature of emotion. In K. Scherer & P. Ekman (Eds.), *Approaches to emotion* (pp. 319–344). Hillsdale, NJ: Erlbaum.

Ekman, P., & Davidson, R. J. (Eds.). (1994). *The nature of emotion: Fundamental questions.* New York: Oxford University Press.

Ekman, P., & Friesen, W. V. (1978). *Facial action coding system: A technique for the measurement of facial movement.* Palo Alto, CA: Consulting Psychologists Press.

Ekman, P., Levenson, R. W., & Friesen, W. V. (1983). Autonomic nervous system activity distinguishes between emotions. *Science, 221,* 1208–1210.

Ewing, J. A., & McCarty, D. (1983). Are the endorphins involved in mediating the mood effects of alcohol? *Alcoholism: Clinical and Experimental Research, 7,* 271–275.

Fanselow, M. S. (1994). Neural organization of the defensive behavior system responsible for fear. *Psychonomic Bulletin and Review, 1,* 429–438.

Finn, P. R., & Pihl, R. O. (1987). Men at high risk for alcoholism: The effect of alcohol on cardiovascular response to unavoidable shock. *Journal of Abnormal Psychology, 96,* 230–236.

Finn, P. R., Zeitouni, N. C., & Pihl, R. O. (1990). Effects of alcohol on psycho-physiological hyperreactivity to nonaversive and aversive stimuli in men at high risk for alcoholism. *Journal of Abnormal Psychology, 99,* 79–85.

Fowles, D. C. (1980). The three-arousal model: Implications of Gray's two-factor learning theory for heart rate, electrodermal activity, and psychopathy. *Psychophysiology, 17,* 87–104.

Gabel, P. C., Noel, N. E., Keane, T. M., & Lisman, S. A. (1980). Effect of sexual versus fear arousal on alcohol consumption in college males. *Behaviour Research and Therapy, 18,* 519–526.

Goldman, M. S., Brown, S. A., & Christiansen, B. A. (1987). Expectancy theory: Thinking about drinking. In H. Blane & K. Leonard (Eds.), *Psychological theories of drinking and alcoholism* (pp. 181–226). New York: Guilford Press.

Graham, F. K., & Clifton, R. K. (1966). Heart rate change as a component of the orienting response. *Psychological Bulletin, 65,* 305–320.

Gray, J. A. (1987). *The psychology of fear and stress* (2nd ed.). Cambridge, UK: Cambridge University Press.

Green, D. P., Goldman, S. L., & Salovey, P. (1993). Measurement error masks bipolarity in affect ratings. *Journal of Personality and Social Psychology, 64,* 1029–1041.

Greenberg, L., & Carpenter, J. (1957). The effect of alcoholic beverages on skin conductance and emotional tension: I. Wine, whiskey and alcohol. *Quarterly Journal of Studies on Alcohol, 18,* 190–204.

Greenwald, M. K., Cook, E. W., III, & Lang, P. J. (1989). Affective judgment and psychophysiological response: Dimensional covariation in the evaluation of pictorial stimuli. *Journal of Psychophysiology, 3,* 51–64.

Grillon, C. (1996). Context and startle: Effect of explicit and contextual cue conditioning following paired versus unpaired training. *Psychophysiology, 33,* S41.

Grillion, C., Ameli, R., Woods, S. W., Merikangas, K., & Davis, M. (1991). Fear-potentiated startle in humans: Effects of anticipatory anxiety on the acoustic blink reflex. *Psychophysiology, 28,* 588–595.

Gusfield, J. (1987). Passage to play: Rituals of drinking time in American society. In M. Douglas (Ed.), *Constructive drinking: Perspectives on drink from anthropology* (pp. 73–90). Cambridge, UK: Cambridge University Press.

Hackley, S. A. (1993). An evaluation of the automaticity of sensory processing using event-related potentials and brain stem reflexes. *Psychophysiology, 30,* 415–428.

Hamm, A. O., Stark, R., & Vaitl, D. (1990). Classical fear conditioning and the startle probe reflex. *Psychophysiology, 27*(Suppl. 1), S37.

Hamm, A. O., & Vaitl, D. (1996). Affective learning: Awareness and aversion. *Psychophysiology, 33,* 698–710.

Heath, D. B. (1995a). An anthropological view of alcohol and culture in international perspective. In D. Heath (Ed.), *International handbook on alcohol and culture* (pp. 328–347). Westport, CT: Greenwood Press.

Heath, D. B. (1995b). Some generalizations about alcohol and culture. In D. Heath (Ed.), *International handbook on alcohol and culture* (pp. 348–361). Westport, CT: Greenwood Press.

Heller, W. (1990). The neuropsychology of emotion: Developmental patterns and implications for psychopathology. In N. L. Stein, B. Leventhal, & T. Trabasso

(Eds.), *Psychological and biological approaches to emotion* (pp. 167–211). Hillsdale, NJ: Erlbaum.

Heller, W. (1993). Neuropsychological mechanisms of individual differences in emotion, personality, and arousal. *Neuropsychology, 7,* 476–489.

Hodgins, D., el-Guebaly, N., & Armstrong, S. (1995). Prospective and retrospective reports of mood states before relapse to substance use. *Journal of Consulting and Clinical Psychology, 63,* 400–407.

Hodgson, R., & Rachman, S. (1978). Desynchrony in measures of fear. *Behaviour Research and Therapy, 12,* 319–326.

Holloway, F. (1994). *Low-dose alcohol effects on human behavior and performance: A review of post-1984 research* (DOT/FAA/AM-94/24 Technical Report). Washington, DC: Office of Aviation Medicine.

Hubert, W., & de Jong-Meyer, R. (1990). Psychophysiological response patterns to positive and negative film stimuli. *Biological Psychology, 31,* 73–93.

Hull, J. G. (1981). A self-awareness model of the causes and effects of alcohol consumption. *Journal of Abnormal Psychology, 90,* 586–600.

Hull, J. G. (1987). Self-awareness model. In H. T. Blane & K. E. Leonard (Eds.), *Psychological theories of drinking and alcoholism* (pp. 272–304). New York: Guilford Press.

Hunt, W. A. (1990a). Biochemical bases for the reinforcing effects of ethanol. In M. Cox (Ed.), *Why people drink: Parameters of alcohol as a reinforcer* (pp. 51–70). New York: Gardner.

Hunt, W. A. (1990b). Brain mechanisms that underlie the reinforcing effects of ethanol. In M. Cox (Ed.), *Why people drink: Parameters of alcohol as a reinforcer* (pp. 71–92). New York: Gardner.

Izard, C. E. (1972). *The face of emotion.* New York: Appleton.

Izard, C. E. (1993). Four systems for emotion activation: Cognitive and noncognitive processes. *Psychological Review, 100,* 68–90.

Jansen, D. M., & Frijda, N. (1994). Modulation of acoustic startle response by film-induced fear and sexual arousal. *Psychophysiology, 31,* 565–571.

Josephs, R. A., & Steele, C. M. (1990). The two faces of alcohol myopia: Attentional mediation of psychological stress. *Journal of Abnormal Psychology, 99,* 115–126.

Keane, T. M., & Lisman, S. A. (1980). Alcohol and social anxiety in males: Behavioral, cognitive and physiological effects. *Journal of Abnormal Psychology, 89,* 213–223.

Kim, J. J., Rison, R. A., & Fanselow, M. S. (1993). Effects of amygdala, hippocampus, and peri-aqueductal gray lesions on short- and long-term contextual fear. *Behavioral Neuroscience, 107,* 1093–1098.

Konorski, J. (1967). *Integrative activity of the brain: An interdisciplinary approach.* Chicago: University of Chicago Press.

Kushner, M. G., MacKenzie, T. B., Fiszdon, J., Valentiner, D. D., Foa, E., Anderson, N., & Wangersteen, D. (1996). The effects of alcohol consumption on laboratory-induced panic and state anxiety. *Archives of General Psychiatry, 53,* 264–270.

Lacey, J. I. (1959). Psychophysiological approaches to the evaluation of psychotherapeutic process and outcome. In E. A. Rubinstein & M. B. Parloff (Eds.), *Research in psychotherapy* (Vol. 1, pp. 160–208). Washington, DC: American Psychological Association Press.

Lacey, J. I. (1967). Somatic response patterning and stress: Some revisions of activation theory. In M. H. Appley & R. Turnbull (Eds.), *Psychological stress: Issues in research* (pp. 14–37). New York: Appleton.

Lamb, M. R., & Robertson, L. C. (1987). Effect of acute alcohol on attention and processing of hierarchical patterns. *Alcoholism: Clinical and Experimental Research, 11*, 243–248.

Lang, P. J. (1968). Fear reduction and fear behavior: Problems in treating a construct. *Research in Psychotherapy, 3*, 90–102.

Lang, P. J. (1971). The application of psychophysiological methods to the study of psychotherapy and behavior modification. In A. E. Bergen & S. L. Garfield (Eds.), *Handbook of psychotherapy and behavior change* (pp. 75–125). New York: Wiley.

Lang, P. J. (1979). A bio-informational theory of emotional imagery. *Psychophysiology, 16*, 495–512.

Lang, P. J. (1994a). The motivational organization of emotion: Affect–reflex connections. In S. Van Goozen, N. E. Van de Poll, & J. A. Sergeant (Eds.), *The emotions: Essays on emotion theory* (pp. 61–93). Hillsdale, NJ: Erlbaum.

Lang, P. J. (1994b). The varieties of emotional experience: A meditation on James–Lange Theory. *Psychological Review, 101*, 211–221.

Lang, P. J. (1995). The emotion probe: Studies of motivation and attention. *American Psychologist, 50*, 372–385.

Lang, P. J., Bradley, M. M., & Cuthbert, B. N. (1990). Emotion, attention, and the startle reflex. *Psychological Review, 97*, 377–395.

Lang, P. J., Bradley, M. M., Cuthbert, B. N., & Patrick, C. J. (1993). Emotion and psychopathology: A startle probe analysis. In L. Chapman & D. Fowles (Eds.), *Progress in experimental personality and psychopathology research* (Vol. 16, pp. 163–199). New York: Springer.

Lang, P. J., Greenwald, M. K., Bradley, M. M., & Hamm, A. O. (1993). Looking at pictures: Affective, facial, visceral, and behavioral reactions. *Psychophysiology, 30*, 261–273.

Lansky, D., & Wilson, G. T. (1981). Alcohol, expectations, and sexual arousal in males: An information processing analysis. *Journal of Abnormal Psychology, 90*, 35–45.

Larsen, R. J., & Diener, E. (1992). Promises and problems with the circumplex model of emotion. In M. S. Clark (Ed.), *Review of personality and social psychology* (Vol. 13, pp. 25–59). Newbury Park, CA: Sage.

LeDoux, J. E. (1989). Cognitive–emotional interactions in the brain. *Cognition and Emotion, 3*, 267–290.

LeDoux, J. E. (1995). Emotion: Clues from the brain. *Annual Review of Psychology, 46*, 209–235.

Levenson, R. W. (1987). Alcohol, affect, and physiology: Positive effects in the early stages of drinking. In E. Gottheil, K. Druley, S. Pasko, & S. Weinstein (Eds.), *Stress and addiction* (pp. 173–196). New York: BrunNer/Mazel.

Levenson, R. W. (1992). Autonomic nervous system differences among emotions. *Psychological Science, 3*, 23–27.

Levenson, R. W., Oyama, O. N., & Meek, P. S. (1987). Greater reinforcement from alcohol for those at risk: Parental risk, personality risk, and sex. *Journal of Abnormal Psychology, 96*, 242–253.

Levenson, R. W., Sher, K. J, Grossman, L. M., Newman, J., & Newlin, D. B. (1980).

Alcohol and stress response dampening: Pharmacological effects, expectancy, and tension reduction. *Journal of Abnormal Psychology, 89,* 528–538.

Lewis, M. J., & June, H. J. (1990). Neurobehavioral studies of ethanol reward and activation. *Alcohol, 7,* 213–219.

Lienert, G. A., & Traxel, W. (1959). The effects of meprobamate and alcohol on galvanic skin response. *Journal of Psychology, 48,* 329–334.

Lister, R. G., Eckhardt, M. J., & Weingartner, H. (1987). Ethanol intoxication and memory: Recent developments and new directions. In M. Galanter (Ed.), *Recent developments in alcoholism* (Vol. 5, pp. 111–126). New York: Plenum.

Lukas, S. E., Mendelson, J. H., Amass, L., Benedikt, R. A., Henry, J. N., Jr., & Kouri, E. M. (1991). Electrophysiological correlates of ethanol reinforcement. In R. E. Meyer, G. F. Koob, M. J. Lewis, & S. M. Paul (Eds.), *Neuropharmacology of ethanol: New approaches* (pp. 201–231). Boston: Birkhäuser.

Lukas, S. E., Mendelson, J. H., Benedikt, R. A., & Jones, B. (1986). EEG alpha activity increases during transient episodes of ethanol-induced euphoria. *Pharmacology Biochemistry and Behavior, 25,* 889–895.

MacAndrew, C., & Edgerton, R. (1969). *Drunken comportment: A social explanation.* Chicago: Aldine.

Marlatt, G. A. (1987). Alcohol, the magic elixir: Stress, expectancy, and the transformation of emotional states. In E. Gottheil, K. Druley, S. Pasko, & S. Weinstein (Eds.), *Stress and addiction* (pp. 302–322). New York: Brunner/Mazel.

Marlatt, G. A., & Rohsenow, D. (1980). Cognitive processes in alcohol use: Expectancy and the balanced-placebo design. In N. Mello (Ed.), *Advances in substance abuse: Behavioral and biological research* (Vol. 1, pp. 159–199). Greenwich, CN: JAI Press.

Martin, C., Earleywine, M., Musty, R., Perrine, M., & Swift, R. (1993). Development and validation of the Biphasic Alcohol Effects Scale (BAES). *Alcoholism: Clinical and Experimental Research, 17,* 140–146.

Mathew, R. J., Wilson, W. J., & Daniel, D. G. (1985). The effect of nonsedating doses of diazepam on regional blood flow. *Biological Psychiatry, 20,* 1109–1116.

Matthews, D. B., Simson, P. E., & Best, P. J. (1995). Acute ethanol impairs spatial memory, but not stimulus/response memory in the rat. *Alcoholism: Experimental and Clinical Research, 19,* 902–909.

Mayford, M., Bach, M. E., Huang, Y., Wang, L., Hawkins, R. D., & Kandel, E. R. (1996). Control of memory formation through regulated expression of a CaMKII transgene. *Science, 274,* 1678–1683.

McCollam, J., Burish, T., Maisto, S., & Sobell, M. (1980). Alcohol's effects on physiological arousal and self-reported affect and sensations. *Journal of Abnormal Psychology, 89,* 224–233.

McGonnell, P. C., & Beach, H. D. (1968). The effects of ethanol on the acquisition of conditioned GSR. *Quarterly Journal of Studies on Alcohol, 29,* 845–855.

McRandle, C., & Goldstein, R. (1973). Effect of alcohol on the early and late components of the averaged electroencephalic response to clicks. *Journal of Speech and Hearing Research, 16,* 353–359.

Melia, K., Corodimas, K., Ryabinin, A., Wilson, M., & LeDoux, J. (1994). Ethanol pre-SA treatment selectively impairs classical conditioning of contextual cues: Possible involvement of the hippocampus. *Society for Neuroscience Abstracts, 24,* 1007.

Mello, N. K. (1968). Some aspects of the behavioral pharmacology of alcohol. In D.

H. Efrow (Ed.), *Psychopharmacology: A review of progress, 1957–1967* (Public Health Service Publication No. 1836, pp. 787–809). Washington, DC: U.S. Government Printing Office.

Miltner, W., Matjak, M., Braun, C., Diekmann, H., & Brody, S. (1994). Emotional qualities of odors and their influence on the startle reflex in humans. *Psychophysiology, 31*, 107–110.

Moruzzi, G., & Magoun, H. W. (1949). Brain stem reticular formation and activation of the EEG. *Electroencephalography and Clinical Neurophysiology, 1*, 455–473.

Nadel, L., & Willner, J. (1980). Context and conditioning: A place for space. *Physiological Psychology, 8*, 218–228.

Naitoh, P. (1972). The effect of alcohol on the autonomic nervous system of humans: Psychophysiological approach. In B. Kissin & H. Begleiter (Eds.), *The biology of alcoholism* (Vol. 2, pp. 367–433). New York: Plenum.

Newlin, D. B., & Thomson, J. B. (1990). Alcohol challenge with sons of alcoholics: A critical review and analysis. *Psychological Bulletin, 108*, 383–402.

Öhman, A., & Soares, J. J. F. (1993). Unconscious anxiety: Phobic responses to masked stimuli. *Journal of Abnormal Psychology, 103*, 231–240.

Orcutt, J. D. (1993). Happy hour and social lubrication: Evidence on mood-setting rituals of drinking time. *Journal of Drug Issues, 23*, 389–407.

Patrick, C. J., Berthot, B., & Moore, J. D. (1996). Diazepam blocks fear-potentiated startle in humans. *Journal of Abnormal Psychology, 105*, 89–96.

Peterson J., & Pihl, R. O. (1990). Information processing, neuropsychological function, and the inherited predisposition to alcoholism. *Neuropsychological Review, 1*, 343–369.

Phillips, R. G., & LeDoux, J. E. (1992). Differential contribution of the amygdala and hippocampus to cued and contextual fear conditioning. *Behavioral Neuroscience, 106*, 274–285.

Pliner, P., & Cappell, H. (1974). Modification of affective consequences of alcohol: A comparison of social and solitary drinking. *Journal of Abnormal Psychology, 83*, 418–425.

Plutchik, R. (1984). Emotions: A general psychoevolutionary theory. In K. Scherer & P. Ekman (Eds.), *Approaches to emotion* (pp. 197–219). Hillsdale, NJ: Erlbaum.

Pohorecky, L. A. (1977). Biphasic action of ethanol. *Biobehavioral Review, 1*, 231–240.

Pohorecky, L. A. (1991). Stress and alcohol interaction: An update of human research. *Alcoholism: Clinical and Experimental Research, 15*, 438–459.

Pohorecky, L. A., Brick, J., & Carpenter, J. A. (1986). Assessment of the development of tolerance to ethanol using multiple measures. *Alcoholism: Clinical and Experimental Research, 10*, 616–622.

Pohorecky, L. A., Cagan, M., Brick, J., & Jaffe, L. S. (1976). The startle response in rats: Effect of ethanol. *Pharmacology Biochemistry and Behavior, 4*, 311–316.

Pohorecky, L. A., & Roberts, P. (1991). Development of tolerance to and physical dependence on ethanol: Daily versus repeated cycles treatment with ethanol. *Alcoholism: Clinical and Experimental Research, 15*, 824–833.

Rassnick, S., Koob, G. F., & Geyer, M. A. (1992). Responding to acoustic startle during chronic ethanol intoxication and withdrawal. *Psychopharmacology, 106*, 351–358.

Rather, B. C., & Goldman, M. S. (1994). Drinking-related differences in the memory organization of alcohol expectancies. *Experimental and Clinical Psychopharmacology, 2,* 167–183.

Rather, B. C., Goldman, M. S., Roehrich, L., & Brannick, M. (1992). Empirical modeling of an alcohol expectancy memory network using multidimensional scaling. *Journal of Abnormal Psychology, 101,* 174–183.

Regier, D. A., Farmer, M. E., Rae, D. S., Locke, B. Z., Keith, S. J., Judd, L. L., & Goodwin, F. K. (1990). Comorbidity of mental disorders with alcohol and other drug abuse. *Journal of the American Medical Association, 264,* 2511–2518.

Routtenberg, A. (1968). The two-arousal hypothesis: Reticular formation and limbic system. *Psychological Review, 75,* 51–80.

Rudy, J. W., & Sutherland, R. J. (1992). Configural and elemental associations and the memory coherence problem. *Journal of Cognitive Neuroscience, 4,* 208–216.

Russell, J. A. (1980). A circumplex model of affect. *Journal of Personality and Social Psychology, 39,* 1161–1178.

Russell, J. A., & Mehrabian, A. (1975). The mediating role of emotions in alcohol use. *Journal of Studies on Alcohol, 36,* 1508–1536.

Russell, J. A., Weiss, A., & Mendelsohn, G. A. (1989). Affect grid: A single-item scale of pleasure and arousal. *Journal of Personality and Social Psychology, 57,* 493–502.

Sayette, M. A. (1993a). Heart rate as an index of stress response in alcohol administration research: A critical review. *Alcoholism: Clinical and Experimental Research, 17,* 802–809.

Sayette, M. A. (1993b). An appraisal-disruption model of alcohol's effects on stress responses in social drinkers. *Psychological Bulletin, 114,* 459–476.

Sayette, M., Breslin, F. C., Wilson, G. T., & Rosenblum, G. (1994). Parental history of alcohol abuse and the effects of alcohol and expectations of intoxication on social stress. *Journal of Studies on Alcohol, 55,* 214–223.

Sayette, M. A., Smith, D. W., Breiner, M. J., & Wilson, G. T. (1992). The effect of alcohol on emotional response to a social stressor. *Journal of Studies on Alcohol, 53,* 541–545.

Sayette, M. A., & Wilson, G. T. (1991). Intoxication and exposure to stress: Effects of temporal patterning. *Journal of Abnormal Psychology, 100,* 56–62.

Sayette, M. A., Wilson, G. T., & Carpenter, J. A. (1989). Cognitive moderators of alcohol's effect on anxiety. *Behaviour Research and Therapy, 27,* 685–690.

Schachter, S., & Singer, J. E. (1962). Cognition, social and physiological determinants of emotion. *Psychological Review, 69,* 379–399.

Schwartz, G. E., Fair, P. L., Salt, P., Mandel, M. R., & Klerman, G. L. (1976). Facial muscle patterning to affective imagery in depressed and nondepressed subjects. *Science, 192,* 489–491.

Schwartz, G. E., Weinberger, D. A., & Singer, J. A. (1981). Cardiovascular differentiation of happiness, sadness, anger and fear following imagery and exercise. *Psychosomatic Medicine, 43,* 343–364.

Sher, K. J. (1987). Stress response dampening. In H. T. Blane & K. E. Leonard (Eds.), *Psychological theories of drinking and alcoholism* (pp. 227–271). New York: Guilford Press.

Sher, K. J., & Levenson, R. W. (1982). Risk for alcoholism and individual differences in the stress-response-dampening effect of alcohol. *Journal of Abnormal Psychology, 91,* 350–367.

Sher, K. J., & Walitzer, K. S. (1986). Individual differences in the stress-response-dampening effect of alcohol: A dose–response study. *Journal of Abnormal Psychology, 95*, 159–167.

Smith, W. W. (1922). *The measurement of emotion.* New York: Harcourt–Brace.

Solomon, R. L. (1977). An opponent–process theory of acquired motivation: The affective dynamics of addiction. In J. Maser & M. Seligman (Eds.), *Psychopathology: Experimental models* (pp. 66–103). San Francisco: Jossey-Bass.

Squire, L. R. (1992). Memory and the hippocampus: A synthesis from findings with rats, monkeys, and humans. *Psychological Review, 99*, 195–231.

Stacy, A. W. (1995). Memory association and ambiguous cues in models of alcohol and marijuana use. *Experimental and Clinical Psychopharmacology, 3*, 183–194.

Stacy, A. W., Leigh, B. C., & Weingardt, K. R. (1994). Memory accessibility and association of alcohol use and its positive outcomes. *Experimental and Clinical Psychopharmacology, 2*, 269–282.

Steele, C. M., & Josephs, R. A. (1988). Drinking your troubles away: II. An attention-allocation model of alcohol's effect on psychological stress. *Journal of Abnormal Psychology, 97*, 196–205.

Steele, C. M., & Josephs, R. A. (1990). Alcohol myopia: Its prized and dangerous effects. *American Psychologist, 45*, 921–933.

Steele, C. M., Southwick, L., & Pagano, R. (1986). Drinking your troubles away: The role of activity in mediating alcohol's reduction of psychological stress. *Journal of Abnormal Psychology, 95*, 173–180.

Stern, R. M., & Sison, C. E. E. (1990). Response patterning. In J. T. Cacioppo & L. G. Tassinary (Eds.), *Principles of psychophysiology: Physical, social, and inferential elements* (pp. 193–215). New York: Cambridge University Press.

Stewart, S. H., Finn, P. R., & Pihl, R. O. (1992). The effects of alcohol on the cardiovascular stress response in men at high risk for alcoholism: A dose response study. *Journal of Studies on Alcohol, 53*, 499–506.

Stewart, S. H., & Pihl, R. O. (1994). Effects of alcohol administration on psychophysiological and subjective-emotional responses to aversive stimulation in anxiety-sensitive women. *Psychology of Addictive Behaviors, 8*, 29–42.

Stritzke, W. G. K., Lang, A. R., & Patrick, C. J. (1996). Beyond stress and arousal: A reconceptualization of alcohol–emotion relations with reference to psychophysiological methods. *Psychological Bulletin, 120*, 376–395.

Stritzke, W. G. K., Patrick, C. J., & Lang, A. R. (1995). Alcohol and human emotion: A multidimensional analysis incorporating startle-probe methodology. *Journal of Abnormal Psychology, 104*, 114–122.

Sutker, P. B., Allain, A. N., Brantley, P. J., & Randall, C. L. (1982). Acute alcohol intoxication, negative affect, and autonomic arousal in women and men. *Addictive Behaviors, 7*, 17–25.

Tassinary, L. G., & Cacioppo, J. T. (1992). Unobservable facial actions and emotion. *Psychological Science, 3*, 28–33.

Tellegen, A. (1985). Structures of mood and personality and their relevance to assessing anxiety, with an emphasis on self-report. In A. H. Tuma & J. D. Maser (Eds.), *Anxiety and the anxiety disorders* (pp. 681–706). Hillsdale, NJ: Erlbaum.

Thyer, B. A., & Curtis, G. C. (1984). The effects of ethanol intoxication on phobic anxiety. *Behaviour Research and Therapy, 22*, 599–610.

Tomkins, S. S. (1984). Affect theory. In K. R. Scherer & P. Ekman (Eds.), *Approaches to emotion* (pp.163–195). Hillsdale, NJ: Erlbaum.

Tranel, D., & Damasio, H. (1994). Neuroanatomical correlates of electrodermal skin conductance responses. *Psychophysiology, 31*, 427–438.

Tucker, J. A., Vuchinich, R. E., & Sobell, M . B. (1982). Alcohol's effects on human emotions: A review of the stimulation/depression hypothesis. *International Journal of the Addictions, 17*, 155–180.

Turkkan, J. S., Stitzer, M. L., & McCaul, M. E. (1988). Psychophysiological effects of oral ethanol in alcoholics and social drinkers. *Alcoholism: Clinical and Experimental Research, 12*, 30–38.

Valins, S. (1966). Cognitive effects of false heart rate feedback. *Journal of Personality and Social Psychology, 4*, 400–408.

Vandergriff, J. L., Matthews, D. B., Best, P. J., & Simson, P. E. (1995). Effect of ethanol and diazepam on spatial and nonspatial tasks in rats on an 8-arm radial arm maze. *Alcoholism: Clinical and Experimental Research, 19*(Suppl.), 64A.

Vrana, S. R. (1993). The psychophysiology of disgust: Differentiating negative emotional context with facial EMG. *Psychophysiology, 30*, 279–286.

Vrana, S. R., & Lang, P. J. (1990). Fear imagery and the startle probe reflex. *Journal of Abnormal Psychology, 99*, 189–197.

Vrana, S. R., Spence, E. L., & Lang, P. J. (1988). The startle probe response: A new measure of emotion? *Journal of Abnormal Psychology, 97*, 487–491.

Vuchinich, R., & Tucker, J. (1996). Alcoholic relapse, life events, and behavioral choice theories: A prospective analysis. *Experimental and Clinical Psychopharmacology, 4*, 19–28.

Vuchinich, R., Tucker, J. A., & Sobell, M. (1979) Alcohol expectancy, cognitive labeling, and mirth. *Journal of Abnormal Psychology, 88*, 641–651.

Watson, D., Clark, L. A., & Tellegen, A. (1988). Development and validation of brief measures of positive and negative affect: The PANAS scales. *Journal of Personality and Social Psychology, 54*, 1063–1070.

Weaver, J. B., Masland, J. L., Kharazmi, S., & Zillman, D. (1985). Effect of alcoholic intoxication on the appreciation of different types of humor. *Journal of Personality and Social Psychology, 49*, 781–787.

West, J. A., & Sutker, P. B. (1990). Alcohol consumption, tension reduction, and mood enhancement. In M. Cox (Ed.), *Why people drink: Parameters of alcohol as a reinforcer* (pp. 93–130). New York: Gardner.

Wilson, G. T. (1988). Alcohol and anxiety. *Behaviour Research and Therapy, 26*, 369–381.

Wilson, G. T., Abrams, D. B., & Lipscomb, T. R. (1980). Effects of intoxication levels and drinking pattern on social anxiety in men. *Journal of Studies on Alcohol, 41*, 250–264.

Wilson, G. T., Niaura, R. S., & Adler, J. L. (1985). Alcohol, selective attention and sexual arousal in men. *Journal of Studies on Alcohol, 46*, 107–115.

Wise, R., & Bozarth, M. (1987). A psychomotor stimulant theory of addiction. *Psychological Review, 94*, 469–492.

Witvliet, C. V., & Vrana, S. R. (1995). Psychophysiological responses as indices of affective dimensions. *Psychophysiology, 32*, 436–443.

Zeichner, A., Allen, J., Petrie, C., Rasmussen, P., & Giancola, P. (1993). Effects of alcohol and information salience on attentional processes in male social drinkers. *Alcoholism: Clinical and Experimental Research, 17*, 727–732.

10

Behavioral Genetic Models of Alcoholism and Drinking

MATT McGUE

INTRODUCTION AND OVERVIEW

For as long as humans have had access to alcohol, the tendency of problem drinking to "run in families" has been noted (Goodwin, 1994). But the familial aggregation of a behavioral characteristic may reflect common environmental as well as common genetic origins. Although psychological researchers have tended to emphasize social and cultural contributions to the familial transmission of alcoholism, and biological researchers have tended to emphasize genetic contributions, there has recently been an effort on both sides to consider how genetic and environmental factors jointly influence alcoholism risk (Zucker, Boyd, & Howard, 1994).

In this chapter, behavioral genetic models of alcohol use and abuse are described and critiqued. While the emphasis is on problem drinking or alcoholism (an emphasis that reflects the major focus of empirical work), behavioral genetic research on nonproblem drinking phenotypes is also considered, especially when that research serves to illustrate a basic behavioral genetic principle. Although behavioral genetics does not at this time offer a comprehensive theory of drinking behavior, it does account for one of the most fundamental aspects of alcoholism etiology—its familial basis. Moreover, behavioral genetics has produced a set of challenging observations that must be reconciled by any valid theory of drinking behavior, and offers a set of principles that are likely to be fundamental to the development of integrative models of alcoholism etiology.

The most salient finding to emerge from the past generation of behavioral genetic research on alcohol is the repeated demonstration that genetic factors contribute fundamentally to individual differences in alcohol-related behaviors. Twin and adoption studies have provided consistent support for the existence of genetic influences on alcoholism risk. Although this evidence is especially compelling in men, recent studies suggest that genetic factors play an important role in the etiology of alcoholism in women also. Moreover, twin studies indicate that a wide range of alcohol-related measures, including ethanol metabolism and sensitivity, drinking quantity and frequency, and even the cognitive factors associated with drinking, are all, in part, heritable.

The strength of the heritability studies on alcohol-related phenotypes has contributed not only to the ascendance of biological models of alcoholism, but also to the justification for initiating the massive research effort that will be required to identify the individual genes affecting alcoholism risk. Progress in molecular genetics has resulted in the development of a powerful set of methodologies for identifying genes for complex disorders such as alcoholism. Nonetheless, other than the alcohol metabolizing genes, the genes underlying alcoholism etiology remain to be identified. There is reason, however, to be optimistic. Systematic large-scale searches of the human genome for alcoholism vulnerability genes are underway, and these efforts, as well as the application of animal models, have helped to identify regions of the human genome that might contain genes influencing alcohol-related behaviors.

Although findings from genetic research have often been viewed as supporting a narrow medical model of alcoholism, genes do not code directly for behavior; there are numerous intervening steps between primary gene product (protein synthesis) and observable behavior. Genetic influences on alcoholism risk might reflect mechanisms ranging from ethanol sensitivity to heritable personality characteristics. Indeed, the heterogeneity of the alcoholism phenotype suggests that no single mediating pathway is likely to account for all, or even the majority, of the heritable effects on alcoholism risk. In the absence of empirically supported mechanistic models that explain how genetic factors exert their distal influence, it is likely counterproductive to adopt rigid conceptualizations that limit the scope of inquiry.

The heritability of alcoholism vulnerability does not imply the genetic determination of alcoholism. The same twin and adoption studies that implicate genetic factors in the etiology of alcoholism also document the fundamental nature of environmental influence. Of interest is the suggestion that the major environmental influences on alcoholism may be those that contribute to differences rather than similarities among reared-together relatives. A major challenge for behavioral genetic research on alcoholism is the development of integrative models of genetic and environmental influence. It is argued here that alcoholism is usefully conceptualized as a developmental disorder, as arising when inherited vulnerability factors interact with experiential risk to influence the progression from adolescent drinking initiation and experimentation to adult problem drinking and dependence. Two behavioral genetic processes, genotype-environment interaction and genotype-environment correlation, are likely to be essential to explicating these developmental pathways.

TWIN AND ADOPTION STUDIES OF ALCOHOLISM AND ALCOHOL-RELATED PHENOTYPES

Twin and Adoption Study Methodology

Behavioral geneticists distinguish three types of influences on individual differences: genetic factors (G), shared environmental factors (C), and nonshared environmental factors (E). Shared environmental factors correspond to those environmental factors that are shared by reared-together relatives, and are thus a potential source of their behavioral similarity. Parents' general orientation toward child rearing, the disordered environment that can be a consequence of parental psychopathology (including alcoholism), and parental conflict are examples of factors that could contribute to behavioral similarity among reared-together individuals. Nonshared environmental factors correspond to those environmental factors that are not shared by reared-together relatives, and are thus a potential source of their behavioral differences. Differential parental treatment, the influence of distinct sets of friends, and differential exposure to traumatic events are examples of environmental factors that could create differences among reared together relatives.

Fundamental to the behavioral genetic analysis of any phenotype is the recognition that both shared environmental and genetic factors can contribute to familial resemblance among reared-together relatives. Consequently, while family studies have convincingly demonstrated the excess risk of alcoholism that exists among the offspring of alcoholics (Cotton, 1979), these studies are unable to determine whether parent–offspring resemblance for alcoholism is genetically or environmentally mediated. Two research strategies, twin and adoption studies, have been used primarily to resolve the separate contribution of genetic and environmental factors to the familial transmission of alcoholism.

In principle, an adoption study provides the most direct method of assessing the separate contribution of genetic and shared environmental factors to alcoholism risk. An individual who was removed from his or her biological parents in infancy and placed with nonbiologically related adoptive parents will share, in principle, only genetic factors with his or her biological relatives and shared environmental factors with his or her adoptive relatives. In practice, however, several factors serve to mitigate the clean separation of the two sources of familial resemblance in an adoption study.

Biological parents contribute to the intrauterine and early postnatal environments of their adopted children, and an excess risk of alcoholism among the reared-away children of alcoholics could be due, at least in part, to the well-known effects of prenatal alcohol exposure (Streissguth et al., 1994) or other intrauterine factors. The practice of selective placement (i.e., matching adoptive family characteristics with biological background) could also reintroduce a correlation between genetic background and rearing circumstances, although it is far from clear that social workers actually attempt to match biological and adoptive backgrounds on psychologically relevant characteristics. Other factors may further limit the utility and generalizability of adoption studies. Because the range of rearing environments is likely restricted, adoption studies may underestimate the importance of shared environmental factors. Use of the adoption study method has also been hampered by the difficulty researchers face in obtaining reliable information on the mental health of birth parents given the confidentiality of adoption records. It is for this latter reason that most adoption research has been undertaken in Scandinavian countries, where national registries of adoption and psychiatric hospitalization or temperance board violations are maintained.

Given these limitations, it is critical that the validity of inferences about the existence of genetic influences on alcoholism risk does not depend exclusively on findings from adoption studies; convergent evidence may be and has been, sought from twin studies. In a twin study, the similarity of reared-together genetically identical, monozygotic (MZ) twins is compared with the similarity of reared-together genetically nonidentical, dizygotic (DZ) twins, who, like ordinary siblings, share on average 50% of their segregating genes. Genetic influences are indicated whenever MZ twins are more similar than DZ twins. The validity of the twin study comparison rests, however, on the assumption that greater phenotypic similarity among MZ as compared to DZ twins cannot be attributed to environmental factors. Given its fundamental nature, it is not surprising that the so-called equal environmental similarity assumption has drawn empirical attention. Two issues are relevant: Are the environments of MZ twins more similar than the environments of DZ twins? And, if yes, does this greater environmental similarity account for the greater phenotypic similarity of MZ relative to DZ twins? Although the relevant research literature is limited, it generally supports the conclusion that while MZ twins do have more similar environments than DZ twins, this greater environmental similarity is more likely a consequence rather than a cause of their greater behavioral similarity (e.g., Kendler, Neale, Kessler, Haeth, & Eaves, 1993; Loehlin & Nichols, 1976; Plomin, DeFries, McClearn, & Rutter, 1997). Nonetheless, the validity of the equal environmental similarity assumption needs to be continually evaluated, especially as concerns the effects of prenatal factors on psychological outcomes (e.g., Sokol et al., 1995).

Twin and Adoption Studies of Alcoholism in Men

Table 10.1 summarizes each of the six published adoption studies of alcoholism in men in terms of the observed rate of alcoholism in the reared-away sons of alcoholics and nonalcoholics. Also given in table 10.1 is the ratio of the odds of alcoholism among the reared-away offspring of alcoholics relative to the odds of alcoholism among the reared-away offspring of nonalcoholics. As can be seen, the relevant studies have been undertaken in several different countries (although the samples are predominantly Cau-

TABLE 10.1. Rate of Alcoholism in the Adopted Sons and Daughters of Alcoholic and Nonalcoholic Biological Parents

Study	Country	Diagnosis	History of alcoholism in biological parents		Odds ratio[a]
			Positive	Negative	(+SE.)
Males					
Roe (1944)	U.S.	Problem drinking; criteria not specified	0.0% (N = 21)	0.0% (N = 11)	Not Defined
Goodwin et al. (1973)	Denmark	Feighner alcoholism[b]	18.0% (N = 55)	5.0% (N = 78)	4.11* (±0.62)
Cloninger et al. (1981)	Sweden	Temperance Board Registration	23.0% (N = 291)	14.7% (N = 571)	1.73* (±0.18)
Cadoret et al. (1985)	U.S.	DSM-III alcohol abuse/dependence	61.1% (N = 18)	23.9% (N = 109)	5.02* (±0.53)
Cadoret et al. (1987)	U.S.	DSM-III alcohol abuse/dependence	62.5% (N = 8)	20.4% (N = 152)	6.51* (±0.57)
Sigvardsson et al. (1996)	Sweden	Temperance Board Registration	24.1% (N = 108)	12.8% (N = 469)	2.16* (±0.26)
Females:					
Roe (1944)	U.S.	Problem drinking; criteria not specified	0.0% (N = 11)	0.0% (N = 14)	Not Defined
Goodwin et al. (1977a)	Denmark	Feighner alcoholism[b]	2.0% (N = 49)	4.0% (N = 47)	0.49 (±1.24)
Bohman et al. (1981)	Sweden	Temperance Board Registrations	4.5% (N = 336)	2.8% (N = 577)	1.64[c] (±0.37)
Cadoret et al. (1985)	U.S.	DSM-III alcohol abuse/dependence	33.3% (N = 12)	5.3% (N = 75)	8.88* (±0.64)
Sigvardsson et al. (1996)	Sweden	Temperance Board Registration	0.9% (N = 114)	1.1% (N = 546)	0.80 (±1.09)

[a]Odds ratio is the ratio of the odds of alcoholism among offspring of alcoholics relative to the odds of alcoholism among the offspring of nonalcoholics.

[b]In Danish adoption studies, alcoholism was diagnosed using criteria that were very similar to but not identical to the criteria of Feighner et al. (1972).

[c]Alcoholism in daughters was significantly associated with maternal but not paternal alcoholism.

*Odds ratio significantly different from null value of 1.0 at $p < .05$.

casian) using alternative diagnostic standards. Against these methodological differences, the consistency of findings is impressive. Except for the early negative study by Roe (1944), which suffers from small sample size and the uncertain documentation of parental alcoholism, in every case, the rate of alcoholism is significantly higher among the reared-away sons of alcoholics than among the reared-away sons of nonalcoholics, with the associated odds ratios generally falling in the moderate (i.e., 2.0) to strong (i.e., 5.0) range, with the largest odds ratios being observed in studies using the broadest definition of alcoholism (DSM-III alcohol abuse or dependence).

Significantly, findings from twin studies converge with findings from adoption studies in implicating a substantial genetic influence on risk of alcoholism in men. Twin studies of alcoholism are summarized in Table 10.2 in terms of the MZ and DZ concordances (i.e., risk of alcoholism among the cotwins of alcoholics) as well as their associated odds ratios (MZ:DZ). While the concordances do vary from study to study (reflecting differences in the diagnostic criteria for alcoholism that were used), the MZ concordance is consistently and, except for a single small study, significantly higher than the DZ concordance. At least two investigators have reported that the zygosity difference in alcoholism concordance could not be accounted for by greater environmental similarity among MZ as compared to DZ twins (Kendler, Heath, Neale, Kessler, & Eaves 1992; Heath, Bucholz, Madden, 1997), thus addressing one of the major assumptions of the twin method. The converging evidence from adoption and twin studies, summarized in Tables 10.1 and 10.2, provides support for the existence of genetic influences on alcoholism risk in men that is as strong as the evidence supporting the existence of a genetic influence on any behavioral disorder.

Twin and Adoption Studies of Alcoholism in Women

Although clinical genetic studies have consistently implicated the existence of genetic influences on risk of alcoholism in men, these same types of studies have produced what appears to be an inconsistent set of findings as concerns the importance of genetic influences on risk of alcoholism in women. Of the five published adoption studies of alcoholism in women, only two report a significant biological parent effect (Table 10.1), one of which (the study by Cadoret, O'Gorman, Troughton, & Heywood, 1985) is notable and exceptional in that it reported a large odds ratio in favor of a biological parent effect (odds ratio = 8.88 $\pm$ .64). A similar pattern of seemingly inconsistent findings is evident in twin studies of alcoholism in women (Table 10.2). Of the six relevant studies, only three reported significantly greater MZ than DZ concordance.

The inconsistent findings from twin and adoption studies of alcoholism in women may indicate that the strength of heritable influences on risk of alcoholism in women is either nonexistent or weak. Alternatively, the inconsistent pattern of findings may reflect the statistical limitations of small

TABLE 10.2. Twin Studies of alcoholism

Study	Country	Diagnosis	Twin Concordance MZ	DZ	Odds Ratio[a]	Heritability
Males:						
Kaij (1960)	Sweden	Chronic alcoholism	.71 (N = 14)	.32 (N = 31)	5.28*	NR
Hrubec & Omenn (1981)	U.S.	ICD-8 alcoholism	.26 (N = 271)	.12 (N = 444)	2.58*	.53
Gurling et al. (1984)	U.K.	WHO alcohol dependence	.33 (N = 15)	.30 (N = 20)	1.15	NR
Pickens et al. (1991)	U.S.	DSM-III alcohol dependence	.59 (N = 39)	.36 (N = 47)	2.56*	.60
Caldwell & Gottesman (1991)	U.S.	DSM-III alcohol dependence	.40 (N = 20)	.13 (N = 15)	4.46*	.49
McGue et al. (1992)	U.S.	DSM-III alcohol abuse/dependence	.77 (N = 85)	.54 (N = 96)	2.85*	.54
Kendler et al. (1997)	Sweden	Temperance Board Registrations	.48 (N = 3185)[b]	.33 (N = 5750)[b]	2.03*	.54
Heath, Bucholz, et al. (1997)	Australia	DSM-III-R alcohol dependence	.56 (N = 396)[b]	.33 (N = 231)[b]	2.58*	.64[c]
Females:						
Gurling et al. (1984)	U.K.	WHO alcohol dependence	.08 (N = 13)	.13 (N = 8)	0.58	NR
Pickens et al. (1991)	U.S.	DSM-III alcohol dependence	.25 (N = 24)	.05 (N = 20)	6.33*	.42
Caldwell & Gottesman (1991)	U.S.	DSM-III alcohol dependence	.29 (N = 7)	.25 (N = 12)	1.23	.10
McGue et al. (1992)	U.S.	DSM-III alcohol abuse/dependence	.39 (N = 44)	.42 (N = 43)	0.88	.00
Kendler et al. (1992)	U.S.	DSM-III-R alcohol dependence	.32 (N = 81)	.24 (N = 79)	1.49*	.56
Heath, Bucholz, et al. (1997)	Australia	DSM-III-R alcohol dependence	.30 (N = 932)[b]	.17 (N = 534)[b]	2.09*	.64[c]

Note. In many twin studies, twin concordance is reported for more than one diagnosis of alcoholism or alcohol abuse; in these cases, concordances for the most restrictive form of diagnosis are given in the table. Heritability values are those given in the original publication and estimate the proportion of liability variance associated with genetic factors; NR = not reported.

[a]Odds ratio is the ratio of the odds of alcoholism among MZ cotwins of alcoholics to the odds of alcoholism among DZ cotwins of alcoholics.

[b]Sample size includes number of pairs concordant for nonalcoholism and is thus not directly comparable to sample sizes reported for other studies which include only pairs where at least one member was alcoholic.

[c]Heritability estimate in this study was constrained to be equal in the male and female samples.

*Odds ratio significantly different from null value of 1.0 at $p < .05$.

samples. While this pattern of results has led several researchers to hypothesize that genetic factors are less important to the etiology of alcoholism in women as compared to men (e.g., McGue & Slutske, 1996), it is important to recognize that in the most recent and best designed adoption and twin studies, significant genetic effects have been observed. Thus, in the largest adoption study of women, the Stockholm Adoption Study, rate of alcohol abuse was significantly greater among the reared-away daughters of alcoholic mothers (9.8%) than among the reared-away daughters of non-alcoholics (2.8%) (Bohman, Sigvardsson, & Cloninger, 1981), but did not vary significantly as a function of paternal diagnosis of alcoholism (3.5% vs. 2.8%), suggesting that genetic effects might be gender-specific (a finding at odds with findings from twin studies that show risk of alcoholism in the unlike-sex cotwins of alcoholic probands is significantly higher than the population prevalence; McGue, Pickens, & Svikis, 1992, Heath, Bucholz, et al., 1997). In the largest twin study of alcoholism in women (Kendler et al., 1992), concordance was significantly greater among MZ (32%) than among DZ (24%) twins, a finding that was replicated in the recent large Australian twin study by Heath, Bucholz, et al. (1997). Although the issue of gender moderation of heritable effects is far from resolved by existing research, in aggregate, there does appear to be some genetic influence on alcoholism risk in women (Heath, Slutske, & Madden, 1997).

The Heritability of Alcoholism Liability

For quantitative phenotypes, the strength of genetic influence is typically quantified in terms of the heritability coefficient, or the proportion of phenotypic variance that is associated with genetic factors. For categorical phenotypes (e.g., alcoholism), the heritability coefficient is defined under the assumptions of the multifactorial threshold (MFT) model. In a MFT model, the categorical diagnosis of alcoholism is assumed to be a manifestation of a latent quantitative liability such that an individual is affected if his or her liability exceeds some fixed threshold value along the liability continuum (Falconer, 1965; Figure 10.1). Genetic and environmental influences on the observed categorical phenotype are mediated by the hypothetical liability variable. Consequently, heritability estimates apply to the underlying continuum, rather than to the categorical phenotype per se.

Table 10.2 gives heritability estimates reported in twin studies of alcoholism (some of the studies did not compute heritability, in which case, no estimate is given). In studies of male twins, heritability estimates are remarkably consistent and suggest that approximately 50%–60% of the variance in alcoholism liability is associated with genetic factors. Further evidence for the consistency of estimates for the heritability of alcoholism liability comes from two recent twin studies (Kendler et al., 1997; Heath, Bucholz, et al., 1997), which both reported stable heritability estimates across multiple 20th-century birth cohorts. The Kendler et al. (1997) study

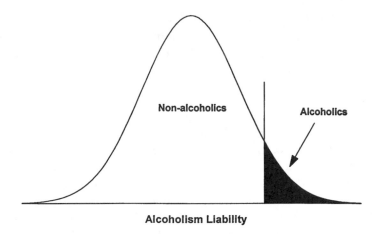

Alcoholism Liability

FIGURE 10.1. Multifactorial Threshold Model (MFT) for Alcoholism. In a MFT model, alcoholism is assumed to be due to quantitative variation in an observed continuously distributed variable termed liability. If an individual's liability exceeds some fixed threshold along the liability continuum, he or she is alcoholic. Heritability calculations apply to the underlying continuum, rather than alcoholism per se.

is especially noteworthy, as it is by far the largest twin study of alcoholism ever undertaken, consisting of nearly 9,000 pairs of male twins born between 1902 and 1949, for whom Swedish Temperance Board registrations were available. In this study, MZ and DZ concordances for alcohol abuse, as well as the resultant heritability estimates, did not vary appreciably by birth cohort, even though per capita income and alcohol consumption had increased substantially in Sweden during the period covered.

In contrast to the consistency of heritability estimates reported in samples of male twins, heritability estimates in studies of female twins vary markedly, ranging from 0% to 64%. The confidence intervals associated with these estimates (not given in the table) are, however, wide and overlapping (Heath, Slutske, et al., 1997). It is noteworthy, nonetheless, that the strongest evidence for genetic influence on alcoholism risk in women comes from the most recent and largest twin studies. Both Kendler et al. (1992) and Heath, Bucholz, et al. (1997) report heritability estimates for women that are comparable to those reported in studies with men (h^2 estimates of .56 and .64, respectively). Given this evidence, it seems most prudent to conclude that behavioral genetic research, when taken in aggregate, supports the existence of a genetic influence on alcoholism risk in women, but does not allow for the precise determination of the magnitude of that influence. In particular, unassailable proof exists neither for the proposition that alcoholism liability is equally heritable in men and women, nor for the proposition that alcoholism liability is less heritable in women than men.

Heterogeneity in the Inheritance of Alcoholism

Although the clinical heterogeneity of alcoholism is well documented (e.g., Babor, 1996), relatively little is known about its etiological heterogeneity. Cloninger (1987) posited the existence of two etiologically distinct forms of alcoholism: Type I alcoholism, which is characterized by a relatively late age of onset, relatively low levels of antisociality, and affects both men and women; and Type II alcoholism, which is characterized by a relatively early age of onset, relatively high levels of antisociality, and primarily affects men only. The Cloninger model overlaps substantially with the Type A/Type B distinction derived empirically by Babor et al. (1992), as well as with other typological models of alcoholism that date back to Jellinck (1960) and earlier, and which all distinguish a reactive late-onset form of alcoholism (akin to Cloninger's Type I) from an essential, early onset form (akin to Type II) (Babor, 1996).

The Cloninger model was deduced from analysis of differential patterns of alcohol abuse inheritance in the Stockholm Adoption Study (Cloninger, Bohman, & Sigvardsson et al., 1981). A distinctive feature of the model is that it is based on etiological as well as clinical considerations. Since the original empirical development, Cloninger (1987) has elaborated the Type I/Type II model by hypothesizing underlying neurobiological mechanisms and associated personality manifestations for the two forms of alcoholism. Although predictions based on the Type I/Type II model have not received consistent empirical support (especially those relating to personality factors; e.g., Schuckit & Irwin, 1989), the model does appear to capture important aspects of the genetic heterogeneity of alcoholism. In the original Stockholm study, the estimated heritability of liability was 90% for Type II alcoholism, but less than 40% for Type I alcoholism. Significantly, the major findings from the Stockholm Adoption Study were recently independently replicated in Gothenburg, Sweden (Sigvardsson, Bohman, & Cloninger et al., 1996). Classification rules developed in the Stockholm study were applied to male adoptees from Gothenburg (although 660 female adoptees were studied in Gothenburg, none met criteria for alcohol abuse based on Temperance Board registrations). As before, a Type II biological background predicted increased risk for Type II but not Type I alcoholism, while a Type I biological background predicted an increased risk for the severe form of Type I alcoholism only when the adoptee was exposed to relatively high levels of environmental risk. Although the corresponding model predictions for mild Type I alcohol abuse were not confirmed, the Swedish studies, when taken together, do suggest that the two forms of alcoholism are etiologically distinct and differentially influenced by genetic factors.

In principle, twin studies provide a powerful methodology for investigating etiological heterogeneity. Twin studies are well suited for investigating the differential heritability of subtypes, and the etiological distinctiveness of subtypes could be confirmed by showing that there is a strong tendency for MZ twins concordant for alcoholism also to be concordant for alcoholism subtype. Unfortunately, only a few twin studies have attempted to identify factors that moderate the heritability of alcoholism liability, and none of these have attempted to use the Type I/Type II classification to evaluate subtype concordance. Consistent with predictions from the Cloninger model, McGue et al. (1992) reported that the age of alcoholism onset significantly moderated the strength of genetic effects on alcoholism. The estimated heritability of liability was greater for male twins whose first alcohol abuse symptom occurred at or before age 20 years (h^2 = .725 $\pm$ .175), than for males twins whose first alcohol abuse symptom occurred after age 20 (h^2 = .295 $\pm$ .264); a similar moderating effect of age of onset was not observed in the female twin sample. In their large study of male twins, however, Kendler et al. (1997) failed to find significant differences in twin concordance as a function of age at first Temperance Board registration, leaving in doubt the significance of age of onset as a marker of differential genetic involvement.

Investigators have also sought to determine whether the strength of genetic influence is moderated by alcoholism severity. In the Danish Adoption studies, Goodwin, Schulsinger, Hermansen, Guze, and Winokur, (1973) reported that paternal alcoholism was not predictive of either problem or heavy drinking in reared-away sons, even though it was predictive of sons' alcoholism. Several twin studies also suggest that genetic effects may be more pronounced for severe as compared to mild problem drinking. For male twins, Pickens et al. (1991) reported a lower heritability of liability estimate for a DSM-III-R diagnosis of alcohol abuse (h^2 = .379 $\pm$ .160) than for a DSM-III-R diagnosis of Alcohol Dependence (h^2 = .595 $\pm$ .213). In Gottesman and Carey's (1983) reanalysis of Kaij's (1960) data on male twins, heritability of liability decreased as the definition of alcoholism in the proband was broadened to include relatively mild forms of alcohol abuse. In their large sample of male twins, Kendler, Prescott, Neale, and Pedersen, (1997) reported that the difference in MZ and DZ concordance (and, consequently, the magnitude of heritability) increased with increasing number of Temperance Board registrations (an indicator of severity). In contrast to the consistent evidence supporting differential heritability as a function of alcoholism severity in men, in the only investigation large enough to reliably investigate the moderating effect of alcoholism severity in women, Kendler et al. (1992) failed to find that more severe forms of alcoholism were more heritable than less severe forms, suggesting again that the inheritance of alcoholism may differ in men and women.

In summary, while there is some support for the differential heritability of alcoholism in the expected directions (i.e., heritability being greatest for severe and early-onset, as compared to mild and late-onset, alcoholism), the empirical evidence is not altogether consistent and moreover, is based almost exclusively on male samples. In general, the issue of differential heritability of alcoholism subtypes has not received the empirical attention it deserves. This failure is largely a consequence of the large and comprehensively characterized samples that are needed to investigate reliably questions of differential heritability and etiological heterogeneity. Few adoption and twin studies meet that standard. Moreover, a sensitive test of etiological heterogeneity or differential heritability requires that the full range of clinical severity be represented in the sample investigated. As severe alcoholics are likely to be underrepresented in volunteer-based twin samples, it is not altogether surprising that the strongest evidence for differential heritability comes from record linkage studies such as those based on the Swedish Temperance Board registration system (e.g., Cloninger, Bohman, & Sigvardsson, 1981; Kendler et al., 1997), where severe alcoholics are not likely to be missed.

Comorbidity of Alcohol and Other Substance Use and Abuse

Given the substantial overlap that exists between the use and abuse of alcohol and the use and abuse of other substances (e.g., Istvan & Matarazzo, 1984), it is important to identify the mechanisms underlying polysubstance use and abuse. In particular, do these associations reflect the predisposing effect of the use of one substance on the other (e.g., as embodied in the concept of "gateway drugs"), or do these associations reflect a common vulnerability factor (e.g., personality risk)? Unfortunately, only a few behavioral genetic studies have investigated the basis of polysubstance use and abuse, with most of the relevant studies focusing on the substantial association that exists between nicotine and alcohol use (Bien & Burge, 1991). Nonetheless, the studies are consistent in showing that common genetic vulnerability is an important contributor to multiple drug use.

The observation that a family history of alcoholism is associated with nicotine dependence independent of its association with alcohol use disorders (Sher, Gotham, Erickson, & Wood, 1996), implicates a common familial vulnerability to nicotine and alcohol abuse. As smoking is itself highly heritable (Heath & Madden, 1995), the familial association between smoking and alcohol use and abuse might be genetically mediated; a possibility that can be evaluated with behavioral genetic methods (Neale & Kendler, 1996). In an adult male twin sample, Reed et al. (1994) reported that the association between smoking and alcohol use was primarily genetically mediated. In a sample of Dutch twins, Koopmans, VanDoornene, and Boomsma, (1997) found that the relationship between smoking and alcohol use was predominantly genetically mediated during young adulthood (ages 17–25 years), but primarily environmentally mediated during early and midadolescence (ages 12–16 years). Genetic mediation of the association is also supported by animal studies, which further suggest that the common use of tobacco and alcohol may have a pharmacological basis. Mouse strains selected for differential ethanol sensitivity also show differential sensitivity to nicotine (De Fiebre & Collins, 1992), and animal studies find partial cross-tolerance between alcohol and nicotine (Collins, Romm, Selvaag, Turner, & Marks, 1993).

A few twin studies have also investigated the association between the use of alcohol and the use of substances other than tobacco. In a sample of middle-aged male twins, Swan, Carmelli, and Cardon (1996) reported that the associations among alcohol use, coffee use, and smoking could all be accounted for by a single genetic vulnerability factor, a factor hypothesized to mediate psychological and physiological reactions to stress. In a sample of male and female 17-year-old twins, Han, McGue, and Iacono (1999) also found evidence for a single-substance use factor underlying the associations among tobacco, alcohol, and other drug (e.g., marijuana, amphetamines) use, although, unlike the earlier study by Swan et al. (1996), the multiple substance-use associations were mediated by both genetic and environmental factors. Pickens, Svikis, McGue, and LaBuda (1995), in a reared-together twin sample, and Grove et al. (1990), in a reared-apart twin sample, both reported substantial genetic contributions to the comorbidity between alcohol use disorders and substance use disorders (other than nicotine), although in both cases the size of the twin samples was modest. Clearly, the use of behavioral genetic methodologies to explicate the mechanisms underlying multiple substance use and abuse is an important area for future research.

Twin Studies of Other Alcohol-Related Phenotypes

The extensive behavioral genetic literature on the heritability of normal-range drinking behavior has been recently and thoroughly reviewed by Heath (1995); findings from these studies are only highlighted here. Large-scale surveys of community samples of twins (in many cases involving thousands of pairs) undertaken in Australia (Heath & Martin, 1994), Finland (Kaprio, Viken, Koskenvuo, Romonov, & Rose, 1992), Sweden (Medlund, Cederlof, Floderus, Myrhed, Friberg, & Sorensen, 1977), the United Kingdom (Clifford, Fulker, Gurling, & Murray, 1984), and the United States (Carmelli, Heath, & Robinette, 1993) have consistently documented the existence of genetic influences on a range of adult drinking behavior, including drinking frequency, heavy drinking, and typical quantity consumed. Estimates of the heritability for these quantitative phenotypes are generally in the moderate to high range (i.e., .40 to .60). In longitudinal twin studies, the heritability of the *stable* variance of drinking measures is generally quite high, in the .70 to .80 range (Heath, 1995), indicating that genetic factors primarily influence the most durable aspects of drinking, and, conversely, that changes in drinking practices are primarily environmentally mediated.

In a large adult twin sample, Heath, Meyer, Eaves, and Martin (1991a, 1991b) investigated the dimensionality of drinking abstinence, frequency, and quantity, seeking to determine whether alcohol consumption could be scaled on a single continuum ranging from abstinence to heavy drinking. These investigators found evidence for independent etiological factors for each of the three drinking measures, with heritability estimates being essentially 0 for abstinence, but moderate to strong for frequency of drinking and quantity consumed (heritability estimates falling generally in the .4 to .6 range). The heritability of drinking measures may also vary by gender, albeit in an unexpected way, given that twin studies of alcoholism suggest that if there is any gender difference, heritability is lower in women than in men. Large studies of adult twins in Finland (Kaprio, Rose, Romanov, & Koskenvuo, 1991), Sweden (Medlund et al. 1977), and Australia (Jardine & Martin, 1984) all report higher heritabilities for alcohol consumption in women than in men, the magnitude of the heritability difference being about 10%–15%.

The heritability of alcohol-related measures other than the standard quantity–frequency indices has also been investigated. In a study of 206 like-sex twin pairs, Martin et al. (1985) reported heritable effects for both ethanol metabolism (heritability estimates in the .50 to .60 range) and ethanol sensitivity, as measured by body sway following an alcohol challenge (heritability estimates in the .44 to .46 range). In a combined twin and adoption study, Wilson and Laffan (1995) failed to find significant genetic influences on objectively assessed reactions to ethanol, perhaps because their measures of ethanol sensitivity had essentially no temporal stability (Nagoshi & Wilson, 1989). Cognitive factors associated with drinking also appear to be, in part, genetically influenced. Perry (1973) reported an MZ twin ($N = 46$) correlation of .66 and a like-sex DZ twin ($N = 38$) correlation of .31 (suggesting substantial heritable influence) for a 20-item scale measuring attitudes toward drinking (e.g., alcohol is risky, alcohol is pleasurable), while Vernon, Lee, Harris, and Jang (1996) reported heritability estimates that ranged from .28 to .45 for the factor scales from the Alcohol Effects Questionnaire.

The finding of moderate to strong genetic effects on alcohol consumption in predominantly middle-aged twin samples does not necessarily apply to other developmental stages. In particular, one might expect weaker genetic effects during adolescence, when drinking is presumably more contextually driven and subject to both social and familial sanction. Nonetheless, large twin studies have generally reported substantial heritable influences on indices of adolescent drinking. Heath and Martin (1988) reported substantial genetic influences on teenage abstinence assessed retrospectively in a large sample of adult Australian twins. Koopmans and Boomsma (1996) reported that genetic factors accounted for 43% of the variability in alcohol use among twins aged 17 years and older, although familial resemblance for alcohol use among twins aged 15–16 years could be accounted for entirely by environmental factors. Maes et al. (1998) and Han et al. (1998) also reported moderate heritabilities for alcohol use in large adolescent twin samples. Although the strength of genetic influences on alcohol use may be weaker in adolescence as compared to adulthood, twin studies are consistent in indicating that adolescent drinking behavior is, in part, heritable.

Conclusions Regarding Twin and Adoption Studies of Alcohol-Related Phenotypes

Twin and adoption studies are consistent in indicating that genetic factors substantially affect men's risk for alcoholism. Although findings are less consistent in studies with women, the most recent and largest twin studies of alcoholism in women also suggest a substantial influence of genetic factors. Estimates of the heritability of alcoholism liability under a MFT model suggest that approximately 50% of the variance in liability can be attributed to genetic factors, the remainder being ascribed to environmental factors. Although prominent typological models posit the existence of differentially heritable forms of alcoholism, and although there is some empirical support for early-onset alcoholism in males being more heritable than late-onset alcoholism, the genetic heterogeneity of alcoholism is poorly understood.

Most alcohol-related phenotypes, like most behavioral phenotypes (McGue & Bouchard, 1998), are partially heritable. Whether it is basic metabolic processes, ethanol sensitivity, or expectations concerning alcohol's effects, genetic factors appear to contribute to individual differences in drinking behaviors. Nonetheless, the strength of genetic influences may vary developmentally and depend upon the specific aspect of drinking being assessed. Thus, drinking measures may be more heritable in adulthood than in adolescence, and whether an individual drinks or not may be less strongly genetically influenced than the typical amount an individual consumes when drinking. Multivariate genetic analyses of the use and abuse of multiple substances have consistently implicated the existence of a common genetic vulnerability to substance use; the nature of this common vulnerability has not as yet been specified, however.

IDENTIFYING THE GENES THAT INFLUENCE ALCOHOLISM RISK

The consistent finding of heritable effects from twin and adoption studies of alcoholism (at least in men) implies that one or more of the 50,000 to 100,000 genes that comprise the human genome affect drinking behavior. Given the complexity and heterogeneity of the alcoholic phenotype, it is unlikely that the genetic diathesis underlying alcoholism reflects the influence of one or two genes. Rather, like most common medical disorders (e.g., diabetes, high blood pressure, epilepsy), heritable effects on alcoholism are likely to owe to the action of multiple genetic loci (e.g., Todd, 1995).

Gene identification is one of the most exciting areas of behavioral genetic research; it is also one of the most frustrating. Nonetheless, the well-publicized early failures to replicate reports of the identification of behaviorally relevant genes have given way to what appear to be more reliable, albeit less dramatic, results (McGue & Bouchard, 1998). There are three general strategies for gene identification; all have been used with alcoholism. These are association studies, linkage studies, and animal models. These methods all make use of recent developments in molecular genetics.

The standard methods for gene identification involve the use of genetic markers, sequences of DNA that vary from individual to individual and whose chromosomal location is known. Prior to the 1980s, the only available genetic markers were those associated with known gene products (e.g., blood group antigens). But, there can be only limited variation in a gene sequence and still produce a functional protein. Consequently, genes that code for protein are not likely to have the substantial between-individual variation that is needed in a good genetic marker. A major breakthrough in the genetic mapping of complex phenotypes came with the discovery that most of the human genome (about 90%–95%) does not code for functional protein. Because it has not been exposed to the homogenizing influence of natural selection, this noncoding DNA is highly variable and, thus, provides a rich source for genetic markers. One of the first goals of the Human Genome Project was the identification of a set of highly informative DNA markers distributed throughout the 22 autosomes and two sex chromosomes (X and Y) in the human genome (Collins & Fink, 1995). Thus far more than 5,000 genetic markers have been identified (Dib, Faure, & Fizames, 1996), making it feasible to search for genes influencing complex phenotypes such as alcoholism.

Association Studies

An association study involves the use of a case-control design, where the frequency of an allele (an alternative form of the gene or genetic marker) is compared among cases (i.e., those having the disorder of interest) and controls (i.e., those not having the disorder). An association study is one of the oldest methods for gene identification, having been used to show, for example, that the frequency of ulcers (stomach and duodenal) is elevated among individuals having an O blood type (Cavalli-Sforza & Bodmer, 1971), and that the HLA region of chromosome 6 is associated with insulin-dependent diabetes (Neiswanger, Kaplan, & Hill, 1995). Apart from artifact, there are two major mechanisms that might produce a genetic association. First, the allele with the higher frequency among cases may code for a protein that is directly involved in the disorder's pathophysiology (i.e., it is a disease-susceptibility gene). Second, the allele having the higher frequency among cases itself may not be directly involved in the pathophysiology of the disorder, but rather may be located in a chromosomal region that is physically near the location of a disease-susceptibility gene. This second mechanism is especially relevant when a disorder is associated with a noncoding genetic marker, as the marker could not be involved directly in the pathophysiology of the disorder but could, nonetheless, be associated with the disorder because it is located near a disease-susceptibility locus. This second way of producing an association, termed "linkage disequilibrium" by geneticists, occurs only when the physical distance between a genetic marker and the disease-susceptibility locus is very small.

Although the logic of an association study is relatively straightforward, geneticists consider this methodology to be fraught with difficulties (Vogel & Motulsky, 1986). The greatest concern is that failure to match carefully the case and control groups, especially on ethnicity, will result in artifactual genetic associations. Specifically, genetic markers having no direct physiological function are likely to vary substantially in frequency across groups with distinct evolutionary histories (i.e., ethnic groups) because DNA sequences not producing a functional protein will not have been exposed to natural selection. If the disorder being investigated also varies by ethnicity, as alcoholism certainly does (Helzer & Canino, 1992), then failure to match cases and controls carefully on ethnicity could produce artifactual genetic associations. Although effective matching for ethnicity can be achieved using family-based controls (Falk & Rubinstein, 1987), only a few studies in the alcohol research field have used these designs.

The Alcohol Metabolizing Genes

The principal metabolic pathway for ethanol elimination is in the liver, where ethanol is converted to acetaldehyde by the enzyme alcohol dehydrogenase (ADH), and acetaldehyde is in turn converted to acetate by the enzyme aldehyde dehydrogenase (ALDH). Elevated levels of acetaldehyde, due either to the rapid conversion of ethanol to acetaldehyde by ADH or the slow conversion of acetaldehyde to ethanol by ALDH, are associated with an acute toxic reaction to alcohol (e.g., disulfiram achieves its aversive therapeutic effect by inhibiting ALDH activity; Lieber, 1994). Consequently, genes that code for functionally different forms of these enzymes are likely candidates for specific genetic influences on drinking behavior.

Both ADH and ALDH exist in different forms, or isoenzymes. Although there are at least nine distinct ALDH isoenzymes, the mitochondrial form, designated ALDH2, is responsible for most of the acetaldehyde breakdown in the cell. A simple point mutation in the ALDH2 gene (the mutant allele being designated ALDH2-2, and the nonmutant allele being designated ALDH2-1) results in deficient ALDH2 activity. ALDH2 deficiency is inherited in an autosomal dominant fashion (i.e., one copy of the ALDH2-2 allele is sufficient to produce ALDH2 deficiency; Crabb, Edenberg, & Borson, 1987), and has a frequency of approximately 30%–50% in individuals of Japanese and Chinese ancestry, but near zero among Europeans, Africans, and Native North Americans (Agarwal & Goedde, 1989). Significantly, ALDH2 deficiency is protective against alcoholism within East Asian populations, as only 2.3% of Japanese alcoholics but nearly 50% of Japanese nonalcoholics are ALDH deficient (Harada, Agarwal, Goedde, Tagaki, & Ishikawa, 1982). ALDH2 deficiency protects against alcoholism by increasing the likelihood of a flushing reaction following the consumption of even small amounts of alcohol (Higuchi, Parrish, Dufour, Towle, & Harford, 1992; Wall, Thomasson, Schuckit, & Ehlers, 1992). Although there has never been a report of an alcoholic who inherited two copies of the ALDH2-2 allele (i.e., homozygotes), the protective effect of inheriting one copy of the ALDH2-2 allele (i.e., of being a heterozygote) is not complete, as a certain, albeit small, percentage of East Asian alcoholics are heterozygous for ALDH2. Genetic variation in the ADH isoenzymes may help to account for some, although clearly not all, of the variability in drinking behavior among ALDH2 heterozygotes (e.g., Thomasson et al., 1991; Shen et al., 1997). Significantly, cultural factors may also moderate the effects of ALDH2 deficiency. Higuchi et al. (1994) investigated the rate of ALDH2 deficiency among Japanese alcoholics at one of three time points selected to span a period of rapid increase in per capita alcohol consumption in Japan. Although none of the Japanese alcoholics at any time point were found to be homozygous for the ALDH2-2 allele, confirming the completely protective effect of inheriting two copies of the mutant allele, the frequency of alcoholics who were heterozygous increased significantly over the three time points (Figure 10.2). Apparently, the inhibitory effect of ALDH2 deficiency has diminished as the Japanese culture has become more accepting of alcohol consumption.

The Dopamine D_2 Receptor Locus (DRD2)

One of the most controversial and perplexing genetic associations in the field of human behavioral genetics involves that between DRD2 and alcoholism. In 1990, Blum and colleagues reported a surprisingly strong association between a genetic marker for DRD2 (having two alleles designated A1 and A2) and alcoholism: 69% of alcoholics, but only 20% of nonalcoholics, carried at least one copy of the marker A1 allele. This finding attracted much scientific and public attention; the news media hailed the discovery of the "alcoholism gene." Given the potential significance of the association, it was not surprising that alcohol researchers quickly sought to replicate the basic observation. The pattern of results they reported, however, was far from what had been expected. A significantly elevated frequency of the A1 allele among alcoholics was reported in at least five

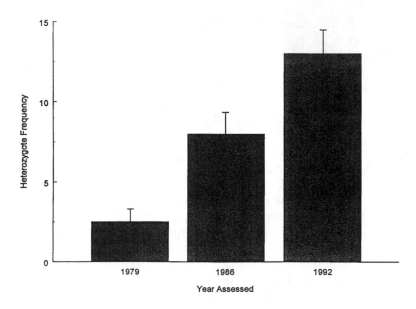

FIGURE 10.2: Rate of ALDH2 deficiency in samples of Japanese alcoholics ascertained at three different time points. ALDH2 deficiency has become less protective as per capita consumption of alcohol has increased in Japan. Data from Higuchi et al. (1994).

independent investigations (Amadeo et al., 1993; Blum et al., 1991; Comings et al., 1991; Neiswanger, Hill, & Kaplan, 1995; Parsian et al., 1991), but an even larger number of studies failed to find evidence for an association (Arinami et al., 1993; Bolos et al., 1990; Cook, Wang, Crowe, Hauser, & Freimer, 1992; Gelernter et al., 1991; Goldman et al., 1992; Schwab et al., 1991; Suarez et al., 1994; Turner et al., 1992). Moreover, even in studies that reported a significant population association between A1 and alcoholism, investigators failed to observe the within-family association (i.e., linkage) that should exist if DRD2 influenced alcoholism risk (Neiswanger et al., 1995; Parsian et al., 1991).

Adding further to the puzzling pattern of results was the observation that, rather than being located within the DRD2 coding region, the A1 marker was located 12 kilobases (thousands of DNA bases) downstream from the DRD2 locus; that is, the non-coding A1 allele has no documented physiological or regulatory function. Nonetheless, because the A1 allele is located very near the DRD2 locus, it could be associated with alcoholism if both (1) DRD2 were a disease-susceptibility locus, and (2) the variant of the DRD2 gene that elevated risk of alcoholism occurred more often with the A1 rather than the A2 allele (i.e., the A1 allele was in linkage disequilibrium with DRD2) Unfortunately, there is little support for either of these propositions. Gejman and colleagues (1994) could not find any functional mutation in the DRD2 gene that was associated with alcoholism, indicating that DRD2 did not appear to be a disease-susceptibility locus; while Suarez and colleagues (1994) concluded that it was unlikely that the A1 site was in linkage disequilibrium with a functional mutation in a gene other than DRD2 in the region that affected risk of alcoholism. In short, the DRD2 association lacks both a consistent pattern of positive findings and a physiological mechanism that might implicate this marker in alcoholism etiology. The research literature relating alcoholism with another dopaminergic polymorphism (the D4 dopamine receptor), although more limited in size, has also produced an inconsistent set of findings (Geijer, et al., 1997; George, Cheng, Nguyen, Israel, & O'Dowd, 1993; Muramatsu, Higuchi, Murayama, Matsushita, & Hayashida, 1996).

Although various explanations for the DRD2 findings have been offered, none appears to have unequivocal support at this time. Positive findings of an association could be the result of poor ethnic matching of cases and controls. The frequency of the A1 allele at DRD2 varies more than eightfold by ethnicity, being relatively low among certain Middle Eastern populations, intermediate among Europeans, and relatively high among certain North American Indian populations (Barr & Kidd, 1993; Goldman et al., 1993). Although the frequency of alcoholism also varies with ethnicity (Helzer & Canino, 1992), it is not clear that these differences parallel ethnic differences in A1 frequency, nor has anyone shown that differential ethnic composition can account for any of the positive DRD2 association findings that have been reported.

Alternatively, it has been noted that most of the positive association studies have involved severe alcoholics and control groups that had been vetted for alcoholism, while most of the negative studies have involved moderate alcoholics and control groups that were unselected for alcoholism (Conneally, 1991). In a meta-analysis of studies of DRD2 associations with alcoholism, Hill and Neiswanger (1997) report that the aggregated frequency of the A1 allele is .24 among 453 alcoholics, .20 among 192 control individuals not screened for alcoholism, and .12 among 213 control individuals screened for alcoholism. Although the frequency of A1 did not differ significantly between alcoholics and unscreened controls it did differ significantly between the alcoholics and the screened controls. Significantly, the distinctive observation was the relatively low frequency of A1 in screened controls, rather than a relatively high frequency of A1 among alcoholics. Given that controls screened for alcoholism were likely also to have been screened for other forms of psychopathology, it may be that rather than the A1 allele being a specific marker for alcoholism risk, the alternative (A2) allele may be a general marker for mental health (Hill & Neiswanger, 1997).

The failure to observe replicable and coherent genetic associations with alcoholism, as well as with other psychiatric disorders, has prompted a critical reassessment of this methodology (Licinio, 1997; Owen, Holmans, & McGuffin, 1997). The need for careful ethnic matching of cases and controls has led some to recommend that only family-based controls be used (Baron, 1997; Berrettini, 1997; Paterson, 1997); none of the positive associations of DRD2 with alcoholism meets this rigorous standard. Another limitation of association studies is that they have a low prior probability of success. As an estimated one-third of the genes in the human genome are expressed in the brain, there may be as many as 10,000–20,000 genes relevant to behavioral disorders and characteristics (Gelernter, 1997). Without some compelling reason for targeting a specific gene system, an unreplicated finding of genetic association is much more likely to be a false positive than a true positive result (Carey, 1994). Concerns over the applicability of association studies with complex phenotypes have led researchers to the use of linkage methods for gene identification.

Linkage Analysis

Two genes that are located near each other on the same chromosome (i.e., are physically linked) will tend to be transmitted together from parents to offspring, while genes located on different chromosomes will be transmitted independently. Linkage analysis is a formal statistical procedure for identifying within-family associations between a genetic marker and a disorder, the finding of which implies the existence of a disease-susceptibility locus located near the marker site. As the tendency for cotransmission is proportional to the distance separating the marker locus and the disease-susceptibility locus, linkage analysis allows researchers to localize disease-susceptibility loci within relatively narrow regions of the human genome, the first step in a process (known as positional cloning) that leads ultimately to the identification and characterization of the disease-susceptibility gene.

A major advantage of a linkage study over an association study is that, while the latter requires a candidate gene that has been motivated by previous research, the former requires no knowledge of the mechanism of genetic influence. With the large number of highly informative genetic markers identified in the early stages of the Human Genome Project, researchers have been able to search for disease-susceptibility loci systematically, using a genome-wide search involving from 300 to 500 genetic markers selected to span most of the human genome. Genome-wide linkage studies have become a standard method for gene identification with complex phenotypes, such as alcoholism, which are etiologically heterogeneous, multigenic, and modulated by environmental factors. Genome-wide searches with schizophrenia (e.g., Moises et al., 1995) and bipolar disorder (e.g., Ginns et al., 1996) have been successful in identifying regions of the human genome that are likely to contain disease-susceptibility loci for these disorders.

It is not altogether surprising that the few linkage studies of alcoholism that have targeted specific chromosomal regions have failed to produce reliable evidence of linkage (Merikangas, 1990). In 1989 the National Institute on Alcohol Abuse and Alcoholism initiated a large-scale research effort to identify the genes influencing alcoholism risk. The Collaborative Study on the Genetics of Alcoholism (COGA) is a multicenter, large, family-based study that uses a genome-wide screening strategy to identify regions of the genome that are likely to contain genes influencing alcoholism risk (Begleiter et al., 1995). The study was designed to ensure that genes having a moderate effect on alcoholism vulnerability would have a reasonable likelihood of being identified. In the first major genetic analysis to emerge from the COGA project, linkage findings from the analysis of 291 genetic markers, in 987 individuals from 105 families, each of which had at least three alcoholic, first-degree relatives were reported (Reich et al., 1998). Although none of the genetic markers met the rigorous criteria proposed by Lander and Kruglyak (1995) for significant linkage in a genome-wide survey, several chromosomal regions showed suggestive linkage with alcoholism. The strongest evidence for regions containing disease-susceptibility loci was found on chromosomes 1 and 7. In addition, a third region, which was associated with a protective effect on alcoholism risk, was provisionally identified on chromosome 4. Interestingly, the ADH locus is included in this latter region.

In the same journal issue in which the initial linkage findings from COGA were published, results from a second genome-wide linkage analysis were reported (Long et al., 1998). This second study involved 172 sibpairs, from a Southwestern American Indian tribe, that had been typed for 517 genetic markers. Because members of this geographically restricted tribe are genetically and environmentally more homogeneous than a general population sample, the sample used in this study was especially well suited for genetic analysis. Suggestive evidence for linkage was reported for chromosomes 4 and 11, with the regions implicated on the former partially overlapping the region identified on chromosome 4 in COGA.

Although neither of the two linkage studies provided unequivocal support for the existence of an alcoholism-susceptibility locus within a specific chromosomal region, and although the regions implicated in the two studies did not entirely overlap, the two studies represent an important first step in the attempt to identify genes contributing to alcoholism vulnerability. Given that alcoholism risk is likely to be affected by multiple genes, different linkage studies are likely to implicate different genetic regions, especially when, as was the case with the linkage studies on alcoholism, the samples used in the multiple studies differ in ethnic composition. The COGA and the American Indian studies have identified genetic regions that can be targeted in future attempts to produce replicable linkage findings for alcoholism. Moreover, the breadth of the COGA assessment (e.g., psychophysiological markers, neuropsychological factors) will allow researchers in that study to increase the power of their study by refining the phenotype (e.g., through subtyping or investigating multivariate phenotypes) used in the linkage analysis.

Animal Models

There is no better demonstration of the existence of genetic influences on individual differences in alcohol-related outcomes than that coming from animal studies, where exact control over breeding patterns and rearing circumstances provides a powerful test for the existence of heritable effects on behavioral phenotypes. Although animal models may not be able to represent accurately all the cognitive and motivational aspects of human drinking, the basic biochemical, physiological, and pharmacological actions of ethanol are likely to be similar across species. It is consequently significant that inbred strain comparisons and selection studies have consistently found that genetic factors influence a wide range of alcohol-related phenotypes, including preference, metabolism, sensitivity, tolerance, and withdrawal sensitivity (Buck, 1995; Crabbe, Belknap, & Buck, 1994).

Ultimately, the greatest benefit of animal models is likely to be in helping to identify and characterize, rather than in merely implying the existence of, specific genes influencing individual differences in behavior. The mouse is an especially well-suited system for research aimed at identifying the multiple genes that underlie quantitative variation in alcohol-related phenotypes (called quantitative trait loci, or QTL, because only a small portion of the overall variation in a quantitative trait is associated with any given genetic locus). Well-characterized mouse models for alcohol sensitivity, preference, and withdrawal severity exist; the mouse genome has been extensively mapped (Silver, 1995). Powerful methods are available for the detection of QTL in mice (Buck, 1995), and, owing to our common evolution, many of the genes expressed in mice are also expressed in humans. QTL identified in mice thus provide strong candidates for linkage or association studies in humans.

Over the past few years, animal researchers have made impressive progress in identifying QTLs for alcohol-related phenotypes in the mouse. Provisional QTL have been identified for alcohol acceptance (Rodriguez et al.,1995), preference (Melo, Shendure, Posciask, & Silver, 1996; Phillips, Crabbe, Metten, & Belknap, 1994; Rodriguez et al.,1995), sensitivity (Cunningham, 1995; Gallaher, Jones, Belknap, & Crabbe, 1996; Rodriguez et al., 1995), tolerance (Phillips, Lessov, Harland, & Mitchell, 1996), and withdrawal severity (Buck, Metten, Belknap, & Crabbe, 1997), with the identified QTL accounting for anywhere from one-fourth to over one-half of the heritable variation in the phenotype studied. Consistent with studies suggesting common genetic etiology, there is partial overlap of the QTL identified across the multiple alcohol phenotypes, as well as partial overlap of loci identified for alcohol phenotypes and those associated with the action of other drugs. Although it seems likely that some of these provisional QTL will not be ultimately confirmed through repeated replication (cf. Belknap, Mitchell, O'Toole, Helms, & Crabbe, 1996), the QTL that have been identified should provide useful targets for human genetic research. Many of the QTL regions that have been identified have homologues in the human genome and contain candidate genes with known neurological expression.

An especially exciting recent trend is the development of methodologies that allow for the manipulation of gene expression in mice. Transgenics refer to mice that have been created through the transfer of foreign DNA in order to over- or underexpress a specific gene product. Knockouts refer to mice in which a specific gene has been completely inactivated. To date, there have been only a limited number of applications of these recently developed methodologies in the alcohol field. For example, mice lacking the gene coding for the serotonin 1B receptor show substantially higher alcohol preference than nonmutant mice (Crabbe et al., 1996), while knocking out the D_4 receptor gene results in increased sensitivity to the activating effects of alcohol, methamphetamine, and cocaine (Rubinstein et al., 1997). It seems likely that these methodologies will see increasing use as alcohol researchers seek to characterize the contribution of individual genes to the heritable variation in alcohol-related phenotypes.

Summary on Gene Identification Efforts

Progress in identifying the genes influencing alcoholism risk is at a stage similar to that in identifying the genes influencing risk for most complex behavioral disorders; that is, despite consistent evidence from twin and adoption studies of the existence of genetic influences, we know precious little about the specific genes that contribute to alcoholism vulnerability. Although this current state of affairs may be disappointing, there is reason to be optimistic. Progress in mapping the human genome has produced a set of powerful methodologies for gene identification with complex phenotypes; there is every reason to believe that the future will see the development of even more powerful methodologies. Moreover, the existence of well-characterized animal models should help in both identifying regions of the human genome to target in searching for alcoholism vulnerability loci, and providing an experimental system for exploring the nature of the effects of identified genes. The next decade should see substantial progress in identifying the genes underlying alcoholism risk.

Although progress in identifying genes that influence individual differences in behavior has generally been slow, there is one gene system that has been unequivocally linked with behavior. A mutation that produces an inactive form of the mitochondrial form of ALDH has been repeatedly shown to protect against the expression of alcoholism. Nonetheless, this protective genetic effect can apparently be overcome by cultural factors. The ALDH association provides a useful model for how genes are likely to influence alcohol-related outcomes. That is, rather than determining alcoholism status, the genes underlying alcoholism risk likely exert their influence by biasing the individual toward or away from problem drinking.

FACTORS THAT MEDIATE HERITABLE INFLUENCES ON ALCOHOLISM

Findings from twin and adoption studies have told us whether, but not necessarily why, alcoholism is heritable. While there may be genes whose effect on alcoholism risk is relatively direct (the alcohol-metabolizing genes being a good example), in all likelihood, genetic influences on alcoholism risk are indirect, mediated by the multiple physiological, pharmacological, and psychological processes that intervene between primary gene product and observed behavior (Figure 10.3). Although genetic findings may be viewed by some as being antagonistic to psychological theories of alcoholism, any viable genetic model of alcoholism must be compatible with what we know about its psychological and social determinants. Indeed, given that virtually all psychological (and, for that matter, nearly all social) characteristics are in part heritable (McGue & Bouchard, 1998), it seems probable that psychological and social factors represent proximal steps in the gene to behavior pathway.

Two strategies for characterizing the gene to behavior pathway have been described (Stent, 1981). The first, and best-known approach, is a bottom-up strategy that begins at the level of the gene and works up through intermediate systems to the behavioral level. Gene identification represents the first step in this effort. The second is a top-down strategy that begins at

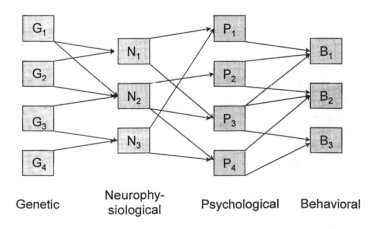

FIGURE 10.3. Gene to behavior pathway is mediated by multiple intervening physiological, pharmacological, and psychological processes.

the behavioral level and attempts to work down through the intermediate systems. The focus of this second approach is to simplify the genetics of a complex and heterogeneous phenotype by identifying etiologically distinct pathways of genetic vulnerability. The two strategies are complementary; the identification of etiologically distinct subtypes of alcoholism will increase the power of gene identification efforts, while identifying the specific genes underlying alcoholism risk will certainly lead to classification systems based on etiology rather than phenomenology.

Those pursuing the top-down approach do so by trying to identify mediators of alcoholism inheritance; that is, the factors that account, at least in part, for heritable effects on alcoholism risk (cf. Baron & Kenny, 1986). An inherited mediator should (1) be associated concurrently and prospectively with alcoholism risk, (2) be heritable, (3) cosegregate within families with alcoholism, and (4) have its familial association with alcoholism owe to common genetic, and not common environmental, effects. Although no single factor meets all of these criteria at this time (primarily, because the fourth has not been systematically evaluated), several risk factors have been implicated as mediating heritable effects on alcoholism risk. These include alcohol sensitivity, personality, psychophysiological markers, and psychopathology. As these factors are the focus of other chapters in this volume, our discussion of each will be brief.

Alcohol Sensitivity

There is wide variation in how individuals respond to alcohol; for some, alcohol is pleasurable and stimulating, while for others, it is nauseating and discomforting. Both selection studies in mice (McClearn & Kakihana, 1981), and twin studies in humans (Martin et al., 1985) indicate that genetic factors influence individual differences in alcohol sensitivity, suggesting that alcohol sensitivity may be an important mediator of alcoholism inheritance. Research with the alcohol-metabolizing genes demonstrate that hypersensitivity to the negative effects of alcohol is an important inherited, protective factor against the manifestation of alcoholism; research on the offspring of alcoholics further suggests that inherited differences in sensitivity to the rewarding effects of alcohol may be important risk factors for alcoholism expression.

Schuckit (1994) hypothesized that reduced sensitivity to alcohol's effects can lead to chronic overconsumption of alcohol, as failure to fully experience alcohol's effects could result in the absence of the feedback mechanisms that normally inhibit continued drinking. In a program of research that has extended over 20 years, Schuckit and his colleagues have reported that, compared to the sons of nonalcoholics, young adult male offspring of alcoholics report a reduced subjective sense of intoxication after a standard dose of alcohol (Schuckit & Gold, 1988). This finding has been consistently replicated in other studies, although expected family-history effects have not always been observed when alcohol sensitivity is assessed objectively (e.g., body sway, hormonal response) rather than subjectively (Sher, 1991). In any case, Schuckit and Smith (1996) recently reported results from an 8-year follow-up of 450 male participants in their original alcohol-challenge studies. Consistent with the mediation hypothesis, reduced alcohol sensitivity at intake was significantly associated with alcoholism risk at follow-up and accounted for much of the family-history effect on alcoholism risk they observed in their study.

Several research groups have also reported findings indicating that a family history of alcoholism is associated with a heightened sensitivity to both the negatively and positively reinforcing effects of alcohol. Finn and his colleagues (Finn & Pihl, 1987, 1988; Finn, Zeitouni, & Pihl, 1990) reported that alcohol was more likely to diminish the cardiovascular response to unavoidable shock in sons of alcoholics as compared to sons of nonalcoholics. Levenson, Oyama, and Meek (1987) reported similar findings of increased sensitivity to alcohol's negative reinforcing properties when comparing daughters of alcoholics and nonalcoholics. Sons of alcoholics appear also to have an increased sensitivity to the positively reinforcing, or activating, effects of alcohol. As compared to the sons of nonalcoholics, the sons of alcoholics show greater levels of beta-endorphin (Gianoulakis, Krishnan, & Thavundayil, 1996), and greater induction of alpha-wave electroencephalography (Cohen, Porjesz, & Begeiter, 1993) following drinking.

The finding by Finn and colleagues that sons of alcoholics have heightened sensitivity to alcohol's effects is not necessarily incompatible with Schuckit and colleagues' finding that the sons of alcoholics show reduced sensitivity to alcohol. The paradigms used by the two research groups are fundamentally different; Finn and colleagues have investigated how alcohol modulates the stress reaction whereas Schuckit and colleagues have studied reactions to alcohol in a nonstressful situation. Moreover, differences between the sons of alcoholics and the sons of nonalcoholics may depend upon when sensitivity is assessed following alcohol ingestion. Newlin and Thomson (1990) have summarized empirical evidence suggesting that sons of alcoholics show hypersensitivity to alcohol's effects during the rising limb of the blood alcohol concentration (BAC) curve, when the pleasurable and activating consequences of drinking dominate, but hyposensitivity to alcohol's effects during the falling limb of the BAC curve, when the negative and depressing effects dominate.

Personality Factors

Although the notion that there are personality characteristics that uniquely characterize the alcoholic has been soundly refuted (e.g., Nathan, 1988), there is growing evidence that personality factors may play an important role in the etiology of at least some forms of alcoholism (e.g., Cloninger,

1987; Tarter, Moss, & Vanyukov, 1995). On average, personality factors differentiate alcoholics from nonalcoholics, both contemporaneously and prospectively, and distinguish the offspring of alcoholics from the offspring of non-alcoholics (Sher, 1991). These findings, along with substantial evidence for the heritability of individual differences in personality (Bouchard, 1994; Loehlin, 1992), suggests that personality may be an important mediator of genetic effects on alcoholism risk.

Two dimensions of personality seem especially relevant to alcoholism risk. The first and most consistently supported dimension is behavioral disinhibition, the inability or unwillingness to inhibit behavioral impulses. On average, alcoholics are more impulsive, more likely to take risks, and more rebellious than nonalcoholics (Graham & Strenger, 1988; McGue, Slutske, Taylor, & Iacono, 1997; Sher & Trull, 1994). Differences in behavioral disinhibition between (future) alcoholics and nonalcoholics exist prior to alcoholism onset (Loper, Kammeier, & Hoffman, 1973; Cloninger, Sigvardsson, Reich, & Bohman, 1988) and, indeed, have been observed as early as age 3 years (Caspi, Moffit, Newman, & Silva, 1996). The finding that behavioral disinhibition differentiates the children of alcoholics from the children of nonalcoholics (Sher, 1991) further indicates that deviations along this dimension of personality are being transmitted within the families of alcoholics. The second personality dimension that has been associated with alcoholism is negative emotionality, the tendency to experience negative mood states and psychological distress. On average, alcoholics rate themselves as being more emotional, neurotic, and aggressive than nonalcoholics (McGue et al., 1997). Nonetheless, negative emotionality has not been consistently associated with either alcoholism risk in prospective studies (e.g., Sieber, 1981) or a family history of alcoholism in studies on the children of alcoholics (Sher, 1991). Relatively high levels of negative emotionality may more likely be a consequence than a cause of alcoholism (cf. Sher, Trull, Bartholow, & Vieth, Chapter 3, this volume).

In their large sample of adult Australian twins, Heath, Bucholz, et al. (1997) investigated whether heritable variation in personality (assessed using scales from the Eysenck Personality Questionnaire and the Tridimensional Personality Questionnaire) could account for genetic influences on alcoholism risk. Modest but statistically significant associations of alcoholism risk with personality scales measuring extraversion, neuroticism, novelty seeking, and social nonconformity were observed. Although twin concordance for alcoholism was reduced after adjustment for these personality factors, sociodemographic factors, and psychopathology, the residual MZ twin concordance remained significantly larger than DZ twin concordance in the male sample, and larger, albeit not significantly larger, than the DZ twin concordance in the female sample. Heritable variation in personality thus appears to have accounted for some, but not all, of the genetic influence on alcoholism risk. Unfortunately, these researchers did not attempt to quantify the degree to which heritable effects on alcoholism were mediated by the personality factors they assessed, nor did their multivariate genetic analyses resolve the causal basis for the personality and alcoholism risk association. A rigorous evaluation of the extent to which personality factors mediate heritable variation in alcoholism-risk remains to be completed.

Comorbidity with Other Mental Disorders

Although comorbidity appears to characterize most behavioral disorders, none appears to co-occur as extensively and as consistently with other behavioral disorders as alcoholism (Helzer & Pryzbeck, 1988). In the National Comorbidity Survey (Kessler et al., 1996), 55.2% of individuals with alcohol dependence also met lifetime diagnostic criteria for either a mood disorder, an anxiety disorder, conduct disorder, or adult antisocial behavior. When disorder onsets were sequenced from retrospective reports in this study, the onset of the comorbid mental disorder preceded the onset of alcoholism in 85.8% of the comorbid cases. Family studies consistently report that the children of alcoholics are at increased risk for a variety of mental disorders (Hill & Hruska, 1992; Reich, Earls, & Powell, 1988), and there is extensive evidence for substantial heritable effects on risk of suffering a mental disorder (McGue & Bouchard, 1998). Nonetheless, there remains much uncertainty regarding the causal mechanisms underlying the co-occurrence of alcoholism with other behavioral disorders. Familial associations between alcoholism and the mood disorders (e.g., Maier, Lichtermann, & Mingas, 1994), anxiety disorders (e.g., Schuckit et al., 1995), and antisocial personality disorder (e.g., Lewis, Robins, & Rice, 1985) have been inconsistently observed, perhaps because there is only a weak common familial etiology between these disorders (e.g., Maier & Merikangas, 1996). In a multivariate analysis of six psychiatric disorders in a large sample of adult female twins, Kendler et al. (1995) reported only modest genetic overlap between alcoholism and anxiety disorders, major depression, and bulimia. Prospective behavioral genetic designs will be needed to determine whether psychopathology is a major mediator of genetic effects on alcoholism.

Psychophysiological Markers of Risk

Two psychophysiological markers have been most consistently associated with alcoholism risk: P3 amplitude and the electroencephalogram (EEG). The amplitude of the P3 event-related potential (ERP), a late positive deflection in the ERP waveform that is thought to reflect allocation of attentional resources during memory update (Polich, Pollock, & Bloom, 1994), has been the most extensively investigated psychophysiological marker of alcoholism risk. P3 amplitude evoked visually is lower on average among abstinent alcoholics as compared to nonalcoholics (Porjesz &

Begleiter, 1996), with the reduction in amplitude being more strongly associated with alcoholics' familial loading for alcoholism than their drinking history (Pfefferbaum, Ford, White, & Mathalon 1991), suggesting that it is a marker of familial risk rather than a consequence of alcohol toxicity. Begleiter, Porjesz, Bihari, and Kissin (1984) were the first to report that reduced P3 amplitude also characterized the preadolescent sons of alcoholics, a finding that has been extensively replicated in other studies of sons of alcoholics (Polich et al., 1994) but has not always been observed in studies of the daughters of alcoholics (Steinhauer & Hill, 1993). Individual differences in P3 amplitude are substantially heritable (O'Connor, Morzorati, Chistian, & Li, 1994; Katsanis, Iacone, McGue, & Carlson, 1997), and longitudinal studies reveal that reduced P3 amplitude predicts early-onset alcohol and drug abuse (Berman, Whipple, Fitch, & Noble, 1993; Hill, Steinhauer, Lowers, & Locke, 1995).

Although research on P3 amplitude suggests that it may well be a marker of genetic vulnerability for alcoholism, there have been only limited attempts to provide a theoretical explanation for why P3 might be implicated in the etiology of alcoholism. Porjesz and Begleiter (1997) have interpreted a relatively low P3 amplitude as reflecting a diminished neurophysiological ability to discriminate significant from nonsignificant stimuli. They go on to speculate that this relative inability to discriminate differentially probable stimuli owes to a failure to inhibit nerve cell response to familiar stimuli (cf. Miller, Li, & Desimone, 1991). Thus, P3 amplitude might reflect an aspect of neurophysiological disinhibition that underlies the behavioral disinhibition that is associated with alcoholism risk. Alternatively, as P3 amplitude changes developmentally (e.g., Katsanis, Iacone, & McGue, 1996) and is more strongly associated with a family history of alcoholism among males aged 17 years and younger than among males aged 18 years and older (Polich et al., 1994), the association of P3 amplitude with alcoholism risk may reflect aspects of neurological development that are related in some unknown way with alcoholism risk. In either case, there is a clear need to articulate and test theoretical models that attempt to account for the association of P3 amplitude with alcoholism risk.

The second neurophysiological marker associated with alcoholism risk is the EEG. Although increased activity in the delta, theta, and beta ranges, and decreased activity in the alpha range distinguish abstinent alcoholics from controls (Begleiter & Platz, 1972), baseline EEG activity has not been consistently associated with a family history of alcoholism (Cohen, Porjesz, & Begleiter, 1991), leaving uncertain its relevance as a marker of familial vulnerability. Findings from studies relating a family history of alcoholism to EEG changes following alcohol ingestion are only somewhat more consistent. Thus, although Pollock et al. (1983) and Cohen et al. (1993) both reported that individuals with a family history of alcoholism showed greater induction of slow alpha activity following an alcohol challenge than individuals not having a family history of alcoholism, both Kaplan,

Hesselbrock, O'Connor, and DePalma, (1988) and Ehlers and Schuckit (1991) failed to observe a family history of alcoholism effect on EEG changes following alcohol consumption. Moreover, contrary to expectations, Volavka et al. (1996) reported that a *diminished* EEG response following alcohol administration at age 19 was associated alcoholism risk 10 years later in a sample of 64 Danish men. Given findings such as these, it is difficult to judge the relevance of baseline EEG and EEG changes following alcohol administration to alcoholism risks.

Summary on Mediators of Genetic Effects on Alcoholism

Genetic influences on alcoholism risk are mediated by the multiple processes and systems that intervene between primary gene product and observable behavior. Psychological models of alcoholism are not precluded by research documenting its heritability. Rather, the heritability of alcoholism vulnerability establishes the existence of a distal cause, the proximal manifestation of which may be psychological processes. Because they have been shown to be heritable and predictive of alcoholism risk, contemporaneously, prospectively, and within families; several psychological factors, including alcohol sensitivity, personality, psychopathology, and psychophysiological markers, constitute probable mediators of inherited influences on alcoholism vulnerability. Each of these factors may mark a distinct etiological pathway to alcoholism and thus help to resolve the heterogeneity of this disorder. The prospective behavioral genetic research needed to explicate the mechanisms underlying each factor's association with alcoholism remains to be undertaken.

THE NATURE OF ENVIRONMENTAL INFLUENCE: A BEHAVIORAL GENETIC PERSPECTIVE

Shared versus Nonshared Environmental Effects

The dominant theoretical and empirical traditions in developmental psychology have tended to emphasize environmental influences that would produce similarities rather than differences among reared-together relatives. Authoritarian parenting style has been hypothesized to contribute to offspring dysfunction, the rearing environment provided by intellectually gifted parents has been claimed to lead to offspring intellectual achievement, and spousal conflict has been thought to provide a model for offspring aggression. Nonetheless, behavioral genetic research is consistent in indicating that, for many psychological characteristics, the major environmental influences are of the unshared rather than the shared variety (Plomin & Daniels, 1987). Twins who were reared in separate homes are not substantially less similar psychologically than twins who were reared together, especially in adulthood (Bouchard, Lykken, McGue, Segal, &

Tellegen, 1990), and family members related only by adoption show little psychological similarity (McGue, Sharma, & Benson, 1996a).

This pattern of greater nonshared than shared environmental influence holds generally, although not completely, for many alcohol-related outcomes. In the Swedish adoption studies (Bohman et al., 1981; Cloninger et al., 1981), the adoptive offspring of alcoholic parents (as determined by Temperance Board registration) were not significantly more likely to be alcoholic than the adoptive offspring of nonalcoholics (13.% vs. 18.0%, respectively, in males, and 3.7% vs. 3.4%, respectively, in females). Similar findings have been reported in the Danish adoption studies. Among offspring of alcoholic biological fathers, the rate of alcoholism was not greater for offspring who had been reared with their alcoholic fathers than among their adopted-away siblings (16.7% vs. 20.0%, respectively, in males [Goodwin et al., 1974], and 2.5% vs. 2.0%, respectively, in females [Goodwin, Schulsinger, Knop, Metnick, & Guze et al., 1997b]).

The adoption studies undertaken in Iowa by Cadoret and colleagues (1985, Cadoret, Troughton, & O'Gorman, 1987), suggest, however, that being reared with alcoholics can be an important shared environmental influence on alcoholism risk. In the 1985 study, rate of alcoholism was significantly higher for those reared in families having other alcoholic members than for those reared in families having no other alcoholic members (17.4% vs. 6.3%, respectively, in female adoptees, and 48.0% vs. 24.5%, respectively, in male adoptees). This finding was independently replicated in a second adoption study in which a higher rate of alcoholism was observed among male adoptees reared with at least one alcoholic as compared to male adoptees reared with nonalcoholics (38.5% vs. 19.4%, respectively; Cadoret et al., 1987). The discrepancy in findings between the Scandinavian and U.S. adoption studies may reflect differences in how a positive adoptive family history of alcoholism was defined. In the former, only adoptive parental alcoholism was considered, whereas in the latter, both sibling and parental alcoholism was considered. It may be that, while parental alcoholism has minimal environmental effect on offspring risk of alcoholism, sibling alcoholism is an important contributor.

A recent adoption study of adolescent alcohol use and abuse provides further support for the proposition that siblings, rather than parents, constitute a major source of familial environmental influence (McGue, Sharma, & Benson, 1996b). Parental problem drinking was significantly correlated with biological but not adoptive offspring alcohol involvement, confirming that genetic factors, but not rearing parents' problem drinking, contribute to individual differences in adolescent alcohol use and abuse. In contrast to the absence of a rearing-parent effect, nonbiologically related adoptive siblings were significantly alike in their degree of involvement with alcohol, especially if the siblings were of the same sex and close in age.

Apart from sibling factors, behavioral genetic research has failed to identify other specific shared environmental factors that have a major influence on alcohol-related outcomes. Surprisingly, the relationship between family atmosphere (e.g., cohesiveness) and adolescent alcohol use and abuse appears to be primarily genetically, not environmentally, mediated (McGue et al., 1996b). Modest, shared environmental influences on adult alcoholism have been found for rearing social class in adoption studies (Bohman et al., 1981; Cloninger et al., 1981), and for marital dissolution in twin studies of women (Kendler et al., 1996). The failure to find evidence of specific, shared environmental effects may reflect the overall minimal impact of these factors on alcohol-related outcomes. In biometrical analysis of twin similarity, the influence of shared environmental factors appears to be near-zero for adult alcoholism (e.g., Heath, Bucholz, et al., 1997; Kendler et al., 1992, 1997), although substantial for alcohol use and abuse in adolescence (e.g. Koopmans & Boomsma, 1996). Apparently, the strength of shared environmental influences on alcohol-related phenotypes, as with other psychological characteristics (McGue & Bouchard, 1998), dissipated once an individual has left his or her rearing home.

By default, nonshared environmental factors must exert a substantial influence on alcoholism risk; they are the only factors that can account for an MZ twin discordance rate that is approximately 50% in men and 70% in women (Table 10.2). Nonetheless, we know virtually nothing about the nature of the specific environmental factors that influence alcoholism risk in particular, and psychological traits in general. Prenatal factors are likely to be important (Bohman et al., 1981; Cloninger et al., 1981), as is a history of abuse, at least in women (Stewart, 1996). It may be that nonshared environmental factors defy easy identification because they are largely unique, idiosyncratic, and of small effect. Nonetheless, there is a clear need for systematic efforts aimed at characterizing the nature of this important contributor to alcoholism risk.

Joint Models for the Influence of Genetic and Environmental Factors

The polarization inherent to the nature–nurture debate perpetuated the erroneous view that genetic and environmental factors represent opposing forces. There is a growing recognition among both biologically and psychosocially oriented researchers that both genetic and environmental factors affect alcoholism risk, even though little is currently known about how these two sets of factors jointly influence behavioral outcomes. Developmental conceptualizations hold great promise for integrating genetic and environmental influences into a comprehensive model of alcoholism etiology. The roots of alcoholism first appear to manifest prior to alcohol exposure (Caspi et al., 1996) and progress from early experimentation to regular drinking, to abusive drinking through a series of transactions between individual-level risk factors and developmental experience (Tarter et al., 1995). Both genotype–environment interaction and correlation processes are likely to be featured prominently in integrative developmental models of alcoholism etiology.

Genotype–environment interaction refers to differential sensitivity of genotypes to environmental influence, which can be documented by showing that the strength of genetic influence (i.e., heritability) varies across environmental circumstances. Thus, for example, in a sample of adult female twins, Heath, Jardine, and Martin (1989) reported that the heritability of amount of alcohol consumed over a 7-day period depended on the respondent's marital status. For married women aged 18-30 years, genetic factors accounted for 31% of variance in amount of alcohol consumed, while for nonmarried women of the same age, the heritability of alcohol consumption was 60%. A similar difference in heritability was found for older women. The difference in heritability presumably reflected the modulating effect of partners' drinking; that is, the strength of genetic influences on alcohol consumption was relatively weak among married women whose drinking behavior was constrained by their partners' drinking practices, but relatively strong among unmarried women who were not exposed to the modulating effect of partners' drinking. The existence of genotype–environment interactions serves to emphasize that genetic effects, rather than being fixed, can be conditioned by environmental circumstance.

The strongest support for genotype–environment interaction effects on alcoholism comes from the Swedish adoption studies (Sigvardsson et al., 1996). Male adoptees' genetic and environmental backgrounds were classified as high or low risk for Type I alcoholism, the more weakly heritable form of alcoholism (no interaction was expected for Type II alcoholism, which is strongly genetically influenced). The classification was derived empirically for adoptees placed in Stockholm and applied independently to adoptees placed in Gothenburg. In both the original Stockholm sample and the replication Gothenburg sample, a significantly elevated rate of severe Type I alcoholism (i.e., multiple Temperance Board registrations or alcoholism treatment) was observed only among adoptees who were both at a relatively high genetic and a relatively high environmental risk for developing Type I alcoholism (Figure 10.4); that is, rearing circumstances were predictive of alcoholism outcome, but only among those adoptees who were genetically vulnerable.

Although the consistency of findings for severe Type I alcoholism across the two samples is impressive, the interaction effect on mild Type I alcohol abuse (one Temperance Board registration and no alcoholism treatment) that was originally observed in the Stockholm sample failed to replicate in the Gothenburg sample. Moreover, other adoption studies of alcoholism have also produced inconsistent findings about the importance of genotype–environment interactions (e.g., Cadoret et al., 1985; Cutrona et al., 1994). Indeed, the research record for detecting and replicating genotype–environment interaction effects on behavioral characteristics is so meager that a group of prominent behavioral geneticists concluded, "The

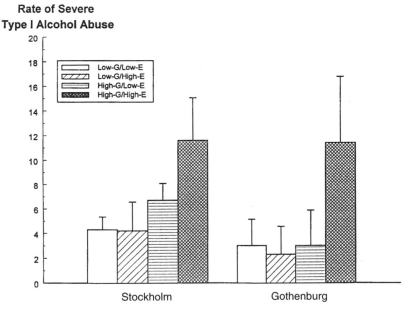

FIGURE 10.4. Rate of severe (i.e., recurrent) Type I alcoholism in Swedish adoption studies of men as a function of genetic and environmental risk. Genetic and environmental risk functions were determined statistically in the Stockholm sample and applied independently to the Gothenburg sample. In both samples, only adoptees at relatively high genetic risk and at relatively high environmental risk develop severe Type I alcoholism at a rate that is significantly higher than the population rate, indicating the existence of a genotype–environment interaction. Data from Sigvardsson et al. (1996).

weakest area in behavioral genetics today is the treatment of genotype–environmental interaction." (Eaves, Eysanck, & Martin, 1989, p. 414).

Despite the weak empirical support, the proposition—that genetic factors establish a level of vulnerability that eventuates in alcoholism only when a vulnerable individual is exposed to provocative circumstances—continues to hold much theoretical appeal. The difficulty in detecting genotype–environment interactions likely owes in large part to measurement problems. Parental alcoholism is an imperfect indicator of both genetic risk when assessed in biological parents, and environmental risk when assessed in rearing parents. Research on complex disorders such as brain trauma (e.g., Jordan et al., 1997) suggest that as molecular geneticists begin to identify the specific genes underlying vulnerability to alcoholism, tests for genotype–environment interaction will become increasingly sensitive.

Genotype–environment correlation refers to a non-independence of genetic and environmental effects that is induced either *passively* (because parents both transmit genes to and influence the rearing circumstances of their children), *evocatively* (because an individual's genetically influenced behavior evokes different responses from teachers, parents, and peers), or *actively* (because an individual's experiential choices are in part a function of his or her genetically influenced abilities, interests, and personality). Although genotype–environment correlational processes have not been much explored for alcohol-related outcomes, the recent adoption study by Ge et al. (1996) on antisocial and hostile behavior provides a useful illustration of how genotype–environment correlational processes might affect complex behavioral phenotypes.

In the Ge et al. (1996) study, a history of psychiatric disorder (either substance abuse/dependency or antisocial personality) in the adoptees' biological parents was related to adoptive parents' disciplinary practices: The reared-away offspring of biological parents with a history of psychiatric disorder were more likely than control adoptees to have adoptive parents who engaged in harsh disciplinary practices, in large part because adoptees with a positive biological background were more likely than control adoptees to be hostile and aggressive; that is, the adoptive parents were apparently reacting to the biologically influenced hostile behavior of their adoptive offspring by becoming more punitive (i.e., an evocative genotype–environment correlation). Significantly, these researchers concluded that the relationship between offspring hostility and parental harsh discipline was reciprocal; hostility evoked harsh discipline, which in turn evoked more hostility. Thus, genetic factors increased the likelihood of hostile behavior in part by increasing the likelihood that an individual prone to hostility was reared in a environment likely to provoke hostile reactions.

Summary on the Nature of Environmental Influence

Behavioral genetic research supports the importance of environmental as well as genetic influences on alcoholism risk. The MZ twin concordance for alcoholism does not approach the 100% value that would be expected if alcoholism risk were entirely genetically mediated, and the rate of alcoholism among the reared-away offspring of alcoholics, although elevated over population levels, falls far short of what would be expected under simple, purely genetic models of etiology. It seems likely that whatever its genetic basis, inherited vulnerability for alcoholism can be moderated by experiential factors (cf. Gauvin et al., 1998).

Behavioral genetic research suggests that the nature of environmental influences on alcoholism vulnerability may differ meaningfully from how they have been conceptualized in many developmental models. Failure to control for genetic factors can lead to heritable contributions to familial resemblance being misinterpreted as shared environmental effects. For alcohol-related outcomes, as for many psychological characteristics, nonshared environmental influences appear to be more important than shared environmental influences, at least in adulthood. Genotype–environment interaction and correlation provide useful conceptualizations for modeling the joint influence of genetic and environmental factors, even though these processes have not been investigated much in the alcohol field. Genotype–environment interaction models posit that only individuals with inherited vulnerability are subject to environmental provocation, and genotype–environment correlation models emphasize the role of heritable behaviors on the nature of individual experience.

CONCLUSIONS

As stated in the introduction, rather than specifying a comprehensive theory of drinking behavior, behavioral genetics offers a set of significant empirical findings and useful theoretical concepts. This is not to conclude that behavioral genetics, as applied in the alcohol field or elsewhere, is an atheoretical enterprise. Behavioral genetics makes many testable predictions, and many of these have been confirmed, and many more are in the process of being empirically evaluated. Behavioral genetic models predict that adoptee risk of alcoholism should be related to biological- and not rearing-parent alcoholism, that MZ twin concordance for alcoholism should exceed DZ twin concordance, and that risk for alcoholism should be related to the density of family loading. All of these predictions have been confirmed. Behavioral genetics also predicts that the genes underlying alcoholism vulnerability should be detectable using recently developed molecular methods; a prediction that will either be confirmed or rejected in the coming decade.

Behavioral genetics has not provided a comprehensive theory of alcoholism etiology in part because behavioral geneticists have been more concerned with determining whether, rather than how, genes affect alcoholism risk. Developing more comprehensive behavioral genetic models of alcoholism etiology will require that (1) the systems and processes that intervene between primary gene product and behavior are identified, and (2) the mechanisms by which environmental factors modulate the effects of these systems and processes are characterized. These goals may be achieved through a bottom-up approach that begins by identifying the relevant vulnerability genes and then goes on to determine their function, or through a top-down approach that attempts to use other theoretical perspectives to identify pathways of genetic influence. In either case, the mechanisms of genetic influence should be compatible, rather than competitive, with the psychological and social determinants of this disorder.

ACKNOWLEDGMENT

Work on this chapter was supported in part by USPHS Grant Nos. AA00175 and AA09367.

REFERENCES

Agarwal, D. P., & Goedde, H. W. (1989). Human aldehyde dehydrogenases: Their role in alcoholism. *Alcohol, 6,* 517–523.

Amadeo, S., Fourcade, M. L., Abbar, M., Leroux, M. G., Castelnau, D., Venisse, J. L., & Mallet, J. (1993). Association between D_2 receptor gene polymorphism and alcoholism. *Psychiatric Genetics, 3,* 130.

Arinami, T., Itokawa, M., Komiyama, T., Mitsushio, H., Mori, H., Mifune, H., Hamaguchi, H., & Toru, M. (1993). Association between the severity of alcoholism and the A1 allele of the dopamine D_2 receptor Taq1 A RFLP. *Biological Psychiatry, 33,* 108–114.

Babor, T. F. (1996). The classification of alcoholics: Typology theories from the 19th century to the present. *Alcohol Health and Research World, 20,* 6–14.

Babor, T. F., Hofmann, M., Del Boca, F., Hesselbrock, V., Meyer, R., Dolinsky, Z., & Rounsaville, B. (1992). Types of alcoholics: I. Evidence for an empirically-derived typology based on indicators of vulnerability and severity. *Archives of General Psychiatry, 49,* 599–608.

Barr, C. L., & Kidd, K. K. (1993). Populations frequencies of the A1 allele at the dopamine D_2 receptor locus. *Biological Psychiatry, 34,* 204–209.

Baron, M. (1997). Association studies in psychiatry: A season of discontent. *Molecular Psychiatry, 2,* 278–281.

Baron, R. M., & Kenny, D. A. (1986). The moderator–mediator variable distinction in social psychological research: Conceptual, strategic, and statistical considerations. *Journal of Personality and Social Psychology, 51,* 1173–1182.

Begleiter, H., & Platz, A. (1972). The effects of alcohol on the central nervous system in humans. In B. Kissin & H. Begleiter (Eds.), *The biology of alcoholism: Vol 2. Physiology and Behavior* (pp. 293–306). New York: Plenum.

Begleiter, H., Porjesz, B., Bihari, B., & Kissin, B. (1984). Event-related brain potential in boys at risk for alcoholism. *Science, 225,* 1493–1496.

Begleiter, H., Reich, T., Hesselbrock, V., Porjesz, B., Li, T.-K., Schuckit, M. A., Edenberg, H. J., & Rice, J. P. (1995). The Collaborative Study on the Genetics of Alcoholism. *Alcohol Health and Research World, 19,* 228–236.

Belknap, J. K., Mitchell, S. R., O'Toole, L. A., Helms, M. L., & Crabbe, J. C. (1996). Type I and Type II error rates for quantitative trait loci (QTL) mapping studies using recombinant inbred strains. *Behavior Genetics, 26,* 149–160.

Berman, S. M., Whipple, S. C., Fitch, R. J., & Noble, E. P. (1993). P300 in young boys as a predictor of adolescent substance use. *Alcohol, 10,* 69–76.

Berrettini, W. (1997). On the interpretation of association studies in the behavioral disorders. *Molecular Psychiatry, 2,* 274–275.

Bien, T. H., & Burge, R. (1990). Smoking and drinking: A review of the literature. *International Journal of the Addictions, 25,* 1429–1454.

Blum, K., Noble, E. P., Sheridan, P. J., Finley, O., Montgomery, A., Ritchie, T., Ozkaragoz, T., Fitch, R. J., Sadlack, F., Sheffield, D., Dahlmann, T., Halbadier, S., & Nogami, H. (1991). Association of the A1 allele of the D_2 dopamine receptor gene with severe alcoholism. *Alcohol, 8,* 409–416.

Blum, K., Noble, E. P., Sheridan, P. J., Montgomery, A., Ritchie, T., Jagadeeswaran, P., Nogami, H., Briggs, A. H., & Cohn, J. B. (1990). Allelic association of human dopamine D_2 receptor gene and alcoholism. *Journal of the American Medical Association, 263,* 2055–2060.

Bohman, M., Sigvardsson, S., & Cloninger, C. R. (1981). Maternal inheritance of alcohol abuse: Cross-fostering analysis of adopted women. *Archives of General Psychiatry, 38*, 965–969.

Bolos, A. M., Dean, M., Lucas-Derse, S., Ramsburg, M., Brown, G. L., & Goldman, D. (1990). Population and pedigree studies reveal a lack of association between the dopamine D_2 receptor gene and alcoholism. *Journal of the American Medical Association, 264*, 3156–3160.

Bouchard, T. J., Jr. (1994). Genes, environment and personality. *Science, 264*, 1700–1701.

Bouchard, T. J., Jr., Lykken, D. T., McGue, M., Segal, N. L., & Tellegen, A. (1990). Sources of human psychological differences: The Minnesota study of twins reared apart. *Science, 250*, 223–228.

Buck, K. J. (1995). Strategies for mapping and identifying quantitative trait loci specifying behavioral responses to alcohol. *Alcoholism: Clinical and Experimental Research, 19*, 795–801.

Buck, K. J., Metten, P., Belknap, J. K., & Crabbe, J. C. (1997). Quantitative trait loci involved in genetic predisposition to acute alcohol withdrawal in mice. *Journal of Neuroscience, 17*, 3946–3955.

Cadoret, R. J., O'Gorman, T., Troughton, E., & Heywood, E. (1985). Alcoholism and antisocial personality: Interrelationships, genetic and environmental factors. *Archives of General Psychiatry, 42*, 161–167.

Cadoret, R. J., Troughton, E., & O'Gorman, T. W. (1987). Genetic and environmental factors in alcohol abuse and antisocial personality. *Journal of Studies on Alcohol, 48*, 1–8.

Caldwell, C. B., & Gottesman, I. I. (1991). Sex differences in risk for alcoholism: A twin study. *Behavior Genetics, 21*, 563–563 (abstract).

Carey, G. (1994). Genetic association study in psychiatry: Analytical evaluation and a recommendation. *American Journal of Medical Genetics, 54*, 311–317.

Carmelli, D., Heath, A. C., & Robinette, D. (1993). Genetic analysis of drinking behavior in World War II veteran twins. *Genetic Epidemiology, 10*, 210–213.

Caspi A., Moffitt, T. E., Newman, D. L., & Silva P. A. (1996). Behavioral observations at age 3 predict adult psychiatric disorders: Longitudinal evidence from a birth cohort. *Archives of General Psychiatry, 53*, 1033–1039.

Cavalli-Sforza, L. L., & Bodmer, W. F. (1971). *The genetics of human populations.* San Francisco: Freeman.

Clifford, C. A., Fulker, D. W., Gurling, H. M. D., & Murray, R. M. (1984). A genetic and environmental analysis of a twin family study of alcohol use, anxiety, and depression. *Genetic Epidemiology, 1*, 47–52.

Cloninger, C. R. (1987). Neurogenetic adaptive mechanisms in alcoholism. *Science, 236*, 410–416.

Cloninger, C. R., Bohman, M., & Sigvardsson, S. (1981). Inheritance of alcohol abuse: Cross-fostering analysis of adopted men. *Archives of General Psychiatry, 38*, 861–868.

Cloninger, C. R., Sigvardsson, S., Reich, T., & Bohman, M. (1988). Childhood personality predicts alcohol abuse in young adults. *Alcoholism: Clinical and Experimental Research, 12*, 494–505.

Cohen, H. L., Porjesz, B., & Begleiter, H. (1991). EEG characteristics in males at risk for alcoholism. *Alcoholism: Clinical and Experimental Research, 15*, 858–865.

Cohen, H. L., Porjesz, B., & Begleiter, H. (1993). The effects of ethanol on EEG activity in males at risk for alcoholism. *Electroencephalography and Clinical Neurophysiology, 86*, 368–376.

Collins A. C., Romm, E., Selvaag, S., Turner, S., & Marks, M. J. (1993). A comparison of the effects of chronic nicotine infusion on tolerance to nicotine and cross-tolerance to ethanol in long- and short-sleep mice. *Journal of Pharmacology and Experimental Therapeutics, 266,* 1390–1397.

Collins, F. S., & Fink, L. (1995). The Human Genome Project. *Alcohol Health and Research World, 19,* 190–194.

Comings, D. E., Comings, B. G., Muhleman, D., Dietz, G., Shahbahrami, B., Tast, D., Knell, E., Kocsis, P., Baumgarten, R., Kovacs, B., Levy, D. L., Smith, M., Borison, R. L., Evans, D. D., Klein, D. N., MacMurray, J., Tosk, J. M., Sverd, J., Gysin, R., & Flanagan, S. D. (1991). The dopamine D_2 receptor locus as a modifying gene in neuropsychiatric disorders. *Journal of the American Medical Association, 266,* 1793–1800.

Conneally, P. M. (1991). Association between D_2 dopamine receptor gene and alcoholism: Continuing controversy. *Archives of General Psychiatry, 48,* 757–759.

Cook, B. L., Wang, Z. W., Crowe, R. R., Hauser, R., & Freimer, M. (1992). Alcoholism and the D_2 receptor gene. *Alcoholism: Clinical and Experimental Research, 16,* 806–809.

Cotton, N. S. (1979). The familial incidence of alcoholism: A review. *Journal of Studies on Alcohol, 40,* 89–116.

Crabb, D. W., Edenberg, H. J., & Borson, W. F. (1987). Genotypes for aldehyde dehydrogenase deficiency and alcohol sensitivity: The inactive $ALDH2_2$ allele is dominant. *Journal of Clinical Investigation, 83,* 314–316.

Crabbe, J. C., Belknap, J. K., & Buck, K. J. (1994). Genetic animal models of alcohol and drug abuse. *Science, 264,* 1715–1723.

Crabbe, J. C., Phillips, T. J., Feller, D. J., Hen, R., Wenger, C. D., Lessov, C. N., & Schafer, G. L. (1996). Elevated alcohol consumption in null mutant mice lacking 5-HT$_{1B}$ sertonin receptors. *Nature Genetics, 14,* 98–101.

Cunningham, C. L. (1995). Localization of genes influencing ethanol-induced conditioned place preference and locomotor activity in BXD recombinant inbred mice. *Psychopharmacology, 120,* 28–41.

Cutrona, C. E., Cadoret, R. J., Suhr, J. A., Richards, C. C., Troughton, E., Schutte, K., & Woodworth, G. (1994). Interpersonal variables in the prediction of alcoholism among adoptees: Evidence for gene–environment interactions. *Comprehensive Psychiatry, 35,* 171–179.

DeFiebre C. M., & Collins, A. C. (1992). Classical genetic analyses of responses to nicotine and ethanol in crosses derived from long- and short-sleep mice. *Journal of Phamacology and Experimental Therapeutics, 261,* 173–180.

Dib, C., Faure, S., & Fizames, C. (1996). A comprehensive genetic map of the human genome based on 5,264 microsatellites. *Nature, 380,* 152–154.

Eaves, L. J., Eysenck, H. J., & Martin, N. G. (1989). *Genes, culture, and personality: An empirical approach.* San Diego: Academic Press.

Ehlers, C. L., & Schuckit, M. A. (1991). Evaluation of EEG alpha activity in sons of alcoholics. *Neuropsychopharmacology, 4,* 199–205.

Falconer, D. S. (1965). The inheritance of liability to certain diseases estimated from the incidence among relatives. *Annals of Human Genetics, 29,* 51–76.

Falk, C. T., & Rubinstein, P. (1987). Haplotype relative risks: An easy reliable way to construct a proper control sample for risk calculations. *Annals of Human Genetics, 51,* 227–233.

Finn, P. R., & Pihl, R. O. (1987). Men at high risk for alcoholism: The effect of alcohol on cardiovascular response to unavoidable shock. *Journal of Abnormal Psychology, 96*, 230–236.

Finn, P. R., & Pihl, R. O. (1988). Risk for alcoholism: A comparison between two different groups of sons of alcoholics on cardiovascular reactivity and sensitivity to alcohol. *Alcoholism: Clinical and Experimental Research, 12*, 742–747.

Finn, P. R., Zeitouni, N. C., & Pihl, R. O. (1990). Effects of alcohol on psychophysiological hyperreactivity to nonaversive and aversive stimuli in men at high risk for alcoholism. *Journal of Abnormal Psychology, 103*, 293–301.

Gainoulakis, C., Krishnan, B., & Thavundayil, J. (1996). Enhanced sensitivity of pituitary β-endorphin to ethanol in subjects at high risk of alcoholism. *Archives of General Psychiatry, 53*, 250–257.

Gallaher, E. J., Jones, G. E., Belknap, J. K., & Crabbe, J. C. (1996). Identification of genetic markers for initial sensitivity and rapid tolerance to ethanol-induced ataxia using quantitative trait locus analysis in BXD recombinant inbred mice. *Journal of Pharmacology and Experimental Therapeutics, 277*, 604–612.

Gauvin, D. V., Vanecek, S. A., Baird, T. J., Briscoe, R. J., Vallett, M., & Holloway, F. A. (1998). Genetic selection of alcohol preference can be countered by conditioning processes. *Alcohol, 15*, 199–206.

Ge, X., Conger, R. D., Cadoret, R. J., Neiderhiser, J. M., Yates, W., Troughton, E., & Stewart, M. A. (1996). The developmental interface between nature and nurture: A mutual influence model of child antisocial behavior and parent behaviors. *Developmental Psychology, 32*, 574–589.

Geijer, T., Jonsson, E., Neiman, J., Persson, M.-L., Brene, S., Gyllander, A., Sedvall, G., Rydberg, U., Wasserman, D., & Terenius, L. (1997). Tyrosine hydroxylase and dopmaine D4 receptor allelic distribution in Scandinavian chronic alcoholics. *Alcoholism: Clinical and Experimental Research, 21*, 35–39.

Gejman, P. V., Ram, A., Gelernter, J., Friedman, E., Cao, Q., Pickar, D., Blum, K., Noble, E. P., Kranzler, H. R., O'Malley, S., Hamer, D. H., Whitsitt, F., Rao, P., DeLisi, L. E., Virkkunen, M., Linnoila, M., Goldman, D., & Gershon, E. S. (1994). No structural mutation in the dopamine D_2 receptor gene in alcoholism or schizophrenia: Analysis using denaturing gradient gel electrophoresis. *Journal of the American Medical Association, 271*, 204–208.

Gelernter, J., O'Malley, S., Risch, N., Kranzler, H. R., Krystal, J., Merikangas, K., Kennedy, J. L., & Kidd, K. K. (1991). No association between an allele at the D_2 dopamine receptor gene (DRD2) and alcoholism. *Journal of the American Medical Association, 266*, 1801–1807.

Gelernter, J. (1997). Genetic association studies in psychiatry: Recent history. In K. Blum & E. P. Noble (Eds.), *Handbook of psychiatric genetics* (pp. 25–36). New York: CRC Press.

George, S. R., Cheng, R., Nguyen, T., Israel, Y., & O'Dowd, B. F. (1993). Polymorphisms of the D4 dopamine receptor alleles in chronic alcoholism. *Biochemical and Biophysical Research Communications, 196*, 107–114.

Ginns, E. I., Ott, J., Egeland, J. A., Allen, C. R., Fann, C. S. J., Pauls, D. L., Weissenbach, J., Carulli, J. P., Falls, K. M., Keith, T. P., & Paul, S. M. (1996). A genome-wide search for chromosomal loci linked to bipolar affective disorder in the Old Order Amish. *Nature Genetic, 12*, 431–435.

Goldman, D., Brown, G. L., Albaugh, B., Robin, R., Goodson, S., Trunzo, M., Akhtar, L., Lucas-Derse, S., Long, J., Linnoila, M., & Dean, M. (1993). DRD2 dopamine receptor genotype, linkage disequilibrium, and alcoholism in American Indians and other populations. *Alcoholism: Clinical and Experimental Research, 17(2),* 199–204.

Goldman, D., Dean, M., Brown, G. L., Bolos, A. M., Tokola, R., Virkkunen, M., & Linnoila, M. (1992). D_2 dopamine receptor genotype and cerebrospinal fluid homovanillic acid, 5-hydroxyindoleacetic acid and 3-methoxy-4-hydroxyphenylglycol in Finland and the United States. *Acta Psychiatrica Scandinavica, 86,* 351–357.

Goodwin, D. W. (1994). *Alcoholism: The facts.* New York: Oxford University Press.

Goodwin, D. W., Schulsinger, F., Hermansen, L., Guze, S. B., & Winokur, G. (1973). Alcohol problems in adoptees raised apart from alcoholic biological parents. *Archives of General Psychiatry, 28,* 238–243.

Goodwin, D. W., Schulsinger, F., Knop, J., Mednick, S., & Guze, S. B. (1977a). Alcoholism and depression in the adopted-out daughters of alcoholics. *Archives of General Psychiatry, 34,* 751–755.

Goodwin, D. W., Schulsinger, F., Knop, J., Mednick, S., & Guze, S. B. (1977b). Psychopathology in adopted and nonadopted daughters of alcoholics. *Archives of General Psychiatry, 34,* 1005–1009.

Goodwin, D. W., Schulsinger, F., Moller, N., Hermansen, L., Winokur, G., & Guze, S. B. (1974). Drinking problems in adopted and nonadopted sons of alcoholics. *Archives of General Psychiatry, 31,* 164–169.

Gottesman, I. I., & Carey, G. (1983). Extracting meaning and direction from twin data. *Psychiatric Developments, 1,* 35–50.

Graham, J. R., & Strenger, V. E. (1988). MMPI characteristics of alcoholics: A review. *Journal of Consulting and Clinical Psychology, 56,* 197–205.

Grove, W. M., Eckert, E. D., Heston, L., Bouchard, T. J. Jr., Segal, N., & Lykken, D. T. (1990). Heritability of substance abuse and antisocial behavior: A study of monozygotic twins reared apart. *Biological Psychiatry, 27,* 1293–1304.

Gurling, H. M. D., Oppenheim, B. E., & Murray, R. M. (1984). Depression, criminality and psychopathology associated with alcoholism: Evidence from a twin study. *Acta Geneticae Medicae et Gemellologiae, 33,* 333–339.

Han, C., McGue, M., & Iacono, W. (1999). *Lifetime tobacco, alcohol and other substance use in adolescent Minnesota twins: Univariate and multivariate behavioural genetic analyses.* Manuscript submitted for publication.

Harada, S., Agarwal, D. P., Goedde, H. W., Tagaki, S., & Ishikawa, B. (1982). Possible protective role against alcoholism for aldehyde dehydrogenase isozyme deficiency in Japan. *Lancet, ii,* 827–827.

Heath, A. C. (1995). Genetic influences on drinking behavior in humans. In H. Begleiter & B. Kissin (Eds.), *The genetics of alcoholism* (pp. 82–121). New York: Oxford University Press.

Heath, A. C., Bucholz, K. K., Madden, P. A. F., Dinwiddie, S. H., Slutske, W. S., Bierut, L. J., Statham, D. J., Dunne, M. P., Whitfield, J. B., & Martin, N. G. (1997). Genetic and environmental contributions to alcohol dependence risk in a national twin sample: Consistency of findings in women and men. *Psychological Medicine, 27,* 1381–1391.

Heath, A. C., Jardine, R., & Martin, N. G. (1989). Interactive effects of genotype and social environment on alcohol consumption in twins. *Journal of Studies on Alcohol, 50,* 38–48.

Heath, A. C., & Madden, P. A. F. (1995). Genetic influences on smoking behavior. In J. R. Turner, L. R. Cardon, & J. K. Hewitt (Eds.), *Behavior genetic approaches in behavioral medicine* (pp. 45–66). New York: Plenum.

Heath, A. C., & Martin, N. G. (1988). Teenage alcohol use in the Australian twin register: Genetic and social determinants of starting to drink. *Alcoholism: Clinical and Experimental Research, 12,* 735–741.

Heath, A. C., & Martin, N. G. (1994). Genetic influences on alcohol consumption patterns and problem drinking: Results from the Australian NH&MRC twin panel follow-up survey. *Annals of the New York Academy of Sciences, 708,* 72–85.

Heath, A. C., Meyer, J., Eaves, L. J., & Martin, N. G. (1991a). The inheritance of alcohol consumption patterns in a general population twin sample: I. Multidimensional scaling of quantity/frequency data. *Journal of Studies on Alcohol, 52,* 345–352.

Heath, A. C., Meyer, J., Eaves, L. J., & Martin, N. G. (1991b). The inheritance of alcohol consumption patterns in a general population twin sample: II. Determinants of consumption frequency and quantity consumed. *Journal of Studies on Alcohol, 52,* 425–433.

Heath, A. C., Slutske, W. S., & Madden, P. A. F. (1997). Gender differences in the genetic contribution to alcoholism risk and to alcohol consumption patterns. In R. W. Wilsnack & S. C. Wilsnack (Eds.), *Gender and alcohol: Individual and social perspectives* (pp. 114–149). New Brunswick, NJ: Rutgers Center of Alcohol Studies.

Helzer, J. E., & Canino, G. J. (1992). *Alcoholism in North America, Europe, and Asia.* New York: Oxford University Press.

Helzer, J. E., & Pryzbeck, T. R. (1988). The co-occurrence of alcoholism with other psychiatric disorders in the general population and its impact on treatment. *Journal of Studies on Alcohol, 49,* 219–224.

Higuchi, S., Matsushita, S., Imazeki, H., Kinoshita, T., Takagi, S., & Kono, H. (1994). Aldehyde dehydrogenase genotypes in Japanese alcoholics. *Lancet, 343,* 741–742.

Higuchi, S., Parrish, K. M., Dufour, M. C., Towle, L. H., & Harford, T. C. (1992). The relationship between three subtypes of the flushing response and DSM-III alcohol abuse in Japanese. *Journal of Studies on Alcohol, 53(6),* 553–560.

Hill, S. Y., & Hruska, D. R. (1992). Childhood psychopathology in families of multigenerational alcoholism. *Journal of the American Academy of Child and Adolescent Psychiatry, 31,* 1024–1030.

Hill, S. Y., & Neiswanger, K. (1997). The value of narrow psychiatric phenotypes and "super" normal controls. In K. Blum & E. P. Noble (Eds.), *Handbook of psychiatric genetics* (pp. 37–46). New York: CRC Press.

Hill, S. Y., Steinhauer, S. R., Lowers, L., & Locke, J. (1995). Eight year follow-up of P300 and clinical outcome in children from high-risk alcoholism families. *Biological Psychiatry, 37,* 823–827.

Hrubec, Z., & Omenn, G. S. (1981). Evidence of genetic predisposition to alcoholic cirrhosis and psychosis: Twin concordances for alcoholism and it biological endpoints by zygosity among male veterans. *Alcoholism: Clinical and Experimental Research, 5,* 207–212.

Istvan, J., & Matarazzo, J. D. (1984). Tobacco, alcohol, and caffeine use: A review of their interrelationships. *Psychological Bulletin, 95,* 301–326.

Jardine, R., & Martin, N. G. (1984). Causes of variation in drinking habits in a large twin sample. *Acta Gemellogicae et Medicae, 33,* 435–450.

Jellinek, E. M. (1960). Alcoholism: A genus and some of its species. *Canadian Medical Association Journal, 83,* 1341–1345.

Jordan, B. D., Relkin, N. R., Ravdin, L. D., Jacobs, A. R., Bennett, A., & Gandy, S. (1997). Apolipoprotein E ε 4 associated with chronic brain injury in boxing. *Journal of the American Medical Association, 278,* 136–140.

Kaij, L. (1960). *Alcoholism in twins.* Stockholm: Almqvist & Wiksell.

Kaplan, R. F., Hesselbrock, V. M., O'Connor, S., & DePalma, N. (1988). Behavioral and EEG responses to alcohol in nonalcoholic men with a family history of alcoholism. *Progress in Neuropsychopharmacology and Biological Psychiatry, 12,* 873–885.

Kaprio, K. S., Rose, R. J., Romanov, K., & Koskenvuo, M. (1991). Genetic and environmental determinants of use and abuse of alcohol: The Finish twin cohort studies. *Alcohol and Alcoholism, 1 (Suppl.),* 131–136.

Kaprio, K. S., Viken, R., Koskenvuo, M., Romanov, K., & Rose, R. J. (1992). Consistency and change in patterns of social drinking: A 6-year follow-up of the Finnish twin cohort. *Alcoholism: Clinical and Experimental Research, 16,* 234–246.

Katsanis, J., Iacono, W. G., & McGue, M. K. (1996). The association between P300 and age from preadolescence to early adulthood. *International Journal of Psychophysiology, 24,* 213–221.

Katsanis, J., Iacono, W. G., McGue, M. K., & Carlson, S. R. (1997). P300 event-related potential heritability in monozygotic and dizygotic twins. *Psychophysiology, 34,* 47–58.

Kendler, K. S., Heath, A. S., Neale, M. C., Kessler, R. C., & Eaves, L. J. (1992). A population based twin study of alcoholism in women. *Journal of the American Medical Association, 268,* 1877–1882.

Kendler, K. S., Neale, M. C., Kessler, R. C., Haeth, A. C., & Eaves, L. J. (1993). A test of the equal-environment assumption in twin studies of psychiatric illness. *Behavior Genetics, 23,* 21–28.

Kendler, K. S., Neale, M. C., Prescott, C. A., Kessler, R. C., Heath, A. C., Corey, L. A., & Eaves, L. J. (1996). Childhood parental loss and alcoholism in women: A causal analysis using a twin-family design. *Psychological Medicine, 26,* 79–95.

Kendler, K. S., Prescott, C. A., Neale, M. C., & Pedersen, N. L. (1997). Temperance Board registration for alcohol abuse in a national sample of Swedish male twins, born 1902 to 1949. *Archives of General Psychiatry, 54,* 178–184.

Kendler, K. S., Walters, E. E., Neale, M. C., Kessler, R. C., Heath, A. C., & Eaves, L. J. (1995). The structure of the genetic and environmental risk factors for six major psychiatric disorders in women. *Archives of General Psychiatry, 52,* 374–383.

Kessler, R. C., Nelson, C. B., McGonagle, K. A., Edlund, M. J., Frank, R. G., & Leaf, P. J. (1996). The epidemiology of co-occuring addictive and mental disorders: Implications for prevention and service utilization. *American Journal of Orthopsychiatry, 66,* 17–31.

Knight, P. R. (1938). Psychoanalytic treatment in a sanatorium of chronic addiction to alcohol. *Journal of the American Medical Association, 111,* 1443–1448.

Koopmans, J. R., & Boomsma, D. I. (1996). Familial resemblances in alcohol use: Genetic or cultural transmission? *Journal of Studies on Alcohol, 57,* 19–28.

Koopmans, J. R., vanDoornen, L. J. P., & Boomsma, D. I. (1997). Association between alcohol use and smoking in adolescent and young adult twins: A bivariate genetic analysis. *Alcoholism: Clinical and Experimental Research, 21,* 537–546.

Lander, E. S., & Kruglyak, L. (1995). Genetic dissection of complex traits: Guidelines for interpreting and reporting linkage results. *Nature Genetics, 11,* 241–247.

Levenson, R. W., Oyama, O. N., & Meek, P. S. (1987). Greater reinforcement from alcohol for those at risk: Parental risk, personality risk, and sex. *Journal of Abnormal Psychology, 96*, 242–253.

Lewis, C. E., Robins, L., & Rice, J. (1985). Association of alcoholism with antisocial personality in urban men. *Journal of Nervous and Mental Disease, 173*, 166–174.

Licinio, J. (1997). Molecular psychiatry: Does a new field need to examine strategy? *Molecular Psychiatry, 2*, 3–4.

Lieber, C. S. (1994). Alcohol and the liver: 1994 update. *Gastroenterology, 106*, 1085–1105.

Loehlin, J. C. (1992). *Genes and environment in personality development.* Newbury Park, CA: Sage Publications.

Loehlin, J. C., & Nichols, R. C. (1976). *Heredity, environment, and personality.* Austin: University of Texas Press.

Long, J. C., Knowler, W. C., Hanson, R. L., Robin, R. W., Urbanek, M., Moore, E., Bennett, P. H., & Goldman, D. (1998). Evidence for genetic linkage to alcohol dependence on chromosomes 4 and 11 from an autosome-wide scan in an American Indian population. *American Journal of Medical Genetics (Neuropsychiatric Genetics), 81*, 216–221.

Loper, R. G., Kammeier, M. I., & Hoffman, H. (1973). MMPI characteristics of college freshman males who later became alcoholics. *Journal of Abnormal Psychology, 82*, 159–162.

Maes, H. H., Woodward, C. E., Murrelle, L., Meyer, J. M., Silberg, J. L., Hewitt, J. K., Rutter, M., Siminoff, E., Pickels, A., Carbonneau, R., Neale, M. C., & Eaves, L. J. (1998). Tobacco, alcohol and drug use in 8–16 year old twins: The Virginia Twin Study of Adolescent Behavioral Development (VTSABD). *Journal of Studies on Alcohol.*

Maier, W., Lichtermann, D., & Minges, J. (1994). The relationship of alcoholism and unipolar depression: A controlled family study. *Journal of Psychiatric Research, 28*, 303–317.

Maier, W., & Merikangas, K. R. (1996). Co-occurrence and cotransmission of affective disorders, anxiety disorders and alcoholism in families. *British Journal of Psychiatry, 168*, 93–100.

Martin, N. G., Oakeshott, J. G., Gibson, J. B., Starmer, G. A., Perl, J., & Wilks, A. V. (1985). A twin study of psychomotor and physiological responses to an acute dose of alcohol. *Behavior Genetics, 15*, 305–347.

McClearn, G. E., & Kakihana, R. (1981). Selective breeding for ethanol sensitivity: Short-sleep versus long-sleep mice. In G. E. McClearn, R. A. Deitrich, & V. G. Erwin (Eds.), *Development of animal models as pharmacologic tools (National Institute on Alcoholism and Alcohol Abuse Research Monograph No. 60, pp. 147–159).* Rockville, MD: National Institute on Alcoholism and Alcohol Abuse.

McGue, M., & Bouchard, T. J., Jr. (1998). Genetic and environmental influences on human behavioral differences. *Annual Review of Neuroscience, 21*, 1–24.

McGue, M., Pickens, R. W., & Svikis, D. S. (1992). Sex and age effects on the inheritance of alcohol problems: A twin study. *Journal of Abnormal Psychology, 101*, 3–17.

McGue, M., Sharma, A., & Benson, P. (1996a). The effect of common rearing on adolescent adjustment: Evidence from a U. S. adoption cohort. *Developmental Psychology, 32*, 604–613.

McGue, M., Sharma, A., & Benson, P. (1996b). Parent and sibling influences on adolescent alcohol use and misuse: Evidence from a U. S. adoption cohort. *Journal of Studies on Alcohol, 57,* 8–18.

McGue, M., & Slutske, W. (1996). The inheritance of alcoholism in women. In J. M. Howard, S. E. Martin, P. D. Mail, M. E. Hilton, & E. D. Taylor (Eds.), *Women and alcohol: Issues for prevention research* (National Institute on Alcohol Abuse and Alcoholism Research Monograph No. 32, pp. 65–91). NIH publication No. 96–3817. Washington DC: NIAAA.

McGue, M., Slutske, W., Taylor, J., & Iacono, W. G. (1997). Personality and substance use disorders. I. Effects of gender and alcoholism subtype. *Alcoholism: Clinical and Experimental Research, 21,* 513–520.

Medlund, P., Cederlof, R., Floderus-Myrhed, B., Friberg, L., & Sorensen, S. (1977). A new Swedish twin registry. *Acta Medica Scandinavica Supplement, 600,* 1–111.

Melo, J. A., Shendure, J., Pociask, K., & Silver, L. M. (1996). Identification of sex-specific quantitative trait loci controlling alcohol preference in C57BL/6 mice. *Nature Genetics, 13,* 1147–153.

Merikangas, K. R. (1990). The genetic epidemiology of alcoholism. *Psychological Medicine, 20,* 11–22.

Miller, E. K., Li, L., & Desimone, R. (1991). A neural mechanism for working and recognition memory in inferior temporal cortex. *Science, 254,* 1377–1379.

Moises, H. W., Yang, L., Kristbjarnarson, H., Wiese, C., Byerly, W., Macciardi, F., Arolt, V., Blackwood, D., Liu, X., Sjogren, B., Aschauer, H. N., Hwu, H.-G., Jang, K., Livesley, W. J., Kennedy, J. L., Zoega, T., Ivarsson, O., Bui, M.-T., Yu, M.-H., Havsteen, B., Commerges, D., Weissenbach, J., Schwinger, E., Gottesman, I. I., Pakstis, A. J., Welterberg, L., Kidd, K. K., & Helgason, T. (1995). An international two-stage genome-wide search for schizophrenia susceptibility genes. *Nature Genetics, 11,* 321–324.

Muramatsu, T., Higuchi, S., Murayama, M., Matsushita, S., & Hayashida, M. (1996). Association between alcoholism and the dopamine D_4 receptor gene. *Journal of Medical Genetics, 33,* 113–115.

Nagoshi, C. T., & Wison, J. R. (1989). Long-term repeatability of human alcohol metabolism, sensitivity and acute tolerance. *Journal of Studies on Alcohol, 50,* 162–169.

Nathan, P. (1988). The addictive personality is the behavior of the addict. *Journal of Consulting and Clinical Psychology, 56,* 183–188.

Neale, M. C., & Kendler, K. S. (1995). Models of comorbidity for multifactorial disorders. *American Journal of Human Genetics, 57,* 935–953.

Neiswanger, K., Hill, S. Y., & Kaplan, B. B. (1995). Association and linkage studies of the TAQI A1 allele at the dopamine D_2 receptor gene in samples of female and male alcoholics. *American Journal of Medical Genetics (Neuropsychiatric Genetics), 60,* 267–271.

Neiswanger, K., Kaplan, K. K., & Hill, S. Y. (1995). What can the DRD2/Alcoholism story teach us about association studies in psychiatric genetics?. *American Journal of Medical Genetics (Neuropsychiatric Genetics), 60,* 272–275.

Newlin, D. B., & Thomson, J. B. (1990). Alcohol challenge with sons of alcoholics: A critical review and analysis. *Psychological Bulletin, 108,* 383–402.

O'Connor, S. J., Morzorati, S., Chistian, J. C., & Li, T. K. (1994). Heritable features of the auditory oddball event-related potential: Peaks, latencies, morphology and topography. *Electroencephalography and Clinical Neurophysiology, 92,* 115–125.

Owen, M. J., Holmans, P., & McGuffin, P. (1997). Association studies in psychiatric genetics. *Molecular Psychiatry, 2,* 270–273.

Parsian, A., Todd, R. D., Devor, E. J., O'Malley, K. L., Suarez, B. K., Reich, T., & Cloninger, C. R. (1991). Alcoholism and alleles of the human D_2 dopamine receptor locus: Studies of association and linkage. *Archives of General Psychiatry, 48,* 655–663.

Paterson, A. D. (1997). Case-control association studies in complex traits— An end of an era? *Molecular Psychiatry, 2,* 277–278.

Perry, A. (1973). The effect of heredity on attitudes toward alcohol, cigarettes, and coffee. *Journal of Applied Psychology, 58,* 275–277.

Pfefferbaum, A., Ford, J. M., White, P. M., & Mathalon, D. (1991). Event-related potentials in alcoholic men: P3 amplitude reflects family history but not alcohol consumption. *Alcoholism: Clinical and Experimental Research, 15,* 839–850.

Phillips, T. J., Crabbe, J. C., Metten, P., & Belknap, J. (1994). Localization of genes affecting alcohol drinking in mice. *Alcoholism: Clinical and Experimental Research, 18,* 931–941.

Phillips, T. J., Lessov, C. N., Harland, R. D., & Mitchell, S. R. (1996). Evaluation of potential genetic associations between ethanol tolerance and sensitization in BXD/Ty recombinant inbred mice. *Journal of Pharmacology and Experimental Therapeutics, 277,* 613–623.

Pickens, R. W., Svikis, D. S., McGue, M., & LaBuda, M. C. (1995). Common genetic mechanisms in alcohol, drug, and mental disorder comorbidity. *Drug and Alcohol Dependence, 39,* 129–138.

Pickens, R. W., Svikis, D. S., McGue, M., Lykken, D. T., Heston, L. L., & Clayton, P. J. (1991). Heterogeneity in the inheritance of alcoholism: A study of male and female twins. *Archives of General Psychiatry, 48,* 19–28.

Plomin, R., & Daniels, D. (1987). Why are children in the same family so different from one another? *Behavior and Brain Sciences, 10,* 1–60.

Plomin, R., DeFries, J. C., McClearn, G. E., & Rutter, M. (1997). *Behavioral genetics: A primer (3rd ed.).* San Francisco: Freeman.

Polich, J., Pollock, V. E., & Bloom, F. E. (1994). Meta-analysis of P300 amplitude from males at risk for alcoholism. *Psychological Bulletin, 115,* 55–73.

Pollock, V. E., Volavka, J., Goodwin, D. W., Mednick, S. A., Gabrielli, W. F., Knop, J., & Schulsinger, F. (1983). The EEG after alcohol administration in men at risk for alcoholism. *Archives of General Psychiatry, 40,* 857–861.

Porjesz, B., & Begleiter, H. (1996). Effects of alcohol on electrophysiological activity of the brain. In H. Begleiter & B. Kissin (Eds.), *Alcohol and alcoholism: Vol. 2. The pharmacology of alcohol and alcohol dependence* (pp. 207–247). New York: Oxford University Press.

Porjesz, B., & Begleiter, H. (1997). Event-related potentials in COA's. *Alcohol Health and Research World, 21,* 236–240.

Reed, T., Slemenda, C. W., Viken, R. J., Christian, J. C., Carmelli, D., & Fabsitz, R. R. (1994). Correlations of alcohol consumption with related covariates and heritability estimates in older adult males over a 14- to 18-year period: The NHLBI Twin Study. *Alcoholism: Clinical and Experimental Research, 18,* 702–710.

Reich, T., Edenberg, H. J., Goate, A., William, J. T., Rice, J. P., Van Eerdewegh, P., Foroud, T., Hesselbrock, V., Schuckit, M. A., Bucholz, K., Porjesz, B., Li, T.-K., Conneally, P. M., Nurnberger, J. J. Jr., Tischfield, J. A., Crowe, R. R., Cloninger, C. R., Wu, W., Shears, S., Carr, K., Crose, C., Willig, C., &

Begleiter, H. (1998). Genome-wide search for genes affecting risk for alcohol dependence. *American Journal of Medical Genetics (Neuropsyhciatric Genetics), 81,* 206–215.

Reich, W., Earls, F., & Powell, J. (1988). A comparison of the home and social environments of children of alcoholic and non-alcoholic parents. *British Journal of Addiction, 83,* 831–839.

Rodriguez, L. A., Plomin, R., Blizard, D. A., Jones, B. C., & McClearn, G. E. (1995). Alcohol acceptance, preference, and sensitivity in mice: II. Quantitative trait loci mapping analysis using BXD recombinant inbred strains. *Alcoholism: Clinical and Experimental Research, 19,* 367–373.

Roe, A. (1944). The adult adjustment of children of alcoholic parents raised in foster homes. *Quarterly Journal of Studies on Alcohol, 5,* 378–393.

Rubinstein, M., Phillips, T. J., Bunzow, J. R., Falzone, T. L., Dziewczapolski, G., Zhang, G., Fang, Y., Larson, J. L., McDougall, J. A., Chester, J. A., Saez, C., Pugsley, T. A., Gershanik, O., Low, M. J., & Grandy, D. K. (1997). Mice lacking dopamine D4 receptors are supersensitive to ethanol, cocaine, and methamphetamine. *Cell, 90,* 991–1001.

Schuckit, M. A., (1994). A clinical model of genetic influences in alcohol dependence. *Journal of Studies on Alcohol, 55,* 5–17.

Schuckit, M. A., Anthenelli, R., Crowe, R., Hesselbrock, V., Nurnberger, J., & Tipp, J. (1995). Prevalence of major anxiety disorder in relatives of alcohol dependent men and women. *Journal of Studies on Alcohol, 56,* 309–317.

Schuckit, M. A., & Gold, E. O. (1988). Simultaneous evaluation of multiple markers of ethanol/placebo challenges in sons of alcoholics and controls. *Archives of General Psychiatry, 45,* 211–216.

Schuckit, M. A., & Irwin, M. (1989). An analysis of the clinical relevance of Type 1 and Type 2 alcoholics. *British Journal of Addiction, 84,* 869–876.

Schuckit, M. A., & Smith, T. L. (1996). An 8–year follow-up of 450 sons of alcoholic and control subjects. *Archives of General Psychiatry, 53,* 202–210.

Schwab, S., Soyka, M., Niederecker, M., Ackenheil, M., Scherer, J., & Wildenauer, D. B. (1991). Allelic association of human D_2-receptor DNA polymorphism ruled out in 45 alcoholics. *American Journal of Human Genetics, 49 (Suppl.), 203 (Abstract).*

Shen, Y.-C., Fan, J.-H., Edenberg, H. J., Li, T.-K., Cui, Y.-H., Wang, Y.-F., Tian, C. H., Zhou, C.-F., Zhou, R.-L., Wang, J., Zhao, Z.-L., & Xia, G.-Y. (1997). Polymorphism of ADH and ALDH genes among four ethnic groups in China and effects upon the risk for alcoholism. *Alcoholism: Clinical and Experimental Research, 21,* 1272–1277.

Sher, K. J. (1991). *Children of alcoholics: A critical appraisal of theory and research.* Chicago: University of Chicago Press.

Sher, K. J., Gotham, H. J., Erickson, D. J., & Wood, P. K. (1996). A prospective, high-risk study of the relationship between tobacco dependence and alcohol use disorders. *Alcoholism: Clinical and Experimental Research, 20,* 485–492.

Sher, K. J., & Trull, T. J. (1994). Personality and disinhibitory psychopathology: Alcoholism and antisocial personality disorder. *Journal of Abnormal Psychology, 103,* 92–102.

Sieber, M. F. (1981). Personality scores and licit and illicit substance use. *Personality and Individual Differences, 2,* 235–241.

Sigvardsson, S., Bohman, M., & Cloninger, C. R. (1996). Replication of the Stockholm Adoption Study of alcoholism: Confirmatory cross-fostering analysis. *Archives of General Psychiatry, 53,* 681–687.

Silver, L. M. (1995). *Mouse genetics: Concepts and application.* New York: Oxford University Press.

Sokol, D. K., Moore, C. A., Rose, R. J., Williams, C. J., Reed, T., & Christian, J. C. (1995). Intra-pair differences in personality and cognitive ability among young monozygotic twins distinguished by chorion type. *Behavior Genetics, 25,* 457–466.

Steinhauer, S. R., & Hill, S. Y. (1993). Auditory event-related potentials in alcoholics and their first-degree relatives. *Journal of Studies on Alcohol, 54,* 408–421.

Stent, G. S. (1981). Strength and weakness of the genetic approach to the development of the nervous system. *Annual Review of Neurology, 4,* 63–94.

Stewart, S. H. (1996). Alcohol abuse in individuals exposed to trauma: A critical review. *Psychological Bulletin, 120,* 83–112.

Streissguth, A. P., Sampson, P. D., Olson, H. C., Bookstein, F. L., Barr, H. M., Scott, M., Feldman, J., & Mirsky, A. F. (1994). Maternal drinking during pregnancy: Attention and short-term memory in 14–year old offspring: A longitudinal prospective study. *Alcoholism: Clinical and Experimental Research, 18,* 202–218.

Suarez, B. K., Parsian, A., Hampe, C. L., Todd, R. D., Reich, T., & Cloninger, C. R. (1994). Linkage disequilibria at the D_2 dopamine receptor locus (DRD2) in alcoholics and controls. *Genomics, 19,* 12–20.

Swan, G. E., Carmelli, D., & Cardon, L. R. (1996). The consumption of tobacco, alcohol, and coffee in Caucasian male twins: A multivariate genetic analysis. *Journal of Substance Abuse, 8,* 19–31.

Tarter, R. E., Moss, H. B., & Vanyukov, M. M. (1995). Behavioral genetics and the etiology of alcoholism. In H. Begleiter & B. Kissin (Eds.), *The genetics of alcoholism* (pp. 294–326). New York: Oxford University Press.

Thomasson, H. R., Edenberg, H. J., Crabb, D. W., Mai, X. L., Jerome, R. E., Li, T. K., Wang, S. P., Lin, Y. T., Lu, R. B., & Yin, S. J. (1991). Alcohol and aldehyde dehydrogenase genotypes and alcoholism in Chinese men. *American Journal of Human Genetics, 48,* 677–681.

Todd, J. A. (1995). Genetic analysis of type I diabetes using whole genome approaches. *Proceedings of the National Academy of Sciences, USA, 92,* 8560–8565.

Turner, E., Ewing, J., Shilling, P., Smith, T. L., Irwin, M., Schuckit, M., & Kelsoe, J. R. (1992). Lack of association between an RFLP near the dopamine D_2 receptor gene and severe alcoholism. *Biological Psychiatry, 31,* 285–290.

Vernon, P. A., Lee, D., Harris, J. A., & Jang, K. L. (1996). Genetic and environmental contributions to individual differences in alcohol expectancies. *Personality and Individual Differences, 21,* 183–187.

Vogel, F., & Motulsky, A. G. (1986). *Human genetics: Problems and approaches.* New York: Springer-Verlag.

Volavka, J., Czobor, P., Goodwin, D. W, Gabrielli, W. F., Penick, E. C., Mednick, S. A., Jensen, P., Knop, J., & Schulsinger, F. (1996). The electroencephalogram after alcohol administartion in high-risk men and the development of alcohol use disorders 10 years later. *Archives of General Psychiatry, 53,* 258–263.

Wall, T. L., Thomasson, H. R., Schuckit, M. A., & Ehlers, C. L. (1992). Subjective feelings of alcohol intoxication in Asians with genetic variations of ALDH2 alleles. *Alcoholism: Clinical and Experimental Research, 16,* 991–995.

Wilson, J. R., & Laffan, E. (1995). Alcohol metabolism, sensitivity, and tolerance: Testing for genetic influences. In H. Begleiter & B. Kissin (Eds.), *The genetics of alcoholism* (pp. 122–135). New York: Oxford University Press.

Zucker, R. A., Boyd, G., & Howard, J. (1994). *The development of alcohol problems: Exploring biopsychosocial matrix of risk* (National Institute on Alcohol Abuse and Alcoholism Research Monograph No. 26). Rockville, MD: NIAAA.

11

Neurobiological Bases of Alcohol's Psychological Effects

KIM FROMME
ELIZABETH J. D'AMICO

INTRODUCTION

The 1990's, known as the "Decade of the Brain," have yielded important knowledge about the cellular, structural, and functional contributions of the central nervous system (CNS) to psychological problems, including addiction. The major neurotransmitters, receptors, and neural circuitry were identified for virtually all abusable drugs (Leshner, 1997). There is, however, a large gap between our understanding of these elegant neurochemical systems and the psychological and behavioral experience of addiction. How, for example, does the release of neurotransmitters and activation of receptor site(s) in particular brain regions cause Joe Smith to drink himself into oblivion after promising his wife he will never touch alcohol again? The answer, unfortunately, is unknown. Despite considerable knowledge about the neurobiological basis of alcohol's effects, we are only beginning to relate neurochemical actions to the psychological effects of addiction. During the next 10 years, we hope that science can bridge the gap between the laboratory and personal experience, and between science and practice in the addictions.

As we enter the new millennium, the National Institutes of Health is heralding the "Decade of Behavior." Funding efforts will be directed toward applying the significant advances that have been made in understanding the neural effects of alcohol to the behavioral and psychological consequences observed in people. We are beginning to learn, for example, that craving for a drug activates different neural pathways and neurotransmitters than does actual drug administration. Using positron emission tomography (PET), Grant and colleagues determined that the brain regions activated during cue-elicited cocaine craving differ from those which are activated during a cocaine high (Grant et al., 1996). Cocaine craving activated those regions associated with memory (e.g.,dorsolateral prefrontal and medial orbiotofrontal cortex), whereas cocaine administration activates neural regions associated with the mesolimbic reward system (e.g., nucleus accumbens, dorsal striatum). These findings provide a possible neurochemical basis for anticipatory reinforcement, or positive outcome expectancies, and more importantly, they imply that pharmacotherapies which block actual drug effects will not necessarily be effective in curtailing desire for the drug.

By educating themselves about the neural mechanisms underlying alcohol's effects, psychologists may begin to refine their psychological theories and to develop more effective interventions. An understanding of alcohol's effects at the neurobiological level may speed the development of pharmacological interventions, and relatedly, may provide an explanation for alcohol-related changes in cognitive processes (e.g., blackouts), expectancy or placebo effects, conditioned cue reactivity, stress-response dampening, emotion regulation, and other psychological and biological responses to alcohol.

This chapter provides the reader with a basic knowledge of the neural systems that are implicated in alcohol's acute and chronic effects. First, we describe the methods used to examine alcohol's effects in the brain, the molecular activity of neurons, and the specific effects of alcohol on primary neurochemicals in the CNS. Next, we propose two relatively distinct neuroanatomical and neurochemical response systems to account for the subjective and behavioral effects of alcohol: (1) a simple reinforcement/motivation system that mediates unconditioned alcohol reinforcement and tolerance, and (2) a complex neurochemical system that mediates higher-order cognitive functions and conditioned effects of alcohol.

Whereas this chapter takes a small step toward bridging the neurochemical–behavioral chasm, there are many links we cannot provide. We have included whatever behavioral correlates of neurochemical processes that are currently known and have offered some speculations about correlates that are likely given the available evidence. Recognizing that this chapter includes terminology that may be unfamiliar to many psychologists, we have included a glossary of terms at the end of the chapter.

OVERVIEW OF THE NEUROBIOLOGICAL BASIS FOR ALCOHOL'S EFFECTS

Basic actions of the CNS underlie the physiological, psychological, and behavioral effects of alcohol. Activity of neurons (i.e., specialized cells of the brain) influences the release of neurochemicals that cause increases or decreases in subsequent cellular activity. These alterations in the firing or inhibition of neurons form the molecular basis for alcohol's effects (e.g., sedation, mood changes), which were described at a molar level in preceding chapters. Chronic exposure to alcohol-induced alterations in neurochemical activity (i.e., neuroadaptation) also contributes to the development of tolerance and possibly dependence. Therefore, efforts to understand the neurobiological basis for alcohol use and dependence focus on the actions of neurochemicals and associated neuroanatomical structures in the brain.

Prior to the 1970s, there was general agreement that alcohol had a nonspecific effect on neuronal membranes and caused diffuse effects on brain functioning. This generalized inhibition of brain function was hypothesized to cause the sedative effects of alcohol, but it could not explain the diverse and sometimes opposite affective and behavioral consequences of alcohol use. Recent neuroscientific studies, however, have revealed the selectivity of alcohol's effects on neurochemical systems and discrete brain regions, thus allowing us to better understand the excitatory as well as inhibitory effects of alcohol on psychological states. Research over the past two decades has therefore begun to unravel the mysteries of how the simple alcohol molecule alters neuronal proteins to cause profound effects on the human organism.

Neurochemicals, which include neurotransmitters (e.g., dopamine) and neuropeptides (e.g., opioids), are key elements in understanding the reinforcing effects of alcohol, as well as the debilitating consequences of chronic use. Neurochemical turnover (i.e., synthesis, release, reuptake, and metabolism) and activity at cellular receptor sites form the basis for the subjective and behavioral consequences of alcohol. Herein, we describe the neurochemical functions and neural systems that are associated with subjective effects of drinking, such as mild euphoria and anxiety reduction, as well as the consequences of alcohol withdrawal following chronic use.

From 30 to 100 neurochemicals have been identified, and a significant number of them have been implicated in alcohol use and dependence. The current review is limited to those neurochemicals that have most consistently been linked with alcohol's effects across both animal and human studies. We include research procedures that have revealed specific neurochemical actions thought to mediate the subjective, physiological, and behavioral effects of drinking. Behavioral studies (e.g., self-administration of alcohol by animals or humans) are included only when they are closely coupled with neurochemical activity.

METHODS USED TO EXAMINE ALCOHOL'S NEUROBIOLOGICAL EFFECTS

A variety of laboratory procedures are used to assess alcohol's effects on neurotransmitter activity at the level of the single cell to whole animal. *In vitro* studies include techniques that examine neurotransmitter and receptor activity in single cells and brain slices. *In vivo* studies examine neuro-transmitter activity in live, typically anethetized, animals, or measure neurotransmitter metabolites (i.e., by-products) in the cerebrospinal fluid (CSF) of humans. For both *in vitro* and *in vivo* research, substances that serve as agonists, antagonists, and inverse agonists (described later) are used to study the characteristics of receptor sites and to understand the effects of psychoactive drugs.

Agonists bind to a receptor and activate it, antagonists occupy receptor sites and either block or reverse the actions of neurochemicals, and inverse agonists cause effects that are the exact opposite of the neurochemical to which they are being compared. By administering agents with these known effects on receptor function, the concomitant physiological and behavioral effects of alcohol can more accurately be characterized. If, for example, administration of a known neurotransmitter antagonist blocks the sedative effects of alcohol, we may infer that alcohol's sedative effects involve that particular neurotransmitter. In contrast, if administration of a known neurotransmitter agonist mimics none of the effects of alcohol, we may infer that the particular neurotransmitter is not involved in alcohol's effects.

Technological advances have opened new windows into the world of neurochemical processes and their behavioral correlates. With micro-dialysis procedures, for example, it is now possible to sample extracellular neurotransmitter levels in the brains of awake and freely moving animals. In microdialysis, a probe and fiber are inserted directly into specific brain regions, and samples of brain extracellular fluid are taken (for a thorough description of the procedure, see DiChiara, 1990). Neurotransmitter levels can then be determined when alcohol is administered or taken ad libitum by the animal (e.g., Imperato & Di Chiara, 1986; Weiss, Lorang, Bloom, & Koob, 1993). Microdialysis has the distinct advantage of directly measuring changes in neurochemical activity in response to acute and chronic alcohol intake.

Electrophysiological techniques are used to assess neuronal electrical activity and to quantify the firing rates of neurons in specific brain regions. These techniques have provided evidence, for example, that alcohol increases the firing rate of dopaminergic neurons in previously identified brain "reward systems." These findings thereby suggest that dopamine in involved in the reinforcing effects of drinking (Gessa, Muntoni, Collu, Vargiu, & Mereu, 1985). Event-related potential (ERP) techniques, which are used to measure brain electrical activity following delivery of a discrete sensory stimulus (Porjesz & Begleiter, 1996), can also be used to evaluate the functional effects of alcohol on attention and other cognitive processes. Alcoholics and sons of alcoholics, for example, show certain aberrant ERP components relative to normal controls (Porjesz & Begleiter, 1996).

Brain imaging techniques, such as positron emission tomography (PET), allow the observation of brain activation when alcohol or other drugs are administered, or when drug cues are presented (e.g., Altura,

Altura, Zhang, & Zakhari, 1996). PET uses radionuclide tracers to evaluate regional brain glucose metabolism or cerebral flood flow (i.e., measures of regional activation) to monitor biochemical pathways (Volkow, Brodie, & Bendriem, 1991).

Together, these relatively recent neurobiological procedures have greatly expanded our understanding of the acute and chronic effects of alcohol on specific neurochemical systems and brain regions. They are a first step toward establishing a functional link between the cellular actions of alcohol and resulting psychological effects in humans. The following section provides a brief overview of the molecular actions of alcohol and the ways in which ion channels alter neuronal activity (for reviews of basic neuronal structure and function, see White, 1991; U.S. Department of Health and Human Services [USDHHS], 1993). We then present a review of predominant findings with regard to alcohol's effects on five ubiquitous CNS neurotransmitters (gamma-aminobutyric acid, glutamate, dopamine, serotonin, and norepinephrine) as well as the opiate peptides that have long been implicated in the rewarding effects of addictive drugs, including alcohol.

CHANGING VIEWS ON THE MECHANISMS OF MOLECULAR ACTION

Scientists agree that alcohol alters the levels or function of neurochemicals and their receptors, but they have disagreed about the mechanisms by which these changes occur. Research by Meyer and Overton in the early 1900s implicated the cellular lipids in causing alcohol's effects (see Hunt, 1993; Peoples, Li, & Weight, 1996), and the theory that followed suggested that alcohol changed the rate and range of motion for cellular lipids in the neuronal membrane (Lee, 1991). This disordering of cellular lipids was thought to alter indirectly the function of membrane proteins (e.g., ion channels), thereby influencing neurotransmission and causing alcohol's psychoactive effects (Peoples et al., 1996).

The lipid theory has been challenged in recent years, because the selectivity of alcohol's effects on neuronal proteins cannot be explained by the simple disordering of membrane lipids (Samson & Harris, 1992; Tabakoff & Hoffman, 1991). The protein theory instead suggests that alcohol and other drugs have direct effects on neuronal proteins with these actions enhancing or inhibiting cellular function (Peoples et al., 1996). Therefore, neurobiological research is now devoted largely to understanding the actions of alcohol on specific neurochemical functions (e.g., ion channel activity) and related effects (e.g., Samson & Harris, 1992).

Ion Channels and Neuronal Activity

When at rest, cell membranes (composed primarily of proteins and lipids, or fatty substances) are relatively impermeable. When activated by a change in electrical voltage or by a neurotransmitter, however, membranes become permeable to ions (i.e., charged atoms) such as sodium, potassium, chloride, and calcium, which enter or leave the cell through specialized ion channels (U.S. Department of Health and Human Services, 1993). These ion channels are essentially pores in the cell membrane that are formed by proteins and function at neurotransmitter release and receptor sites. Voltage-gated ion channels respond to changes in electrical potential, whereas ligand-gated ion channels respond to neurotransmitter actions (see Hunt, 1993, for review). The opening of ion channels allows movement of ions into and out of the cell, thereby altering the cell's firing potential.

If an ion channel allows positively charged ions to enter the cell, the cell is "excited" and its firing is more likely. For example, because sodium is positively charged, its entry into the cell facilitates the generation of electrical impulses and neuronal firing that enhance neurotransmitter release. Conversely, entry of negatively charged ions (e.g., chloride) decreases the neuron's firing potential and inhibits the release of neurotransmitters. As we will describe, alcohol's effects on chloride ion channels are especially important in producing certain biological consequences of drinking (Hunt, 1993).

When a neurotransmitter is released, it may be broken down by enzymes in the synaptic cleft, taken back up into the cell (i.e., reuptake) for later use, or attached to a receptor site on an adjacent or nearby neuron. Each receptor site is coupled or paired with a particular biochemical system. When a neurotransmitter attaches (or binds) to the receptor, it may excite or inhibit the activity of the cell, depending upon the type of receptor(s) to which it binds. If the receptor activates an ion channel that facilitates inward movement of positively charged ions, it enhances the activity of the neuron, and the neurotransmitter is said to be "excitatory." Conversely, if the receptor activates an ion channel that facilitates inward movement of negatively charged ions, it decreases the activity of the neuron, and the neurotransmitter is said to be "inhibitory." Thus, neurotransmitters serve excitatory or inhibitory functions in the CNS, depending upon the particular type(s) of receptor sites (and associated ion channels) they affect.

ALCOHOL'S EFFECTS ON NEUROTRANSMITTERS

Without its own receptor system, alcohol instead alters brain function by changing the level, activity, and receptor function of a number of endogenous neurochemicals (Hunt, 1993; Samson & Harris, 1992). In general, alcohol acutely enhances inhibitory neurotransmission and inhibits excitatory neurotransmission. Thus, the overall acute effect of alcohol is sedation, despite an initial arousal at low doses (USDHHS, 1993). Repeated suppression of excitatory neurotransmitters with chronic alcohol exposure, however, can result in an increase (i.e., upregulation) in the number or density of excitatory neurotransmitter receptors (see Buck & Harris, 1991, for review). As a consequence, chronic use involves tolerance to the sedative effects of alcohol, whereas alcohol withdrawal is associated with hyperexcitability. Consistent with the principle of homeostasis, whenever alcohol acutely enhances neurotransmission, withdrawal from chronic administration decreases it. The acute and chronic effects of alcohol on important neurotransmitters are described in the following sections.

Gamma-Aminobutyric Acid (GABA)

Acute Effects

GABA is the major inhibitory amino acid neurotransmitter in the CNS and plays a fundamental role in regulating the inhibition of neuronal activity, specifically, those involved in motor activity, sensory function, and cognition (Buck & Harris, 1991). Activation or potentiation of GABA is thought to mediate the locomotor depressant and anxiety-reducing (i.e., anxiolytic) effects of alcohol (Hunt, 1993; Lewis, 1996; Tabakoff & Hoffman, 1996).

GABA has at least two receptor subtypes, $GABA_A$ and $GABA_B$ (see Tabakoff & Hoffman, 1996). The $GABA_A$ receptor complex is the primary site of an alcohol–GABA interaction, although activation of the $GABA_B$ receptor may be involved in the locomotor stimulation effects of low alcohol doses (Humeniuk, White, & Ong, 1993). Activation of the $GABA_A$ receptor allows chloride ions to enter the cell, and the neuron becomes less excitable (Hunt, 1993). The result is sedation and decreased muscle tone (Buck & Harris, 1991). The ability of $GABA_A$ to alter chloride uptake is highly correlated with intoxication potency, providing additional support for the GABA receptor complex as a partial mediator of the psychoactive properties of alcohol (Morrow, Montpied, & Paul, 1991).

The $GABA_A$ receptor complex comprises five subunits, and various combinations of these subunits mediate sensitivity to different drugs. Combinations that confer sensitivity to alcohol, for example, differ from those that confer sensitivity to benzodiazepines or barbiturates (Tabakoff & Hoffman, 1996). Selective subunit sensitivity may explain why only certain $GABA_A$-containing cells respond to alcohol, whereas all cells containing $GABA_A$ receptors have been shown to respond to benzodiazepines and barbiturates (Aguayo, 1990; Reynolds & Prasad, 1991). Shared receptor subunits, in contrast, may account for similarities among the sedative effects of alcohol, benzodiazepines, and barbiturates.

Administration of benzodiazepine inverse agonists (e.g., Ro15-2513) and GABA antagonists (e.g., picrotoxin) decrease alcohol intake (June, Lin, Greene, Lewis, & Murphy, 1995; Rassnick, D'Amico, Riley, & Koob, 1993) and reverse the locomotor and anxiolytic effects of alcohol in rats (Suzdak, Schwartz, Skolnick, & Paul, 1986). Although the precise mechanisms for these effects are unknown, benzodiazepine inverse agonists and

GABA antagonists possibly diminish the reinforcing effects of alcohol (Morrow et al., 1991; Rassnick et al., 1993).

Chronic Effects

Chronic alcohol intoxication is associated with decreased GABAergic inhibitory neurotransmission as tolerance develops to alcohol's potentiation of GABA-stimulated chloride movement (Sanna et al., 1992). This decrease in GABA activity is hypothesized to explain the development of tolerance to the sedative and intoxicating effects of alcohol (Allan & Harris, 1987; Hunt, 1983).

The effects of chronic alcohol administration on the number or density of GABA$_A$ receptors are inconsistent. Some studies find a decrease in the density of certain GABA$_A$ receptors, whereas others find no change (see Nevo & Hamon, 1995, for review). A decrease in GABA$_A$ receptors would contribute to ethanol dependence and seizure susceptibility during withdrawal by affecting overall inhibition of CNS activity (Buck & Harris, 1991). Because GABA$_A$ receptors are widely distributed throughout the brain, a decrease could also affect cognition, motor activity, and sensory function. Alternatively, changes in subunit composition (e.g., decreases in alpha$_1$) of the GABA$_A$ receptor may account for aspects of tolerance to alcohol in the absence of overall change in GABA$_A$ receptor number or density (Tabakoff & Hoffman, 1996).

By enhancing the binding of GABA to receptor sites, benzodiazepines appear to counteract the cellular adaptations to chronic alcohol use. Thus, benzodiazepines offer a relatively safe treatment for alcohol withdrawal syndrome (Ozdemir, Bremner, & Naranjo, 1994).

Summary

GABA plays an important role in both the acute and chronic effects of alcohol, primarily through its sedative and anxiety-reducing properties. The anxiolytic effects of enhanced GABA function with acute alcohol intake may be perceived as rewarding and motivate alcohol-seeking behavior. As tolerance develops to alcohol's anxiolytic effects, however, increased doses are needed to provide the same anxiety-reducing effects. To the extent that chronic alcohol exposure results in fewer GABA receptors or decreased receptor function, alcohol withdrawal may be characterized by heightened anxiety and seizure susceptibility.

Glutamate

Acute Effects

Glutamate, the major excitatory neurotransmitter in the brain, is associated with three ligand-gated, ion-channel receptor types: N-methyl-D-aspartate acid (NMDA), alpha-amino-3-hydroxy-5-methyl-4-isoxazole propionic acid (AMPA), and kainate (Tsai, Gastfriend, & Coyle, 1995). Ion channels associated with these receptors allow positively charged ions (i.e., calcium, sodium, and potassium) to enter the cell and thus potentiate neuronal excitation. Kainate and AMPA receptors mediate fast excitatory neurotransmission, whereas NMDA receptors mediate slower excitatory responses (Hunt, 1993). The NMDA receptor is the focus of this review, as recent research suggests it may mediate the acutely intoxicating effects of alcohol, as well as the cognitive deficits observed with chronic alcohol use.

NMDA receptors modulate the release of glutamate, dopamine, and norepinephrine (Gonzales & Woodward, 1990; Smirnova et al., 1993; Tabakoff & Hoffman, 1996). When glutamate is released into the synapse, it interacts with non-NMDA receptors to cause rapid depolarization of the postsynaptic neuron. Depolarization releases a magnesium blockade of postsynaptic NMDA receptors and activates the voltage-gated calcium ion channels with which they are coupled (Tabakoff & Hoffman, 1996).

Activation of this NMDA receptor complex has a number of pharmacological and clinical implications. Most importantly, it is crucial for initiation of long-term potentiation (LTP) (Morrisett & Swartzwelder, 1993). LTP is evidenced by an increase in the strength of synaptic transmission that results from repetitive high frequency synaptic activation (Collingridge & Bliss, 1987). Because of its lasting changes in synaptic function, LTP is thought to provide the neural mechanism of memory formation (Browning, Hoffer, & Dunwiddie, 1992) and associative conditioning (Collingridge & Bliss, 1987) at the cellular level.

Even low doses of alcohol have been shown to alter LTP in the hippocampus, a region closely associated with learning and memory (Blitzer, Gil, & Landau, 1990). Alcohol appears to have this effect via multiple indirect mechanisms, which include interference with the glycine–NMDA interaction (Tabakoff & Hoffman, 1996). Glycine acts as an NMDA coagonist and has been found to reverse the inhibitory effects of alcohol on NMDA-stimulated calcium uptake in cerebellar granule cells (Rabe & Tabakoff, 1990), but not in cerebral cortical or hippocampal slices (Gonzales & Woodward, 1990; Woodward, 1994). Thus, consistent with evidence that brain regions differ in sensitivity to alcohol's effects, NMDA receptor function may be differentially affected by alcohol depending on the cell type and brain region (Tabakoff & Hoffman, 1996).

Chronic Effects

Tolerance does not develop to the effects of alcohol on glutamate release (Brown, Leslie, & Gonzales, 1991), and early reports suggested no involvement of the glutamatergic system in the development of physiological tolerance (Buck & Harris, 1991; Tabakoff & Hoffman, 1996). Recent evidence, however, shows NMDA receptors are intricately involved in the development of conditioned or behavioral tolerance. Animals with blockade of NMDA receptors by the NMDA antagonist dizocilpine (MK-801) demonstrated an impaired acquisition of conditioned tolerance to the effects of alcohol (Khanna, Weiner, Kalant, Chau, & Shah, 1992; Szabo, Tabakoff, & Hoffman, 1994). These effects probably relate to the general role of NMDA receptors in learning and memory (Tabakoff & Hoffman, 1996).

Chronic alcohol exposure leads to an upregulation of NMDA receptors (Grant, Valverius, Hudspith, & Tabakoff, 1990) which results in increased activity and sensitivity of the glutamatergic system upon alcohol withdrawal (Sanna et al., 1992). This increase in excitatory neurotransmission contributes to at least two pathological processes (Tsai et al., 1995). First, enhanced glutamatergic activity has been associated with the expression, and perhaps the development, of alcohol withdrawal seizures (Lovinger, 1993). Administration of MK 801 reduced the severity of withdrawal seizures in rats and mice by antagonizing the NMDA receptor (Grant et al., 1990; Morrisett et al., 1990). Genetic studies provide additional support for the role of enhanced glutamatergic functioning in withdrawal seizures. Mice bred to be seizure-prone have more binding sites for MK-801 than mice bred to be seizure-resistant (Valverius, Crabbe, Hoffman, & Tabakoff, 1990). Consequently, recent research has suggested that the hyperexcitability of alcohol withdrawal may be treated effectively with NMDA receptor antagonists (Grant, Snell, Rogawaski, Thurkauf, & Tabakoff, 1992).

Markedly enhanced postsynaptic glutamatergic activity following chronic alcohol exposure may also contribute to neuronal cell death (Lovinger, 1993). Excessive glutamatergic activity causes large increases in intracellular calcium, which contribute to destruction of the cell (i.e., excitotoxicity) (Choi, 1992). Glutamate-induced excitotoxicity has been observed in cells from the cerebellum, hippocampus, and cerebral cortex, which were chronically exposed to, and then withdrawn from, alcohol (Chandler, Newsom, Sumners, & Crews, 1993; Iorio, Tabakoff, & Hoffman, 1993). Loss or degeneration of neurons associated with alcohol withdrawal contributes to the neurological deficits of chronic alcohol dependence. These include impairments in memory and complex reasoning abilities.

Summary

Evidence suggests that inhibition of NMDA receptor function underlies alcohol-related impairments in learning and memory (Lister, Eckardt, & Weingartner, 1987). By inhibiting NMDA receptor–mediated LTP, alcohol may contribute to impaired cognitive processes such as blackouts. Compensatory overactivity of the glutamate system leads to neuronal cell death, which contributes to the cognitive deficits associated chronic alcohol use (Nevo & Hamon, 1995).

Dopamine (DA)

Acute Effects

Dopamine (dihydroxyphenylethyl amine) is one of three monoamine (also called catecholamine) neurotransmitters. Unlike GABA and glutamate, which act directly on ion-coupled receptor sites and alter the generation of action potentials, DA acts indirectly as a neuromodulator (Tabakoff & Hoffman, 1996); that is, DA's major role is to change the activity of other neurotransmitters. Presynaptically, DA modulates the release of neurotransmitters such as glutamate and GABA, as well as regulates increases and decreases in its own release via autoreceptors (Di Chiara, 1995). Postsynaptically, DA receptors modify the voltage dependence of the cell membrane and thereby alter neurotransmission (Di Chiara, 1995). For example, DA modifies the voltage sensitivity of potassium (K^+) ion channels (Kitai & Surmeier, 1993) making depolarization more likely in response to excitatory input.

The presence of DA can facilitate or inhibit neurotransmission, depending on the type and location of dopamine receptor. Acting on D_1 receptors, for example, DA causes the neuronal membrane to become more sensitive to depolarizing influences (as described for K^+), thereby facilitating neuronal activity. Conversely, stimulation of D_2 receptors makes the neuron more stable by inhibiting the excitatory responses of AMPA receptors (Di Chiara, 1995), thereby inhibiting neuronal transmission.

Brain self-stimulation studies provided early evidence that DA mediates pleasurable experience (see Lewis, 1991, for review). During the ensuing decades, DA has been established as a key component in the locomotor stimulation and pleasurable effects of psychostimulant drugs (Wise & Bozarth, 1987), and perhaps alcohol (Weiss & Koob, 1991). A recent and controversial body of evidence, however, has questioned the role of DA in the experience of pleasure, suggesting instead that DA is more generally involved in attention. Specifically, DA may function to draw attention to significant and unexpected events, which include (but are not limited to) those that provide reinforcement (see Wickelgren, 1997, for review). Additional evidence has also shown that DA release following reward may help consolidate memory for the reinforcing event by inhibiting depotentiation at the DA synapse (Otmakhova & Lisman, 1998).

Whether DA is found to mediate pleasure or attention, it is clearly involved in alcohol's acute and chronic effects. Low doses of alcohol increase the firing of dopaminergic neurons *in vivo* in the ventral tegmental area (Gessa et al., 1985) and result in an increase in extracellular DA, particularly in the nucleus accumbens (De Witte, 1996). Similarly, intracranial administration of alcohol (Yoshimoto, McBride, & Li, 1991) as well as alcohol self-administration (Weiss et al., 1996), produced increases in extracellular DA in the nucleus accumbens.

The effects of alcohol on DA appear to be dose- and region-dependent.

Low doses increase DA release in the nucleus accumbens, whereas high doses are required to increase firing of dopaminergic neurons in the substantia nigra (Mereu, Fadda, & Gessa, 1984) and ventral tegmental area (Gessa et al., 1985). This dose response effect of alcohol may relate to the fact that other neurotransmitters mediate alcohol's effects on DA. Specifically, activation of GABA, NMDA, serotonin, and opioid receptors appear to alter the release of DA (Tabakoff & Hoffman, 1996).

Paradoxically, both dopaminergic agonists (amphetamine) and antagonists (haloperidol and pimozide) reduce alcohol self-administration in rats (see Samson, Tolliver, & Schwarz-Steven, 1990, for review). Whereas agonists may substitute for the reinforcing effects of alcohol, antagonists may prevent the postsynaptic stimulation of dopamine by alcohol (Weiss & Koob, 1991). Interactions between DA and other neurotransmitters may also help explain these paradoxical effects.

Chronic Effects

Chronic alcohol intake leads to a reduction in available DA, which is restored by alcohol intake (Weiss et al., 1996). Withdrawal from alcohol is associated with decreased firing of DA neurons in the ventral tegmental area and decreased DA release in the nucleus accumbens (Diana, Pistis, Carboni, Gessa, & Rosetti, 1993). This inhibition of activity in the DA system may serve as the neurochemical basis for the dysphoric symptoms of alcohol withdrawal (Nevo & Hamon, 1995; Koob, 1992) and appears to contribute to continued alcohol self-administration (Weiss et al., 1996).

The search for possible genetic markers for alcoholism have focused on the D_2 receptor. Reports first identified a positive correlation between alcoholism and a polymorphism in the A1 allele of the D_2 receptor gene (Blum et al., 1990). Later research disputed the findings (e.g., Bolos et al., 1990), claiming, for example, that they resulted from inappropriate selection of controls and failure to consider severity of disease. A subsequent collaborative project among the scientists involved in this controversy failed to find an association between alcoholism and a structural coding abnormality in the D_2 receptor gene (Gejman et al., 1994). Further evidence of no association between D_2 allele variant and DA receptor sensitivity or treatment outcome among inpatient alcoholics contributes to the view that this receptor abnormality is a state, rather than trait, marker for alcoholism (Heinz et al., 1996).

Summary

The acutely reinforcing effects of alcohol are thought to result from enhanced dopaminergic activity. Recent evidence also suggests that DA mediates attention to any behaviorally significant event, including those that signal possible reinforcement, and that DA functions to consolidate memories for the reinforcing event. Consequently, DA release may provide the neural basis for the formation of positive expectancies. Chronic alcohol consumption and decreased dopaminergic activity may, however, underlie the dysphoria of alcohol withdrawal. The dependent individual may therefore drink in anticipation of regaining the pleasurable acute effects of alcohol-stimulated DA release (Weiss et al., 1996).

Norepinephrine (NE)

Acute Effects

Norepinephrine (also called noradrenaline) is a metabolic by-product of dopamine (Cooper, Bloom, & Roth, 1996). Previously identified in the peripheral nervous system, NE is now recognized as an important neurotransmitter in the CNS with concentrations in the locus coeruleus (Tabakoff & Hoffman, 1991). At the cellular level, NE inhibits the spontaneous firing rate of affected neurons but increases the cell's responsiveness to other inputs (Segal & Bloom, 1976). Behaviorally, NE increases arousal and helps direct attention to salient aspects of a situation (see Wolkowitz, Tinklenberg, & Weingartner, 1985, for a review of pharmacology and cognitive function).

Some have argued that NE contributes more significantly to alcohol reinforcement than does DA (Socaransky, Aragon, Rusk, Amit, & Ogren, 1985; Weiss & Koob, 1991). Early evidence for this came from research showing neurochemical lesions or inhibition of NE neurons decreased alcohol self-administration in rats (Brown & Amit, 1977; Davis, Smith, & Werner, 1978). Later research showed that inhibition of NE neurons in the locus coeruleus stimulated the release of DA, which was thought to account for alcohol reinforcement (Wise & Bozarth, 1985).

Alcohol has an acute biphasic effect on NE. Low doses increase NE release, which mediates an increased alertness and arousal (Borg, Kvande, & Sedvall, 1983). High doses decrease NE release, thereby contributing to the sedative–hypnotic effects of alcohol (Rossetti, Longu, Mercuro, Hmaidan, & Gessa, 1992). Decreased levels of NE have also been associated with impairments in the acquisition of novel responses via associative learning (Frith, Dowdy, Ferrier, & Crow, 1985).

Chronic Effects

Similar to the biphasic, acute effects of alcohol on NE, chronic alcohol use and withdrawal have opposite effects on NE. During chronic use, the alcoholic is consistently exposed to the increases and decreases in NE that are associated with acute intake. This results in a new homeostatic level of NE (Hawley et al., 1994), decreased NE turnover, and lower levels of NE metabolites in the CSF (Tabakoff & Hoffman, 1996). Because NE metabolites are negatively correlated with craving (Borg, Czarnecka, Kvande, Mossberg, & Sedvall, 1983), alcohol-seeking behavior may be motivated, in part, by chronically low levels of NE.

Decreased NE activity in response to chronic alcohol intake has also been associated with neurological deficits such as those exhibited by Korsakoff's patients (Wolkowitz, Tinklenberg, & Weingartner, 1985). Interestingly, retrieval from semantic memory is relatively unaffected in Korsakoff's patients, indicating a selective effect of NE on memorial processes.

Withdrawal from chronic alcohol use is marked by increased levels of NE in rat prefrontal cortex (Rossetti et al., 1992) and hippocampus (Huttunen, 1991), and increased NE metabolites in the CSF of humans (Borg et al., 1983). Enhanced release of NE, combined with an increase in NE receptor density, is thought to contribute to increased blood pressure and heart rate, delirium tremens, and hallucinations during acute alcohol withdrawal (Borg et al., 1983; Hawley et al., 1994).

Alcohol tolerance is associated with an impaired ability of NE to stimulate formation of the secondary messenger cyclic adenosine monophosphate (cAMP) in the cerebral cortex. A complete discussion of second messenger systems is beyond the scope of this chapter, but second messengers facilitate neurotransmission through interactions with other neurochemicals. The inability to produce cAMP may therefore alter interactions between NE and other neurotransmitters (e.g., DA). Although the specific subjective and behavioral effects of this process are currently unknown, they are expected to have long-term effects on brain function (Cooper et al., 1996).

Summary

Norepinephrine may help explain the biphasic acute effects of alcohol that have been observed in a number of studies (e.g., Earleywine & Erblich, 1996). Low doses of alcohol contribute to enhanced NE levels, which have an arousal effect, whereas larger doses reduce NE levels, thereby contributing to alcohol's sedative effects. Reductions in NE have also been shown to impair associative learning (Frith et al., 1985), perhaps by inhibiting the formation of conditioned signals of reward or punishment.

Chronic alcohol use results in reduced NE levels and altered secondary messenger systems in the cerebral cortex. These effects may help explain craving and certain neurological deficits that result from chronic alcohol use. Acute withdrawal from chronic alcohol intake is associated with increased NE activity, which contributes to sympathetic arousal (i.e., increased blood pressure and heart rate) as well as the delirious features of withdrawal (i.e., hallucinations, delirium tremens).

Serotonin (5-HT)

Acute effects

Serotonin (5-hydroxytryptamine) is a modulatory neurotransmitter that alters the release and function of other neurochemicals. Serotonin appears to be involved in both behavioral activation/inhibition and higher order information processing (Spoont, 1992). It has been suggested that serotonergic activity serves to inhibit signal propogations that are not sufficiently intense or psychologically important to the organism, thereby enhancing attention to salient cues (Spoont, 1992). Serotonin may therefore be involved in the transmission of such salient cues as those that signal punishment and nonreward (LeMarquand, Pihl, and Benekelfat, 1994a). Consequently, reduced serotonergic functioning has been related to impulsive responding (LeMarquand et al., 1994a). Serotonin is also involved in the regulation of consumption, with increased 5-HT levels contributing to decreased food and fluid intake (Nevo & Hamon, 1995).

Early research suggested alcohol preference was decreased by pharmacological depletion of cerebral 5-HT or elimination of 5-HT neurons (Myers & Veale, 1968), but current evidence supports an inverse relation between 5-HT levels and alcohol self-administration (see Sellers, Higgins, & Sobel, 1992, for review). In both animals and humans, alcohol intake is decreased by pharmacological manipulations that increase available 5-HT at the synapse. Specifically, 5-HT_{1A} receptor agonists (e.g., buspirone) and 5-HT_3 antagonists (e.g., zacopride, MDL 72222) reduce alcohol self-administration (Bruno, 1989; Knapp & Pohorecky, 1992; Toneatto, Romach, Sobell, Somer, & Sellers, 1991). It therefore appears that 5-HT precursors, agonists, and uptake inhibitors decrease alcohol intake by facilitating serotonergic functioning (LeMarquand, Pihl, & Benkelfat, 1994b).

Acute alcohol intake has been associated with increased levels of 5-HT and its metabolite 5-HIAA, suggesting increased serotonergic release or turnover, respectively (LeMarquand et al., 1994b). The effects of alcohol on 5-HT receptor binding, however, are less well understood. As with glutamate and GABA, serotonin has multiple receptor sites and differing effects depending upon the receptor that is activated. Of at least 13 5-HT receptors that have been identified (Petroutka, 1994), the 5-HT_3 receptor is the only one that directly controls ion channels and, consequently, has shown the greatest promise in understanding alcohol's effects (Grant, 1995).

Low doses of alcohol activate the 5-HT_3 receptor (Lovinger & White, 1991; Samson & Harris, 1992) which, in turn, increases DA release in the nucleus accumbens (Jiang, Ahsby, Kasser, & Wang, 1990). Conversely, antagonism of 5-HT_3 receptors attenuates alcohol-related DA release in the nucleus accumbens (Nevo & Hamon, 1995). This dynamic association between serotonergic activity and DA release provides a potential modulatory mechanism for the reinforcing effects of alcohol (Nevo & Hamon, 1995; LeMarquand et al., 1994a).

The use of 5-HT$_3$ antagonists such as ondansetron has provided further support for the role of 5-HT in mediating the subjective and behavioral effects of alcohol. In addition to decreasing alcohol self-administration in both animal and human, antagonism of 5-HT$_3$ receptors by ondansetron attenuated the pleasurable subjective effects of alcohol when administered to healthy human volunteers (Johnson, Campling, Griffiths, & Cowen, 1993; see Grant, 1995, for review). 5-HT$_3$ antagonists therefore appear to reduce the motivation to consume alcohol (see Le, Tomkins, & Sellers, 1996, for review).

Serotonin reuptake inhibitors such as fluoxetin (Prozac) have also demonstrated short-term success in decreasing the alcohol use of problem drinkers (Naranjo & Bremner, 1994; Naranjo, Poulos, Bremner, & Lanctot, 1992). In controlled clinical trials, the short-term efficacy of fluoxetin was found to reduce participants' alcohol use in nondependent (Naranjo & Bremner, 1994) and dependent individuals (Gorelick & Paredes, 1992). These effects, however, were modest (i.e., 14.5–17% decrease in consumption) and transient (see Lejoyeux, 1996, for review). Subsequent trials showed that the efficacy of pharmacotherapy with 5-HT reuptake inhibitors was enhanced when combined with psychotherapy (Naranjo et al., 1992).

Some have suggested that the efficacy of 5-HT reuptake inhibitors results from a general suppression of consummatory behaviors, rather than from a selective effect on alcohol self-administration (Nevo & Hamon, 1995). Conversely, research with 5-HT$_{1A}$ receptor agonists has shown a specific effect on decreased alcohol intake, without altering general food or fluid consumption (Bruno, 1989; see Le et al., 1996, for review). Further research on agents that target specific 5-HT receptors may provide avenues for the development of new pharmacological interventions for alcohol abuse.

Chronic Effects

Whereas acute alcohol administration is clearly associated with increased levels of 5-HT, the effects of chronic alcohol exposure on 5-HT functioning are uncertain. Some studies find a decrease in 5-HT turnover, whereas others suggest an increase in 5-HT with chronic intoxication (LeMarquand et al., 1994a, 1994b). There are similarly mixed research findings on the effects of chronic alcohol exposure on 5-HT receptor density or number. Both increases and decreases have been reported, depending on the particular receptor subtype, experimental procedures, and brain region investigated (see Nevo & Hamon, 1995, for review). A reduction in 5-HT$_{2A}$ receptors in the platelets of male alcoholics was first thought to be a trait marker for alcoholism (Simonsson & Alling, 1988) but was later found to be a state effect associated with alcohol withdrawal (Simonsson, Berglund, Oreland, Moberg, & Alling, 1992).

The development of tolerance to alcohol's effects appears to be related to 5-HT levels. When the 5-HT levels of rats were increased through administration of tryptophan (a serotonin precursor), development of tolerance was enhanced (Le, Khanna, Kalant, & Le Blanc, 1979). Conversely, when brain 5-HT was lowered by facilitating the breakdown of tryptophan, acquisition of tolerance was impaired (Frankel, Khanna, Le Blanc, & Kalant, 1975). Research further found that alcoholics had lower CSF levels of 5-HAAA (a 5-HT metabolite), suggesting that a hypofunctioning serotonin system may be a predisposing factor for alcoholism (Beck et al., 1984).

Summary

With widespread serotonergic projections throughout the brain, alcohol-related changes in serotonin may have significant effects on cognitive processes. Recall that a key function of 5-HT is to inhibit weak or unimportant neural signals and to serve a constraining influence on information flow. Consequently, acute alcohol-related excesses in 5-HT may inhibit all but highly salient signals and inappropriately reduce information flow. Such an effect is consistent with the concept of "alcohol myopia" (Steele & Josephs, 1990) whereby intoxicated individuals are said to focus only on the most salient cues in their environment.

Alcohol-seeking behavior has also been hypothesized as reflecting an attempt to correct deficient levels of 5-HT (Nevo & Hamon, 1995). At least some alcoholics (i.e., those with early onset and histories of violent and impulsive behavior) have lowered 5-HT neurotransmission (LeMarquand et al., 1994b). The consequences of chronic alcohol use on serotonin and associated functions, however, are less well understood. To the extent that 5-HT levels may be reduced with long-term drinking, deficits in information processing, and perhaps in the ability to terminate nonrewarded behavior may be observed (Spoont, 1992). Self-defeating behaviors may eventually be traced to a dysregulation in serotonergic projections to frontal cortex.

Opioid Peptides

Acute Effects

The endorphins, enkephalins, and dynorphins belong to a family of opioid peptides that act on the same receptors as opiate drugs and are known to be involved in analgesia, reward, and reinforcement (Olson, Olson, & Kastin, 1990). Because alcohol demonstrates certain similarities in neuropharmacological response and behavioral effects to opiates (e.g., hypothermia, analgesia), the reinforcing effects of alcohol are thought to be mediated, at least in part, by the opioid peptides (see Nevo & Hamon, 1995, for review).

Acute alcohol exposure increases beta-endorphin and met-enkephalin

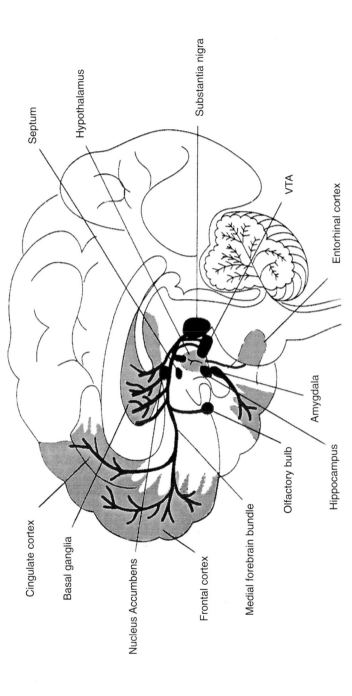

PLATE 11.1. Hypothesized neural system mediating alcohol reinforcement and tolerance. Dopaminergic cell bodies are illustrated in pink and opioid concentrations that overlap with dopamine are illustrated in blue. Neurochemical terminals are represented by lighter shaded areas. GABA is distributed widely throughout this neural system (not shown). Adapted from Julien (1996, p. 478). Copyright 1996 by W.H. Freeman. Adapted by permission.

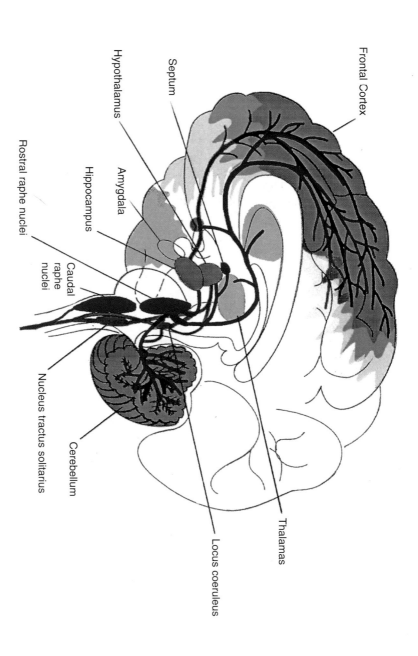

PLATE 11.2. Hypothesized neural system mediating alcohol's effects on cognition and information processing. Serotonergic cell bodies and tracts are illustrated in red, whereas norepinephrine cell bodies and tracts are illustrated in blue. Neurotransmitter terminals are represented by lighter shaded areas, and regions of overlap for the two neurotransmitters are illustrated in purple. Glutamate is widely distributed throughout this neural system (not shown). Adapted from Julien (1996, pp. 380 and 477). Copyright 1996 by W.H. Freeman. Adapted by permission.

Frontal Cortex

Septum

Hypothalamus

Amygdala

Hippocampus

Rostral raphe nuclei

Caudal raphe nuclei

Nucleus tractus solitarius

Cerebellum

Locus coeruleus

Thalamus

levels in the blood of humans and rats *in vitro* (see Weiss & Koob, 1991) and increases beta-endorphin release from the hypothalamus and pituitary gland *in vivo* (Gianoulakis, 1996). Alcohol may also alter the rate of synthesis or processing of opioid peptides, as well as their density in certain brain regions (Gianoulakis, 1996). These acute increases in opioid peptides are thought to contribute to the intoxicating and rewarding effects of alcohol (Gianoulakis, De Waele, & Thavundayil, 1996).

In addition to a direct effect of alcohol on beta-endorphin levels, acetaldehyde (an intermediatory by-product of alcohol) reacts with certain neurotransmitters to form tetrahydroisoquinolines (TIQs). TIQs are structurally similar compounds to the precursors for morphine. Consequently, it has been suggested that alcohol indirectly alters the levels of endogenous opioid peptides through the production of TIQs (see Weiss & Koob, 1991, for review). The alcohol–TIQ hypothesis is supported by findings that the administration of TIQs elicits alcohol self-administration that is reversed by the nonspecific opiate antagonists naloxone and naltrexone.

Two opioid receptor subtypes, mu and delta, are regarded as critical to alcohol's acutely reinforcing effects. Alcohol-related activation of both these receptor subtypes enhances DA activity: delta by directly facilitating DA release in nucleus accumbens, and mu by decreasing the inhibitory effect of GABA neurons on DA activity (Di Chiara, Acquas, & Tanda, 1996; Di Chiara & Imperato, 1988). Thus, the net effect of alcohol-related activation of mu and delta opioid receptors is an increase in available DA. Activation of these opioid receptors may therefore mediate alcohol reward and self-administration by increasing DA levels.

Chronic Effects

Following chronic alcohol exposure, beta-endorphin and met-enkephalin levels are reduced in the rat hypothalamus (Patel & Pohorecky, 1989). Similarly, CSF levels of beta-endorphin are reduced among human alcoholics 3–10 days after detoxification (Genazzani et al., 1982). A reduction in function of the mu opiate receptor subtype (Hoffman, Chung, & Tabakoff, 1984) and an upregulation of the delta receptor are further consequences of chronic alcohol exposure (see Nevo & Hamon, 1995, for review).

The opioid deficiency hypothesis, like the serotonin deficiency hypothesis, suggests that alcoholics drink to compensate for an insufficient number or function of opioid peptides (Nevo & Hamon, 1995). Consistent with this hypothesis, individuals at high risk for alcoholism (based on a two-generation family history of alcoholism) demonstrated lower basal levels of beta-endorphin, but a greater release of beta-endorphin with alcohol than low-risk individuals (Gianoulakis, 1996).

Recent clinical trials have shown that naltrexone, in combination with psychotherapy, reduced the alcohol consumption of problem drinkers (see O'Brien, Volpicelli, & Volpicelli, 1996, for review; Volpicelli, Alterman, Hayashida, & O'Brien, 1992). Consistent with research on the delta and mu opioid receptors, naltrexone may decrease alcohol reinforcement, in part, by preventing alcohol-induced DA release (Acquas, Meloni, & Di Chiara, 1993). Animal research, however, casts doubt on the selective effect of opioid antagonists on alcohol self-administration, suggesting that the suppression of alcohol is secondary to a general inhibition of food and fluid intake (Weiss & Koob, 1991). To date, the precise means whereby opioid antagonists reduce alcohol consumption are unknown.

Summary

Activation of opioid receptor peptides appears to be important for the acutely rewarding effects of drinking (e.g., mild euphoria), whereas reduction in function of the opioid receptors with chronic alcohol abuse may contribute to anhedonia. It is unclear whether alcohol reward is directly mediated by opioid activity, or whether the stimulation of DA by opioid peptides is solely responsible for the rewarding effects of alcohol. Further research on the efficacy of specific opioid receptor antagonists may enhance our understanding of the effects of alcohol on opioid peptides and associated reinforcement.

Summary of Alcohol's Effects on Neurochemicals

As illustrated in Table 11.1, alcohol reliably alters neural transmission by acutely augmenting certain neurotransmitters (i.e., GABA, 5-HT, DA, opioid peptides) and inhibiting others (i.e., glutamate, norepinephrine). Consequently, the overall acute effect of alcohol on neurotransmission is inhibitory, with the resulting effects including mild euphoria, anxiety reduction, sedation, and impaired coordination and cognitive abilities. Conversely, chronic alcohol exposure results in an upregulation of those receptor systems that are inhibited by acute alcohol administration (e.g., NMDA) and diminished neurotransmission in those receptor systems that are augmented by alcohol (e.g., GABA). Consequently, chronic alcohol exposure is associated with development of tolerance, neuronal damage, and cognitive impairments, whereas withdrawal from chronic use is associated with hyperexcitability and seizures. The following section proposes an organizational system whereby the primary neurochemicals (i.e., GABA, DA, 5-HT, NE, glutamate, and opioid peptides), operating via their neural circuitry, may account for alcohol's psychological effects.

NEURAL SYSTEMS THAT MEDIATE
ALCOHOL'S EFFECTS

The various neurotransmitters are not evenly distributed throughout the brain, but are instead concentrated within particular neural pathways or

TABLE 11.1. Acute and Chronic Effects of Alcohol

Neurochemical	Acute effects	Behavioral correlates	Withdrawal and chronic effects	Behavioral correlates
GABA	Increase	Sedation; anxiety reduction	Decrease	Heightened anxiety
Glutamate	Decrease	Impaired memory formation	Increase	Seizures
Dopamine	Increase	Reward; exploratory behavior; attention	Decrease	Craving; dysphoria
Norepinephrine	Increase[a]	Arousal	Decrease[b]	Cognitive deficits; craving
	Decrease[a]	Sedation; decreased anxiety; impaired associative learning	Increase[b]	Increased blood pressure and heart rate; delirium tremens
Serotonin	Increase	Behavioral activation; attention to salient cues	Decrease[c]	Deficits in cognitive processing
			Increase[c]	Tolerance
Opioid peptides	Increase	Reward; self-administration of alcohol	Decrease	Anhedonia

[a]At low doses, alcohol increases norepinephrine, whereas at higher doses, alcohol decreases norepinephrine.
[b]Chronic alcohol use is associated with decreased norepinephrine levels, whereas acute withdrawal from chronic alcohol use is associated with increased norepinephrine levels.
[c]Alcohol increases or decreases serotonin activity depending on the receptor subtype and brain region involved.

systems. These neural systems, composed of neuroanatomical structures densely innervated with a particular type or types of neurotransmitters, provide the pathways through which neurochemicals affect neuronal communication and subsequent behavioral experience.

Although there are many converging and intermingling neural pathways, there is reason to believe that relatively distinct neural response systems mediate many of the acute and chronic effects of psychoactive drugs. Separate neural mechanisms may, for example, mediate the effects of alcohol on arousal/sedation and on judgment/reasoning.

From studies of anxiety and benzodiazepines, Gray (1990, 1991) hypothesized separate neural systems that mediate behavioral activation and behavioral inhibition. Not surprisingly, the behavioral activation system is associated with exploratory, appetitive behavior and would correspond to the dopaminergic, reward pathways. The behavioral inhibition system includes the septum–hippocampus and other memory-related structures that

Gray suggested inhibit responses when environmental cues deviate from those expected. Gray's behavioral inhibition system might correspond, for example, with those neural structures innervated by serotonin.

We propose that two relatively distinct neuroanatomical and neurochemical response systems mediate many of the psychological effects of alcohol. The first system (see Plate 11.1), involves DA, opioid peptides, and GABA to account for the positive and negative reinforcing effects of drinking and the development of tolerance to these effects. The second system (see Plate 11.2) involves serotonin, glutamate, and norepinephrine to account for alterations in cognitive processes and impaired associative learning, which may help explain alcohol-seeking behavior in the absence of drug reinforcement.

Alcohol Reinforcement and Tolerance

Classic indices of reinforcement are euphoria and anxiety reduction. Euphoria is thought to provide positive reinforcement or reward, whereas anxiety reduction provides negative reinforcement. DA and opioid peptides are central to the rewarding effects of alcohol, whereas alcohol-enhanced GABA mediates the locomotor depressant and anxiolytic effects of drinking.

The limbic area is well established as the center of drug reward (Wise, 1990). Dopaminergic neurons of the mesolimbic region begin in the ventral tegmental area (VTA) and have projections into the nucleus accumbens, amygdala, olfactory bulb, and hippocampus. The mesocortical DA projections also link the VTA with prefrontal cortex, cingulate, and entorhinal areas (Cooper et al., 1996). Whereas mesolimbic DA is involved in emotional experience and reward, prefrontal DA is believed to mediate attention (Wolkowitz et al., 1985). Thus, activation of the mesocorticolimbic system and DA release may mediate alcohol self-administration via its positively rewarding properties (Weiss & Koob, 1991; Weiss et al., 1993), as well as through enhanced attention to, and memories for, cues that signal reward. Brain imaging techniques confirm the activation of mesocorticolimbic regions at low doses of alcohol (Williams-Hemby & Porrino, 1994).

Concentrations of neurons containing opioid peptides are also found in the VTA and other limbic structures (Gianoulakis, 1996; Harris, Brodie, & Dunwiddie, 1992). Although some have questioned whether DA and opioid reinforcement operate through the same or different neural mechanisms, there is considerable evidence to suggest the two neurochemicals work together to produce mild euphoria and pleasant mood alterations that motivate alcohol-seeking behavior (Harris et al., 1992).

Positive reinforcement mediated by DA and opioid peptides is complemented by the negative reinforcement provided by GABAergic systems. People often report they drink alcohol to relax or to relieve anxiety, and these GABA-mediated anxiolytic effects contribute to alcohol-seeking behavior. GABA, however, is not limited to anxiety reduction. Like 5-HT, GABA is widely distributed across a number of circuits in the brain, including the hippocampus, septum, cerebral cortex, and cerebellum. Consequently, in addition to mediating alcohol's locomotor depressant, muscle relaxation, and anxiety-reduction effects, the GABAergic system functions to reduce overall arousal and to temper emotional responses (Bond & Lader, 1979). Through GABA activation, alcohol may thus exert its more general effect on mood modulation.

Cognition and Information-Processing Systems

Many of the complex cognitive and behavioral consequences of alcohol use and abuse cannot be explained by a simple reinforcement model. For example, drinking is often maintained in the absence of reward (Berridge & Robinson, 1995). Moreover, alcohol expectancy or cues associated with alcohol produce important neurochemical reactions without actual drug administration. Consequently, we propose a second neurochemical response system whereby alcohol affects learning and memory, therefore mediating alcohol-seeking behavior via alterations in information processing. With concentrations of glutamate, norepinephrine, and serotonin, the proposed system comprises, primarily, the hippocampus, septum, amygdala, locus coeruleus, raphe nuclei, frontal cortex, and cerebellum.

The molecular foundations of learning are found within the glutamatergic system, with glutamate and the NMDA receptor necessary for long-term potentiation (LTP). This is particularly true in the hippocampus, a region known to be involved in learning and memory (Blitzer et al., 1990; Collingridge & Bliss, 1987). Alcohol intoxication inhibits NMDA receptor function and, consequently, impairs memorial functions. Whereas serotonin and norepinephrine appear to be highly sensitive to low doses of alcohol, glutamate and the NMDA receptor are sensitive to higher doses (e.g., Grant & Colombo, 1993). Thus, the amnesic effects of high doses of alcohol are thought to be mediated by impairments in glutamatergic functioning and associated LTP.

Recent evidence also documents the importance of NMDA receptor function in associative learning, with dose-dependent alcohol impairment evident in the formation of conditioned associations. As a consequence, memories for conditioned associations to low doses of alcohol may be unaffected, whereas memories for conditioned associations to high doses of alcohol may show considerable impairment. Thus, the alcohol–NMDA link may help explain the durability of positive alcohol expectancies in the face of substantial negative consequences (Brown, Goldman, & Christiansen, 1985).

Norepinephrine, implicated in the regulation of arousal states and behavioral tendencies, also contributes to the proposed response system mediating learning and memory. Noradrenergic cell bodies are densely clustered in the locus coeruleus, with five major tracts (including dorsal and medial forebrain bundles) innervating thalamic and hypothalamic nuclei, the olfactory bulb, cerebellar cortex, cerebral cortex, and hippocampus. These brain structures are involved broadly in the regulation of behavior and emotion, motor coordination, thinking, reasoning, and memory. Even the cerebellum, long thought to mediate only motor behavior, has recently been implicated in sensory discrimination (Gao et al., 1996) and cognition (Fiez, 1996).

Decreased NE impairs associative learning and reduces the individual's ability to distinguish relevant from irrelevant stimuli. Consequently, alcohol's acute suppression of NE is hypothesized as contributing to impulsivity and a failure to benefit from previous experiences. A compensatory overreactivity in noradrenergic functioning with chronic alcohol exposure may result in cognitive deficits and the arousal associated with acute withdrawal. Alterations in the NE system may therefore contribute to the cognitive impairments that are often associated with both acute intoxication and chronic use.

Serotonin is the third hypothesized component in the neurochemical response system that governs alcohol's effects on cognitive processes. Serotonergic neurons originate predominately in the raphe nuclei and have widespread projections via the dorsal and median raphe tracts. Following along the medial forebrain bundle, the dorsal raphe nuclei innervate the amygdala, nucleus accumbens, and basal ganglia, whereas the median raphe nuclei innervate the septum, hippocampus, and cingulate cortex (Spoont, 1992). Together, these serotonergic tracts serve a broad homeostatic function (Cooper et al., 1996). Extensive 5-HT projections throughout the brain provide a modulatory role in coordinating complex sensory and motor patterns, and constraining information flow (Spoont, 1992).

The increase in 5-HT associated with acute alcohol intake may alter the organism's attentional processes and contribute to a focus on only the most salient cues when intoxicated. Chronic alcohol exposure has been associated with both increases and decreases in 5-HT levels, which may, respectively, mediate cognitive deficits and craving for alcohol. Through an effect on 5-HT, alcohol can have far-ranging effects on complex cognitive processes that are involved in social behaviors. For example, decreased 5-HT is associated with increased sexual behavior and aggression (Spoont, 1992).

In summary, alcohol-seeking behavior is mediated by at least two neurochemical systems. Although we suggested these systems might be organized according to simple reinforcement functions and effects on higher order cognitive processes, shared neuroanatomical structures (e.g., amygdala, cerebral cortex) make it impossible to completely separate the two systems. Moreover, functional relations among the neurotransmitters make it unlikely that a single neurotransmitter will be identified as the "cause" of alcohol dependence. For example, serotonergic neurons demonstrate a reciprocal functional relation with the noradrenergic system whereby lesions in the raphe nuclei result in increased NE, whereas lesions in the locus coeruleus result in an increase in 5-HT (Le, Khanna, Kalant, & LeBlanc, 1981). Consequently, drugs that alter 5-HT also impact the noradrenergic system. Research must therefore continue to explore the reciprocal, inverse, and facilitory relations among the many neurochemicals involved in alcohol's effects.

Finally, the hypothesized neural systems are likely to shift in prominence as alcohol use proceeds to alcohol abuse and dependence. For naive drinkers, the primary reinforcement system dominates in the absence of conditioned alcohol experiences. As social drinkers garner alcohol experiences, both the primary reinforcement system and the conditioned associations of the information-processing system govern the use of alcohol. As the individual develops dependence on alcohol, however, a dysregulation may occur in the two neural response systems. Tolerance to the reinforcing effects of alcohol is combined with impaired functioning of the information-processing system. As a consequence, the powerful craving for alcohol overrides judgment, and use is continued despite significant negative consequences. This shift may contribute to alcohol-seeking behavior in the absence of significant reinforcement and is akin to the distinction made by Berridge and Robinson (1995) in "wanting versus liking."

SUMMARY AND CONCLUSIONS

Virtually everything we do, think, feel, and consume is associated with changes in neurochemicals. The magnitude and unique pattern of responses elicited by psychoactive drugs such as alcohol, however, make them particularly interesting. Whereas it is seductive to believe a "magic bullet" will be discovered to correct neurochemical imbalances and thereby eliminate alcohol abuse and dependence, many complex social and behavioral aspects of alcohol use cannot be readily explained by neurochemical actions. Multidisciplinary approaches that take into account both the neurochemical and social aspects of alcohol abuse hold the greatest promise for success.

Psychologists, neuroscientists, and pharmacologists must work together to relate neurochemical processes to the psychological effects of alcohol on people. Only through multidisciplinary dialogue and an appreciation of the molecular and molar aspects of alcohol's effects will we develop effective treatment and prevention strategies. Such strategies will result from an understanding of the effects of alcohol at all levels: from cells, to neural systems, to human behavior.

GLOSSARY OF TERMS

Affinity: A measure of the binding strength of endogenous and exogenous substances, determined by the structure and charge of the molecules.

Agonist: Substance that mimics or increases the activity of neurochemicals.

Antagonist: Substance that decreases or blocks the activity of neurochemicals.

Dopamine: A neurotransmitter that may mediate pleasurable experience or attention to salient cues, and acts indirectly by changing the activity of other neurotransmitters.

Depolarization: A reduction in membrane potential that causes an increase in a cell's ability to generate a transmittable signal.

Event-related potentials: Time-locked neuroelectric signals that allow the observation of cellular activation in response to discrete stimuli.

Excitotoxic damage/Excitotoxicity: Neuronal death related to overactivity of excitatory neurotransmitters, for example, glutamate.

GABA (gamma-aminobutyric acid): The major inhibitory amino acid neurotransmitter in the central nervous system.

Glutamate: The major excitatory amino acid neurotransmitter in the brain that is associated with three primary receptor types: NMDA, AMPA, and kainate.

In vitro studies: Methods to examine cellular and neurotransmitter activity in nonintact organisms (e.g., dissociated cells, cell cultures, or brain slices).

Inverse agonist: Substance that produces effects opposite to those of the particular neurochemical to which it is compared.

In vivo studies: Methods to examine cellular and neurotransmitter activity in live, typically anesthetized animals, or to measure neurotransmitter metabolites in the cerebrospinal fluid of humans.

Ligand-gated ion channel: Ion channel that is part of a receptor protein complex and is altered (e.g., opened) when a neurotransmitter binds to it.

Lipids: Any of the free fatty acid fractions in the cell. Lipids are stored in the body and serve as energy reserve (e.g., cholesterol, fatty acids, triglycerides).

Long-term potentiation: An increase in the strength of synaptic transmission due to repetitive high frequency synaptic activation; possible molecular mechanism of memory formation.

Metabolite: By-products of neurochemical activity through which levels of that substance are estimated (e.g., in cerebrospinal fluid).

Microdialysis: A procedure in which a tube is implanted in a particular brain region so that neurotransmitter levels may be measured in an awake, freely moving animal.

Neurochemical: Term that includes both neurotransmitters and other chemicals typically associated with neurotransmission.

Neurons: Cells in the nervous system.

Neuropeptide: Small molecule made up of amino acids; found in the nervous system and acts at some type of recognition site (e.g., opioid peptides). Some neuropeptides function as neurotransmitters and some do not.

Neurotransmitter: Chemical that is released from neurons and triggers a series of chemical and electrical impulses; the chemical messengers of the brain.

Norepinephrine/Noradrenaline: Neurochemical that is the metabolic by-product of dopamine and is responsible for the inhibition of the spontaneous firing rate of affected neurons and the subsequent increase of the cell's responsiveness to other inputs.

Positron emission tomography (PET): A noninvasive tracer technique that examines *in vivo* concentrations of positron-labeled compounds in the brain.

Potentiation: When an electrical charge or a difference in potential occurs and the neuron is activated.

Precursors: A chemical or compound that leads to the production of another chemical or compound (e.g., tryptophan is a precursor of serotonin).

Proteins: A large group of naturally occurring, complex, organic, nitrogenous compounds composed of combinations of amino acids.

Release: When a neurochemical is discharged from a neuron.

Reuptake: When a neurochemical is released into the synaptic cleft and then is taken back up into the neuron from which it was released.

Serotonin: Neurotransmitter that alters the release and function of other neurochemicals and appears to be involved in both behavioral activation/inhibition and higher-order information processing.

Synapse: Junction where two neurons meet.

Synthesis: Formation of complex chemical compounds such as neurochemicals from simpler units of amino acids.

Tetrahydroisoquinolines (TIQs): Compounds that are structurally related to morphine precursors and are formed by an interaction between monoamine neurotransmitters and acetaldehyde (by-product in the breakdown of alcohol).

Uptake inhibitors: Chemicals or compounds which inhibit the reuptake of a neurochemical, thus making more of that particular neurochemical available in the synapse.

Voltage-gated ion channel: Ion channels that respond to changes in electrical potential.

ACKNOWLEDGMENT

We are grateful to Reuben Gonzales and Tim Schallert for comments on drafts of this chapter. Writing of this chapter was partially funded by grants from the National Institute of Alcohol Abuse and Alcoholism (R29AA09135 and 5T32AA07471).

REFERENCES

Aquas, E., Meloni, M., & Di Chiara, G. (1993). Blockade of d-opioid receptors in the nucleus accumbens prevents ethanol- induced stimulation of dopamine release. *European Journal of Pharmacology, 230,* 239–241.

Aguayo, L. G. (1990). Ethanol potentiates the GABA$_A$-activated Cl$^-$ current in mouse hippocampal and cortical neurons. *European Journal of Pharmacology, 187,* 127–130.

Allan, A. M., & Harris, R. A. (1987). Acute and chronic ethanol treatments alter GABA receptor-operated chloride channels. *Pharmacology, Biochemistry, and Behavior, 27*, 665–670.

Altura, B. M., Altura, B. T., Zhang, A., & Zakhari, S. (1996). Effects of alcohol on overall brain metabolism. In H. Begleiter & B. Kissin (Eds.), *The pharmacology of alcohol and alcohol dependence* (pp. 145–180). Oxford, UK: Oxford University Press.

Beck, O., Borg, S., Edman, G., Fyro, B., Oxenstierna, G., & Sedvall, G. (1984). 5-hydroxytryptophol in human cerebrospinal fluid: Conjugation, concentration gradient, relationship to 5-hydroxyindoleactic acid, and influence of hereditary factors. *Journal of Neurochemistry, 43*, 58–61.

Berridge, K. C., & Robinson, T. E. (1995). The mind of an addicted brain: Neural sensitization of wanting versus liking. *Current Directions in Psychological Science, 4*, 71–76.

Blitzer, R. D., Gil, O., & Landau, E. M. (1990). Long-term potentiation in rat hippocampus is inhibited by low concentrations of ethanol. *Brain Research, 537*, 203–208.

Blum, K., Noble, E. P., Sheridan, P. J., Montgomery, A., Ritchie, T., Jagadeeswaran, P., Nogami, H., Briggs, A. H., & Cohn, J. B. (1990). Allelic association of human dopamine D_2 receptor gene in alcoholism. *Journal of American Medical Association, 263*, 2055–2060.

Bolos, A. M., Dean, M., Lucas-Derse, S., Ramsburg, M., Brown, G. L., & Goldman, D. (1990). Population and pedigree studies reveal a lack of association between the dopamine D_2 receptor gene and alcoholism. *Journal of American Medical Association, 264*, 3156–3160.

Bond, A., & Lader, M. L. (1979). Benzodiazepine and aggression. In M. Sandler (Ed.), *Psychopharmacology of aggression* (pp. 173–182). New York: Raven Press.

Borg, S., Czarnecka, A., Kvande, H., Mossberg, D., & Sedvall, G. (1983). Clinical conditions and concentrations of MOPEG in the cerebrospinal fluid and urine of male alcoholic patients during withdrawal. *Alcoholism: Clinical and Experimental Research, 7*, 411–415.

Borg, S., Kvande, H., & Sedvall, G. (1983). Monoamine metabolites in lumbar cerebro-spinal fluid and urine in alcoholic patients before and after treatment with disulfiram. *Alcohol and Alcoholism, 18*, 61–65.

Brown, L. M., Leslie, S. W., & Gonzales, R. A. (1991). The effects of chronic ethanol exposure on N-methyl-D-aspartate-stimulated overflow of [^{3}H]catecholamines from rat brain. *Brain Research, 547*, 289–294.

Brown, S. A., Goldman, M. S., & Christiansen, B. A. (1985). Do alcohol expectancies mediate drinking patterns of adults? *Journal of Consulting and Clinical Psychology, 53*, 512–519.

Brown, Z. W., & Amit, Z. (1977). The effects of selective catecholamine depletions by 6-hydroxydopamine on ethanol preference in rats. *Neuroscience Letters, 5*, 333–336.

Browning, M. D., Hoffer, B. J., & Dunwiddie, T. V. (1992). Alcohol, memory, and molecules. *Alcohol, Health and Research World, 16*, 280–284.

Bruno, F. (1989). Buspirone in the treatment of alcoholic patients. *Psychopathology, 22*(Suppl. 1), 49–59.

Buck, K. J., & Harris, A. (1991). Neuroadaptive responses to chronic ethanol. *Alcoholism: Clinical and Experimental Research, 15*, 460–470.

Chandler, L. J., Newsom, H., Sumners, C., & Crews, F. T. (1993). Chronic ethanol exposure potentiates NMDA in cerebral cortical neurons. *Journal of Neurochemistry, 60,* 1578–1581.

Choi, D. W. (1992). Excitotoxic cell death. *Journal of Neurobiology, 23,* 1261–1276.

Collingridge, G. L., & Bliss, T. V. P. (1987). NMDA receptors-their role in long-term potentiation. *Trends in Neurosciences, 10,* 288–293.

Cooper, J. R., Bloom, F. E., & Roth, R. H. (1996). *The biochemical basis of neuropharmacology* (7th ed.). Oxford, UK: Oxford University Press.

Davis, W. M., Smith, S. G., & Werner, T. E. (1978). Noradrenergic role in self-administration of ethanol. *Pharmacology, Biochemistry, and Behavior, 9,* 369–374.

De Witte, P. (1996). Role of neurotransmitters in alcohol dependence: Animal research. *Alcohol and Alcoholism, 31*(Suppl. 1), 13–16.

Diana, M., Pistis, M., Carboni, S., Gessa, G. L., & Rossetti, Z. L. (1993). Profound decrement of mesolimbic dopaminergic neuronal activity during ethanol withdrawal syndrome in rats: Electrophysiological and biochemical evidence. *Proceedings of the National Academy of Sciences of the USA, 90,* 7966–7969.

Di Chiara, G. (1990). *In-vivo* brain dialysis of neurotransmitters. *Trends in Pharmacological Science, 11,* 116–121.

Di Chiara, G. (1995). The role of dopamine in drug abuse viewed from the perspective of its role in motivation. *Drug and Alcohol Dependence, 38,* 95–137.

DiChiara, G., Acquas, E., & Tanda, G. (1996). Ethanol as a neurochemical surrogate of conventional reinforcers: The dopamine–opioid link. *Alcohol, 13,* 13–17.

Di Chiara, G., & Imperato, A. (1988). Drugs abused by humans preferentially increase synaptic dopamine concentrations in the mesolimbic system of freely moving rats. *Proceedings of the National Academy of Sciences of the USA, 85,* 5274–5278.

Earlywine, M., & Erblich, J. (1996). A confirmed factor structure for the biphasic alcohol effects scale. *Experimental and Clinical Psychopharmacology, 4,* 107–113.

Fiez, J. A. (1996). Cerebellar contributions to cognition. *Neuron, 16,* 13–15.

Frankel, D., Khanna, J. M., LeBlanc, A. E., & Kalant, H. (1975). Effect of *p*-chlorophenylalanine on the acquisition of tolerance to ethanol and pentobarbital. *Psychopharmacology, 44,* 246–252.

Frith, C. D., Dowdy, J., Ferrier, I. N., & Crow, T. J. (1985). Selective impairment of paired associate learning after administration of a centrally-acting adrenergic agonist (clonidine). *Psychopharmacology, 87,* 490–493.

Gao, J.-H., Parsons, L. M., Bower, J. M., Xiong, J., Li, J., & Fox, P. T. (1996). Cerebellum implicated in sensory acquisition and discrimination rather than motor control. *Science, 272,* 545-547.

Gejman, P. V., Ram, A., Gelernter, J., Friedman, E., Cao, Q., Pickar, D., Blum, K., Noble, E. P., Kranzler, H. R., O'Malley, S., Hamer, D. H., Whitsitt, F., Rao, P., DeLisi, L. E., Virkkunen, M., Linnoila, M., Goldman, D., & Gershon, E. S. (1994). No structural mutation in the dopamine D_2 receptor gene in alcoholism or schizophrenia: Analysis using denaturing gradient gel electrophoresis. *Journal of the American Medical Association, 271,* 204–208.

Gennazzani, A. R., Nappi, G., Facchinetti, F., Mazella, G. L., Parrin, D., Sinforiani, E., Petraglia, F., & Savoldi, F. (1982). Central deficiency of *ß*-endorphin in alcohol addicts. *Journal of Clinical Endocrinology and Metabolism, 55,* 583–586.

Gessa, L. G., Muntoni, F., Collu, M., Vargiu, L., & Mereu, G. (1985). Low doses of ethanol activate dopaminergic neurons in the ventral tegmental area. *Brain Research, 348,* 201–203.

Gianoulakis, C. (1996). Implications of endogenous opioids and dopamine in alcoholism: Human and basic science studies. *Alcohol and Alcoholism, 31*(Suppl.), 33–42.

Gianoulakis, C., De Waele, J.-P., & Thavundayil, J. (1996). Implication of the endogenous opioid system in excessive ethanol consumption. *Alcohol, 13,* 19–23.

Gonzales, R. A., & Woodward, J. J. (1990). Ethanol inhibits N-methyl-D-aspartate [³H]norepinephrine from rat cortical slices. *Journal of Pharmacology and Experimental Therapeutics, 253,* 1138–1144.

Gorelick, D. A., & Paredes, A. (1992). Effect of fluoxetine on alcohol consumption in male alcoholics. *Alcoholism: Clinical and Experimental Research, 16,* 261–265.

Grant, K. A. (1995). The role of 5-HT₃ receptors in drug dependence. *Drug and Alcohol Dependence, 38,* 155–171.

Grant, K. A., & Colombo, G. (1993). Substitution of the 5-HT1 agonist trifluoromethylphenylpiperazine (TFMPP) for the discriminative stimulus effects of ethanol: Effect of training dose. *Psychopharmacology, 113,* 26–30.

Grant, K. A., Snell, L. D., Rogawaski, M. A., Thurkauf, A., Tabakoff, B. (1992). Comparison of the effects of the uncompetitive N-methyl-D-aspartate antagonist (+)-5-aminocarbonyl-10,11-dihydro-5H-dibenzo[a,d]cyclohepten-5,10-imine (ADCI) with its structural analogs dizocilpine (MK-801) and carbamazeppine on ethanol withdrawal seizures. *Journal of Pharmacology and Experimental Therapeutics, 260,* 1017–1022.

Grant, K. A., Valverius, P., Hudspith, M., & Tabakoff, B. (1990). Ethanol withdrawal seizures and the NMDA receptor complex. *European Journal of Pharmacology, 176,* 289–296.

Grant, S., London, E. D., Newlin, D. B., Villemagne, V. L., Liu, X., Contoreggi, C., Phillips, R. L., Kimes, A. S., & Margolin, A. (1996). Activation of memory circuits during cue-elicited cocaine craving. *Proceedings of the National Academy of Sciences USA, 93,* 12040–12045.

Gray, J. A. (1990). Brain systems that mediate both emotion and cognition. *Cognition and Emotion, 4,* 269–288.

Gray, J. A. (1991). Neural systems, emotion, and personality. In J. Madden, IV (Ed.), *Neurobiology of learning, emotion, and affect* (pp. 273–306). New York: Raven Press.

Harris, R. A., Brodie, M. S., & Dunwiddie, T. V. (1992). Possible substrates of ethanol reinforcement: GABA and dopamine. In P. W. Kalivas & H. H. Samson (Eds.), *Annals of the New York academy of sciences: Vol. 654. The neurobiology of drug and alcohol addiction* (pp. 61–69). New York: New York Academy of Sciences.

Hawley, R. J., Nemeroff, C. B., Bissette, G., Guidotti, A., Rawlings, R., & Linnoila, M. (1994). Neurochemical correlates of sympathetic activation during severe alcohol withdrawal. *Alcoholism: Clinical and Experimental Research, 18,* 1312–1316.

Heinz, A., Sander, T., Harms, H., Finckh, U., Kuhn, S., Dufeu, P., Dettling, M., Graf, K., Rolfs, A., Rommelspacher, H., & Schmidt, L. G. (1996). Lack of allelic association of dopamine D_1 and D_2 (*TacIA*) receptor gene polymorphisms with reduced dopaminergic sensitivity in alcoholism. *Alcoholism: Clinical and Experimental Research, 20,* 1109–1113.

Hoffman, P. L., Chung, C. T., & Tabakoff, B. (1984). Effects of ethanol, temperature, and endogenous regulatory factors on the characteristics of striatal opiate receptors. *Journal of Neurochemistry, 43,* 1003–1010.

Humeniuk, R. E., White, J. M., & Ong, J. (1993). The role of $GABA_B$ receptors in mediating the stimulatory effects of ethanol in mice. *Psychopharmacology, 111,* 219–224.

Hunt, W. A. (1983). The effect of ethanol on GABAergic transmission. *Neuroscience and Biobehavioral Reviews, 7,* 87–95.

Hunt, W. A. (1993). Neuroscience research: How it has contributed to our understanding of alcohol abuse and alcoholism: A review. *Alcoholism: Clinical and Experimental Research, 17,* 1055–1065.

Huttunen, P. (1991). Microdialysis of extracellular noradrenaline in the hippocampus of the rat after long-term alcohol intake. *Brain Research, 560,* 225–228.

Imperato, A., & Di Chiara, G. (1986). Preferential stimulation of dopamine release in the nucleus accumbens of freely moving rats by ethanol. *Journal of Pharmacology and Experimental Therapeutics, 239,* 219–228.

Iorio, K. R., Tabakoff, B., & Hoffman., P. L. (1993). Glutamate-induced neurotoxicity is increased in cerebellar granule cells exposed chronically to ethanol. *European Journal of Pharmacology, 248,* 209–212.

Johnson, B. A., Campling, G. M., Griffiths, P., & Cowen, P. J. (1993). Attenuation of some alcohol-induced mood changes and the desire to drink by 5-HT_3 receptor blockade: A preliminary study in healthy male volunteers. *Psychopharmacology, 112,* 142–144.

Julien, R. M. (1996). *A primer of drug action.* New York: Freeman.

June, H. L., Lin, M., Greene, T. L., Lewis, M. J., & Murphy, J. M. (1995). Effects of negative modulators of GABAergic efficacy on ethanol intake: Correlation of biochemical changes with pharmacological effect using a behavior paradigm. *Experimental and Clinical Psychopharmacology, 3,* 252–260.

Khanna, J. M., Weiner, J., Kalant, H., Chau, A., & Shah, G. (1992). Ketamine blocks chronic but not acute tolerance to ethanol. *Pharmacology, Biochemistry, and Behavior, 42,* 347–350.

Kitai, S. T., & Surmeier, D. (1993). Cholinergic and dopaminergic modulation of potassium conductances in neostriatal neurons. *Advances in Neurology, 60,* 40–52.

Knapp, D. J., & Pohorecky, L. A. (1992). Zacopride, a 5-HT_3 receptor antagonist, reduces voluntary ethanol consumption in rats. *Pharmacology, Biochemistry, and Behavior, 41,* 847–850.

Koob, G. F. (1992). Neural mechanisms of drug reinforcement. In P. W. Kalivas & H. H. Samson (Eds.), *The neurobiology of drug and alcohol addiction* (pp. 171–191). New York: New York Academy of Sciences.

Le, A. D., Khanna, J. M., Kalant, H., & LeBlanc, A. E. (1979). Effect of tryptophan on the acquisition of tolerance to ethanol-induced motor impairment and hypothermia. *Psychopharmacology, 61,* 125–129.

Le, A. D., Khanna, J. M., Kalant, H., & LeBlanc, A. E. (1981). Effect of modification of brain serotonin (5-HT), norepinephrine (NE) and dopamine (DA) on ethanol tolerance. *Psychopharmacology, 75,* 231–235.

Le, A. D., Tomkins, D. M., & Sellers, E. M. (1996). Use of serotonin (5-HT) and opiate-based drugs in the pharmacotherapy of alcohol dependence: An overview of the preclinical data. *Alcohol and Alcoholism, 31*(Suppl. 1), 27–32.

Lee, A. G. (1991). Lipids and their effects on membrane proteins: Evidence against a role for fluidity. *Progress in Lipid Research, 30,* 323–348.

Lejoyeux, M. (1996). Use of serotonin (5-hydroxytryptamine) reuptake inhibitors in the treatment of alcoholism. *Alcohol and Alcoholism, 31*(Suppl. 1), 69–75.

LeMarquand, D., Pihl, R. O., & Benkelfat, C. (1994a). Serotonin and alcohol intake, abuse, and dependence: Findings of animal studies. *Biological Psychiatry, 36,* 395–421.

LeMarquand, D., Pihl, R. O., & Benkelfat, C. (1994b). Serotonin and alcohol intake, abuse, and dependence: Clinical evidence. *Biological Psychiatry, 36,* 326–337.

Leshner, A. I. (1997). Addiction is a brain disease, and it matters. *Science, 278,* 45–47.

Lewis, M. J. (1991). Alcohol effects on brain-stimulation reward: Blood alcohol concentration and site specificity. In R. E. Meyer, G. F. Koob, M. J. Lewis, & S. M. Paul (Eds.), *Neuropharmacology of ethanol* (pp. 164–178). Boston: Birkhauser.

Lewis, M. J. (1996). Alcohol reinforcement and neuropharmacological therapeutics. *Alcohol and Alcoholism, 31*(Suppl. 1), 17–25.

Lister, R. G., Eckardt, M. J., & Weingartner, H. (1987). Ethanol intoxication and memory: Recent developments and new directions. In M. Galanter (Ed.), *Recent developments in alcoholism* (Vol. 5, pp. 111–126). New York: Plenum.

Lovinger, D. M. (1993). Excitotoxicity and alcohol-related brain damage. *Alcoholism: Clinical and Experimental Research, 17,* 19–27.

Lovinger, D. M., & White, G. (1991). Ethanol potentiation of 5-hydroxytryptamine$_3$ receptor mediated ion current in neuroblastoma cells and isolated adult mammalian neurons. *Molecular Pharmacology, 40,* 263–270.

Mereu, G. P., Fadda, F., & Gessa, G. L. (1984). Ethanol stimulates the firing rate of nigral dopaminergic neurons in unanesthetized rats. *Brain Research, 292,* 62–69.

Morrisett, R. A., Rezvani, A. H., Overstreet, D., Janowsky, D. S., Wilson, W. A., & Swartzwelder, H. A. (1990). MK-801 potently inhibits alcohol withdrawal seizures in rats. *European Journal of Pharmacology, 176,* 103–105.

Morrisett, R. A., & Swartzwelder, H. S. (1993). Attenuation of hippocampal long-term potentiation by ethanol: A path-clamp analysis of glutamatergic and GABAergic mechanism. *Journal of Neuroscience, 13,* 2264–2272.

Morrow, L., Montpied, P., & Paul, S. M. (1991). Ethanol and the GABA$_A$ receptor-gated chloride ion channel. In R. E. Meyer, G. F. Koob, M. J. Lewis, & S. M. Paul (Eds.), *Neuropharmacology of ethanol* (pp. 50–76). Boston: Birkhauser.

Myers, R. D., & Veale, W. L. (1968). Alcohol preference in the rat: Reduction following depletion of brain serotonin. *Science, 160,* 1469–1471.

Naranjo, C. A., & Bremner, K. E. (1994). Serotonin-altering medications and desire, consumption and effects of alcohol-treatment implications. In B. Jansson, H. Jornvall, U. Rydberg, L. Terenius, & B. L. Vallee (Eds.), *Toward a molecular basis of alcohol use and abuse* (pp. 209–219). Basel, Switzerland: Birkhauser Verlag.

Naranjo, C. A., Poulos, C. X., Bremner, K. E., & Lanctot, K. (1992). Citalopram decreases desirability, liking, and consumption of alcohol in alcohol-dependent drinkers. *Clinical Pharmacology and Therapeutics, 51,* 729–739.

Nevo, I., & Hamon, M. (1995). Neurotransmitter and neuromodulatory mechanisms involved in alcohol abuse and alcoholism. *Neurochemistry International, 26,* 305–336.

O'Brien, C. P., Volpicelli, L. A., & Volpicelli, J. R. (1996). Naltrexone in the treatment of alcoholism: A clinical review. *Alcohol, 13,* 35–39.

Olson, G. A., Olson, R. D., & Kastin, A. J. (1990). Endogenous opiates: 1989. *Peptides, 11,* 1277–1304.

Otmakhova, N. A., & Lisman, J. E. (1998). D1/D5 dopamine receptors inhibit depotentiation at CA1 synapses via cAMP-dependent mechanism. *Journal of Neuroscience, 18,* 1270–1279.

Ozdemir, V., Bremner, K. E., & Naranjo, C. A. (1994). Treatment of alcohol withdrawal syndrome. *Annals of Medicine, 26,* 101–105.

Patel, V. A., & Pohorecky, L. A. (1989). Acute and chronic ethanol treatment on beta-endorphin and catecholamine levels. *Alcohol, 6,* 59–63.

Peoples, R. W., Li, C., & Weight, F. F. (1996). Lipid vs. protein theories of alcohol action in the nervous system. *Annual Review of Pharmacology and Toxicology, 36,* 185–201.

Petroutka, S. J. (1994). 5-Hydroxytryptamine receptors. In S. J. Petroutka (Ed.), *Handbook of receptors and channels* (pp. 209–236). Ann Arbor, MI: CRC Press.

Porjesz, B., & Begleiter, H. (1996). Effects of alcohol on electrophysiological activity of the brain. In H. Begleiter & B. Kissin (Eds.), *The pharmacology of alcohol and alcohol dependence* (pp. 207–247). Oxford, UK: Oxford University Press.

Rabe, C. S., & Tabakoff, B. (1990). Glycine site directed agonists reverse ethanol's actions at the NMDA receptor. *Molecular Pharmacology, 38,* 753–757.

Rassnick, S., D'Amico, E., Riley, E., & Koob, G. F. (1993). GABA antagonist and benzodiazepine partial inverse agonist reduce motivated responding for ethanol. *Alcoholism: Clinical and Experimental Research, 17,* 124–130.

Reynolds, J. N., & Prasad, A. (1991). Ethanol enhances $GABA_A$ receptor-activated chloride currents in chick cerebral cortical neurons. *Brain Research, 564,* 138–142.

Rossetti, Z. L., Longu, G., Mercuro, G., Hmaidan, Y., & Gessa, G. L. (1992). Biphasic effect of ethanol on noradrenaline release in the frontal cortex of awake rats. *Alcohol and Alcoholism, 27,* 477–480.

Samson, H. H., & Harris, R. A. (1992). Neurobiology of alcohol abuse. *Trends in Pharmacological Science, 13,* 206–211.

Samson, H. H., Tolliver, G. A., & Schwarz-Stevens, K. (1990). Oral ethanol self-administration: A behavioral pharmacological approach to SND control mechanisms. *Alcohol, 7,* 187–191.

Sanna, E., Serra, M., Cossu, A., Columbo, G., Follesa, P., & Biggio, G. (1992). $GABA_A$ and NMDA receptor function during chronic administration of ethanol. In G. Biggio, A. Concas, & E. Costa (Eds.), *GABAergic synaptic transmission* (pp. 317–324). New York: Raven Press.

Segal, M., & Bloom, F. E. (1976). The action of norepinephrine in the rat hippocampus: IV. The effects of a locus coeruleus stimulation on evoked hippocampal unit activity. *Brain Research, 107,* 513–525.

Sellers, E. M., Higgins, G. A., & Sobel, M. B. (1992). 5-HT and alcohol abuse. *Trends in Pharmacological Science, 13,* 69–75.

Simonsson, P., & Alling, C. (1988). The 5-hydroxytryptamine stimulated formation of inositol monophosphate is inhibited in platelets from alcoholics. *Life Science, 42,* 385–391.

Simonsson, P., Berglund, M., Oreland, L., Moberg, A. L., & Alling, C. (1992). Serotonin-stimulated phosphoinositide hydrolysis in platelets from post-withdrawal alcoholics. *Alcohol and Alcoholism, 27,* 607–612.

Smirnova, T., Laroche, S., Errington, M. L., Hicks, A. A., Bliss, T. V. P., & Mallet, J. (1993). Transsynaptic expression of a presynaptic glutamate receptor during hippocampal long-term potentiation. *Science, 262,* 433–436.

Socaransky, S. M., Aragon, C. M. G., Rusk, I., Amit, Z., & Ogren, S. O. (1985). Norepinephrine turnover and voluntary consumption of ethanol in the rat. *Alcohol, 2,* 339–342.

Spoont, M. R. (1992). Modulatory role of serotonin in neural information processing: Implications for human psychopathology. *Psychological Bulletin, 112,* 330–350.

Steele, C. M., & Josephs, R. A. (1990). Alcohol myopia: Its prized and dangerous effects. *American Psychologist, 45,* 921–933.

Suzdak, P. D., Schwartz, R. D., Skolnick, P., & Paul, S. M. (1986). Ethanol stimulates gamma-aminobutyric acid receptor-mediated chloride transport in rat brain synaptoneurosomes. *Proceedings of the National Academy of Sciences of the USA, 83,* 4071–4075.

Szabo, G., Tabakoff, B., & Hoffman, P. L. (1994). The NMDA receptor antagonist dizocilpine differentially affects environment-dependent and environment-independent ethanol tolerance. *Psychopharmacology, 113,* 511–517.

Tabakoff, B., & Hoffman, P. L. (1991). The changing view of ethanol's actions: From generalities to specifics. In T. N. Palmer (Ed.), *Alcoholism: A molecular perspective* (pp. 167–174). New York: Plenum.

Tabakoff, B., & Hoffman, P. L. (1996). Effect of alcohol on neurotransmitters and their receptors and enzymes. In H. Begleiter & B. Kissin (Eds.), *The pharmacology of alcohol and alcohol dependence* (pp. 356–430). Oxford, UK: Oxford University Press.

Toneatto, T., Romach, M. K., Sobell, L. C., Somer, G. R., & Sellers, E. M. (1991). Ondansetron, a 5-HT$_3$antagonist, reduces alcohol consumption in alcohol abusers. *Alcohol: Clinical and Experimental Research, 15,* 382.

Tsai, G., Gastfriend, D. R., & Coyle, J. T. (1995). The glutamatergic basis of human alcoholism. *American Journal of Psychiatry, 152,* 332–340.

U. S. Department of Health and Human Services. (1993). *Eighth Special Report to the U. S. Congress on Alcohol and Health.* Rockville, MD: Author.

Valverius, P., Crabbe, J. C., Hoffman, P. L., & Tabakoff, B. (1990). NMDA receptors in mice bred to be prone or resistant to ethanol withdrawal seizures. *European Journal of Pharmacology, 184,* 185–189.

Volkow, N. D., Brodie, J., & Bendriem, B. (1991). Positron Emission Tomography: Basic principles and applications in psychiatric research. *Annals New York Academy of Sciences, 620,* 128–144.

Volpicelli, J. R., Alterman, A. I., Hayashida, M., & O'Brien, C. P. (1992). Naltrexone in the treatment of alcohol dependence. *Archives of General Psychiatry, 49,* 876–880.

Weiss, F., & Koob, G. F. (1991). The neuropharmacology of ethanol self-administration. In R. E. Meyer, G. F. Koob, M. J. Lewis, & S. M. Paul (Eds.), *Neuropharmacology of ethanol* (pp. 125–162). Boston: Birkhauser.

Weiss, F., Lorang, M. T., Bloom, F. E., & Koob, G. F. (1993). Oral self-administration stimulates dopamine release in the rat nucleus accumbens: Genetic and motivational determinants. *Journal of Pharmacology and Experimental Therapeutics, 267,* 250–258.

Weiss, F., Parsons, L. H., Schulteis, G., Hyytia, P., Lorang, M. T., Bloom, F. E., & Koob, G. F. (1996). Ethanol self-administration restores withdrawal-associated deficiencies in accumbal dopamine and 5-hydroxytryptamine release in dependent rats. *Journal of Neuroscience, 16,* 3474–3485.

White, J. M. (1991). *Drug dependence.* New Jersey: Prentice Hall.

Wickelgren, I. (1997). Getting the brain's attention. *Science, 278,* 35–37.

Williams-Hemby, L., & Porrino, L. J. (1994). Low and moderate doses of ethanol produce distinct patterns of cerebral metabolic changes in rats. *Alcoholism: Clinical and Experimental Research, 18,* 982–988.

Wise, R. A. (1990). The role of reward pathways in the development of drug dependence. In D. J. K. Balfour (Ed.), *Psychotropic drugs of abuse* (pp. 23–57). Oxford, UK: Pergamon Press.

Wise, R. A., & Bozarth, M. A. (1987). A psychomotor stimulant theory of addiction. *Psychological Review, 94,* 469–492.

Wise, R. A., & Bozarth, M. A. (1985). Actions of abused drugs on reward systems in the brain. In K. Blum & L. Manzo (Eds.), *Neurotoxicology* (pp. 111–133). New York: Marcel Dekker.

Wolkowitz, O. M., Tinkleberg, J. R., & Weingartner, H. (1985). A psychopharmacological perspective of cognitive functions. *Neuropsychobiology, 14,* 135–156.

Woodward, J. J. (1994). A comparison of the effects of ethanol and the competitive glycine antagonist 7-chlorkynurenic acid on N-methyl-D-aspartic acid–induced neurotransmitter release from rat hippocampal slies. *Journal of Neurochemistry, 62,* 987–991.

Yoshimoto, K., McBride, W. J., & Li, T.-K. (1991). Alcohol stimulates the release of dopamine and serotonin in the nucleus accumbens. *Alcohol, 9,* 17–22.

12
Conclusion

KENNETH E. LEONARD
HOWARD T. BLANE

I find that the great thing in this world in not so much where we
stand as in what direction we are moving; to reach the port of heaven,
we must sail sometimes with the wind and sometimes against it—but
we must sail, and not drift, nor lie at anchor.
—OLIVER WENDELL HOLMES

The tremendous excitement and activity in the psychology of drinking and
alcoholism that we described in the first edition of this book has fueled
continued and impressive progress over the past decade. The intensive focus on psychological processes and the awareness that, ultimately, a
biopsychosocial approach was required to understand the development of
alcoholism have fostered sophisticated experimental and longitudinal developmental research and have created the opportunity for a major expansion of integrative research, both within psychological frameworks, as well
as truly interdisciplinary integrations. While one criterion of success of a
psychological theory is the generation of further empirical research, a more
important criterion is the value of the theory in addressing the conditions
that necessitated and motivated the psychological theory initially. In this regard, the recent success of psychological theories of drinking and alcoholism in penetrating into the design of prevention and treatment programs
has been an important advancement in the past decade.

The increasingly sophisticated experimental and longitudinal research
is evident in many of the chapters in this volume. This sophistication is

nowhere more apparent than in the advances of cognitive-psychological approaches to addiction. Mirroring the advances in the study of psychopathology more generally, the basic research in social cognition that exploded in the 1980s has exerted an enormous influence on theoretical development in alcoholism and addictions. Although this trend toward cognition was apparent in development of the social learning perspective throughout the late 1970s and 1980s, as documented in Chapter 4 by Maisto, Carey, and Bradizza, the tremendous advances in computer technology and the inexpensive availability of this technology has been a major element in growth of cognitive research. Goldman, Del Boca, and Darkes (Chapter 6) show how alcohol expectancy theory has progressed over the past decade from an approach that on the surface appeared to be an attitude model of heavy drinking and alcoholism to a model that integrates cognitive processes and content to explain these phenomena. Vogel-Sprott and Fillmore's (Chapter 8) review of learning perspectives is imbued with cognitive language, and these authors explicitly tie learning models to alcohol expectancies. Even within the broad tension-reduction theory, the chapter Greeley and Oei (Chapter 2) document the explicit cognitive direction that this approach has taken. Nonetheless, the extent to which the contributions of social-cognitive approaches to addictions have grown beyond their presence in these perspectives required the addition of Chapter 7 by Sayette, devoted entirely to cognitive models of drinking and alcoholism.

The increasing sophistication of research is also evident in the derivation and accessibility of statistical analyses that enable the more detailed examination of models of interrelationships among variables and the more appropriate analysis of longitudinal developmental data. The value of these statistical advances is described in Chapter 5 by Windle and Davies as important to the advancement of developmental-psychology approaches to psychopathology. These statistical models have also played a vital role in the explication of the importance of genetic factors in alcoholism as described by McGue in Chapter 10, and may be of further importance in the untangling of the interrelationships among alcoholism and other psychopathologies described in Chapter 3 by Sher, Trull, Bartholow, and Vieth.

A second major trend that has continued over the past decade has been a continuing attempt by psychologists to integrate biological and neurocognitive findings into their theoretical approaches. At a general level, McGue's chapter demonstrates that heredity does have an influence on the development of drinking and alcohol problems, a proposition that certainly was not accepted by a majority of psychologists a decade ago. The translation from genotype to phenotype is unknown, and as McGue points out, the unambiguous identification of genes associated with alcoholic disorders opens the way for a more sensitive methodology for understanding the psychological contributions. At the most detailed level, Fromme and D'Amico (Chapter 11) point to neurological substrates that appear to be activated when alcohol is consumed. The significance of these neurological substrates is illustrated in Chapter 9 by Lang, Patrick, and Stritzke, in which alcohol's psychological impact on the processing of emotional material is linked to the neurological impact of alcohol.

This continuing trend of integration of knowledge of the biological underpinnings has not signaled a retreat from the importance of psychological processes. Chapter 8 by Vogel-Sprott and Fillmore convincingly demonstrates that psychological processes (classical conditioning, expectancies) influence the physiological impact of different substances. The demonstration that animals administered a drug in a novel situation are more likely to die than animals with the same drug-administration history, who are administered the drug under familiar circumstances, is a stunning example. The cognitive approaches to craving described by Sayette also illustrate the impact of psychological factors on biological processes. Clearly, the psychological and biological realms influence each other in subtle, but sometimes powerful ways.

In 1987, one of the areas that we highlighted as important was the application of psychological theories and basic research to the development of prevention and treatment approaches. At that time, we noted that, with the exception of social learning theory, none of the theories had engendered intervention techniques. Given the early stage of many of the psychological theories, this state of affairs was not surprising. The recent research described in the current volume is very encouraging in terms of the transference of theoretically derived knowledge from the laboratory to the clinic. Goldman, Del Boca, and Darkes (Chapter 6) describe their work in challenging the expectancies that individuals hold with respect to alcohol, and the impact that this has on subsequent drinking. Given that alcohol expectancies have developed prior to drinking and that they are associated with heavy drinking in adolescence, the possibility of dampening expectancies among adolescents holds considerable promise as a prevention tool. Expectancies also predict heavy drinking in adulthood and present a useful target for secondary prevention and treatment, though the malleability of positive alcohol expectancies may be less among the older, more experienced drinkers. Social learning theory has continued to inform and be informed by clinical practice. Although social learning theory has been influential in the development of treatments for alcoholism, there is a growing trend toward applications in adolescent prevention. These applications have focused on stress and coping, and the influence of peers, but have typically targeted a broader range of problem behaviors, rather than simply alcohol use. With respect to theories that informed alcoholism treatment, the impact of learning theory and, to a lesser extent, cognitive theory, on treatment has also become more apparent. Although seminal studies in this area in the 1980s demonstrated that exposure to alcohol elicitied reactions that could undermine successful abstinence, more recently, there has been increasing interest in using exposure to alcohol cues to reduce cravings and urges for alcohol. Although these prevention/treatment applications are still in the early phases of development, they are potentially of great importance in our attempts to ameliorate alcohol problems. They are also important as a stage in theory development/refinement. The ability to change the behavior of a clinical population in accordance with the precepts of the theory serves to strengthen the theory tremendously. The inability to do so may speak to a need for further theoretical/empirical analysis.

Although the direction of theoretical and empirical inquiry can be abruptly altered by one or more advances in technology, or through the discovery of a key piece of information, the direction of psychological approaches to drinking and alcoholism seems clear at this point. There has always been a transmission of ideas and knowledge about drinking and alcoholism within psychology. This transmission was apparent in the first volume, with many of the theories returning to the same empirical base for support. It has become even more obvious in this volume. However, the information interchange has not necessarily led to integrative frameworks. It is our belief that the ensuing years will see more thorough attempts at integration among the different psychological perspectives such that the overlap among the construct systems that we see now will become theoretical/empirical linkages.

As we argued in the first edition (Blane & Leonard, 1987), psychological theories of drinking and alcoholism have fostered a "growing recognition that integrative, multivariate models aimed at highly specific aspects of alcohol use will provide a better understanding of the problems associated with such use" (p. 392). This theme clearly conflicted with models that argued for the "primacy of physiologic dependence, alcoholism as a unitary phenomenon, and alcoholism as a progressive disease" (p. 389). Instead, the theories incorporated the biological and pharmacological impact of ethanol as factors that interact with and are mediated by psychological processes, as well as factors that have independent effects; it suggested that the heterogeneity among alcoholics was as important as, if not more important than, the similarity; and it espoused the view that alcoholism should be viewed as a variety of different process components with different etiologies rather than a single progressive disease. The view that we see emerging from the current volume is similar. Drinking, alcohol problems, and alcoholism clearly emerge from biological, pharmacological, psychological, and social factors. However, in the earlier volume, this approach represented, for the most part, a heuristic perspective. In the current volume, we see this heuristic perspective in the early stages of implementation. Just as we see integration among psychological approaches, we believe that the conditions are ripe for an explosion of interdisciplinary research and theoretical visions that begin to cross levels of analysis.

Finally, the past decade has been marked by the need to translate the vast theoretical and empirical literature for the purposes of ameliorating the extensive problems associated with drinking and alcoholism. This force has been fostered by sociopolitical events and enabled by the growing maturity of the field, and the momentum in this direction shows no signs of abatement, nor should it. Although there has been progress in the integration of psychological approaches in the area of alcoholism treatment, there is a continued need in this regard. However, the need to integrate psychological knowledge of drinking and alcoholism in the development of prevention programs and public policy is even greater. This represents the next great opportunity for psychological approaches to drinking and alcoholism.

REFERENCES

Blane, H. T., & Leonard, K. E. (1987). *Psychological theories of drinking and alcoholism.* New York: Guilford Press.

Index